Clinical Toxicology: Principles and Mechanisms

Clinical Toxicology: Principles and Mechanisms

Edited by Bradley Delk

hayle
medical

New York

Hayle Medical,
750 Third Avenue, 9th Floor,
New York, NY 10017, USA

Visit us on the World Wide Web at:
www.haylemedical.com

ISBN: 978-1-63241-795-4

Cataloging-in-Publication Data

Clinical toxicology : principles and mechanisms / edited by Bradley Delk.
    p. cm.
Includes bibliographical references and index.
ISBN 978-1-63241-795-4
1. Clinical toxicology. 2. Drugs--Toxicology. 3. Toxicology.
4. Pharmacology. I. Delk, Bradley.
RA1238 .C55 2019
615.704 072 4--dc23

Table of Contents

Preface

Toxicology is the field of science that is focused on the study of the symptoms, making a diagnosis and developing a treatment strategy for the individuals exposed to toxins and venoms. Some of the factors that contribute to the exposure and its consequences are route of exposure, the dosage, age, sex and environment. Medical toxicologists in intensive care units, emergency departments and other inpatient units, provide direct treatment and consultation to acutely poisoned children and adults. Providing advanced evidence-based patient care is also under the scope of clinical toxicology. Evaluating the health impact from chronic and acute exposure to toxic substances in the workplace or outside is also under the scope of this field. This book unravels the recent studies in the field of clinical toxicology. Also included herein is a detailed explanation of the various principles and mechanisms of clinical toxicology. The extensive content of this book provides the readers with a thorough understanding of the subject.

Various studies have approached the subject by analyzing it with a single perspective, but the present book provides diverse methodologies and techniques to address this field. This book contains theories and applications needed for understanding the subject from different perspectives. The aim is to keep the readers informed about the progresses in the field; therefore, the contributions were carefully examined to compile novel researches by specialists from across the globe.

Indeed, the job of the editor is the most crucial and challenging in compiling all chapters into a single book. In the end, I would extend my sincere thanks to the chapter authors for their profound work. I am also thankful for the support provided by my family and colleagues during the compilation of this book.

Editor

1

Tomatidine and analog FC04–100 possess bactericidal activities against *Listeria*, *Bacillus* and *Staphylococcus* spp

Isabelle Guay[1†], Simon Boulanger[1†], Charles Isabelle[1], Eric Brouillette[1], Félix Chagnon[2], Kamal Bouarab[1], Eric Marsault[2*] and François Malouin[1*] (iD)

Abstract

Background: Tomatidine (TO) is a plant steroidal alkaloid that possesses an antibacterial activity against the small colony variants (SCVs) of *Staphylococcus aureus*. We report here the spectrum of activity of TO against other species of the *Bacillales* and the improved antibacterial activity of a chemically-modified TO derivative (FC04–100) against *Listeria monocytogenes* and antibiotic multi-resistant *S. aureus* (MRSA), two notoriously difficult-to-kill microorganisms.

Methods: *Bacillus* and *Listeria* SCVs were isolated using a gentamicin selection pressure. Minimal inhibitory concentrations (MICs) of TO and FC04–100 were determined by a broth microdilution technique. The bactericidal activity of TO and FC04–100 used alone or in combination with an aminoglycoside against planktonic bacteria was determined in broth or against bacteria embedded in pre-formed biofilms by using the Calgary Biofilm Device. Killing of intracellular SCVs was determined in a model with polarized pulmonary cells.

Results: TO showed a bactericidal activity against SCVs of *Staphylococcus aureus*, *Bacillus cereus*, *B. subtilis* and *Listeria monocytogenes* with MICs of 0.03–0.12 μg/mL. The combination of an aminoglycoside and TO generated an antibacterial synergy against their normal phenotype. In contrast to TO, which has no relevant activity by itself against *Bacillales* of the normal phenotype (MIC > 64 μg/mL), the TO analog FC04–100 showed a MIC of 8–32 μg/mL. Furthermore, FC04–100 showed a strong bactericidal activity against *L. monocytogenes* SCVs in kill kinetics experiments, while TO did not. The addition of FC04–100 (4 μg/mL) to a cefalexin:kanamycin (3:2) combination improved the activity of the combination by 32 fold against cefalexin and kanamycin-resistant MRSA strains. In combination with gentamicin, FC04–100 also exhibited a strong bactericidal activity against biofilm-embedded *S. aureus*. Also, FC04–100 and TO showed comparable intracellular killing of *S. aureus* SCVs.

Conclusions: Chemical modifications of TO allowed improvement of its antibacterial activity against prototypical *S. aureus* and of its bactericidal activity against *L. monocytogenes*. Antibacterial activities against such prominent pathogens could be useful to prevent *Listeria* contamination in the food chain or as treatment for MRSA infections.

Keywords: Tomatidine, Aminoglycoside, Synergy, SCV, *Bacillales*, *S. aureus*, *L. monocytogenes*, Foodborne disease, Cystic fibrosis

* Correspondence: Eric.Marsault@USherbrooke.ca;
Francois.Malouin@USherbrooke.ca
[†]Equal contributors
[2]Département de pharmacologie, Faculté de médecine et des sciences de la santé, Université de Sherbrooke, 3001, 12 th avenue Nord, Sherbrooke, QC J1H 5N4, Canada
[1]Centre d'Étude et de Valorisation de la Diversité Microbienne (CEVDM), Département de biologie, Faculté des sciences, Université de Sherbrooke, 2500 Boul. Université, Sherbrooke, QC J1K 2R1, Canada

Background

The *Bacillales* are divided into the genus of *Staphylococcus*, *Listeria* and *Bacillus*. A number of bacterial species such as *Listeria* spp. and *Bacillus* spp. can contaminate food and cause infections in humans [1]. To name a few, *Listeria monocytogenes*, *L. ivanovii*, and *Bacillus cereus* can cause listeriosis [2] and food poisoning [3]. *Bacillus subtilis*, *B. coagulans*, *B. licheniformis* and *B. sphaericus* are also known to cause illnesses. *Bacillus anthracis* causes anthrax and can often be acquired by contact with food producing animals and cattle (beef cattle, sheep, etc.) and this bacterium is also well-known for its endospores that have been used as biological weapons [4]. Staphylococci are divided in coagulase-positive species, *Staphylococcus aureus* being the most clinically relevant of this group, and coagulase-negative species, such as *S. epidermidis*, the most prevalent pathogen associated with infections of implanted medical devices [5]. The emergence and spread of resistance to multiple antibiotics in staphylococci is now considered a real health treat and impaired therapeutic endeavor to combat these bacteria [6]. Notably, the prevalence of methicillin-resistant *S. aureus* (MRSA) has steadily increased over the recent years, not only in hospitals but also in the community [7], and in veterinary medicine and livestock [8–10].

Staphylococcus aureus small-colony variants (SCVs) have attracted a great deal of interest over the past recent years. *S. aureus* SCVs often present a dysfunctional oxidative metabolism causing a slow growth and a change in the expression of virulence factors [11]. This dysfunctional oxidative metabolism is also responsible for a decreased susceptibility to aminoglycoside antibiotics because this class of molecules requires the proton-motive force in order to penetrate the bacterium [12]. This respiratory deficiency is often caused by mutations affecting the electron transport system, and several SCV isolates can recover normal growth with supplemental hemin or menadione, which are needed to synthesize electron transport system components. *S. aureus* SCVs often are isolated from chronic infections, such as lung infections in cystic fibrosis (CF) patients, osteomyelitis, septic arthritis, bovine mastitis, and from infections associated with orthopedic devices [11, 13, 14]. The ability of *S. aureus* to switch back and forth from the prototypic to the SCV phenotypes in vivo is an integral part of the pathogenesis of *S. aureus* and may be responsible for the establishment of chronic infections [15, 16].

Tomatidine (TO) is a steroidal alkaloid produced by the *Solanaceae* plant family such as the tomato [17, 18]. We showed previously the antibacterial activity of TO against *S. aureus* SCVs and also documented a strong synergic activity of TO in combination with aminoglycoside antibiotics against prototypic *S. aureus* [19, 20]. Recently, we synthesized a variety of TO analogs in

order to explore the structure-activity relationship of this new class of antibiotics able to act on SCVs [21]. One analog, FC04–100, showed the same steroidal backbone as the natural molecule but with an additional carbon chain and amines on the A cycle (Fig. 1). Preliminary characterization of FC04–100 revealed an antibacterial activity that was similar to that of TO against *S. aureus* SCVs and also preserved the synergic activity with aminoglycosides against prototypic *S. aureus* [21]. However, contrary to TO, FC04–100 showed notable antibiotic activity by itself against prototypic *S. aureus* with a MIC of 8–16 µg/mL, whereas that of TO was > 64 µg/mL.

The aim of this study was to further describe the spectrum of activity of TO and FC04–100. It was of great interest to see if the discovered antibacterial activity of FC04–100 against prototypical *S. aureus* modifies or improves its spectrum of antibacterial activity. The susceptibility of several species among the *Bacillales* to TO and FC04–100 alone or in combination with other antibiotics was investigated. The improved antibacterial activity of FC04–100 was demonstrated against *Listeria monocytogenes* and methicillin-resistant *S. aureus* (MRSA).

Methods

Chemical reagents and antibiotics

Tomatidine (TO) (Sigma Aldrich, Oakville, Ontario, Canada) (Fig. 1a) was solubilised in dimethylsulfoxide (DMSO) at a concentration of 2 mg/mL. The TO analog, FC04–100 (Fig. 1b) was synthesized [21] and solubilised in DMSO at 20 mg/mL. Cefalexin, kanamycin, gentamicin (GEN) (all from Sigma Aldrich), were solubilised in water at a concentration of 10 mg/mL. Menadione was solubilized in DMSO, hemin in 1.4 M NH_4OH and thymidine in water (all from Sigma Aldrich) and were prepared at a concentration of 10 mg/mL.

Bacterial strains and growth conditions

Staphylococcus aureus ATCC 29213, *S. aureus* Newbould (ATCC 29740), *S. epidermidis* ATCC 12228, *Listeria monocytogenes* ATCC 13932, *Bacillus subtilis* ATCC 6333 and *Bacillus cereus* ATCC 11778 were used as prototypic strains. Methicillin-resistant *S. aureus* (MRSA) strains COL and USA100 (hospital acquired-MRSA, ATCC BAA-41) and strain USA300 (community acquired-MRSA, ATCC BAA-1556), were also used in this study. The reference laboratory strain *S. aureus* SH1000, an isogenic mutant strain derived from *S. aureus* 8523–4 but with a functional *rsbU* allele [22], was used for its good yield of biofilm production. The *S. aureus* strains CF07-L (prototypic) and CF07-S (SCV phenotype) are genetically related clinical strains originally isolated from a cystic fibrosis patient [19]. Strain CF07-S was used in the intracellular infection model. *Staphylococcus* and *Bacillus*

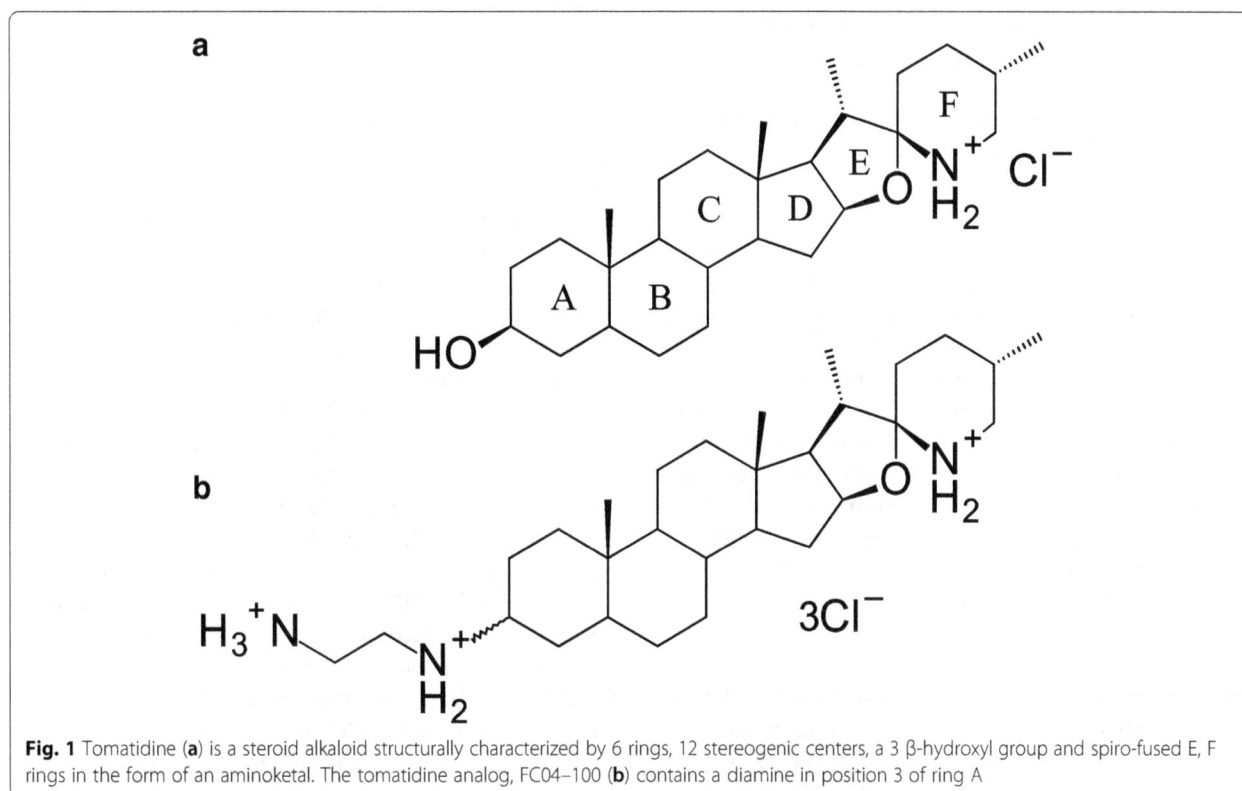

Fig. 1 Tomatidine (**a**) is a steroid alkaloid structurally characterized by 6 rings, 12 stereogenic centers, a 3 β-hydroxyl group and spiro-fused E, F rings in the form of an aminoketal. The tomatidine analog, FC04–100 (**b**) contains a diamine in position 3 of ring A

were maintained on Tryptic Soy agar (TSA, BD, Mississauga, Ontario, Canada), whereas *L. monocytogenes* was grown on brain-heart infusion (BHI) agar (BD, Mississauga, Ontario, Canada).

Small colony variants (SCVs)

For *S. aureus*, strain Newbould*ΔhemB* was used as the reference SCV. Newbould*ΔhemB* was generated from strain Newbould (ATCC 29740) by disrupting the *hemB* gene with the *ermA* cassette by homologous recombination [23]. Another SCV *hemB* mutant was similarly constructed from *S. aureus* ATCC 29213 [24]. SCVs from *B. cereus*, *B. subtillis* and *L. monocytogenes* were generated by growth in presence of a subinhibitory concentration of GEN. Briefly, overnight broth cultures (18–20 h) were used to inoculate BHI broths at a dilution of 1:100, supplemented or not with 0.25 to 1X the MIC of GEN. Cultures were incubated 18 h at 35 °C with shaking (225 rpm) and then adjusted to an $A_{595\ nm}$ of 2.0 in PBS at 4 °C. Determination of CFU and SCV colonies was done by serial dilution plating. SCVs were obtained by plating on TSA (BHI agar for *L. monocytogenes*) containing GEN at a concentration of 8 to 16 times the induction concentration followed by an incubation of 48 h at 35 °C. The pinpoint colonies selected by this method were confirmed to be SCVs by streaking several of them on agar plates without antibiotic. SCV that conserved their phenotype after two passages were

considered to have a stable phenotype and were used in subsequent experiments. Selected SCVs had a colony size a tenth of the size of a normal colony and showed no pigmentation or hemolytic activity on blood agar plates. The SCV species were confirmed by rDNA 16S sequencing after PCR amplification using universal primers [25].

Auxotrophy assays

For SCVs, auxotrophism is defined as the requirement of specific compounds in order to regain a normal growth phenotype [26]. An agar diffusion method was used to characterize the auxotrophism of SCVs using hemin or menadione (1–10 μg each/well) or thymidine (100 μg/well) on an inoculated Mueller-Hinton agar (MHA) or Brain-heart infusion agar (BHIA) plate [27]. Auxotrophy for specific supplements was detected by a zone of normal growth surrounding the well after 18 h of incubation at 35 °C. The results were confirmed by two independent experiments.

Antibiotic susceptibility testing

MICs were determined by a broth microdilution technique following the recommendations of the Clinical and Laboratory Standards Institute (CLSI) [28], except that the incubation period was extended to 48 h and the medium used was BHI to allow SCVs to reach maximal growth as previously described [29]. As recommended by the CLSI, *L. monocytogenes* (and its SCVs) were grown in cation-adjusted Muller-Hinton broth (CAMHB, BD) containing 3% lysed horse blood (LHB, Remel, Hartford, CT, USA). The reported results were obtained from three independent experiments.

Time-kill experiments

Kill kinetics were performed to determine whether the effect of compounds alone or in combination with an aminoglycoside was bacteriostatic or bactericidal. Bacteria were inoculated at 10^5–10^6 CFU/mL in the appropriate medium in the absence or presence of the different antibiotic compounds at concentrations specified in figure legends. At several points in time at 35 °C (225 rpm), bacteria were sampled, serially diluted, and plated on TSA for CFU determinations. Plates were incubated for 24 or 48 h at 35 °C for normal and SCV strains, respectively. The data were collected from a minimum of three independents experiments.

Antibiotic activity in biofilms

The viability of bacteria in biofilms was evaluated based on previously described protocols [30–32]. For these assays, 96-peg lids and corresponding 96-well plates were used (Thermo Scientific, Ottawa, ON, Canada). Wells were inoculated with a suspension of *S. aureus* SH-1000 adjusted to a 0.5 McFarland standard in TSB (150 µL per wells) and plates with 96-well lids were incubated at 35 °C with an agitation of 120 rpm for 24 h. The biofilms on pegs were then washed three times with 200 µL PBS. Biofilms on pegs were further incubated in fresh 96-well plates containing 200 µL of TSB containing or not antibiotic compounds or a combination of molecules at 35 °C, 120 rpm for 24 h. The treated biofilms on pegs were washed three times in PBS and bacteria in biofilms were recovered by sonication in a new microtiter plate containing 200 µL of PBS per wells using an ultrasonicator bath for 10 min followed by centrifugation for 5 min at 1000 RPM. The bacteria recovered in each well were suspended, serially diluted, plated on TSA and incubated at 35 °C for 24 h before CFU determination.

Cell invasion and measurement of intracellular antibiotic activity

The Calu-3 cell line (ATCC HTB 55, *Homo sapiens* lung adenocarcinoma), was cultured in Eagle's Minimum Essential Medium (EMEM) supplemented with 0.1 mM MEM nonessential amino acids, 1 mM of sodium pyruvate, 100 U/mL penicillin, 100 µg/mL streptomycin, 2.5 µg/mL of Fungizone and 10% fetal bovine serum (FBS) at 37 °C in 5% CO_2. For routine culture, 4 µg/mL of puromycin was added to culture media. All cell culture reagents were purchased from Wisent (St-Bruno, QC, Canada).

The cell invasion assay was performed with the Calu-3 cells in an air-liquid interface as previously described with few modifications [19]. Briefly, cells were seeded at 1.5×10^5 cells per insert in a 12-well Transwell plate (Corning, Tewksbury, MA) and cultured for 10 days with the apical medium replaced each day. The complete medium in the basal compartment was replaced by the invasion medium (1% FBS and no antibiotics) 18 h before invasion assays. Inocula were prepared by suspending bacteria grown 20 h on BHI agar plates in ice-cold PBS. Bacteria were then washed three times in ice-cold PBS and suspended in the invasion medium supplemented with 0.5% BSA at a density of approximately 4.0×10^8 CFU/mL. Cells were washed twice with PBS and 250 µL of bacterial suspension (multiplicity of infection [MOI] of 10, i.e., the ratio bacteria/cells) were apically added to each insert. Invasion of cells by bacteria was allowed for 3 h, inserts were emptied and washed three times with PBS. The basal medium was changed for the invasion medium with 20 µg/mL of lysostaphin (Sigma) to kill extracellular bacteria and with or without the tested antibiotic compounds. The infected cells were incubated for a total of 48 h with a change of medium at 23 h (invasion medium with lysostaphin with or without the tested antibiotic compounds). The invasion medium with lysostaphin but without tested compound was also apically added 1 h before cell lysis to ensure that only intracellular bacteria were counted. At 48 h, following three washes with PBS, the apical and basal media were removed and cells were detached with 100 µL of trypsin 0.25% and lysed for 10 min by the addition of 400 µL of water containing 0.05% of Triton X-100. Then, 50 µL of PBS (10X) was added and mixed. Lysates were serially diluted 10-fold and plated on TSA for CFU determination. Plates were incubated at 35 °C for 48 h.

Statistical analysis

Statistical analyses were carried out with the GraphPad Prism software (v.6.02). Bacterial CFUs were transformed in base 10 logarithm values before being used for statistical analyses. One-way ANOVA and post-tests were used as appropriate for the analysis of data as specified in each of the figure legends.

Results

Emergence the SCV phenotype

The SCV phenotype is characterized by a slow growth yielding a small colony size on agar plates (i.e., typically 1/5 to 1/10 of the normal colony size). Two prototypic *S. aureus*, Newbould and CF07-L, and their SCV counterparts, Newbould$\Delta hemB$ and CF07-S, respectively, were used as control strains (Fig. 2a and b). Figure 2 shows the colony sizes of the parental strains compared to that of the SCV derivatives. A subinhibitory

Tomatidine and analog FC04–100 possess bactericidal activities against Listeria, Bacillus...

5

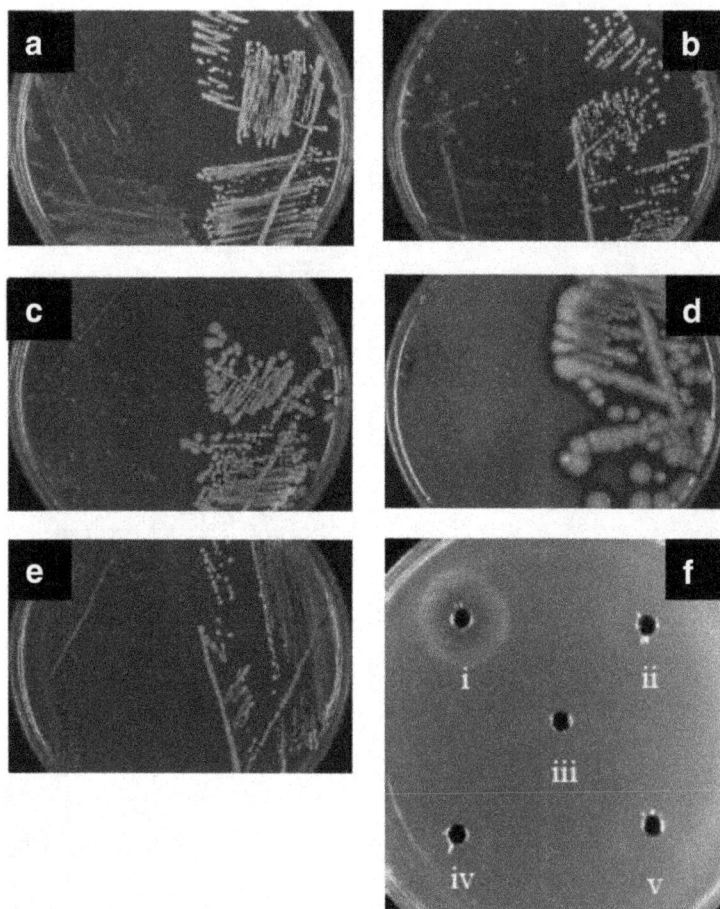

Fig. 2 Typical colony sizes for SCV and prototypic strains (left and right sides of the plates, respectively) for (**a**) *S. aureus* CF07-S and CF07-L, (**b**) *S. aureus* NewbouldΔ*hemB* and Newbould, (**c**) *B. cereus* ATCC 11778 (SCV#1 and prototypic), (**d**) *B. subtilis* ATCC 6333 (SCV#2 and prototypic), and (**e**) *L. monocytogenes* ATCC 13932 (SCV#1 and prototypic). In (**f**), a TSA plate was inoculated with *L. monocytogenes* ATCC 13932 SCV#2 and wells were filled with (i) 10 μg hemin, (ii) 10 μg menadione, (iii) 100 μg thymidine, and diluents (iv) DMSO, and (v) NH₄OH 1.4 N. A zone of enhanced growth is observed around (i). The enhanced growth appears white and surrounds a small zone of growth inhibition

concentration of GEN was used to promote the emergence of the SCV phenotype for *B. cereus*, *B. subtilis* and *L. monocytogenes*. The *B. cereus* SCVs were obtained at an inducing concentration of 1 X MIC of GEN (Fig. 2c), *B. subtilis* SCVs at 0.5 X MIC (Fig. 2d), and *L. monocytogenes* SCVs at 0.25 X MIC (Fig. 2e). The SCV isolates selected for the rest of the study were stable and kept their small-colony phenotype without a GEN selection pressure. The *B. cereus* SCVs showed auxotrophy for menadione (Table 1), some of the *L. monocytogenes* SCVs showed auxotrophy for hemin (Fig. 2f, Table 1), while the *B. subtilis* SCVs showed no apparent auxotrophy to hemin, menadione or thymidine (i.e., unknown auxotrophy, Table 1). These results show that SCVs with defects in their respiratory chain (i.e., hemin or menadione auxotrophy) can indeed emerge from a selective pressure with aminoglycosides.

Antibacterial activity of TO and analog FC04–100 against *Bacillales* spp

The MICs of TO and FC04–100 against a panel of prototypic and SCV strains of the *Bacillales* are reported in Table 1. The MICs for TO ranged from 0.03 to 0.12 μg/mL against all the SCVs tested from the species *S. aureus*, *L. monocytogenes*, *B. cereus* and *B. subtilis*, whereas TO showed no activity (MIC > 64 μg/mL) against the prototypic strains including *S. epidermidis* (Table 1). Noteworthy, strains of the normal phenotype were more susceptible to GEN compared to their SCV derivatives; this was expected because aminoglycosides (e.g., GEN) require an active respiratory chain and the proton-motive force in order to penetrate the bacterium. Besides, the MICs of analog FC04–100 against the SCV strains (MIC of 1–2 μg/mL, Table 1) were slightly higher than that found for TO. On the other hand, the MICs of

Table 1 Susceptibility of prototypic and SCV strains and species to TO, FC04–100, GEN or the combination of GEN with one of either steroidal alkaloids

Species and strains	Auxo[a]	MIC (µg/mL)				
		TO	FC	GEN	GEN + TO (fold)[b]	GEN + FC (fold)[c]
Staphylococcus ssp.						
S. aureus ATCC 29213	–	> 64	8–16	0.5	0.06 (8)	0.06–0.12 (4–8)
S. aureus ATCC 29213 ΔhemB (SCV)	H	0.06	2	8	–	–
S. aureus Newbould	–	> 64	8–16	0.5	0.06 (8)	0.12 (4)
S. aureus Newbould ΔhemB (SCV)	H	0.06	2	8	–	–
S. aureus CF07-L	–	> 64	8	0.5	0.06(8)	0.12 (4)
S. aureus CF07-S (SCV)	M	0.12	2	8	–	–
S. aureus SH1000	–	> 64	8–16	0.5	0.06 (8)	0.06–0.12 (4–8)
S. aureus MRSA USA100 ATCC BAA-41	–	> 64	16	0.5	0.12 (4)	0.12 (4)
S. aureus MRSA USA300 ATCC BAA-1556	–	> 64	16	0.5	0.06 (8)	0.06 (8)
S. aureus MRSA COL	–	> 64	16	0.25	0.06 (4)	0.06 (4)
S. epidermidis ATCC 12228	–	> 64	8	0.5	0.12 (4)	0.12 (4)
Bacillus ssp.						
B. cereus ATCC 11778	–	> 64	8	1	0.25 (4)	0.25 (4)
B. cereus ATCC 11778 (SCV#1)	M	0.03	2	16	–	–
B. cereus ATCC 11778 (SCV#2)	M	0.03	2	16	–	–
B. subtilis ATCC 6333	–	> 64	8	0.12	0.03 (4)	0.06 (2)
B. subtilis ATCC 6333 (SCV#1)	U	0.03	2	2	–	–
B. subtilis ATCC 6333 (SCV#2)	U	0.03	2	4	–	–
B. subtilis ATCC 9372	–	> 64	8	0.12	0.015 (8)	0.06 (2)
B. subtilis ATCC 9372 (SCV#1)	U	0.03	1	1	–	–
B. subtilis ATCC 9372 (SCV#2)	U	0.03	1	1	–	–
Listeria						
L. monocytogenes ATCC 13932	–	> 64	32	0.5	0.12 (4)	0.12 (4)
L. monocytogenes ATCC 13932 (SCV#1)	U	0.03	1	> 64	–	–
L. monocytogenes ATCC 13932 (SCV#2)	H	0.03	1	> 64	–	–

Abbreviations: TO tomatidine, FC FC04–100, GEN gentamicin, Auxo auxotrophy, SCV small-colony variant, H hemin, M menadione, T thymidine, U unknown
[a]For SCVs, auxotrophism is defined as the requirement of specific compounds in order to regain a normal growth phenotype. An agar diffusion method was used to characterize the auxotrophism of SCVs using H, M or T. If none of these compounds restored normal growth, the auxotrophy was unknown (U)
[b]GEN was used in combination with TO at a sub-MIC of 8 µg/mL. The fold increase in GEN susceptibility is the ratio of the MIC of GEN used alone vs GEN in the presence of TO
[c]GEN was used in combination with FC at a sub-MIC of 4 µg/mL. The fold increase in GEN susceptibility is the ratio of the MIC of GEN used alone vs GEN in the presence of FC

FC04–100 against all prototypic *Bacillales* were lower than that of TO (8–32 µg/mL for FC04–100 vs. > 64 µg/mL for TO). Furthermore, a synergy of TO or FC04–100 with GEN against all the prototypic strains tested was also observed (Table 1). Indeed, the addition of either TO or FC04–100 to GEN in the susceptibility tests provoked a 2 to 8-fold decrease of GEN MIC against all species tested (Table 1).

These results show that the spectrum of activity of TO and FC04–100 is similarly directed against the *Bacillales* (*Staphylococcus, Bacillus, Listeria*).

The interesting antibacterial activity of FC04–100 against prototypic strains was therefore noted against antibiotic

multi-resistant MRSA strains (MICs of 16 µg/mL, Table 1) and such an activity was further investigated. Although the multi-resistant *S. aureus* MRSA USA100, USA300 and COL are resistant to cefalexin (beta-lactam antibiotic, MIC of 256 µg/mL) and to the aminoglycoside kanamycin (MIC of 256 µg/mL and > 1024 µg/mL, for USA100 and USA300, respectively, Table 2), the combination of both cefalexin and kanamycin decreased their respective MICs (Table 2). Indeed, the combination of cefalexin and kanamycin in a proportion of 3:2 (commercialized under the name Ubrolexin™) decreased the MIC of one or both antibiotics. This is as expected for the combination of a beta-lactam with an aminoglycoside [33]. However, the synergy

Table 2 Synergistic activity of FC04–100 with the combination cefalexin:kanamycin

Species and strains	MIC (µg/mL)				
	CEF	KAN	CEF:KAN[a]	CEF:KAN (+FC)[b]	Fold[c]
S. aureus MRSA USA100 ATCC BAA-41	256	256	128:86	4:3	32
S. aureus MRSA USA300 ATCC BAA-1556	256	>1024	256:171	8:6	32
S. aureus MRSA COL	256	4	4:3	0.5:0.35	8

Abbreviations: CEF cefalexin, KAN kanamycin, FC FC04–100
[a]CEF:KAN was used at a proportion of 3:2
[b]FC04–100 was used at a sub-MIC of 4 µg/mL
[c]The fold increase in susceptibility is the ratio of the MIC of CEF:KAN alone vs CEF:KAN in the presence of FC04–100

is weak with MRSA strains that are resistant to one or the other or both antibiotics and the addition of 4 µg/mL of FC04–100 further improved by 8 to 32 fold the MIC of the cefalexin:kanamycin combination against these strains (Table 2).

Bactericidal activity of TO and analog FC04–100 against SCVs and bactericidal synergy in combination with GEN against prototypic strains

As was shown in Table 1, the addition of 8 µg/mL of TO to GEN reduced the MIC of GEN against all prototypic Bacillales. In this section, kill kinetics also show that the TO-GEN combination importantly improves the bactericidal effect of GEN against prototypic B. subtilis and B. cereus with a > 4 log10 reduction in viable bacteria at 24 h compared to the no drug control (Fig. 3a and b, respectively). However, although the MIC of GEN was improved when in combination with TO against

L. monocytogenes (Table 1), time-kill experiments failed to demonstrate a bactericidal synergy with an improvement of at most 1 $\log_{10}$ in killing compared to that achieved with GEN alone (Fig. 3c). Similarly, the effect of TO used alone against SCVs was strongly bactericidal against S. aureus, B. subtilis and B. cereus, but not against the L. monocytogenes SCV (Fig. 3d), and this even if the MIC of TO against L. monocytogenes SCVs was 0.03 µg/mL (Table 1).

On the other hand, the addition of 8 µg/mL of FC04–100 to GEN (2 µg/mL) decreased by an average of 5 $\log_{10}$ the viable counts (CFU/mL) of prototypic L. monocytogenes, after 24 h of treatment, in comparison to GEN alone (Fig. 4a). Also, the bactericidal activity of FC04–100 used alone against the L. monocytogenes SCV was shown to be better than that observed for TO. To quantitate and facilitate such a comparison between TO and FC04–100, Fig. 4b shows the residual CFU of the L. monocytogenes SCV strain after treatment with TO or FC04–100 and

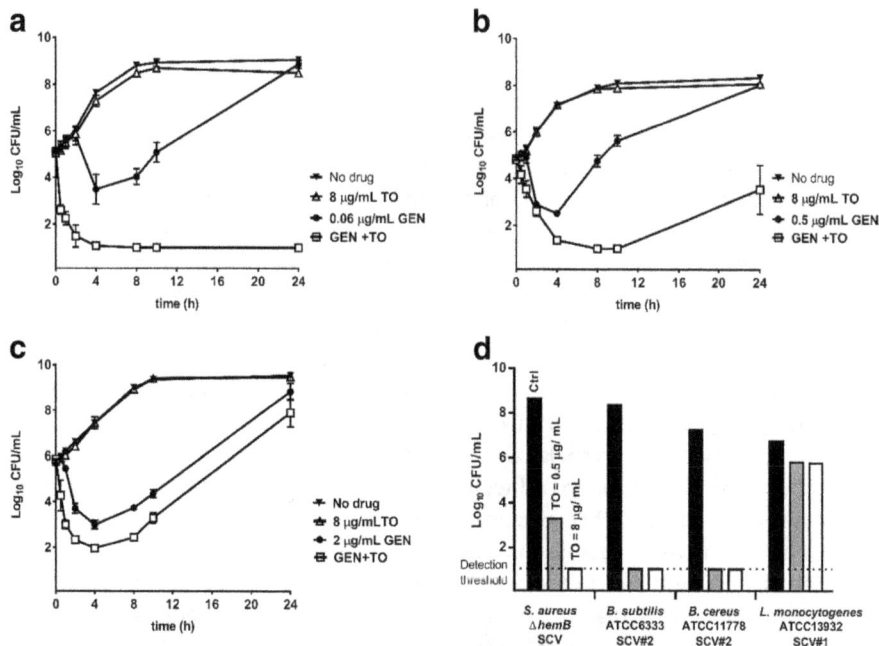

Fig. 3 Kill kinetics of TO, GEN or the combination of both (GEN + TO) against (**a**) prototypic B. subtilis ATCC 6333, (**b**) B. cereus ATCC 11778, and (**c**) L. monocytogenes ATCC 13932. The bactericidal effect of TO against SCVs at 0, 0.5 and 8 µg/mL at 24 h is also shown (**d**). The results were obtained from at least three independent experiments

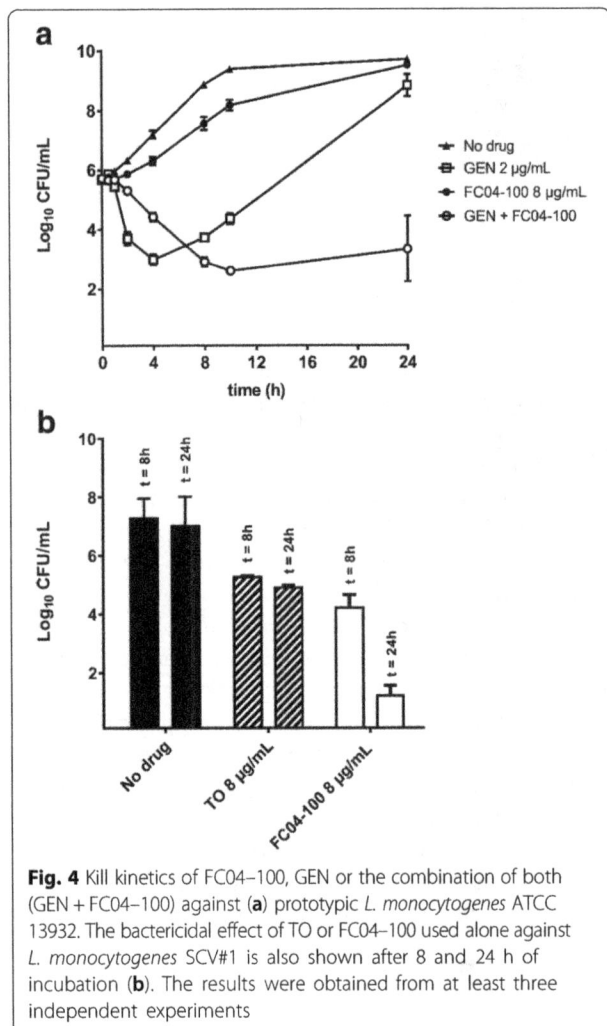

Fig. 4 Kill kinetics of FC04–100, GEN or the combination of both (GEN + FC04–100) against (**a**) prototypic *L. monocytogenes* ATCC 13932. The bactericidal effect of TO or FC04–100 used alone against *L. monocytogenes* SCV#1 is also shown after 8 and 24 h of incubation (**b**). The results were obtained from at least three independent experiments

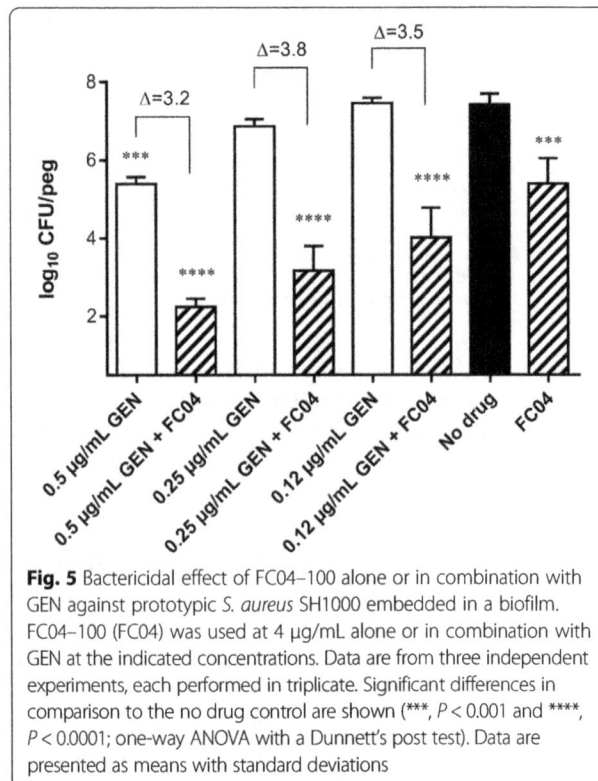

Fig. 5 Bactericidal effect of FC04–100 alone or in combination with GEN against prototypic *S. aureus* SH1000 embedded in a biofilm. FC04–100 (FC04) was used at 4 μg/mL alone or in combination with GEN at the indicated concentrations. Data are from three independent experiments, each performed in triplicate. Significant differences in comparison to the no drug control are shown (***, $P < 0.001$ and ****, $P < 0.0001$; one-way ANOVA with a Dunnett's post test). Data are presented as means with standard deviations

calculated as the percentage of live CFU in comparison with untreated *L. monocytogenes* SCVs after 24 h of incubation. These results show that TO can be chemically modified (e.g., derivative FC04–100) to improve its antibacterial activity against *L. monocytogenes*.

FC04–100 potentiates the activity of GEN against *S. aureus* embedded in biofilm

The interesting bactericidal properties of FC04–100, notably against *Listeria* (Fig. 4) prompted us to further investigate the bactericidal activity of this steroidal alkaloid in other instances where *Bacillales* spp. are difficult to kill. For example, strain *S. aureus* SH1000 produces copious amounts of biofilm and is thus suitable for use in an assay measuring the intrabiofilm bactericidal activity of antibiotics. Figure 5 demonstrates that compound FC04–100 can also kill prototypical *S. aureus* SH1000 embedded in a biofilm. Indeed, FC04–100 used alone at 4 μg/mL (i.e., 0.25–0.5 × MIC) significantly reduced the number of viable bacteria remaining in the biofilm as

compared to the no drug control ($P < 0.001$). Furthermore, when FC04–100 (4 μg/mL) was used in combination with GEN, the antibacterial activity of GEN (used at either 0.25, 0.5 or 1 × MIC) was significantly improved ($P < 0.0001$). In other words, addition of FC04–100 to GEN improved its intrabiofilm bactericidal activity by more than 3 log10 at all tested GEN concentrations (Fig. 5).

FC04–100 inhibits the intracellular replication of SCVs

Another instance where some *Bacillales* spp. are difficult to kill by antibiotics is when they hide within host cells. Indeed, intracellular replication of *S. aureus* SCVs is an important contributor to the establishment of chronic infections such as those occurring in the lungs of cystic fibrosis patients. Hence, to mimic the human pulmonary epithelium, Calu-3 cells were cultivated in an air-liquid interface and were subsequently infected with the *S. aureus* SCV strain CF07-S. Strain CF07-S was originally isolated from a patient with cystic fibrosis. After invasion of cells by CF07-S, remaining extracellular bacteria were removed and Calu-3 cells were exposed to TO or FC04–100 to evaluate their ability to kill intracellular bacteria. Figure 6 shows that FC04–100 (used at 8 μg/mL), like TO, can significantly decrease the intracellular population of *S. aureus* CF07-S by at least 3 log10 compared to the no drug control ($P < 0.0001$).

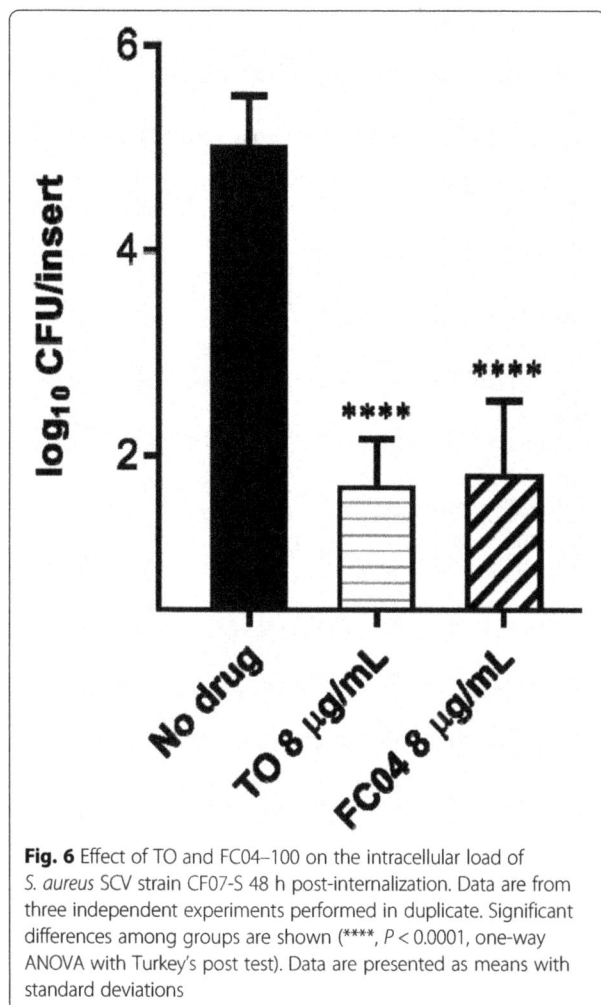

Fig. 6 Effect of TO and FC04–100 on the intracellular load of *S. aureus* SCV strain CF07-S 48 h post-internalization. Data are from three independent experiments performed in duplicate. Significant differences among groups are shown (****, $P < 0.0001$, one-way ANOVA with Turkey's post test). Data are presented as means with standard deviations

Discussion

In previous studies, we have demonstrated that TO has a strong inhibitory activity against *S. aureus* SCVs and improves the bactericidal activity of aminoglycoside antibiotics against prototypic *S. aureus*, and also more broadly, against staphylococci. The mode of action of TO and its analog FC04–100 against *S. aureus* has yet to be understood. Our initial work suggested that TO inhibits the biosynthesis of macromolecules, with a pronounced effect on protein synthesis and that when used in combination, the aminoglycoside or TO could help each other to reach their respective intracellular target through cell permeabilization [19, 20]. However, more recently, we have putatively identified the cellular target of TO as the bacterial ATP synthase using genomic analysis of TO-resistant mutants [34]. Such a cellular target would explain both the action of TO against the already impaired respiratory-deficient SCVs, the reduction in macromolecular biosyntheses resulting from a reduction in ATP production, and the synergy with an aminoglycoside which action is also linked to the

respiratory chain and proton motive force. The TO-aminoglycoside synergy was documented for several prototypical strains of diverse clinical origins including aminoglycoside-resistant *S. aureus* carrying aminoglycoside modifying enzymes. This effect occurring by a mechanism that has yet to be understood was documented for several strains of diverse clinical origins including aminoglycoside-resistant *S. aureus* carrying aminoglycoside modifying enzymes. TO showed however no synergistic effect on the activity of aminoglycosides against *P. aeruginosa*, *E. coli* or *Enterococcus spp.* In the present study, we showed that the antibacterial spectrum of TO can be extended to species of the *Bacillales* order having very low MICs against *L. monocytogenes*, *B. cereus* and *B. subtillis* SCVs (0.03 to 0.12 µg/mL). Time-kill kinetics showed that the combination of TO and GEN creates a bactericidal synergy against prototypic strains of *B. subtilis* and *B. cereus*, similarly to that previously demonstrated against *S. aureus*. However, the mixture of TO and GEN did not demonstrate much improvement over the activity of GEN alone against prototypic *L. monocytogenes* in time-kill experiments. Likewise, investigations with *Bacillales* SCVs showed that TO efficiently killed *S. aureus*, *B. cereus* and *B. subtillis* but not *L. monocytogenes* SCVs despite its very low MIC and TO was thus bacteriostatic against that species. *L. monocytogenes* SCVs are indeed quite tolerant to the bactericidal effects of many classes of antibacterial agents [35]. Therefore, amelioration of the bactericidal activity of TO against this important pathogen, as seen with its derivative FC04–100, is an important breakthrough.

TO is a steroid alkaloid found in the *Solanaceae* plants [20, 21] and is structurally characterized by 6 rings, 12 stereogenic centers, a 3β-hydroxyl group on ring A and spiro-fused E, F rings in the form of an aminoketal (Fig. 1). Although we previously documented some interesting antibacterial activity for TO, the absence of an identified cellular target makes difficult the establishment of a structure-activity relationship (SAR). In initial attempts to elucidate SAR, we prepared analogs bearing modifications on ring A of TO [21]. The addition of two ammonium groups in position C3 on ring A was highly beneficial for antibiotic activity against normal non-SCV strains and the antibacterial spectrum of activity of one of such analogs, FC04–100, is detailed in the present work. On the other hand, although FC04–100 increased its antibacterial activity against prototypical strains of the *Bacillales* compared to TO (Table 1), it presents a reduced activity against *S. aureus* SCVs (from a MIC of 0.03–0.12 µg/mL for TO to a MIC of 1–2 µg/mL for FC04–100). The study of Chagnon et al. [21] also demonstrated that the stereochemistry of the 3 position substitution moderately affected activity against *S. aureus* SCVs and since FC04–100 is a mixture of stereoisomers for that position, separation and purification of FC04–100 stereoisomers will need to be done in future studies to see if one or the other stereoisomer drives the antibacterial activity against prototypical or SCV strains.

Here we demonstrated that FC04–100 was able to kill both *L. monocytogenes* SCVs as well as the normal phenotype, alone and in the presence of GEN, respectively (Fig. 4). Furthermore, FC04–100 showed a noticeable antibacterial activity on its own (MIC of 16 µg/mL) against the MRSA strains USA100, USA300 and COL (Table 1). FC04–100 was also synergistic in combination with an aminoglycoside against such MRSA strains with a 4 to 8 fold gain in the MIC of GEN. Because MRSA strains are often multi-resistant to antibiotics and often carry aminoglycoside-modifying enzymes (AMEs), we examined the possibility of using a triple antibiotic combination. Indeed, the combination of cefalexin and kanamycin in a proportion 3:2 is already approved to treat bovine mastitis pathogens under the brand name of Ubrolexin™ [36]. This antibiotic combination offers an extended spectrum of activity compared to each individual drug and is expected to cover both *S. aureus*, *Streptococcus uberis*, and *E. coli* [36–38]. Unfortunately, the increased frequency of livestock-associated MRSA [8–10] and frequent incidence of strains and species carrying AMEs [39] may limit the spectrum of activity of the combination of a beta-lactam and an aminoglycoside. With this in mind, we showed that the use of FC04–100 in combination with cefalexin and kanamycin improves by 32 fold the activity of this mixture against MRSA strains carrying AMEs (Table 2). Overall the addition of FC04–100 to the aminoglycoside-beta-lactam combination decreased the MICs of cefalexin and kanamycin below their resistance breakpoints, and this for all the MRSA strains tested.

S. aureus, although not primarily recognized as a typical intracellular pathogen, is able to enter and survive in host cells [40]. Moreover, the ability of *S. aureus* to convert to the SCV phenotype showing increased biofilm production, improved adherence to host cells and tissues as well as increased intracellular persistence allows this pathogen to cause chronic and difficult to treat infections [41, 42]. Discovering antibacterial drugs able to act in the intracellular compartment is generally recognized as a difficult challenge. Previously, we demonstrated that steroidal alkaloids such as TO had such an ability and could act on intracellular *S. aureus* SCVs [19], and here, we demonstrated that this was also the case for the TO analog FC04–100 (Fig. 6). Since FC04–100 showed a good bactericidal activity against *L. monocytogenes* in vitro, it will be interesting to see if it can also kill this highly specialized intracellular pathogen [43], in future studies. In addition, we also show in the present study that FC04–100 greatly improves the bactericidal activity

of aminoglycosides such as GEN against bacteria embedded in biofilms. Biofilms are recognized to be a major hindrance to antibiotic action and are responsible for persistent colonization in many diseases [44] and in the food industry [45]. The important intracellular and intrabiofilm bactericidal properties of FC04–100 certainly provides further justifications for a continued interest for this class of molecules in general.

Conclusion

We showed in this study that the spectrum of activity of TO is related to the *Firmicutes* division, and more precisely, to the order of the *Bacillales*. TO possesses an antibacterial activity against SCVs and a synergistic activity with aminoglycoside antibiotics against prototypic strains. The novel TO analog FC04–100 showed very promising new characteristics that include a much improved bactericidal activity against *L. monocytogenes* and killing of *S. aureus* when embedded in biofilms as well as when bacteria are within host cells.

Abbreviations
AME: Aminoglycoside-modifying enzyme; Auxo: Auxotrophy; BHI: Brain-heart infusion; BHIA: Brain-heart infusion agar; CAMHB: Cation-adjusted Mueller-Hinton broth; CEF: Cefalexin; CF: Cystic fibrosis; FBS: Fetal bovine serum; FC: FC04–100; GEN: Gentamicin; KAN: Kanamycin; MHA: Mueller-Hinton agar; MHB: Mueller-Hinton broth; MIC: Minimal inhibitory concentration; MRSA: Methicillin-resistant *S. aureus*; PBS: Phosphate-buffered saline; SAR: Structure-activity relationship; SCV: Small colony variant; TO: Tomatidine; TSA: Tryptic soy agar; TSB: Tryptic soy broth

Acknowledgements
Not applicable.

Funding
This study was supported by an operation grant from Cystic Fibrosis Canada to FM and EM and by a team grant from the *Fonds Québécois de la Recherche sur la Nature et les Technologies* (FQRNT) to FM, KB and EM. FM also acknowledges funding for this project from the *Regroupement de recherche pour un lait de qualité optimale* (Op+Lait, St-Hyacinthe, Québec, Canada), which is supported by the FRQNT.

Authors' contributions
Conception of idea and research design: FM, EM, KB. Conduct of research and experimentation: IG, SB, CI, FC. Data analyses: IG, SB, EB, FC, EM, FM. Drafting of manuscript: IG, FM. Review and edition of final manuscript: FM, EB. All authors read and approved the final manuscript.

Competing interests
The authors declare that they have no competing interests.

References

1. Magalhães LNM. Antimicrobial activity of rhamnolipids against Listeria monocytogenes and their synergistic interaction with nisin. Food Control. 2013;1:138–42.
2. Guillet C, Join-Lambert O, Le Monnier A, Leclercq A, Mechaï F, Mamzer-Bruneel M-F, et al. Human Listeriosis caused by Listeria ivanovii. Emerg Infect Dis. 2010;16:136–8.
3. Food and Drug Administration. Bad Bug Book, Foodborne pathogenic microorganisms and natural toxins. Gram-positive bacteria. Second edition. Lampel K, Al-Khaldi S, Cahill S, editors. Silver Spring: Center for Food Safety and Applied Nutrition of the Food and Drug Administration (FDA), U.S. Department of Health and Human Services; 2012.
4. Beierlein JM, Anderson AC. New developments in vaccines, inhibitors of anthrax toxins, and antibiotic therapeutics for bacillus anthracis. Curr Med Chem. 2011;18:5083–94.
5. Vuong C, Otto M. Staphylococcus Epidermidis infections. Microbes Infect. 2002;4:481–9.
6. Witte W, Strommenger B, Stanek C, Cuny C. Methicillin-resistant Staphylococcus Aureus ST398 in humans and animals, Central Europe. Emerg Infect Dis. 2007;13:255–8.
7. Hiramatsu K, Ito T, Tsubakishita S, Sasaki T, Takeuchi F, Morimoto Y, et al. Genomic basis for Methicillin resistance in Staphylococcus Aureus. Infect Chemother. 2013;45:117–36.
8. García-Álvarez L, Holden MTG, Lindsay H, Webb CR, Brown DFJ, Curran MD, et al. Methicillin-resistant Staphylococcus Aureus with a novel mecA homologue in human and bovine populations in the UK and Denmark: a descriptive study. Lancet Infect Dis. 2011;11:595–603.
9. Graveland H, Duim B, van Duijkeren E, Heederik D, Wagenaar JA. Livestock-associated methicillin-resistant Staphylococcus Aureus in animals and humans. Int J Med Microbiol. 2011;301:630–4.
10. Leonard FC, Markey BK. Meticillin-resistant Staphylococcus Aureus in animals: a review. Vet J. 2008;175:27–36.
11. Proctor RA, von Eiff C, Kahl BC, Becker K, McNamara P, Herrmann M, et al. Small colony variants: a pathogenic form of bacteria that facilitates persistent and recurrent infections. Nat Rev Microbiol. 2006;4:295–305.
12. Bryan LE, Kwan S. Aminoglycoside-resistant mutants of Pseudomonas Aeruginosa deficient in cytochrome d, nitrite reductase, and aerobic transport. Antimicrob Agents Chemother. 1981;19:958–64.
13. Moisan H, Brouillette E, Jacob CL, Langlois-Bégin P, Michaud S, Malouin F. Transcription of virulence factors in Staphylococcus Aureus small-colony variants isolated from cystic fibrosis patients is influenced by SigB. J Bacteriol. 2006;188:64–76.
14. Atalla H, Gyles C, Jacob CL, Moisan H, Malouin F, Mallard B. Characterization of a Staphylococcus Aureus small colony variant (SCV) associated with persistent bovine mastitis. Foodborne Pathog Dis. 2008;5:785–99.
15. Tuchscherr L, Medina E, Hussain M, Völker W, Heitmann V, Niemann S, et al. Staphylococcus Aureus phenotype switching: an effective bacterial strategy to escape host immune response and establish a chronic infection. EMBO Mol Med. 2011;3:129–41.
16. Mitchell G, Grondin G, Bilodeau G, Cantin AM, Malouin F. Infection of polarized airway epithelial cells by normal and small-colony variant strains of Staphylococcus Aureus is increased in cells with abnormal cystic fibrosis transmembrane conductance regulator function and is influenced by NF-κB. Infect Immun. 2011;79:3541–51.
17. Ruiz-Rubio M, Pérez-Espinosa A, Lairini K, Roldàn-Arjona T, Dipietro A, Anaya N. Metabolism of the tomato saponin α-tomatine by phytopathogenic fungi. In: Rahman A, editor. Stud. Nat. Prod. Chem. 25. Oxford: Elsevier; 2001. p. 293–326.
18. Simons V, Morrissey JP, Latijnhouwers M, Csukai M, Cleaver A, Yarrow C, et al. Dual effects of plant steroidal alkaloids on Saccharomyces Cerevisiae. Antimicrob Agents Chemother. 2006;50:2732–40.
19. Mitchell G, Gattuso M, Grondin G, Marsault E, Bouarab K, Malouin F. Tomatidine inhibits replication of Staphylococcus Aureus small-Colony variants in cystic fibrosis airway epithelial cells. Antimicrob Agents Chemother. 2011;55:1937–45.
20. Mitchell G, Lafrance M, Boulanger S, Séguin DL, Guay I, Gattuso M, et al. Tomatidine acts in synergy with aminoglycoside antibiotics against multiresistant Staphylococcus Aureus and prevents virulence gene expression. J Antimicrob Chemother. 2012;67:559–68.
21. Chagnon F, Guay I, Bonin M-A, Mitchell G, Bouarab K, Malouin F, et al. Unraveling the structure-activity relationship of tomatidine, a steroid alkaloid with unique antibiotic properties against persistent forms of Staphylococcus aureus. Eur J Med Chem. 2014;80:605–20.
22. Horsburgh MJ, Aish JL, White IJ, Shaw L, Lithgow JK, Foster SJ. sigmaB modulates virulence determinant expression and stress resistance: characterization of a functional rsbU strain derived from Staphylococcus aureus 8325-4. J Bacteriol. 2002;184:5457–67.
23. Brouillette E, Martinez A, Boyll BJ, Allen NE, Malouin F. Persistence of a Staphylococcus aureus small-colony variant under antibiotic pressure in vivo. FEMS Immunol Med Microbiol. 2004;41:35–41.
24. Côté-Gravel J, Brouillette E, Obradović N, Ster C, Talbot BG, Malouin F. Characterization of a vraG mutant in a genetically stable Staphylococcus aureus small-colony variant and preliminary assessment for use as a live-attenuated vaccine against intrammamary infections. Huber VC, editor. PLoS One. 2016;11:e0166621.
25. Gomaa OA, Momtaz OA. 16 rRNA characterization of bacillus isolate and its tolerence profile after subsequent subculturing. Arab J Biotech. 2007;10:107–16.
26. Sendi P, Proctor RA. Staphylococcus aureus as an intracellular pathogen: the role of small colony variants. Trends Microbiol. 2009;17:54–8.
27. Besier S, Smaczny C, von Mallinckrodt C, Krahl A, Ackermann H, Brade V, et al. Prevalence and clinical significance of Staphylococcus aureus small-colony variants in cystic fibrosis lung disease. J Clin Microbiol. 2007;45:168–72.
28. Clinical and Laboratory Standards Institute.
29. Mitchell G, Séguin DL, Asselin A-E, Déziel E, Cantin AM, Frost EH, et al. Staphylococcus aureus Sigma B-dependent emergence of small-colony variants and biofilm production following exposure to Pseudomonas aeruginosa 4-hydroxy-2-heptylquinoline-N-oxide. BMC Microbiol. 2010;10:33.
30. Ceri H, Olson M, Morck D, Storey D, Read R, Buret A, et al. The MBEC assay system: multiple equivalent biofilms for antibiotic and biocide susceptibility testing. Methods Enzymol. 2001;337:377–85.
31. Moskowitz SM, Foster JM, Emerson J, Burns JL. Clinically feasible biofilm susceptibility assay for isolates of Pseudomonas aeruginosa from patients with cystic fibrosis. J Clin Microbiol. 2004;42:1915–22.
32. Harrison JJ, Stremick CA, Turner RJ, Allan ND, Olson ME, Ceri H. Microtiter susceptibility testing of microbes growing on peg lids: a miniaturized biofilm model for high-throughput screening. Nat Protoc. 2010;5:1236–54.
33. Davis BD. Bactericidal synergism between beta-lactams and aminoglycosides: mechanism and possible therapeutic implications. Rev Infect Dis. 1982;4:237–45.
34. Lamontagne Boulet M, Guay I, Rodrigue S, Jacques P-É, Brzezinski R, Bouarab K, et al. Identification of mutations associated with a reduced susceptibility of Staphylococcus aureus small-colony variants to tomatidine. European Society for Clinical Microbiology and Infectious Diseases, Geneva, Switzerland. European Congress of Clinical Microbiology and Infectious Diseases, ECCMID, Abst. P0729, Copenhagen; 2015.
35. Curtis TD, Gram L, Knudsen GM. The small Colony variant of Listeria monocytogenes is more tolerant to antibiotics and has altered survival in RAW 264.7 Murine macrophages. Front Microbiol. 2016;7:1056.
36. Ganière JP, Denuault L. Synergistic interactions between cefalexin and kanamycin in Mueller-Hinton broth medium and in milk. J Appl Microbiol. 2009;107:117–25.
37. Maneke E, Pridmore A, Goby L, Lang I. Kill rate of mastitis pathogens by a combination of cefalexin and kanamycin. J Appl Microbiol. 2011;110:184–90.
38. Silley P, Goby L, Pillar CM. Susceptibility of coagulase-negative staphylococci to a kanamycin and cefalexin combination. J Dairy Sci. 2012;95:3448–53.
39. Ramirez MS, Tolmasky ME. Aminoglycoside modifying enzymes. Drug Resist Updat. 2010;13:151–71.
40. Lowy FD. Is Staphylococcus aureus an intracellular pathogen? Trends Microbiol. 2000;8:341–3.
41. Garcia LG, Lemaire S, Kahl BC, Becker K, Proctor RA, Denis O, et al. Antibiotic activity against small-colony variants of Staphylococcus aureus: review of in vitro, animal and clinical data. J Antimicrob Chemother. 2013;68:1455–64.
42. Mitchell G, Malouin F. Outcome and prevention of Pseudomonas aeruginosa-Staphylococcus aureus interactions during pulmonary infections in cystic fibrosis. In: Sriramulu D, editor. Cyst. Fibros. - renewed hopes through res: InTech; 2012.
43. Hamon M, Bierne H, Cossart P. Listeria monocytogenes: a multifaceted model. Nat Rev Microbiol. 2006;4:423–34.
44. Costerton JW, Stewart PS, Greenberg EP. Bacterial biofilms: a common cause of persistent infections. Science. 1999;284:1318–22.
45. Srey S, Jahid I, Ha S-D. Biofilm formation in food industries: a food safety concern. Food Control. 2013;31:572–85.

2

Causality and preventability assessment of adverse drug events of antibiotics among inpatients having different lengths of hospital stay

Anum Saqib[1†], Muhammad Rehan Sarwar[1,2*†] (iD), Muhammad Sarfraz[3] and Sadia Iftikhar[2]

Abstract

Background: A large number of hospital admissions are attributed to adverse drug reactions (ADRs) and they are the fifth leading cause of death worldwide. The present study aimed to assess the causality and preventability of adverse drug events (ADEs) of antibiotics among inpatients having different lengths of hospital stay.

Methods: A prospective, observational study was conducted in four tertiary-care public sector hospitals of Lahore, Pakistan. Study population consisted of hospitalized patients who were prescribed one or more antibiotics. Data were collected between 1st January, 2017 and 30th June, 2017 from 1249 patients. Naranjo score, modified Schumock and Thornton scale were used for causality and preventability assessments, respectively. Medication errors (MEs) were assessed by MEs tracking form. SPSS and Microsoft Excel were used for data analysis.

Results: A total of 2686 antibiotics were prescribed to 1249 patients and 486 ADEs were found. The preventability assessment revealed that most of the ADEs (78.8%) were found among patients having long length of stay (LOS) in hospital and were preventable (59.3% of the ADEs were definitely preventable while 44.7% were probably preventable) and caused by MEs including wrong drug (40.1%) and monitoring errors (25%). The errors were caused due to non-adherence of policies (38.4%) and lack of information about antibiotics (32%). Most of the non-preventable ADEs or ADRs among patients having long and short LOS in hospital were "probable" (35.5%) and "possible" (35.8%), respectively. Logistic regression analysis revealed that ADEs were significantly less among females (OR = 0.047, 95% CI = 0.018—0.121, *p-value* = < 0.001), patients aged 18—52 years (OR = 0.041, 95% CI = 0.013—0.130, *p-value* = < 0.001), patients with ARTIs (OR = 0.004, 95% CI = 0.01–0.019, *p-value* = < 0.001), patients prescribed with 2 antibiotics per prescription (OR = 0.455, 95% CI = 0.319—0.650, *p-value* = < 0.001) and patients with long LOS (OR = 14.825, 95% CI = 11.198—19.627, *p-value* = < 0.001).

Conclusion: Antibiotics associated definitely preventable ADEs were more commonly found in patients having long LOS in the inpatient departments because of MEs and lack of proper pharmacovigilance system. The ADRs showed a probable and possible causal association with both β-lactams and non β-lactams antibiotics.

Keywords: Antibiotics, Adverse drug reactions, Adverse drug events, Length of stay, Causality, Preventability

* Correspondence: rehansarwaralvi@gmail.com
†Anum Saqib and Muhammad Rehan Sarwar contributed equally to this work.
[1]Department of Pharmacy, The Islamia University of Bahawalpur, Bahawalpur, Punjab, Pakistan
[2]Akhtar Saeed College of Pharmaceutical Sciences, Lahore, Pakistan
Full list of author information is available at the end of the article

Background

According to the World Health Organization (WHO) adverse drug reactions (ADRs) are defined as, "any response to a drug which is noxious, unintended, and that occurs at doses normally used in man for the prophylaxis, diagnosis, or therapy of disease" [1]. On the basis of the National Coordinating Council for Medication Error Reporting and Prevention (NCC MERP) recommendations, adverse drug events (ADEs) can be termed as injuries which are either related to the medical interventions or the dose of the drugs [2]. As ADEs are not always associated with the use of drugs, so all ADRs can be attributed as ADEs but all ADEs can never be the result of ADRs. The risk of ADRs is associated with almost all the prescribed therapeutic agents. But these untoward effects may vary in terms of severity level i.e., from minor to severe or lethal [3].

The duration of a single episode of hospitalization i.e., length of stay (LOS) can be considered as one of the risk factors of ADEs. The stay of patient for each additional day in hospital increases the probability of developing ADEs because this provides more time for an ADE to occur [4]. According to a study if the LOS in hospital is prolonged then there will be an increment of 6% in the development of ADEs with the stay for each additional day [5]. Similarly, a Swedish study demonstrated ADRs as one of the most recurrent causes of mortality because one out of every seventh inpatient suffers from ADR during hospital stay [6]. A study demonstrated the prevalence rate of ADEs among hospitalized patients of England as 3.2%, Germany as 4.8% and the United States of America (USA) as 5.6% [7]. Furthermore, it is estimated that the incidence of life threatening ADRs during hospital stay ranges from 0.05 to 0.09% [8, 9]. Besides LOS, a meta-analysis revealed age, gender and drug exposure as the major contributing factors towards ADRs [8].

The prime role of pharmacovigilance system is to ensure patient safety due to its involvement in comprehension, recognition and prevention of ADEs [10]. The identification of ADEs still remains a major challenge for physicians. The causal association of ADRs with the drug is mandatory to evaluate in pharmacovigilance because it gives an insight about risk to benefit ratio of a particular drug on individual level [11]. Thus, poor monitoring and reporting system of ADEs has dramatically increase the patient's LOS in hospital and economically burdened the healthcare system [12].

Antibiotics are among the most frequently prescribed therapeutic agents among hospitalized patients of all age groups [13]. It is estimated that more than half of the hospitalized patients are prescribed with antibiotics [14, 15]. It has been reported that the excessive use of antibiotics is associated with problems like antibiotic resistance [16]. Moreover, the higher rate of prescribing these agents has increased the chances of MEs up to several folds which in turn leads to the development of preventable ADEs [17]. In correspondence to this fact, a study conducted in Netherland report the incidence of preventable ADEs among 0.2% of the hospitalized patients [18]. A study conducted by Shehab, et al. documented that 19% patients visited emergency department due to antibiotics-associated ADRs [19]. Multiple reasons make inpatients more prone to ADRs which may include; 1) the trend of administering multiple antibiotics among inpatients. and 2) mostly, the inpatients comprises of pediatrics, geriatrics or patients having various co-morbidities and all these patients have high risk of developing ADRs [20, 21]. There is a dearth of proper pharmacovigilance surveillance system in Pakistan on regional, provincial and national level which leads to poor availability of data regarding antibiotic associated ADEs and its association with the LOS. Previously published studies do not give insight on this issue. The present study aims to assess the causality and preventability of adverse drug events of antibiotics (β-lactams and non β-lactams) among inpatients having different lengths of hospital stay.

Methods

Study design and settings

A prospective, cross-sectional, observational study was conducted in four public tertiary care hospitals (Mayo hospital, Jinnah hospital, General hospital, and Services hospital) of Lahore, Punjab province of Pakistan. According to latest Pakistani census, the total population living in Pakistan is 201,995,540 [22]. Lahore is the most populous city of Punjab province of Pakistan, with a total population of 11,126,285 [23]. The study settings lack pharmacovigilance centers and ADEs registers. The characteristics of the selected hospitals are summarized in Table 1.

Study inclusion criteria

The study population included the patients of all age groups, admitted in general internal medicine ward and pediatric ward, prescribed with antibiotics on the basis of differential diagnosis for ≥24 h.

Study exclusion criteria

All the patients with medical history of cardiac diseases, hepatic and renal insufficiencies, ear, nose and throat (ENT) disorders and unavailability of information regarding LOS in the hospital were excluded from this study.

Table 1 Characteristics of selected hospitals

Sr. no.	Characteristics	Mayo hospital	Jinnah hospital	General hospital	Services hospital
1	Number of beds	2400	1500	1300	1196
2	Inpatients visit last year	343, 114	217, 245	134, 491	125, 868
3	Prescribers/Medical officers	550	348	300	274
4	Nurses	500	313	271	249
5	Pharmacists/Dispensers	30	19	16	14
8	a Other paramedical staff	671	445	382	304
10	Existence of pharmacovigilance center in hospital	No	No	No	No
11	Maintenance of ADR registers	No	No	No	No

aOther Paramedical staff includes; medical technicians, ward boys, and sweepers

Data collection

A data collection form was developed which consisted of seven parts: 1) characteristics of the patients, 2) diagnosis, 3) recommended antibiotics, 4) medication errors, 5) causality assessment by Naranjo score, 6) preventability assessment and 7) the effect of ADRs on organ system (if any). The Anatomical Therapeutic Chemical (ATC) classification system [24] was used for the coding of antibiotics. SPSS version 21.0 was used for calculation of reliability coefficients. Internal consistency was measured by Cronbach's alpha, while reproducibility was evaluated by using intra-class correlation for each item in the scales, with acceptable values ≥0.6. Calculation for Cronbach's alpha was set at 0.76 for Schmuck and Thornton scale, 0.74 for ME tracking form, and 0.78 for Naranjo score. A pilot study was undertaken between November and December 2016 for pre-testing the study instrument. Data were collected between 1st January, 2017 and 30th June, 2017 according to the objectives of the study. The investigational team included a medical practitioner, pharmacist and a nurse. A total of 8 investigational teams were made. Two investigational teams were assigned to each hospital; one for internal medicine ward and other for pediatric ward.

The review of medical record was conducted on daily basis until the patient was discharged from the respective ward. This enables the investigators to scrutinize data from pertinent lab reports, physician's progress notes, patient's medication records (dose, dosage form, frequency and duration of prescribed antibiotics), physician's order, multidisciplinary progress notes and discharge summaries. All the sign and symptoms that appeared after the use of antibiotics were also recorded. The team also participated in ward rounds and checked the presence of any alerts for MEs and ADEs. The expert opinions of physicians and clinical pharmacists were also taken in account before reaching the final decision about the occurrence of ADEs. The LOS in hospital was evaluated by measuring the difference between date of admission from the date of discharge [25]. Although it was difficult to evaluate whether the prolonged LOS in

hospital was the contributing factor of ADEs or any underlying disease, so the assessment was made by taking into account the clinical judgments, nature and severity of underlying disease and social factors that may contribute in lengthening the patient's stay time in hospital.

Note: In this study ADEs refers to injuries which are either caused by the drug (i.e., ADRs or non-preventable ADEs) or by the use of the therapeutic agents (i.e., medication errors or preventable ADEs) while ADRs refer to

Table 2 Characteristics of patients (N = 1249)

Characteristics	n (%)a
Gender	
Male	716 (57.3)
Female	533 (42.7)
Age	
Adults (> 18 years)	865 (69.3)
Children (≤18 years)	384 (30.7)
Co-morbidities	
Diabetes	526 (42.1)
Asthma	424 (33.9)
Tuberculosis	137 (11.0)
Cystic fibrosis	162 (13.0)
Reasons of prescribing antibiotics	
Acute respiratory tract infections	362 (29.0)
Urinary tract infections	462 (37.0)
Soft tissue infections	287 (23.1)
Skin infections	138 (11.0)
Number of antibiotics prescribed per prescription	
1	229 (18.3)
2	603 (48.3)
3	417 (33.4)
LOS in the hospital	
Long (≥5 days)	536 (42.9)
Short (< 5 days)	713 (57.1)

aPercentages have been calculated with respect to the total sample size (n = 1249)

Table 3 Antibiotics prescribed among study population

Antibiotics Class	ATC code	Number of patients received antibiotics, N = 1249, n (%)	Number of prescribed antibiotics, N = 2686, n (%)
β – Lactams			
Penicillins	J01C	194 (15.5)	261 (9.7)
Carbapenem	J01DH	106 (8.5)	234 (8.7)
Cephalosporins	J01D	223 (17.9)	292 (10.9)
Non- β Lactams			
Flouroquinolones	J01 M	291 (23.3)	316 (11.8)
Aminoglycosides	J01G	192 (15.4)	226 (8.4)
Tetracyclines	J01AA	193 (15.5)	221 (8.2)
Lincosamide	J01FF	127 (10.2)	209 (7.8)
Macrolides	J01FA	252 (20.2)	311 (11.6)
Glycopeptide	J01XA	91 (7.3)	214 (7.9)
Oxazolidones	J01XX	102 (8.2)	186 (6.9)
Imidazole derivatives	G01AF	113 (9.5)	216 (8.0)

ATC Anatomical Therapeutic Chemical Classification System

the definition given by Edwards and Aronson i.e., unpleasant or harmful reactions that have causal relation with the medicinal product and predicts untoward outcomes from future administration and demands withdrawal from therapy, alteration of dosage regimen and specific treatments [26]. British National Formulary was used for confirming the ADRs [27]. MEs are those that occur during the processing of medication i.e., prescribing, transcribing, dispensing, administering, adherence, or monitoring a drug [28]. MEs were identified through the standard guidelines of Current Medical Diagnosis AND Treatment (CMDT) [29], National Institute of Health and Clinical Excellence (NICE) guidelines [30], British National Formulary (BNF) for children [31] and Infectious Diseases Society of Pakistan (IDSP) guidelines for antibiotic use [32].

Outcome variables

The outcome variables included causality assessment and preventability assessment. The cases in which ADEs appeared were further analyzed for assessing the preventability by Schumock and Thornton Scale. Medication errors were determined by using medication error tracking form among definitely preventable and probably preventable ADEs. Naranjo scale was used for determining the causal relationship between non-preventable ADEs and antibiotics.

Schumock and Thornton scale

The Schumock and Thornton criteria [33] was established for assessing the preventability of ADRs. The modified form of this criterion has been used in various studies [34, 35]. It has three sections namely definitely preventable, probably preventable and non-preventable. Section A comprises of five questions

while section B has four questions. All the answers are categorized as "Yes" or "No". ADRs were "definitely preventable" if answer was "yes" to one or more questions in section A. If answers were all negative then we proceeded to section B. ADRs were "probably preventable" if answer was "yes" to one or more questions in section B. If answers were all negative then we proceeded to section C. In Section C the ADRs were non-preventable.

Naranjo scale

The Naranjo Scale was developed by Naranjo and co-workers from the University of Toronto [36] for assessing the likelihood of whether an ADR is due to some particular drug or due to other factors. This validated tool has been used in multiple studies [37, 38]. This scale comprises of 10 questions that are answered "Yes", "No", or "Do not know". Different point values (– 1, 0, + 1 or + 2) are assigned to each answer. Total scores range from – 4 to + 13; the reaction is considered definite if the score is 9 or higher, probable if 5 to 8, possible if 1 to 4, and doubtful if 0 or less.

Medication error tracking form

This tool was prepared for addressing MEs in hospitals for the California Health Care Foundation Data [39]. It consisted of three sections: 1) patient information, 2) medication order information and 3) medication error categorization. The third section comprised of "medication class", "categories" and "possible causes" of MEs. It also classified MEs into five categories: A) prescribing, B) transcribing, C) dispensing, D) administering and E) monitoring.

Table 4 Effect of antibiotics on organ systems of study participants (N = 486)

Antibiotics	Total ADEs n (%)	LOS n (%)	Cardiac[a] n (%)	GIT[b] n (%)	Ototoxicity[c] n (%)	Hematology[d] n (%)	Hepatobiliary[e] n (%)	Renal[f] n (%)	Neurotoxicity[g] n (%)	Others[h] n (%)
β - Lactams										
Penicillins	62 (12.8)	Short LOS 0 (0.0)	0 (0.0)	0 (0.0)	0 (0.0)	0 (0.0)	0 (0.0)	0 (0.0)	0 (0.0)	0 (0.0)
		Long LOS 62 (100.0)	0 (0.0)	34 (54.8)	0 (0.0)	2 (3.2)	5 (8.1)	2 (3.2)	10 (16.1)	9 (14.5)
Carbapenem	34 (6.9)	Short LOS 9 (26.5)	0 (0.0)	2 (22.2)	0 (0.0)	0 (0.0)	7 (77.8)	0 (0.0)	0 (0.0)	0 (0.0)
		Long LOS 25 (73.5)	0 (0.0)	14 (56.0)	0 (0.0)	10 (40.0)	1 (4.0)	0 (0.0)	0 (0.0)	0 (0.0)
Cephalosporins	66 (13.6)	Short LOS 15 (22.7)	0 (0.0)	4 (26.7)	0 (0.0)	6 (40.0)	2 (13.3)	1 (6.7)	1 (6.7)	1 (6.7)
		Long LOS 51 (77.3)	0 (0.0)	10 (19.6)	0 (0.0)	18 (35.3)	17 (33.3)	5 (9.8)	1 (1.9)	0 (0.0)
Total β – Lactams	*162 (33.3)*	*Short LOS 24 (14.8)*	*0 (0.0)*	*6 (25.0)*	*0 (0.0)*	*6 (25.0)*	*9 (37.5)*	*1 (4.2)*	*1 (4.2)*	*1 (4.2)*
		Long LOS 138 (85.2)	*0 (0.0)*	*58 (42.0)*	*0 (0.0)*	*30 (21.7)*	*23 (16.7)*	*7 (5.1)*	*11 (7.9)*	*9 (6.5)*
Non- β Lactams										
Aminoglycosides	37 (7.6)	Short LOS 5 (13.5)	0 (0.0)	0 (0.0)	1 (20.0)	0 (0.0)	0 (0.0)	1 (20.0)	1 (20.0)	2 (40.0)
		Long LOS 32 (86.5)	0 (0.0)	5 (15.6)	10 (31.3)	2 (6.3)	0 (0.0)	10 (31.3)	2 (6.3)	3 (9.4)
Macrolides	61 (12.6)	Short LOS 5 (8.2)	0 (0.0)	1 (20.0)	1 (20.0)	1 (20.0)	1 (20.0)	0 (0.0)	0 (0.0)	1 (20.0)
		Long LOS 56 (91.8)	8 (14.3)	17 (30.4)	10 (17.9)	2 (3.4)	8 (14.3)	0 (0.0)	1 (1.8)	10 (17/9)
Fluoroquinolones	61(12.6)	Short LOS 17 (27.9)	0 (0.0)	0 (0.0)	6 (35.3)	2 (11.8)	6 (35.3)	1 (5.9)	0 (0.0)	2 (11.8)
		Long LOS 44 (72.1)	7 (15.9)	8 (18.2)	3 (6.8)	3 (6.8)	9 (20.5)	5 (11.4)	8 (18.2)	1 (2.3)
Tetracyclines	36 (7.4)	Short LOS 7 (19.4)	0 (0.0)	3 (42.9)	0 (0.0)	0 (0.0)	0 (0.0)	0 (0.0)	2 (28.6)	2 (28.6)
		Long LOS 29 (80.6)	0 (0.0)	16 (55.2)	0 (0.0)	0 (0.0)	0 (0.0)	0 (0.0)	4 (13.8)	9 (31.0)
Lincosamide	26 (5.4)	Short LOS 5 (19.2)	0 (0.0)	4 (80.0)	0 (0.0)	1 (20.0)	0 (0.0)	0 (0.0)	0 (0.0)	0 (0.0)
		Long LOS 21 (80.8)	0 (0.0)	15 (71.4)	0 (0.0)	3 (14.3)	0 (0.0)	0 (0.0)	0 (0.0)	3 (14.3)
Glycopeptide	37 (7.6)	Short LOS 18 (48.6)	0 (0.0)	4 (22.2)	0 (0.0)	0 (0.0)	0 (0.0)	8 (44.4)	0 (0.0)	6 (33.3)
		Long LOS 19 (51.4)	0 (0.0)	0 (0.0)	8 (42.1)	7 (36.8)	0 (0.0)	2 (10.5)	0 (0.0)	2 (10.5)
Oxazolidones	29 (5.9)	Short LOS 9 (31.0)	0 (0.0)	2 (22.2)	0 (0.0)	0 (0.0)	0 (0.0)	0 (0.0)	4 (44.4)	3 (33.3)
		Long LOS 20 (68.9)	0 (0.0)	7 (35.0)	0 (0.0)	1 (5.0)	0 (0.0)	0 (0.0)	5 (25.0)	7 (35.0)
Imidazole derivative	37 (7.6)	Short LOS 13 (35.1)	0 (0.0)	5 (38.5)	0 (0.0)	0 (0.0)	0 (0.0)	0 (0.0)	0 (0.0)	8 (61.5)
		Long LOS 24 (64.9)	0 (0.0)	11 (40.8)	0 (0.0)	0 (0.0)	0 (0.0)	0 (0.0)	13 (54.2)	0 (0.0)
Total non β – Lactams	*324 (66.7)*	*Short LOS 79 (24.4)*	*0 (0.0)*	*19 (24.1)*	*8 (10.1)*	*4 (5.1)*	*7 (8.9)*	*10 (12.7)*	*7 (8.9)*	*24 (30.4)*
		Long LOS 245 (75.6)	*15 (6.1)*	*79 (32.3)*	*31 (12.7)*	*18 (7.4)*	*17 (6.9)*	*17 (6.9)*	*33 (13.5)*	*35 (14.3)*

Table 4 Effect of antibiotics on organ systems of study participants (N = 486) (Continued)

Antibiotics	Total ADEs n (%)	LOS n (%)		Cardiac[a] n (%)	GIT[b] n (%)	Ototoxicity[c] n (%)	Hematology[d] n (%)	Hepatobiliary[e] n (%)	Renal[f] n (%)	Neurotoxicity[g] n (%)	Others[h] n (%)
Total (β – Lactams + Non β – Lactams)	486 (38.9)	Short LOS	103 (21.2)	0 (0.0)	25 (24.3)	8 (7.8)	10 (9.7)	16 (15.5)	11 (10.7)	8 (7.8)	25 (24.3)
		Long LOS	383 (78.8)	15 (3.9)	137 (35.8)	31 (8.1)	48 (12.5)	40 (10.4)	24 (6.3)	44 (11.5)	44 (11.5)

[a]QTc > 440 millisecond (ms) in males or > 460 ms in females in the absence of preexisting arrhythmias, based on ≥2 electrocardiograms

[b]Abdominal discomfort, nausea and vomiting associated with antibiotic administration, in the absence of an alternate explanation

[c]The ability of speech discrimination was diminished upon administration of antibiotics

[d]Developed in the absence of myelosuppressive drugs and characterized as thrombocytopenia (decrease in platelet count < 150 × 103/μL), anemia (decrease in hemoglobin level < 10 g/dL) and leukopenia (decrease in white blood cells level < 4500 cells/ μL)

[e]Characterized as increase in total bilirubin (> 3 mg/dL) or alanine transaminase (> 3 times patient's baseline) or aspartate transaminase (> 3 times patient's baseline) when there was no preexisting hepatobiliary disease

[f]Characterized as high level of serum creatinine i.e. > 1.5 time baseline when there was no preexisting acute kidney injury (e.g. sepsis) or exposure to nephrotoxic drug or intravenous contrast

[g]Demonstrated as antibiotic associated toxicity, peripheral neuropathy, seizures (when there was no preexisting neurologic condition) or altered mental condition

[h]Other ADRs among children may include penicillins-associated hypersensitivity; macrolides-associated rashes and Stevens-Johnson syndrome; flouroquinolones-associated arthralgia and tendon disorders; tetracyclines-associated tooth discoloration and enamel defects; Lincosamide-associated metallic taste; Glycopeptide-associated flushing and maculopapular rash; Oxazolidones-associated red man syndrome, pruritus and oral candidiasis; imidazole-associated taste disturbance. Other ADRs among adults may include penicillins-associated hypersensitivity; aminoglycosides-associated stomatitis; macrolides-associated pancreatitis; cephalosporins-associated Stevens-Johnson syndrome, pruritus and urticaria; Fluoroquinolones-associated hypotension; Tetracyclines-associated rash, dermatitis and angioedema; Glycopeptide-associated red man syndrome and phlebitis; Oxazolidones-associated taste disturbance and polyuria; imidazole-associated taste disturbance and neuropathy

Statistical analysis

A convenient sampling technique was used to select the study participants. All the patients, admitted in internal medicine and pediatric departments during the 6 months of study period were considered as study population. Among them, patients met the inclusion criteria were taken as a sample size for this study. Statistical Package for Social Sciences (IBM Corp. Released 2012. IBM SPSS Statistics for Windows Version 21.0. Armonk, NY: IBM Corp.) and Microsoft Excel (MS Office 2010) were used for data analysis. Like previously published studies [40–42], descriptive statistics such as frequencies and percentages were used to present the data. And logistic regression analysis was performed to figure out the factors associated with ADEs. Results were expressed as Odds Ratio (OR) accompanied by 95% Confidence Intervals (95% CI) and a p-value < 0.05 was used for statistical significance of differences.

Results

Characteristics of the patients

According to hospitals records, 14,592 patients were admitted in internal medicine and pediatric departments during the 6 months of study period. A total of 1249 patients (age range 6 to 52 years) met the inclusion criteria of this study. Among them, 57.3% were male and 69.3% were aged > 18 years. 37% patients ($n = 462$) were prescribed antibiotics for urinary tract infections, 29% ($n = 362$) for acute respiratory tract infections, 23% ($n = 287$) for soft tissue infections and 11% ($n = 137$) for skin

infections. Overall the LOS of 42.9% ($n = 536$) patients in the hospital was ≥ 5 days while 57.1% ($n = 713$) patients stayed for < 5 days in the healthcare settings (Table 2).

Prescribing pattern of antibiotics

A total of 2686 antibiotics were prescribed among 1249 patients. Among β – Lactams, cephalosporins (10.9%, $n = 292$) while in non β – Lactams, fluoroquinolones (11.8%, $n = 316$) and macrolides (11.6%, $n = 311$) were the most frequently prescribed antibiotics (Table 3).

Organ system affected by ADEs

The proportion of ADEs was 486 (38.9%) among the total study participants. Overall, the most affected organ system by both β-lactams and non β-lactams antibiotics was GIT (long LOS = 35.8%, short LOS = 24.3%) as shown in Table 4.

Preventability assessment

More than half ($n = 383$, 78.8%) of the ADEs were found among patients having long LOS in hospital. Among them, most of the ADEs were preventable i.e., the proportion of definitely preventable ADEs was 171 (44.7%); whereas, the proportion of probably preventable ADEs was 56 (14.6%) according to modified Schumock and Thornton criteria (Table 5).

Overall most of the definitely preventable (63.7%, $n = 109$), probably preventable (69.6%, $n = 39$) and

Table 5 Preventability assessment ($N = 486$)

Schumock and Thornton criteria	Long LOS, $N = 383$, n (%)	Short LOS, $N = 103$, n (%)	Total, $N = 486$, n (%)
Section A: Definitely preventable ADEs			
Was there a history of allergy or previous reaction to the drug?	4 (1.0)	5 (4.9)	9 (1.9)
Was the drug involved inappropriate for the patient's clinical condition?	100 (26.1)	14 (13.6)	114 (23.5)
Was the dose, route, or frequency of administration inappropriate for patient's age, weight or disease state?	53 (13.8)	11 (10.7)	64 (13.2)
Was toxic serum drug concentration or lab monitoring test documented?	7 (1.8)	9 (8.7)	16 (3.3)
Was there a known treatment for ADEs?	7 (1.8)	2 (1.9)	9 (1.9)
Total	171 (44.7)	41 (39.8)	212 (43.6)
Section B: Probably preventable ADEs			
Was therapeutic drug monitoring or other necessary lab test not performed?	31 (8.1)	7 (6.8)	38 (7.8)
Was the drug interaction involved in ADEs?	4 (1.0)	2 (1.9)	6 (1.2)
Was poor compliance involved in ADE?	13 (3.4)	4 (3.9)	17 (3.5)
Were preventative measures not prescribed or administered to the patient?	8 (2.1)	3 (2.9)	11 (2.3)
Total	56 (14.6)	16 (15.5)	72 (14.8)
Total (preventable ADEs)	227 (59.3)	57 (55.3)	284 (58.4)
Section C: Non-preventable ADEs or ADRs			
If all the above criteria not fulfilled.	156 (40.7)	46 (44.7)	202 (41.6)

LOS Length of stay ADEs Adverse drug events ADRs Adverse drug reactions

Table 6 Adverse drug events with respect to class of prescribed antibiotics (N = 486)

Antibiotics	ATC code	Definitely preventable ADEs			Probably preventable ADEs			Non-preventable ADEs		
		Long LOS, N = 171, n (%)	Short LOS, N = 41, n (%)	Total, N = 212, n (%)	Long LOS, N = 56, n (%)	Short LOS, N = 16, n (%)	Total, N = 72, n (%)	Long LOS, N = 156, n (%)	Short LOS, N = 46, n (%)	Total, N = 202, n (%)
β - Lactams										
Penicillins	J01C	25 (14.6)	0 (0.0)	25 (11.8)	9 (16.1)	0 (0.0)	9 (12.5)	28 (17.9)	0 (0.0)	28 (13.9)
Carbapenem	J01DH	11 (6.4)	7 (17.1)	18 (8.5)	2 (3.6)	0 (0.0)	2 (2.8)	12 (7.7)	2 (4.4)	14 (6.9)
Cephalosporins	J01D	26 (15.2)	5 (12.2)	31 (14.6)	6 (10.7)	0 (0.0)	6 (8.3)	19 (12.2)	10 (21.7)	29 (14.4)
Total β – Lactams		62 (36.2)	12 (29.3)	74 (34.9)	17 (30.4)	0 (0.0)	17 (23.6)	59 (37.8)	12 (26.1)	71 (35.2)
Non- β Lactams										
Flouroquinolones	J01 M	18 (10.5)	3 (7.3)	21 (9.9)	7 (12.5)	6 (37.5)	13 (18.1)	19 (12.2)	8 (17.4)	27 (13.4)
Aminoglycosides	J01G	13 (7.6)	3 (7.3)	16 (7.6)	6 (10.7)	0 (0.0)	6 (8.3)	13 (8.3)	2 (4.4)	15 (7.4)
Tetracyclines	J01AA	12 (7.0)	1 (2.4)	13 (6.1)	5 (8.9)	3 (18.8)	8 (11.1)	12 (7.7)	3 (6.5)	15 (7.4)
Macrolides	J01FA	27 (15.8)	4 (9.8)	31 (14.6)	4 (7.1)	0 (0.0)	4 (5.6)	25 (16.0)	1 (2.2)	26 (12.9)
Lincosamide	J01FF	4 (2.3)	1 (2.4)	5 (2.4)	10 (17.8)	0 (0.0)	10 (13.9)	7 (4.5)	4 (8.7)	11 (5.5)
Glycopeptide	J01XA	9 (5.3)	8 (19.5)	17 (8.0)	2 (3.6)	2 (12.5)	4 (5.6)	8 (5.1)	8 (17.4)	16 (7.9)
Oxazolidones	J01XX	13 (7.6)	3 (7.3)	16 (7.6)	1 (1.8)	3 (18.8)	4 (5.6)	6 (3.9)	3 (6.5)	9 (4.5)
Imidazole derivatives	G01AF	13 (7.6)	6 (14.6)	19 (8.9)	4 (7.1)	2 (12.5)	6 (8.3)	7 (4.5)	5 (10.9)	12 (5.9)
Total Non β – Lactams		109 (63.7)	29 (70.7)	138(65.1)	39 (69.6)	16(100.0)	55 (76.4)	97 (62.2)	34 (73.9)	131(64.9)

ATC Anatomical Therapeutic Chemical Classification System, ADEs Adverse drug events, LOS Length of stay

non-preventable ADEs (62.2%, $n = 92$) were most commonly caused by non β-Lactams as compared to β-Lactams class of antibiotics especially among patients having long LOS in hospital (Table 6).

Medication errors

Among 284 cases of preventable ADEs, the wrong drug errors ($n = 114$, 40.1%) and monitoring errors ($n = 71$, 25%) were more commonly found among study population. The antibiotics administered through oral route had greater ADEs (proportion of ADEs = 4 out of 5) as compared to the antibiotics administered through parental route (proportion of ADEs = 1 out of 5). Physician ordering (22.2%, $n = 63$) and patient monitoring (21.1%, $n = 60$) were the most common stages of medication errors. These errors were caused due to non-adherence of policies and procedures (38.4%, $n = 109$) and lack of information about antibiotics (32%, $n = 91$) (Table 7).

Causality assessment

156 (77.2%) ADEs were detected among patients having long LOS (> 5 days) and 46 (22.3%) among patients having short LOS (≤ 5 days). Overall, most of the ADRs were "probable" (long LOS = 35.3%, short LOS = 34.8%) and "possible" (long LOS = 33.9%, short LOS = 30.4%) and occurred more frequently due to non β lactams as compared to β lactams antibiotics (Table 8).

Determinants associated with ADEs among study respondents

Logistic regression analysis was used to examine the association between ADEs and the independent variables. Results of this analysis revealed that females had 95.3% less ADEs (OR = 0.047, 95% CI = 0.018—0.121, *p-value* = < 0.001) as compared to males. Among the age groups, patients aged > 18 years (OR = 0.041, 95% CI = 0.013—0.130, *p-value* = < 0.001) were likely to have less ADEs as compared to patients aged ≤18 years. While examining the association between co-morbidities and

Table 7 Antibiotic associated errors in study population ($N = 284$)

Variables	Long length of stay, $N = 227$, n (%)	Short length of stay, $N = 57$, n (%)	Total, $N = 284$, n (%)
Type of medication errors			
Wrong drug	100 (44.1)	14 (24.6)	114 (40.1)
Wrong dose	35 (15.4)	6 (10.5)	41 (14.4)
Wrong route	2 (0.9)	3 (5.3)	5 (1.8)
Wrong time	13 (5.7)	2 (3.5)	15 (5.3)
Deteriorated drug	3 (1.3)	0 (0.0)	3 (1.1)
Omission	12 (5.3)	3 (5.3)	15 (5.3)
Wrong dosage form	3 (1.3)	0 (0.0)	3 (1.1)
Non-adherence	13 (5.7)	4 (7.0)	17 (5.9)
Monitoring error	46 (20.3)	25 (43.9)	71 (25.0)
Stages of errors			
Physician ordering	59 (25.9)	4 (7.0)	63 (22.2)
Transcribing	41 (18.1)	7 (12.3)	48 (16.9)
Dispensing pharmacist	36 (15.9)	14 (24.6)	50 (17.6)
Nurse administering	37 (16.3)	9 (15.8)	46 (16.2)
Patient monitoring	37 (16.3)	23 (40.4)	60 (21.1)
Others[a]	17 (7.5)	0 (0.0)	17 (5.9)
Causes of errors			
Lack of knowledge about the patients[b]	46 (20.3)	2 (3.5)	48 (16.9)
Lack of information about antibiotics[c]	77 (33.9)	14 (24.6)	91 (32.0)
Non-adherence to policies and procedures[d]	73 (32.2)	36 (63.2)	109 (38.4)
Miscellaneous[e]	31 (13.7)	5 (8.8)	36 (12.7)

[a]Medication errors due to patient non-adherence
[b]Information about allergy, lab tests results, concomitant medications and conditions either not available or noted
[c]Indication for antibiotic use, compatibility, available dosage form, dosing guidelines and route of administration
[d]Use of abbreviation in medication ordering, incomplete medication order processed, deviation from treatment protocols, delay in dispensing, use of non-standard dosing schedule, and drug preparation errors
[e]Illegible handwriting of physicians, memory lapse, and unavailability of drugs

Table 8 Causality assessment with respect to antibiotics class (N = 202)

Antibiotics Class	ATC code	Long length of stay					Short length of stay				
		Naranjo score				Total ADRs	Naranjo score				Total ADRs
		Definite[a] n (%)	Probable[b] n (%)	Possible[c] n (%)	Doubtful[d] n (%)		Definite[a] n (%)	Probable[b] n (%)	Possible[c] n (%)	Doubtful[d] n (%)	
β – Lactams											
Penicillins	J01C	1 (3.6)	15 (53.6)	4 (14.3)	8 (28.6)	28	0 (0.0)	0 (0.0)	0 (0.0)	0 (0.0)	0
Carbapenem	J01DH	0 (0.0)	5 (41.7)	3 (25.0)	4 (33.3)	12	1 (50.0)	1 (50.0)	0 (0.0)	0 (0.0)	2
Cephalosporins	J01D	0 (0.0)	7 (36.8)	9 (47.4)	3 (15.8)	19	3 (30.0)	1 (10.0)	1 (10.0)	5 (50.0)	10
Total β - Lactams		*1 (1.7)*	*27 (45.8)*	*16 (27.1)*	*15 (25.4)*	*59*	*4 (33.3)*	*2 (16.7)*	*1 (8.3)*	*5 (41.7)*	*12*
Non- β Lactams											
Flouroquinolones	J01 M	4 (21.1)	6 (31.6)	7 (36.8)	2 (10.5)	19	0 (0.0)	5 (62.5)	2 (25.0)	1 (12.5)	8
Aminoglycosides	J01G	2 (15.4)	4 (30.8)	5 (38.5)	2 (15.4)	13	0 (0.0)	1 (50.0)	0 (0.0)	1 (50.0)	2
Macrolides	J01FA	2 (7.1)	5 (20.0)	12 (48.0)	6 (24.0)	25	0 (0.0)	0 (0.0)	1 (100.0)	0 (0.0)	1
Tetracyclines	J01AA	0 (0.0)	3 (25.0)	4 (33.3)	5 (41.7)	12	2 (66.7)	0 (0.0)	1 (33.3)	0 (0.0)	3
Lincosamide	J01FF	0 (0.0)	2 (28.6)	2 (28.6)	3 (42.9)	7	1 (25.0)	3 (75.0)	0 (0.0)	0 (0.0)	4
Glycopeptide	J01XA	2 (25.0)	3 (37.5)	1 (12.5)	2 (25.0)	8	0 (0.0)	2 (25.0)	5 (62.5)	1 (12.5)	8
Oxazolidones	J01XX	0 (0.0)	2 (33.3)	4 (66.7)	0 (0.0)	6	0 (0.0)	1 (33.3)	1 (33.3)	1 (33.3)	3
Imidazole derivatives	G01AF	1 (14.3)	3 (42.9)	2 (28.6)	1 (14.3)	7	0 (0.0)	2 (40.0)	3 (60.0)	0 (0.0)	5
Total Non β - Lactams		*11 (11.3)*	*28 (28.9)*	*37 (38.1)*	*21 (21.7)*	*97*	*3 (8.8)*	*14 (41.2)*	*13 (38.2)*	*4 (11.8)*	*34*
Total (β – Lactams + Non β – Lactams)		12 (7.7)	55 (35.3)	53 (33.9)	36 (23.1)	156	7 (15.2)	16 (34.8)	14 (30.4)	9 (19.6)	46

[a]Definite (≥ 9 score) ADRs are (1) followed a chronological sequence after the administration of drug or in which the drug had achieved a toxic concentration in the tissues or physiological fluid, and (3) could show improvement when the drug was withdrawal but reappeared on exposure

[b]Probable (5–8 score) ADRs are (1) followed a chronological sequence after the administration of drug, (2) were in accordance to a recognized pattern of reactions, (3) were not confirmed by the exposure to the suspected drug but by the withdrawal of that drug, and (4) could not be described by features of the patient's disease

[c]Possible (1–4) ADRs are (1) could be described by features of the patient's disease, (2) followed a chronological sequence after the administration of drug, and (3) were in accordance to a recognized pattern of reactions

[d]Doubtful (≤0) are factors other than a drug are associated with the reactions

ADEs, asthmatic patients (OR = 0.808, 95% CI = 0.598—1.093, *p-value* = 0.167), tuberculosis patients (OR = 0.304, 95% CI = 0.186—0.497, *p-value* = < 0.001) and cystic fibrosis patients (OR = 0.527, 95% CI = 0.334—0.829, *p-value* = 0.006) were likely to have less ADEs as compared to diabetic patients. According to diagnosis, patients with acute respiratory tract infections had 99.6% less ADEs (OR = 0.004, 95% CI = 0.01–0.019, *p-value* = < 0.001) and patients with soft tissue infections had 95.1% less ADEs (OR = 0.49, 95% CI = 0.018–0.133, *p-value* = < 0.001) as compared to the patients having urinary tract infections. Among the number of antibiotics prescribed per prescription, 2 antibiotics prescribed per prescription had 54.5% less ADEs (OR = 0.455, 95% CI = 0.319—0.650, *p-value* = < 0.001) while 3 antibiotics prescribed per prescription had 1.529 times more ADEs (OR = 1.529, 95% CI = 1.063—2.198, *p value* = 0.022) as compared to those which had 1 antibiotic prescribed per prescription. According to LOS in hospital, patients with long LOS had 14.825 times more ADEs (OR = 14.825, 95% CI = 11.198—19.627, *p-value* = < 0.001) as compared to patients who had short LOS (Table 9).

Discussion

The current study set out to determine the causality and preventability of ADEs associated with the use of antibiotics among inpatients having different LOS in hospital. It was revealed that overall 38.9% of the patients were detected with ADEs upon administering β-lactams and non β-lactams antibiotics. ADRs were less commonly observed as compared to preventable ADEs. MEs especially wrong drug selection might be the possible reason for preventable ADEs. The disobedience of international guidelines and non-availability of national formularies are the biggest hurdles in provision of optimal patient care and thus raise the risk of inappropriate prescribing and MEs [43–48]. This finding is in line with a previously published study where inappropriate prescribing trend of antibiotics had been the cause of majority of the non-preventable ADEs [49]. A study conducted in an Indian healthcare setting also predicted that less than half of the total ADEs were non-preventable and caused by β-lactams. Most of these non-preventable ADEs had a probable or possible causal relationship with the antibiotics [50]. In Pakistan, the high rate of preventable ADEs is the result of several factors which mainly include, (a)

Table 9 Logistic regression analysis of factors associated with Adverse drug events (N = 1249)

Characteristics	ADEs		OR	95% CI	p-value
	Yes n (%)	No n (%)			
Gender					
Male	293 (23.5)	423 (33.9)	1.0	–	–
Female	193 (15.5)	340 (27.2)	0.047	0.018—0.121	**< 0.001**
Age					
Children (≤18 years)	184 (14.7)	200 (16.0)	1.0	–	–
Adults (> 18 years)	302 (24.2)	563 (45.1)	0.041	0.013—0.130	**< 0.001**
Co-morbidities					
Diabetes	210 (16.8)	316 (25.3)	1.0	–	–
Asthma	169 (13.5)	255 (20.4)	0.808	0.598—1.093	0.167
Tuberculosis	37 (3.0)	100 (8.0)	0.304	0.186—0.497	**< 0.001**
Cystic fibrosis	70 (5.6)	92 (7.4)	0.527	0.334—0.829	**0.006**
Reasons of prescribing antibiotics					
Urinary tract infections	198 (15.9)	264 (21.1)	1.0	–	–
Acute respiratory tract infections	157 (12.6)	205 (16.4)	0.004	0.001—0.019	**< 0.001**
Soft tissue infections	131 (10.5)	156 (12.5)	0.049	0.018—0.133	**< 0.001**
Skin infections	0 (0.0)	138 (11.0)	0.000	0.000—0.000	0.994
Number of antibiotics prescribed per prescription					
1	101 (8.1)	128 (10.2)	1.0	–	–
2	153 (12.2)	450 (36.0)	0.455	0.319—0.650	**< 0.001**
3	232 (18.6)	185 (14.8)	1.529	1.063—2.198	**0.022**
LOS					
Short (< 5 days)	103 (30.7)	610 (48.8)	1.0	–	–
Long (≥5 days)	383 (8.2)	153 (12.2)	14.825	11.198—19.627	**< 0.001**

ADEs Adverse drug events, OR Odd Ratio, CI Confidence Interval, LOS Length of stay. The variables with p-value <0.05 are significantly associated with adverse drug events

non-availability of clinical pharmacist during ward rounds and prescription evaluation, (b) improper monitoring and reporting of ADRs, ADEs and MEs due to unestablished pharmacovigilance centers, (c) high patient load in public hospitals, and (d) low budget allocation for healthcare systems by the government [51–56].

Findings also suggested that ADEs associated with the use of β-lactams and non β-lactams antibiotics had mainly affected the GIT, hematologic system and skin. These results are in line with the previously published studies that predict the GIT as the most affected organ system by the antibiotic associated ADEs [57, 58]. The prime reason of it might be the suppression of normal flora of gut upon oral administration of antibiotics that may lead to the pathogenic and non-pathogenic colonization in GIT [59]. Thus, it is the need of the hour to establish a proper pharmacovigilance surveillance system under Drug Regulatory Authority of Pakistan (DRAP) for the proper monitoring and reporting of ADEs in all the primary, secondary and tertiary care settings. This initiative of provincial and

federal government will be fruitful in making statistical analysis of ADEs at national level.

Like the previously published studies [58, 60], most of the non-preventable ADEs or ADRs were "probable" and observed in patients having long LOS in hospital. As the under lying diseases may lead to poly pharmacy, so an ADR cannot be designated to have a definite causal association with the single therapeutic agent [61]. The causality assessment of antibiotics with ADRs is helpful in providing optimal care, establishing safety measures and preventing the risk of reoccurrence and iatrogenic complications [62].

The statistically significant association was established between ADEs and several risk factors by using logistic regression analysis. These factors mainly include age, gender, co-morbidities, number of drugs which were being exposed to the patient and LOS in hospital. It was found that factors like adult age group, female patients, under lying diseases (tuberculosis and acute respiratory infections), prescribing 2 antibiotics per prescription and short LOS (> 5 days) were significantly less associated with the development of ADEs. Similar association of age and prescribing antibiotics with ADEs was also significantly found in a previously published study [63]. The physiological and pharmacological differences may cause drugs to respond differently among different age groups [64]. Another study revealed significant association of ADEs with the number of drugs exposed but insignificant association was found with the age and gender [65]. As the risk of drug interactions is directly proportional to the number of drugs prescribed per prescription, so it may lead to the development of ADEs [66]. The significant correlation of male gender with the development of ADEs found in the present study is also in line with the previously published literature [50, 67]. This is in contrast with other studies which showed significant correlation of female gender with the development of ADEs [68, 69]; however, some studies declared no significant association of ADEs with gender [65, 70]. The prime reason of this divergence is that besides biologic differences several social, behavioral, cultural and physiological dissimilarities may have an impact on factors like gender [71]. It was also found that co-morbidities like diabetes mellitus (DM) had a significant association with ADEs because this metabolic disease may negatively affect the renal function and cause the undesired metabolism of drugs which makes the patients more prone towards the development of ADEs [72]. Long LOS in hospital is also found to be significantly associated with the ADEs which is consistent with the results of previously study wherein most of the preventable ADEs caused an increase in LOS in healthcare settings [73–77]. This is because of the fact that more number of prescribed drugs may increases the risk of drug interactions and MEs and thus leading to increased LOS in the healthcare settings.

This study has some limitations. First, the effects of prescribing multiple drugs at the same time or switching between drugs (bacterial resistance, or changing the medication after a full course treatment) have not been determined. Second, since the data was collected for short period of time and no follow up could be performed after the discharge of patients, so the long term effects of ADEs on organ systems (e.g., liver and kidney) and its risk factors could not be determined. However, future longitudinal studies could address these aspects. Third, the outcomes of treatment interventions like rechallenge and dechallenge were not measured in this study, therefore very few had shown a definite causal association of ADEs with the antibiotics. Last, the Hawthorne effect could have affected the result because physicians, nurses and other paramedical staff were well aware of the study.

Conclusion

The current study concluded that non β-lactams were among the most frequently prescribed antibiotics and most of the ADEs caused an increase in LOS in hospital. As per preventability assessment, most of the ADEs were preventable because these were caused due to MEs during the stages of medication processing like physician ordering and patient monitoring. Most of the non-preventable ADEs were having probable causal relationship with the antibiotics and found in patients having prolonged LOS. Gastrointestinal system, hematologic system and skin rashes were commonly found in patients prescribed with both β-lactams and non β-lactams. Moreover, the logistic regression showed significant association between ADEs and its risk factors like age, gender, co-morbidities, number of prescribed antibiotics and LOS in hospital. The present findings are beneficial as they give an insight about the current pharmacovigilance system and open the doorsteps for stakeholders in making strategies to overcome these issues.

Abbreviations

ADEs: Adverse drug events; ADRs: Adverse drug reactions; DRAP: Drug Regulatory Authority of Pakistan; LOS: Length of stay; MEs: Medication errors; WHO: World Health Organization

Acknowledgements

We would like to express wholehearted thankfulness to the administration of all the selected settings of Lahore, Pakistan. We wish to express gratitude to Dr. Muhammad Atif (Assistant Professor, Islamia University of Bahawalpur) and Dr. Fahad Saleem (Assistant Professor, University of Balochistan), for reviewing and editing the paper and for valuable comments. Also, a note of thanks to all pharmacy students who acted as data collectors.

Authors' contributions

MRS conceptualized and designed the study. AS, MS and SI analyzed and interpreted the data. MRS and AS drafted the manuscript. SI, MS and MRS critically revised the manuscript. All authors read and approved final version of the manuscript.

Competing interests

The authors declare that they have no competing interests.

Author details

[1]Department of Pharmacy, The Islamia University of Bahawalpur, Bahawalpur, Punjab, Pakistan. [2]Akhtar Saeed College of Pharmaceutical Sciences, Lahore, Pakistan. [3]College of Pharmacy, Al Ain University of Science and Technology, Al Ain, Abu Dhabi, UAE.

References

1. McDonnell PJ, Jacobs MR. Hospital admissions resulting from preventable adverse drug reactions. Ann Pharmacother. 2002;36(9):1331–6.

2. Prevention, N.C.C.f.M.E.R.a., Contemporary view of medication– related harm. A new paradigm. 2015.

3. Curtin F, Schulz P. Assessing the benefit: risk ratio of a drug-randomized and naturalistic evidence. Dialogues Clin Neurosci. 2011;13(2):183.

4. Bates DW, et al. Patient risk factors for adverse drug events in hospitalized patients. Arch Intern Med. 1999;159(21):2553–60.

5. Andrews LB, et al. An alternative strategy for studying adverse events in medical care. Lancet. 1997;349(9048):309–13.

6. Wester K, et al. Incidence of fatal adverse drug reactions: a population based study. Br J Clin Pharmacol. 2008;65(4):573–9.

7. Stausberg J. International prevalence of adverse drug events in hospitals: an analysis of routine data from England, Germany, and the USA. BMC Health Serv Res. 2014;14(1):125.

8. Lazarou J, Pomeranz BH, Corey PN. Incidence of adverse drug reactions in hospitalized patients: a meta-analysis of prospective studies. Jama. 1998; 279(15):1200–5.

9. Zoppi M, et al. Incidence of lethal adverse drug reactions in the comprehensive hospital drug monitoring, a 20-year survey, 1974–1993, based on the data of Berne/St. Gallen. Eur J Clin Pharmacol. 2000;56(5):427–30.

10. Khan LM, et al. Impact of pharmacovigilance on adverse drug reactions reporting in hospitalized internal medicine patients at Saudi Arabian teaching hospital. Saudi Med J. 2012;33(8):863–8.

11. Macedo AF, et al. Causality assessment of adverse drug reactions: comparison of the results obtained from published decisional algorithms and from the evaluations of an expert panel. Pharmacoepidemiol Drug Saf. 2005;14(12):885–90.

12. Pathak AK, et al. A retrospective analysis of reporting of adverse drug reactions in a tertiary care teaching hospital: one year survey. J Clin Diagn Res. 2016;10(8):FC01.

13. Routledge PA, O'mahony M, Woodhouse K. Adverse drug reactions in elderly patients. Br J Clin Pharmacol. 2004;57(2):121–6.

14. Hecker MT, et al. Unnecessary use of antimicrobials in hospitalized patients: current patterns of misuse with an emphasis on the antianaerobic spectrum of activity. Arch Intern Med. 2003;163(8):972–8.

15. Magill SS, et al. Prevalence of antimicrobial use in US acute care hospitals, May–September 2011. Jama. 2014;312(14):1438–46.

16. Bell BG, et al. A systematic review and meta-analysis of the effects of antibiotic consumption on antibiotic resistance. BMC Infect Dis. 2014;14(1):13.

17. Pharmacists, A.S.o.H.-S. Suggested definitions and relationships among medication misadventures, medication errors, adverse drug events, and adverse drug reactions. Am J Health Syst Pharm. 1998;55(2):165–6.

18. Hoonhout LH, et al. Nature, occurrence and consequences of medication-related adverse events during hospitalization. Drug Saf. 2010;33(10):853–64.

19. Shehab N, et al. Emergency department visits for antibiotic-associated adverse events. Clin Infect Dis. 2008;47(6):735–43.

20. Martin RM, et al. Age and sex distribution of suspected adverse drug reactions to newly marketed drugs in general practice in England: analysis of 48 cohort studies. Br J Clin Pharmacol. 1998;46(5):505–11.

21. Pretorius RW, et al. Reducing the risk of adverse drug events in older adults. Am Fam Physician. 2013;87(5):331–6.

22. Factbook, C.W. Population of Pakistan 2017; Available from: http://stats.pk/population-of-pakistan/.

23. Review, W.P. Population of Lahore Census 2017; Available from: http://www.pakinformation.com/population/lahore.html.

24. World Health Organization. The anatomical therapeutic chemical classification system with defined daily doses (ATC/DDD). Oslo: WHO; 2006.

25. Government of Pennsylvenia. *Average Length of Stay in Hospitals.* USA. http://www.statistics.health.pa.gov/StatisticalResources/UnderstandingHealthStats/ToolsoftheTrade/Documents/Average_Length_of_Stay_in_Hospitals.pdf.

26. Edwards IR, Aronson JK. Adverse drug reactions: definitions, diagnosis, and management. Lancet. 2000;356(9237):1255–9.

27. Committee, J.F. British national formulary (online). London: BMJ Group and Pharmaceutical Press; 2016. URL: www.medicinescomplete.com. Accessed 1 Aug 2015

28. Hepler CD, Segal R. Preventing medication errors and improving drug therapy outcomes: a management systems approach. Boca Raton: CRC Press; 2003.

29. McPhee SJ, Papadakis MA, Tierney LM. Current medical diagnosis & treatment 2010. New York: McGraw-Hill Medical; 2010.

30. Tan T, et al. Antibiotic prescribing for self limiting respiratory tract infections in primary care: summary of NICE guidance. BMJ. 2008;337:a437.

31. Committee, P.F. BNF for children 2014–2015 (BNFC). London: Pharmaceutical Press; 2014.

32. Pakistan, T.I.D.S.o. Guidelines for the use of antmicrobials. Pakistan; 2007. http://www.mmidsp.com/wp-content/uploads/2012/06/Guidelines-for-Antimicrobial-Use-2.pdf.

33. Schumock GT, Thornton JP. Focusing on the preventability of adverse drug reactions. Hosp Pharm. 1992;27(6):538.

34. Kurian J, et al. Adverse drug reactions in hospitalized pediatric patients: a prospective observational study. Indian J Pediatr. 2016;83(5):414–9.

35. Doshi K, Yegnanarayan R, Gokhale N. A retrospective study of drug induced cutaneous adverse reactions (CADR) in patients attending a tertiary care hospital. Curr Drug Saf. 2017;12(1):46–50.

36. Naranjo CA, et al. A method for estimating the probability of adverse drug reactions. Clin Pharmacol Ther. 1981;30(2):239–45.

37. Anderson M, et al. A prospective study of adverse drug reactions to antiepileptic drugs in children. BMJ Open. 2015;5(6):e008298.

38. Trubiano JA, et al. A comparative analysis between antibiotic-and nonantibiotic-associated delayed cutaneous adverse drug reactions. J Allergy Clin Immunol Pract. 2016;4(6):1187–93.

39. Sciences, P. Addressing medication errors in hospitals-ten tools; 2001. p. 47.

40. Padmavathi S, Manimekalai K, Ambujam S. Causality, severity and preventability assessment of adverse cutaneous drug reaction: a prospective observational study in a tertiary care hospital. J Clin Diagn Res. 2013;7(12):2765–7.

41. Leendertse AJ, et al. Frequency of and risk factors for preventable medication-related hospital admissions in the Netherlands. Arch Intern Med. 2008;168(17):1890–6.

42. Pirmohamed M, et al. Adverse drug reactions as cause of admission to hospital: prospective analysis of 18 820 patients. Bmj. 2004;329(7456):15–9.

43. Khalil S, K.M.T, Khan HS. Irrational use of antibiotics in children. Pak Pediatr J. 2015;39:131–39.

44. Atif M, et al. Assessment of core drug use indicators using WHO/INRUD methodology at primary healthcare centers in Bahawalpur, Pakistan. BMC Health Serv Res. 2016;16(1):684.

45. Atif M, et al. Evaluation of prescription errors and prescribing indicators in the private practices in Bahawalpur, Pakistan. J Chin Med Assoc. 2018;81(5):444–9.

46. Atif M, et al. WHO/INRUD prescribing indicators and prescribing trends of antibiotics in the Accident and Emergency Department of Bahawal Victoria Hospital, Pakistan. SpringerPlus. 2016;5(1):1928.

47. Atif M, et al. Assessment of WHO/INRUD core drug use indicators in two tertiary care hospitals of Bahawalpur, Punjab, Pakistan. J Pharm Policy Pract. 2016;9(1):27.

48. Atif M, et al. Drug utilization patterns in the global context: a systematic review. Health Policy Technol. 2017;6:457–70.

49. Trubiano JA, et al. The prevalence and impact of antimicrobial allergies and adverse drug reactions at an Australian tertiary centre. BMC Infect Dis. 2015;15(1):572.

50. Shamna M, et al. A prospective study on adverse drug reactions of antibiotics in a tertiary care hospital. Saudi Pharm J. 2014;22(4):303–8.

51. Nazir S. Adverse drug reaction reporting system at different hospitals of Lahore-An evaluation and patient outcome analysis. Value Health. 2014; 17(3):A166.

52. Shamim S, et al. Adverse drug reactions (ADRS) reporting: awareness and reasons of under-reporting among health care professionals, a challenge for pharmacists. SpringerPlus. 2016;5(1):1778.

53. Atif M, Azeem M, Sarwar MR. Potential problems and recommendations regarding substitution of generic antiepileptic drugs: a systematic review of literature. SpringerPlus. 2016;5(1):182.

54. Atif M, et al. A review indicating the migraine headache as a prevalent neurological disorder: still under-estimated, under-recognized, under-diagnosed and under-treated. J Pharm Pract Community Med. 2017;3(1):3–11.

55. Sarwar MR, et al. Drug utilization patterns among elderly hospitalized patients on poly-pharmacy in Punjab, Pakistan. J Pharm Policy Pract. 2017;10(1):23.

56. Sarwar MR, et al. Knowledge of community pharmacists about antibiotics, and their perceptions and practices regarding antimicrobial stewardship: a cross-sectional study in Punjab, Pakistan. Infect Drug Resist. 2018;11:133.

57. de Araújo Lobo MGA, et al. Adverse drug reaction monitoring: support for

pharmacovigilance at a tertiary care hospital in Northern Brazil. BMC Pharmacol Toxicol. 2013;14(1):5.

58. Khan, F.A., et al., A prospective study on prevalence of adverse drug reactions due to antibiotics usage in otolaryngology department of a tertiary care hospital in North India. 2013.

59. Hadjibabaie M, et al. The adverse drug reaction in the gastrointestinal tract: an overview. Int J Pharmacol. 2005;1(1):1–8.

60. Issac AJ, Yogananda R, Shehin M. Assessment of prescription pattern and monitoring adverse drug reaction of antibiotics in paediatric inpatients. Int J Contemp Pediatr. 2016;3(3):1071–5.

61. Kaur S, et al. Monitoring of incidence, severity, and causality of adverse drug reactions in hospitalized patients with cardiovascular disease. Indian J Pharm. 2011;43(1):22–6.

62. Varallo FR, et al. Imputation of adverse drug reactions: causality assessment in hospitals. PLoS One. 2017;12(2):e0171470.

63. Silva DC, et al. Adverse drug events in a paediatric intensive care unit: a prospective cohort. BMJ Open. 2013;3(2):e001868.

64. Kearns GL, et al. Developmental pharmacology—drug disposition, action, and therapy in infants and children. N Engl J Med. 2003;349(12):1157–67.

65. Ji H-h, et al. Adverse drug events in Chinese pediatric inpatients and associated risk factors: a retrospective review using the global trigger tool. Sci Rep. 2018;8(1):2573.

66. Fushiki Y, Kinoshita K, Tokuda Y. Polypharmacy and adverse drug events leading to acute care hospitalization in Japanese elderly. J Gen Fam Med. 2014;15(2):110–6.

67. Jose J, Rao PG, Jimmy B. Adverse drug reactions to fluoroquinolone antibiotics–analysis of reports received in a tertiary care hospital. Int J Risk Saf Med. 2008;20(3):169–80.

68. Hussain MM, et al. Incidence of adverse drug reactions in a tertiary care hospital: a systematic review and meta-analysis of prospective studies. Pharm Lett. 2010;2(3):358–68.

69. Stavreva G, et al. Detection of adverse drug reactions to antimicrobial drugs in hospitalized patients. Trakia J Sci. 2008;6(1):7–9.

70. Macy E, Ho NJ. Adverse reactions associated with therapeutic antibiotic use after penicillin skin testing. Perm J. 2011;15(2):31.

71. Alomar MJ. Factors affecting the development of adverse drug reactions. Saudi Pharm J. 2014;22(2):83–94.

72. Haile DB, Ayen WY, Tiwari P. Prevalence and assessment of factors contributing to adverse drug reactions in wards of a tertiary care hospital, India. Ethiop J Health Sci. 2013;23(1):39–48.

73. Davies EC, et al. Adverse drug reactions in hospital in-patients: a prospective analysis of 3695 patient-episodes. PLoS One. 2009;4(2):e4439.

74. Amelung S, et al. Association of preventable adverse drug events with inpatients' length of stay—a propensity-matched cohort study. Int J Clin Pract. 2017;71(10). https://doi.org/10.1111/ijcp.12990.

75. Dedefo MG, Mitike AH, Angamo MT. Incidence and determinants of medication errors and adverse drug events among hospitalized children in West Ethiopia. BMC Pediatr. 2016;16(1):81.

76. Gallo M, et al. Active surveillance of adverse drug reactions in children in five Italian paediatric wards. Open J Pediatr. 2012;2(02):111.

77. Montané E, Arellano AL, Sanz Y, Roca J, Farré M. Drug-related deaths in hospital inpatients: a retrospective cohort study. Br J Clin Pharmacol. 2018;84(3):542–52.

3

Sulforaphane attenuates pulmonary fibrosis by inhibiting the epithelial-mesenchymal transition

Sun Young Kyung[1†], Dae Young Kim[2†], Jin Young Yoon[1], Eun Suk Son[1], Yu Jin Kim[1], Jeong Woong Park[1] and Sung Hwan Jeong[1*]

Abstract

Background: Idiopathic pulmonary fibrosis (IPF) is a progressive and fatal disease with no effective treatment. The epithelial-mesenchymal transition (EMT) is a critical stage during the development of fibrosis. To assess the effect of sulforaphane (SFN) on the EMT and fibrosis using an in vitro transforming growth factor (TGF)-β1-induced model and an in vivo bleomycin (BLM)-induced model.

Methods: In vitro studies, cell viability, and cytotoxicity were measured using a Cell Counting Kit-8. The functional TGF-β1-induced EMT and fibrosis were assessed using western blotting and a quantitative real-time polymerase chain reaction. The lungs were analyzed histopathologically in vivo using hematoxylin and eosin and *Masson's trichrome* staining. The BLM-induced fibrosis was characterized by western blotting and immunohistochemical analyses for fibronectin, TGF-β1, E-cadherin (E-cad), and α-smooth muscle actin (SMA) in lung tissues.

Results: SFN reversed mesenchymal-like changes induced by TGF-β1 and restored cells to their epithelial-like morphology. The results confirmed that the expression of the epithelial marker, E-cadherin, increased after SFN treatment, while expression of the mesenchymal markers, N-cadherin, vimentin, and α-SMA decreased in A549 cells after SFN treatment. In addition, SFN inhibited TGF-β1-induced mRNA expression of the EMT-related transcription factors, Slug, Snail, and Twist. The SFN treatment attenuated TGF-β1-induced expression of fibrosis-related proteins, such as fibronection, collagen I, collagen IV, and α-SMA in MRC-5 cells. Furthermore, SFN reduced the TGF-β1-induced phosphorylation of SMAD2/3 protein in A549 cells and MRC-5 cells. BLM induced fibrosis in mouse lungs that was also attenuated by SFN treatment, and SFN treatment decreased BLM-induced fibronectin expression, TGF-β1 expression, and the levels of collagen I in the lungs of mice.

Conclusions: SFN showed a significant anti-fibrotic effect in TGF-β-treated cell lines and BLM-induced fibrosis in mice. These findings showed that SFN has anti-fibrotic activity that may be considered in the treatment of IPF.

Keywords: Idiopathic pulmonary fibrosis, Bleomycin, Sulforaphane, Epithelial-mesenchymal transition

* Correspondence: jsw@gilhospital.com
†Equal contributors
[1]Department of Internal Medicine, Gachon University Gil Medical Center, 21 Namdong-daero 774, Namdong-gu, Incheon 21565, Republic of Korea
Full list of author information is available at the end of the article

Background

Idiopathic pulmonary fibrosis (IPF) is a chronic, progressive, fibrotic lung disease characterised by expansion of fibroblast/myofibroblast populations and aberrant remodelling, which can lead to respiratory failure and death [1]. The major pathological findings of IPF are the expressional upregulation of connective tissue growth factor and transforming growth factor (TGF)-β1, fibroblast migration and proliferation, and extracellular matrix deposition [2, 3]. In IPF, the ability of alveolar epithelial cells to repair against recurrent microinjury is impaired and they secrete fibrogenic growth factors, such as TGF-β, and exhibit fibroblast/myofibroblast proliferation and activation. Furthermore, myofibroblast activation induces excessive accumulation of extracellular matrix components, which destroy the alveolar structure. Resident mesenchymal cell proliferation, epithelial mesenchymal transition (EMT), and circulating fibroblasts are likely sources of myofibroblasts [4].

EMT is a process whereby epithelial cells transition into cells of the mesenchymal phenotype, such as fibroblasts or myofibroblasts [5–7]. Recently, it has been recognised that EMT has important roles in embryogenesis, cancer progression, and organ fibrosis [5]. During fibrogenesis of several organs, EMT may be a major provider of pathogenic mesenchymal cell types, such as myofibroblasts [7]. EMT can be induced by various factors. For example, a wealth of evidence indicates that TGF-β is a major inducer of EMT [6, 8]. Growth factors downregulate genes expressed in epithelial cells, such as E-cadherin (E-cad), and upregulate genes normally expressed in mesenchymal cells, such as N-cadherin (N-cad), vimentin, and α-smooth muscle actin (α-SMA) [8, 9]. At the molecular level, EMT is characterised by downregulation of E-cad and cytokeratins. This process is controlled by a group of transcription factors referred to as EMT regulators, which include Snail, Slug, Twist, ZEB1, SIP1, and E12/47 [7, 8, 10, 11].

Although many immunomodulatory and anti-inflammatory drugs have been used to treat IPF, they do not prevent its progression [11, 12]. Recently, pirfenidone and nintedanib were found to be partially effective against IPF, and were approved by the Food and Drug Administration for mild-to-moderate IPF [1, 13, 14]. Unlike nintedanib, which is an inhibitor of multiple tyrosine kinases, pirfenidone has anti-inflammatory and antifibrotic effects, although no specific molecular target has been identified [15]. However, additional treatment trials are needed, because current treatments for IPF have limited efficacy.

Sulphoraphane (SFN) is a phytochemical that is mainly found in cruciferous vegetables, such as broccoli, cabbage, and Brussels sprouts, and its antioxidative effects are known to involve nuclear factor, erythroid-derived 2-related factor 2 (Nrf2)-mediated induction of phase II detoxifying enzymes [16, 17]. The chemopreventative effects of SFN are known to involve the induction of cell cycle arrest and apoptosis [18, 19]. Furthermore, recent studies have shown that it modulates various signalling pathways associated with oncogenic EMT [20, 21]. Several studies have reported that SFN has anti-fibrotic activity in hepatic fibrosis and airway smooth muscles [22, 23]. Nrf2 activation by SFN attenuates TGF-β signalling in hepatic fibrosis, and SFN treatment was found to induce Nrf2 expression and myofibroblastic dedifferentiation in IPF fibroblasts [22, 24]. Moreover, SFN was recently reported to prevent bleomycin-induced pulmonary fibrosis by inhibiting oxidative stress [25].

We hypothesised that SFN might show an anti-fibrotic efficacy in pulmonary fibrosis by inhibiting EMT. We assessed the effects of SFN on TGF-β1-induced EMT and fibrosis in a lung alveolar epithelial (A549) cell line and a fibroblast (MRC-5) cell line. In addition, we assessed the effects of SFN on a BLM-induced pulmonary fibrosis model in C57BL/6 mice followed by treatment with SFN for 4 weeks.

Methods

In vitro cell culture and sample treatment

The human type II alveolar epithelial A549 cell line (ATCC° CCL-185™) and the human fibroblast MRC-5 cell line (ATCC° CCL-171™) were purchased from the American Type Culture Collection (Manassas, VA, USA). The A549 cells were cultured in RPMI medium (Welgene, Seoul, Republic of Korea) supplemented with 100 U/mL penicillin, 100 μg/mL streptomycin, and 10% foetal bovine serum (Gibco, Grand Island, NY, USA). The MRC-5 cells were cultured in Dulbecco's Modified Eagle's Medium (Welgene) supplemented with 100 U/mL penicillin, 100 μg/mL streptomycin, and 10% foetal bovine serum (Gibco). The cells were treated with various concentrations of SFN (10 and 20 μM) for the indicated times. Cells were also treated with 0.1% ultrapure water as a vehicle control.

In vivo BLM-induced pulmonary fibrosis in mice

Male C57BL/6 mice (3 weeks of age; body weight, 20–25 g) were purchased from Dae Han Biolink (Umsung, Republic of Korea). This animal study was approved by the Panel on Laboratory Animal Care of Gachon University (GIACUCR-011). The mice were fed a commercial diet (Cargill Agri Purina, Sungnam, Republic of Korea) together with tap water ad libitum. They were housed in an animal facility maintained at 20 ± 2 °C with 40 ± 10% humidity under a 12/12 h light/dark cycle. The mice were cared for according to the Guidelines of the Korean Food and Drug Administration and the United States National Institutes of Health Guidelines for the Care and Use of Laboratory Animals. BLM was purchased from Sigma-Aldrich (St.

Louis, MO, USA). Twenty male mice were divided randomly into three experimental groups and a control group, with five mice per group, as follows: (1) treatment with distilled water (DW) (control), (2) treatment with BLM (5 units, twice) (BLM group), and (3) treatment with BLM and SFN (50 μg/kg) (BLM + SFN group). The control mice received only DW on days 0 and 14. BLM (5 units) was instilled intratracheally in a DW suspension on days 0 and 14. Intratracheal administration was performed using the "tongue-pull" method. SFN (50 μg/kg body weight) was or-ally administered three times a week for 28 days. At the end of the experiments, mice were sacrificed by euthanasia using isoflurane inhalation and lung tissue was collected.

Histopathological analyses

The right lungs were embedded in paraffin wax, fixed in 10% formalin, and processed into sections. The sections were stained with haematoxylin and eosin (H&E) or sub-jected to Masson's trichrome (M-T) staining and immu-nohistochemical (IHC) staining. The histopathological evaluation of pulmonary fibrosis was scored according to the density of M-T staining (the M-T score) and IHC staining using an image J analysis program.

Hydroxyproline assay

To assess collagen accumulation, the hydroxyproline content in lung tissues was measured according to the protocol provided with a hydroxyproline test kit (BioVi-sion, Milpitas, CA, USA). 10 mg of tissues were homog-enized in 100 μl of DW. 100 μl of 12 M HCl were added to 100 μl of sample and hydrolyzed for overnight at 120 °C. The samples were centrifuged at 14,000 rpm for 20 min, and 10 μl of supernatant was transferred to a 96-well plate. 100 μl of chloramine-T reagent was added to the samples and incubated for 5 min at room temperature. After 100 μl of dimethylaminobenzalde-hyde reagent was added to each sample and incubated for 90 min at 60 °C. The absorbance of the samples was measured using a microplate reader (Thermo LabSystems, Helsinki, Finland) at 560 nm.

Cell viability assay

This assay method was based on the ability of a mito-chondrial dehydrogenase enzyme from viable cells to reduce 3-(4,5-dimethylthiazol-2-yl)-2,5-diphenyltetrazol ium bromide (MTT) into a dark blue formazan crystal that accumulated in cells. The A549 and MRC-5 cells were seeded at a density of 5×10^3 cells/well in a 96-well plate and incubated at 37 °C for 24 h under a humidified 5% CO_2 atmosphere. The cells were treated with various concentrations of SFN (10, 20, and 40 μM) for the indi-cated times with or without TGF-β1. At the end of the incubation, 10 μL of MTT solution (5 mg/mL in phosphate-buffered saline) was added to each well. After

additional incubation at 37 °C for 4 h, the medium was gently removed and 100 μL of dimethylsulphoxide was added. The absorbance of samples was then measured using a microplate reader (Thermo LabSystems, Helsinki, Finland) at 550 nm.

Western blot analyses

The protein was extracted from MRC-5 cells, A549 cells, and mouse lung tissue using a radioimmunoprecipitation assay buffer according to the manufacturer's protocol. Then, 20–40 μg protein from each sample was separated by 10% sodium dodecyl sulphate-polyacrylamide gel elec-trophoresis and transferred to a polyvinylidene difluoride membrane (Millipore, Bedford, MA, USA). The mem-brane was blocked with 5% (w/v) non-fat skim milk for 60 min at room temperature and then incubated with the following primary antibodies: anti-p-SMAD2/3, anti-SMAD2/3, anti-TGF-β1, anti-E-cad, anti-N-cadherin, or anti-vimentin (Cell Signaling Technology, Danvers, MA, USA); anti-fibronectin or anti-type 1 collagen (Santa Cruz Biotechnology, Santa Cruz, CA, USA); or anti-α-SMA or anti-type 1 collagen (Abcam, Cambridge, UK) overnight at 4 °C. The membrane was then incubated with a 1:5000 di-lution of horseradish peroxidase-conjugated secondary antibody for 1 h at room temperature. Each protein was detected using a chemiluminescence detection system ac-cording to the manufacturer's protocol (Amersham ECL, Little Chalfont, UK). The band intensity was quantified by densitometric analyses using ImageJ software (National Institutes of Health, Bethesda, MD, USA).

RNA extraction and quantitative real-time-polymerase chain reaction (qRT-PCR)

Expression levels of fibrosis-related genes and EMT related-transcription factors were determined by qRT-PCR. Total RNA was extracted using the RNAiso Plus reagent (Takara Bio, Dalian, China) according to the manufacturer's instructions. The concentrations of all RNA samples were determined spectrophotometrically. The cDNA was produced from the total RNA (1 μg) using a Prime Script RT reagent kit (Takara Bio) accord-ing to the manufacturer's protocol. The qRT-PCR was performed on a Bio-Rad iQ5 RT-PCR detection system (Bio-Rad, Hercules, CA, USA) using a SYBR Premix Ex Taq II kit (Takara Bio). All samples were run in tripli-cate, and glyceraldehyde 3-phosphate dehydrogenase (GAPDH) was used as an internal control. The expres-sion levels were calculated from the PCR profiles of each sample using the threshold cycle (Ct), corresponding to the cycle with a statistically significant increase in fluor-escence. To correct for differences in the amount of total cDNA in the starting reaction, the Ct values for the endogenous control (GAPDH) were subtracted from those of the corresponding sample.

Statistical analysis

Values were expressed as means ± standard deviation (SD). A one-way analysis of variance was used to identify differences among groups. Tukey's test was used to determine specific mean differences. All statistical analyses were performed using GraphPad Prism software (ver. 4.0; GraphPad, La Jolla, CA, USA). A value of $p < 0.05$ was considered to be significant.

Results

The effects of SFN on the TGF-β1-induced EMT in alveolar epithelial A549 cells

Cell viability of A549 cells did not significant decrease at the concentration of 10 or 20 μM SFN (Fig. 1b). TGF-β1 treatment of A549 lung epithelial-like cells resulted in a spindle-like mesenchymal phenotype and the loss of cell-cell contact. Treatment with SFN caused reversion to the mesenchymal-like changes induced by TGF-β1 and restored the cells to their epithelial-like morphology (Fig. 1a). To investigate whether SFN could influence EMT-related protein expression, western blot analyses of A549 cell lysates showed that the expression of the epithelial marker, E-cad, increased after SFN treatment, while expression of the mesenchymal markers, N-cad, vimentin, and a-SMA, decreased in A549 cells (Fig. 1c). The effects of SFN treatment on EMT-related transcription factors were also analysed using RT-PCR. SFN treatment inhibited TGF-β1-

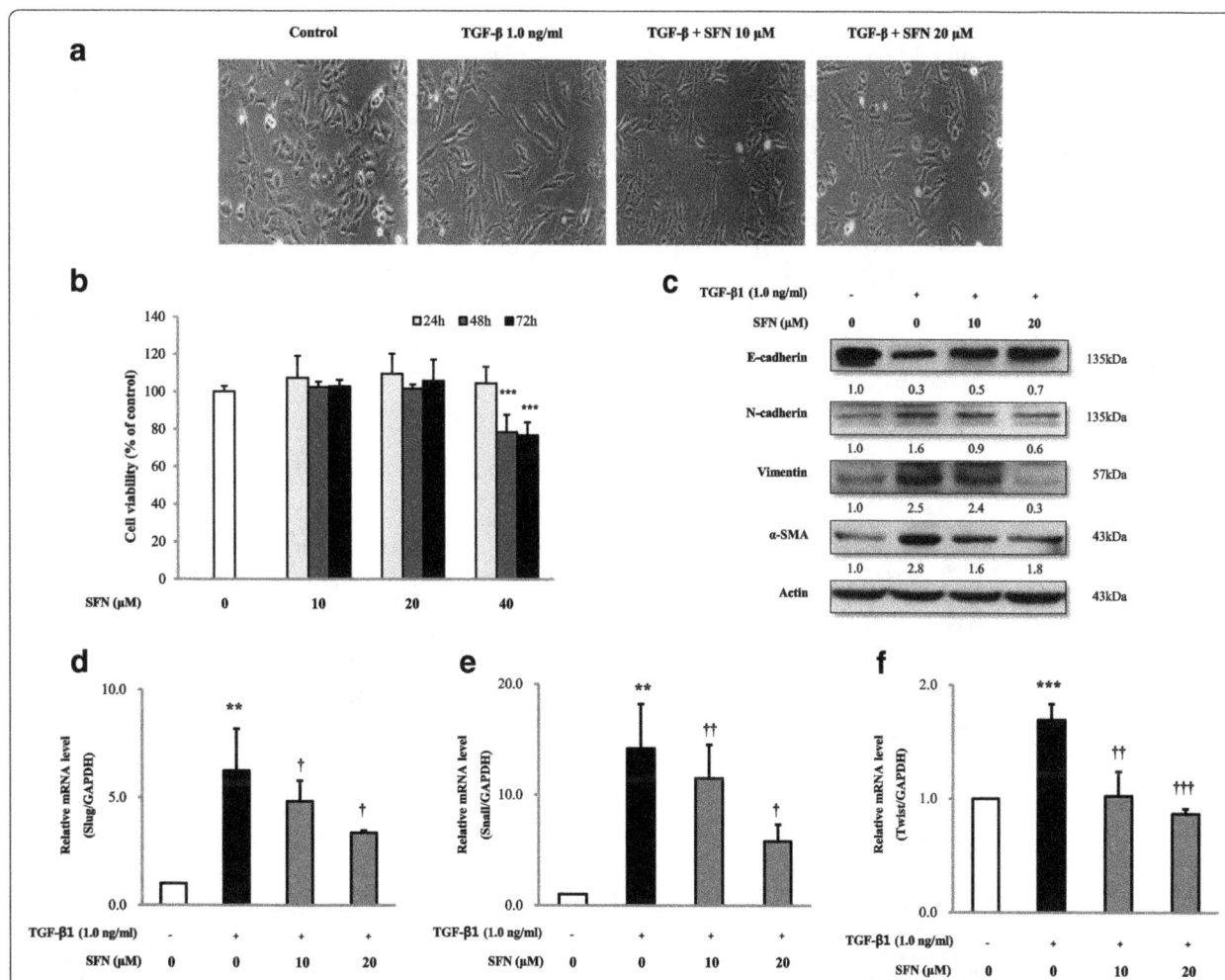

Fig. 1 The effect of sulphoraphane (SFN) treatment on the morphology and protein markers in the transforming growth factor (TGF)-β1-induced epithelial-mesenchymal transition (EMT) in A549 epithelial cells. The cells were pre-treated with the indicated concentrations of SFN for 1 h and then stimulated with TGF-β1 (1.0 ng/ml) for 24 h except a-smooth muscle actin for 72 h. The effects of SFN on cell viability for 24, 48, and 72 h (**b**). SFN treatment restored the TGF-β1-induced changes in epithelial morphology with original magnification, ×200 (**a**). Western blot analysis of the epithelial cell marker (E-cadherin), and the mesenchymal markers (N-cadherin, vimentin, and a-smooth muscle actin) (**c**). The mRNA levels of EMT-related transcription factors including Slug (**d**), Snail (**e**), and Twist (**f**) were measured by the quantitative real-time polymerase chain reaction (qRT-PCR). The data are expressed as means ± standard deviation of at least three different experiments. $^*p < 0.05$, $^{**}p < 0.01$, $^{***}p < 0.001$ versus the control; $^†p < 0.05$, $^{††}p < 0.01$, $^{†††}p < 0.001$ versus TGF-β1 induction

induced mRNA expression of the EMT-related transcription factors, Slug, Snail, and Twist (Fig. 1d, e, f). These results suggested that transcription factors were involved in the TGF-β1-induced EMT inhibition after SFN treatment.

The effects of SFN on TGF-β1-induced fibrosis in fibroblast MRC-5 cells

To test the effect of SFN on cell viability, MRC-5 cells were incubated with various concentrations of SFN (0, 10, 20, and 40 μM) for 24, 48, or 72 h. At a concentration of 20 μM SFN, the cell viability was 85% of the control values. In our present study, treatment with ≥40 μM SFN resulted in a significant reduction over 20% in the viability of MRC-5 cells (Fig. 2a). TGF-β1 stimulation induced proliferation of MRC-5 cells significantly and SFN treatment showed anti-proliferative effects in TGF-β1-induced proliferation (Additional file 1). TGF-β1 stimulation significantly increased fibronectin, type I collagen, type IV collagen, and α-SMA protein expression ($p < 0.05$), which was inhibited by SFN treatment (Fig. 2b). Fibronectin, type I collagen, type IV collagen, and α-SMA mRNA expression levels in MRC-5 cells were also measured by qRT-PCR (Fig. 2c, d, e, f). The expression of fibronectin and α-SMA in the TGF-β1-stimulated cells was significantly higher than that in the control cells ($p < 0.05$). SFN treatment significantly inhibited TGF-β1-induced fibronectin and α-SMA mRNA expression in fibroblasts. Western blotting and qRT-PCR showed similar results: SFN treatment attenuated TGF-β1-induced fibronectin, type I collagen, type IV collagen and α-SMA expression in fibroblasts.

The effects of SFN on the TGF-β/SMAD signalling pathway

We characterised the effects of SNF treatment on TGF-β1-induced SMAD2/3 phosphorylation in an alveolar epithelia cell line and a fibroblast cell line. As shown in Fig. 3, expression of SMAD2/3 phosphorylation increased after TGF-β1 treatment, and SFN significantly reduced the TGF-β1-induced phosphorylation of SMAD2/3 protein expression in epithelial and fibroblast cells. These results suggested that the inhibition of the TGF-β-1/SMAD signalling pathway was involved in the TGF-β1-induced EMT and fibrosis. The inhibition of SFN in TGF-β1-induced phosphorylation of SMAD2/3 started in early time point within 1 h and maintained to 24 h persistently (Additional file 2).

The effects of SFN on BLM-induced pulmonary fibrosis in an in vivo model

BLM instillation into mouse lungs induced significant pulmonary fibrosis. H&E and M-T staining of lung specimens showed that BLM instillation induced severe distortions of lung structure and accumulation of collagen fibres in the lungs. Furthermore, the expression of fibronectin and hydroxyproline significantly increased in the BLM group compared with the control group.

Histopathological results showed that the BLM + SFN group showed significantly attenuated BLM-induced

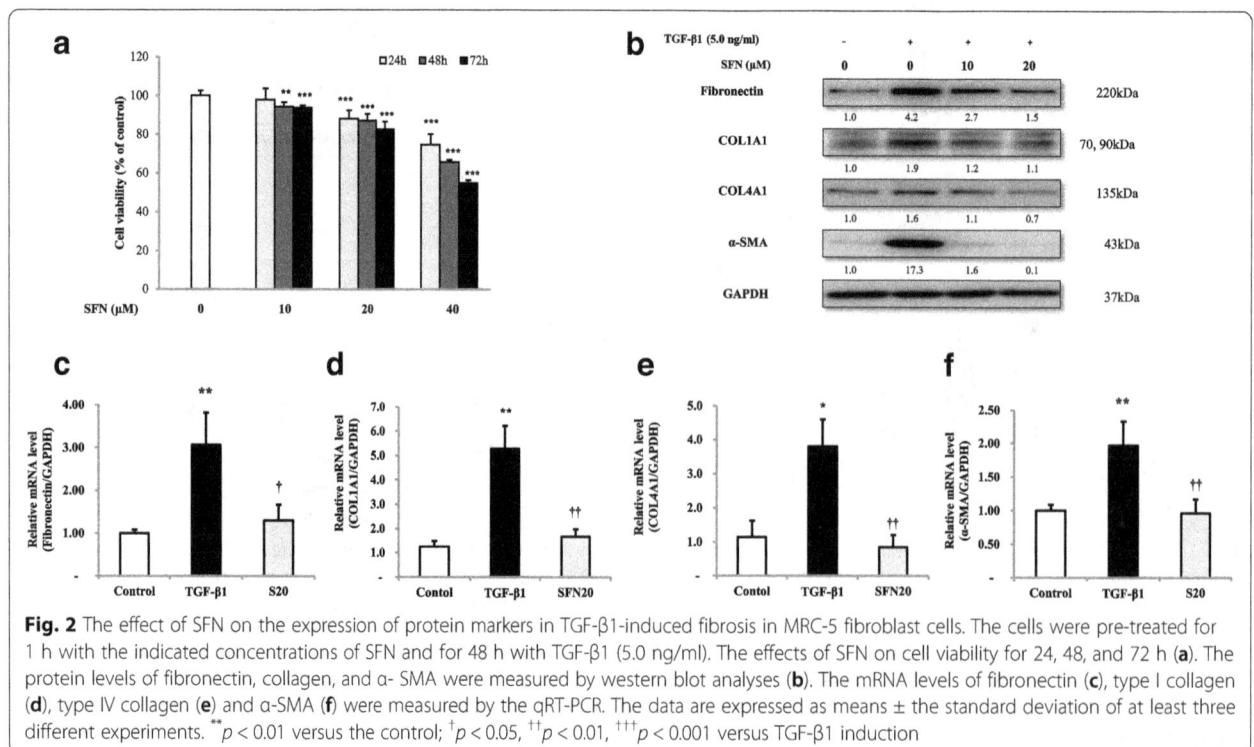

Fig. 2 The effect of SFN on the expression of protein markers in TGF-β1-induced fibrosis in MRC-5 fibroblast cells. The cells were pre-treated for 1 h with the indicated concentrations of SFN and for 48 h with TGF-β1 (5.0 ng/ml). The effects of SFN on cell viability for 24, 48, and 72 h (**a**). The protein levels of fibronectin, collagen, and α-SMA were measured by western blot analyses (**b**). The mRNA levels of fibronectin (**c**), type I collagen (**d**), type IV collagen (**e**) and α-SMA (**f**) were measured by the qRT-PCR. The data are expressed as means ± the standard deviation of at least three different experiments. **$p < 0.01$ versus the control; †$p < 0.05$, ††$p < 0.01$, †††$p < 0.001$ versus TGF-β1 induction

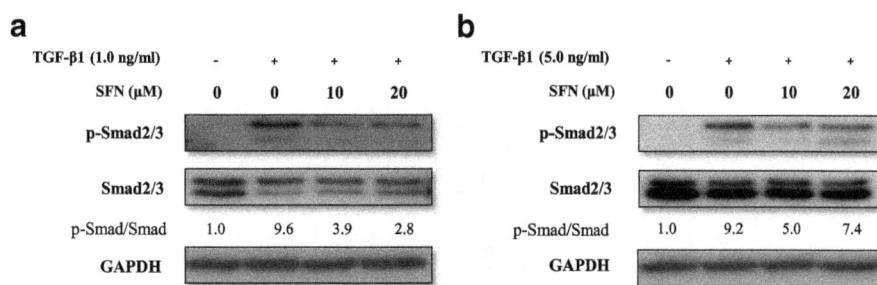

Fig. 3 The effect of SFN on TGF-β/SMAD signalling in A549 epithelial cells and MRC-5 fibroblast cells. The cells were pre-treated for 1 h with the indicated concentrations of SFN and for 24 h with TGF-β1 (1.0 or 5.0 ng/ml). Western blotting for phosphorylated and total form of SMAD 2/3 was performed using the cell lysates of A549 epithelial cells (**a**) and MRC-5 cells (**b**). The data are expressed as means ± standard deviation of at least three different experiments

fibrotic lesions and collagen accumulation in the lungs of mice (Fig. 4a). To confirm the effects of SFN on the histopathological changes during BLM-induced pulmonary fibrosis, the overall grade of the fibrotic changes in the lungs was scored by imaging analyses of M-T staining (M-T score). The scores of the BLM + SFN group were significantly lower than those of the BLM group (Fig. 4b).

The collagen content in lung tissues was assessed by measuring the hydroxyproline content. Compared with the BLM group, the hydroxyproline content decreased in the BLM + SFN group (Fig. 4c). Because they are important components in pulmonary fibrosis, fibronectin and TGF-β1 were assessed by western blotting. BLM significantly increased fibronectin and TGF-β1 protein expression in lung tissues, which was attenuated by SFN treatment (Fig. 5a, b).

Immunohistochemistry was used to characterise epithelial (E-cad) and mesenchymal markers (α-SMA) from lung samples of mice treated with distilled water (control), BLM, and BLM + SFN (Fig. 4a). As expected, the control group contained many stained E-cad-positive cells on the surface of the bronchus and the alveolar wall epithelial layer. In contrast, there were decreased E-cad-positive cells in the BLM group, and more E-cad-positive cells were found in the BLM + SFN group than the BLM group (Fig. 4d). The α-SMA expression was mostly found in interstitial fibrotic areas and sporadically in epithelial tissue. The expression of α-SMA was also significantly decreased in the BLM + SFN group compared with the BLM group (Fig. 4e).

Discussion

SFN is a natural isothiocyanate found in cruciferous vegetables with reported anti-inflammatory, bactericidal, anti-helminthic, and anti-fibrotic properties, and has been tested as an anti-tumour agent [16, 17]. Several studies have examined the efficacy of SFN in the treatment of fibrosis. In IPF fibroblasts, Artaud-Macari et al.

[24] reported that SFN decreased oxidants and induced the production of Nrf2 and antioxidants, as well as the dedifferentiation of myofibroblasts. Oh et al. [22] reported that SFN inhibited the development and progression of early-stage hepatic fibrosis induced by bile duct ligation in mice. In that study, SFN was also reported to have an anti-fibrotic effect during hepatic fibrosis involving Nrf2-mediated inhibition of TGF-β/SMAD signalling and subsequent suppression of hepatic stellate cell activation and fibrogenic gene expression [22]. Under hyperglycaemic and oxidative conditions, SFN treatment prevented nephropathy, diabetes-induced fibrosis, and vascular complications [26]. Several studies have concluded that the anti-fibrotic effect of SFN involves the suppression of oxidative stress [24, 25, 27, 28]. In the present study, the anti-fibrotic effect of SFN on TGF-β1-stimulated MRC-5 cells, A549 cells, and on BLM-induced pulmonary fibrosis was found to involve the inhibition of EMT. In a previous study, SFN was reported to have inhibitory activity during oncogenic EMT [20, 21]. Shan et al. [18] reported that SFN inhibited the EMT process involving E-cad induction via the transcriptional repressors ZEB1 and Snail in bladder cancer cells.

In the present study, SFN inhibited BLM-induced pulmonary fibrosis in mice. BLM causes alveolar cell damage and pulmonary inflammation, and has been used to produce experimental pulmonary fibrosis models in different animals [29]. In the present study, BLM (5 units on days 1 and 14) was introduced intratracheally into mouse lungs to induce pulmonary fibrosis because repetitive intratracheal administration of BLM more effectively induces the chronic pulmonary fibrosis [30]. We demonstrated fibronectin overexpression and collagen overproduction after BLM treatment and found that SFN attenuated these upregulations in the mouse model. The histological changes observed by H&E and M-T staining after BLM stimulation showed massive inflammation, fibrosis, and structural distortion. In the

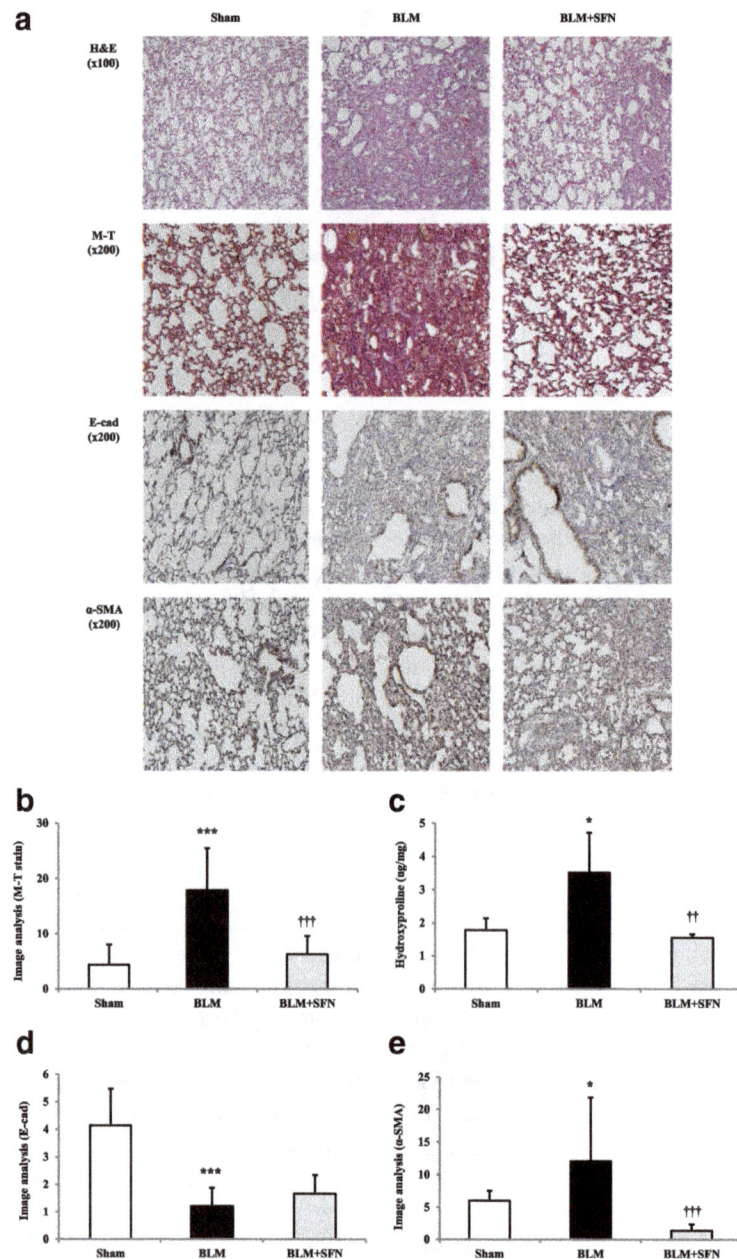

Fig. 4 The effect of SFN on bleomycin (BLM)-induced pulmonary fibrosis. The histological results of haematoxylin and eosin, Masson's trichrome (M-T) staining, immunohistochemistry staining of E-cad and α-SMA in lung sections (**a**). BLM induced extensive pulmonary inflammation and fibrosis. SFN treatment attenuated BLM-induced pulmonary fibrosis. M-T scores of lung histology (**b**). The M-T score increased significantly in the BLM group, and SFN treatment decreased the M-T score compared with the BLM group. The hydroxyproline assay of lung tissues (**c**). Collagen contents were evaluated by the hydroxyproline assay. The results were similar to the M-T scores. Image analysis of immunohistochemistry for E-cad (**d**) and α-SMA (**e**). SFN treatment restored E-cad expression and decreased the expression of α-SMA. The data are expressed as means ± standard deviation, $n = 4$ in each group. $^*p < 0.05$, $^{***}p < 0.001$ versus the control; $^{\dagger\dagger}p < 0.01$, $^{\dagger\dagger\dagger}p < 0.001$ versus the BLM group

present study, BLM was introduced into lungs, and the animals were then treated with SFN three times a week for 4 weeks. This treatment inhibited pulmonary fibrosis progression. BLM was observed to induce strong M-T staining versus the controls, and SFN significantly attenuated the severity of this staining.

Moreover, we observed that SFN inhibited BLM-induced TGF-β1 protein expression. TGF-β is a potent profibrogenic mediator and has been reported to be expressionally upregulated in many fibrotic diseases, including pulmonary fibrosis [31]. Thus, reports on the effects of TGF-β on fibrogenesis during pulmonary fibrosis

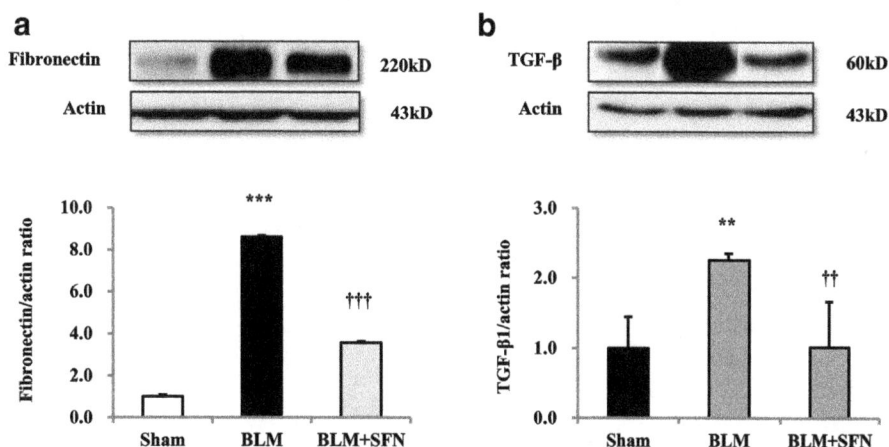

Fig. 5 The effect of SFN on TGF-β, fibronectin expression in BLM-induced pulmonary fibrosis. The protein levels of fibronectin (**a**) and TGF-β (**b**) were measured by western blot analyses. Each experiment was performed in triplicate and repeated three times. The data are expressed as means ± standard deviation, $n = 4$ in each group. $^{**}p < 0.01$, $^{***}p < 0.001$ versus the control; $^{††}p < 0.01$, $^{†††}p < 0.001$ versus the BLM group

have suggested that the disruption of TGF-β production or blocking of TGF-β signalling be considered as therapeutic targets of IPF [3]. TGF-β acts on multiple cell types during pulmonary fibrosis, for example, to induce EMT in alveolar or airway epithelial cells, and proliferation and differentiation into myofibroblasts in fibroblasts [3, 4, 6, 8]. TGF-β-induced EMT is an important component of the mechanisms of fibrotic pulmonary diseases [5–8]. In the present study, we observed that SFN inhibited TGF-β1-induced EMT in alveolar epithelial cells. Furthermore, immunohistochemical analysis showed that BLM downregulated E-cad and upregulated α-SMA, which are markers of EMT. In addition, SFN prevented BLM-induced changes in the expression of EMT markers in the lungs of mice. SFN also inhibited the proliferation of MRC-5 cells (a pulmonary fibroblast cell line) and suppressed the TGF-β1-induced overexpression of fibrogenic proteins (fibronectin, collagen I, and α-SMA) in these cells. The results of the mRNA assays also showed that SFN decreased the levels of TGF-β1-induced fibronectin, collagen I, and α-SMA mRNA in MRC-5 cells. In A549 alveolar epithelial cells, western blotting showed that SFN treatment resulted in TGF-β1-induced EMT, reduced E-cad expression, and increased expression of N-cad, vimentin, and α-SMA. We also observed that SFN treatment reduced the mRNA levels of TGF-β1-induced EMT-related transcriptional factors (Slug, Snail, and Twist) in A549 cells. Moreover, SFN suppressed the TGF-β1-induced phosphorylation of SMAD2/3 in MRC-5 and A549 cells, and showed a significant anti-fibrotic effect. These results suggest that the anti-fibrotic activity of SFN in pulmonary fibrosis involves the inhibition of TGF-β signalling by SMAD2/3.

In pulmonary fibroblasts, fibrous proteins, such as fibronectin, collagen I, and α-SMA, were induced by TGF-β1,

and SFN treatment inhibited TGF-β1-induced fibrous protein expression. Fibronectin is a glycoprotein of the extracellular matrix and has major roles in cell adhesion, growth, migration, and differentiation, and in wound healing [32]. Altered fibronectin expression has been associated with the pathogenesis of various conditions, including cancer and fibrosis [3, 32]. Collagen is another major fibrous protein of the extracellular matrix, and its excessive deposition contributes to the pathogenesis of pulmonary fibrosis [3, 32]. In the present study, we evaluated α-SMA (a commonly used marker of myofibroblast formation), fibronectin, and collagen I levels in TGF-β1-stimulated fibroblasts in the presence or absence of SFN.

The intracellular transcriptional pathway of TGF-β including SMAD and non-SMAD pathways is well established [31]. When TGF-β receptors are activated, they undergo conformational changes that allow direct binding with SMADs and their phosphorylated products. This results in the accumulation of SMADs in the nucleus to regulate target gene transcription. When we investigated how SFN treatment affected the TGF-β1/SMAD2/3 signalling pathway, we found that it inhibited the TGF-β1-induced phosphorylation of SMAD2/3. Interestingly, Yan et al. [25] reported recently that the anti-fibrotic efficacy of SFN in BLM-induced pulmonary fibrosis involved amelioration of oxidative stress. Thus, we hypothesise that the major mechanism underlying the action of SFN probably involves inhibition of the TGF-β1-induced SMAD2/3 signalling pathway and the subsequent suppression of EMT. In the studies about antifibrotic efficacy of SFN, the dose of SFN is variable according to the route of administration such as subcutaneous injection, intraperitoneal injection, or gavage (0.5–25.0 mg/kg) [22, 25, 26]. In this study, we used SFN with minimal dose (50 µg/kg) and demonstrated anti-fibrotic effect in pulmonary fibrosis mice model.

Conclusion

In summary, we found that SFN attenuated TGF-β1-induced fibrosis in MRC-5 cells, TGF-β1-induced EMT in A549 cells, and BLM-induced pulmonary fibrosis in a mouse model. These findings indicate that the major mechanism responsible for the effects of SFN involves inhibition of the TGF-β1-induced SMAD2/3 signalling pathway and subsequent EMT suppression. Based on these results, we suggest that SFN may be considered a potential treatment for IPF. Future studies should determine the optimal dosage of SFN and identify other mechanisms that contribute to pulmonary fibrosis.

Abbreviations

BLM: Bleomycin; COL1A1: Type I collagen; COL4A1: Type IV collagen; E-cad: E-cadherin; EMT: Epithelial-to-mesenchymal transition; FN: Fibronectin; IPF: Idiopathic pulmonary fibrosis; N-cad: N-cadherin; Nrf2: Nuclear factor erythroid-derived 2-related factor 2; qRT-PCR: Quantitative real-time polymerase chain reaction; SFN: Sulphoraphane; TGF-β: Transforming growth factor-β; α-SMA: α-smooth muscle actin

Acknowledgements

Not applicable

Funding

This study was supported by the Gachon University Gil Medical Center Research Fund [2013–34]. Authors are grateful to the Gachon University for the financial support.

Authors' contributions

SYK, DYK, and SHJ designed the study, developed the methodology, performed the animal experiments, analysed the data and wrote the manuscript. JYY and ESS performed the in vitro experiments, analysed the data and wrote the revised manuscript. YJK, and JWP offered technical support and wrote the manuscript. All authors have read and approved the final manuscript. SYK and DYK are equally contributed in this work as first author.

Competing interests

The authors declare that they have no competing interests.

Author details

[1]Department of Internal Medicine, Gachon University Gil Medical Center, 21 Namdong-daero 774, Namdong-gu, Incheon 21565, Republic of Korea. [2]Department of Biological Science, College of Bio-nano Technology, Gachon University, Seongnam-daero 1342, Seongnam, South Korea.

References

1. Raghu G, Collard HR, Egan JJ, Martinez FJ, Behr J, Brown KK, Colby TV, Cordier JF, Flaherty KR, Lasky JA, et al. An official ATS/ERS/JRS/ALAT statement: idiopathic pulmonary fibrosis: evidence-based guidelines for diagnosis and management. Am J Respir Crit Care Med. 2011;183(6):788–824.
2. King TE, Pardo A, Selman M. Idiopathic pulmonary fibrosis. Lancet. 2011; 378(9807):1949–61.
3. Selman M, King TE, Pardo A. Idiopathic pulmonary fibrosis: prevailing and evolving hypotheses about its pathogenesis and implications for therapy. Ann Intern Med. 2001;134(2):136–51.
4. Richeldi L, Collard HR, Jones MG. Idiopathic pulmonary fibrosis. Lancet. 2017;389(10082):1941–52.
5. Thiery JP, Acloque H, Huang RY, Nieto MA. Epithelial-mesenchymal transitions in development and disease. Cell. 2009;139(5):871–90.
6. Willis BC, Liebler JM, Luby-Phelps K, Nicholson AG, Crandall ED, du Bois RM, Borok Z. Induction of epithelial-mesenchymal transition in alveolar epithelial cells by transforming growth factor-β1: potential role in idiopathic pulmonary fibrosis. Am J Pathol. 2005;166(5):1321–32.
7. Nieto MA, Huang RY, Jackson RA, Thiery JP. EMT: 2016. Cell. 2016;166(1):21–45.
8. Willis BC, Borok Z. TGF-β-induced EMT: mechanisms and implications for fibrotic lung disease. Am J Physiol Lung Cell Mol Physiol. 2007;293(3):L525–34.
9. Zhong Q, Zhou B, Ann DK, Minoo P, Liu Y, Banfalvi A, Krishnaveni MS, Dubourd M, Demaio L, Willis BC, Kim KJ, et al. Role of endoplasmic reticulum stress in epithelial-mesenchymal transition of alveolar epithelial cells: effects of misfolded surfactant protein. Am J Respir Cell Mol Biol. 2011; 45(3):498–509.
10. Kim KK, Wei Y, Szekeres C, Kugler MC, Wolters PJ, Hill ML, Frank JA, Brumwell AN, Wheeler SE, Kreidberg JA, et al. Epithelial cell α3β1 integrin links β-catenin and Smad signaling to promote myofibroblast formation and pulmonary fibrosis. J Clin Invest. 2009;119(1):213–24.
11. Behr J. Evidence-based treatment strategies in idiopathic pulmonary fibrosis. Eur Respir Rev. 2013;22(128):163–8.
12. Richeldi L. Clinical trials of investigational agents for IPF: a review of a Cochrane report. Respir Res. 2013;14(Suppl 1):S4.
13. King TE Jr, Bradford WZ, Castro-Bernardini S, Fagan EA, Glaspole I, Glassberg MK, Gorina E, Hopkins PM, Kardatzke D, Lancaster L, et al. A phase 3 trial of pirfenidone in patients with idiopathic pulmonary fibrosis. N Engl J Med. 2014;370(22):2083–92.
14. Richeldi L, du Bois RM, Raghu G, Azuma A, Brown KK, Costabel U, Cottin V, Flaherty KR, Hansell DM, Inoue Y, et al. Efficacy and safety of nintedanib in idiopathic pulmonary fibrosis. N Engl J Med. 2014;370(22):2071–82.
15. Schaefer CJ, Ruhrmund DW, Pan L, Seiwert SD, Kossen K. Antifibrotic activities of pirfenidone in animal models. Eur Respir Rev. 2011;20(120):85–97.
16. Keum YS, Khor TO, Lin W, Shen G, Kwon KH, Barve A, Li W, Kong AN. Pharmacokinetics and pharmacodynamics of broccoli sprouts on the suppression of prostate cancer in transgenic adenocarcinoma of mouse prostate (TRAMP) mice: implication of induction of Nrf2, HO-1 and apoptosis and the suppression of Akt-dependent kinase pathway. Pharm Res. 2009;26(10):2324–31.
17. Elbarbry F, Elrody N. Potential health benefits of sulforaphane: a review of the experimental, clinical and epidemiological evidences and underlying mechanisms. J Med Plant Res. 2011;5(4):473–84.
18. Chaudhuri D, Orsulic S, Ashok BT. Antiproliferative activity of sulforaphane in Akt-overexpressing ovarian cancer cells. Mol Cancer Ther. 2007;6(1):334–45.
19. Gamet-Payrastre L, Li P, Lumeau S, Cassar G, Dupont MA, Chevolleau S, Gasc N, Tulliez J, Tercé F. Sulforaphane, a naturally occurring isothiocyanate, induces cell cycle arrest and apoptosis in HT29 human colon cancer cells. Cancer Res. 2000;60(5):1426–33.
20. Shan Y, Zhang L, Bao Y, Li B, He C, Gao M, Feng X, Xu W, Zhang X, Wang S. Epithelial-mesenchymal transition, a novel target of sulforaphane via COX-2/MMP2, 9/snail, ZEB1 and miR-200c/ZEB1 pathways in human bladder cancer cells. J Nutr Biochem. 2013;24(6):1062–9.
21. Illam SP, Narayanankutty A, Mathew SE, Valsalakumari R, Jacob RM, Raghavamenon AC. Epithelial mesenchymal transition in Cancer progression: preventive phytochemicals. Recent Pat Anticancer Drug Discov. 2017;12(3):234–46.
22. Oh CJ, Kim JY, Min AK, Park KG, Harris RA, Kim HJ, Lee IK. Sulforaphane attenuates hepatic fibrosis via NF-E2-related factor 2-mediated inhibition of

transforming growth factor-beta/Smad signaling. Free Radic Biol Med. 2012; 52(3):671–82.

23. Michaeloudes C, Chang PJ, Petrou M, Chung KF. Transforming growth factor-β and nuclear factor E2 related factor 2 regulate antioxidant responses in airway smooth muscle cells: role in asthma. Am J Respir Crit Care Med. 2011;184(8):894–903.

24. Artaud-Macari E, Goven D, Brayer S, Hamimi A, Besnard V, Marchal-Somme J, Ali ZE, Crestani B, Kerdine-Römer S, Boutten A, et al. Nuclear factor erythroid 2-related factor 2 nuclear translocation induces myofibroblastic dedifferentiation in idiopathic pulmonary fibrosis. Antioxid Redox Signal. 2013;18(1):66–79.

25. Yan B, Ma Z, Shi S, Hu Y, Ma T, Rong G, Yang J. Sulforaphane prevents bleomycin-induced pulmonary fibrosis in mice by inhibiting oxidative stress via nuclear factor erythroid 2-related factor-2 activation. Mol Med Rep. 2017; 15(6):4005–14.

26. Bai Y, Cui W, Xin Y, Miao X, Barati MT, Zhang C, Chen Q, Tan Y, Cui T, Zheng Y, et al. Prevention by sulforaphane of diabetic cardiomyopathy is associated with up-regulation of Nrf2 expression and transcription activation. J Mol Cell Cardiol. 2013;57:82–95.

27. Cho HY, Reddy SP, Yamamoto M, Kleeberger SR. The transcription factor NRF2 protects against pulmonary fibrosis. FASEB J. 2004;18(11):1258–60.

28. Kikuchi N, Ishii Y, Morishima Y, Yageta Y, Haraguchi N, Itoh K, Yamamoto M, Hizawa N. Nrf2 protects against pulmonary fibrosis by regulating the lung oxidant level and Th1/Th2 balance. Respir Res. 2010;11:31.

29. Moeller A, Ask K, Warburton D, Gauldie J, Kolb M. The bleomycin animal model: a useful tool to investigate treatment options for idiopathic pulmonary fibrosis? Int J Biochem Cell Biol. 2008;40(3):362–82.

30. Mouratis MA, Aidinis V. Modeling pulmonary fibrosis with bleomycin. Curr Opin Pulm Med. 2011;17(5):355–61.

31. Derynck R, Zhang YE. Smad-dependent and Smad-independent pathways in TGF-β family signalling. Nature. 2003;425(6958):577–84.

32. Nakamura T, Matsushima M, Hayashi Y, Shibasaki M, Imaizumi K, Hashimoto N, Shimokata K, Hasegawa Y, Kawabe T. Attenuation of transforming growth factor-β–stimulated collagen production in fibroblasts by quercetin-induced Heme oxygenase–1. Am J Respir Cell Mol Biol. 2011;44(5):614–20.

4

Antimicrobial resistance profile of *Staphylococcus aureus* isolated from patients with infection at Tikur Anbessa Specialized Hospital, Addis Ababa, Ethiopia

Sileshi Tadesse[1], Haile Alemayehu[2], Admasu Tenna[3], Getachew Tadesse[4], Tefaye Sisay Tessema[5], Workineh Shibeshi[6] and Tadesse Eguale[2*] (iD)

Abstract

Background: *Staphylococcus aureus* is one of the major pathogens of public health importance responsible for various forms of infection. Development of resistance to commonly used antimicrobials limited treatment options against infections due to this pathogen. Antimicrobial resistance profile of *Staphylococcus aureus* isolated from patients with surgical site infection and ear infection and corresponding nasal swab was investigated in Tikur Anbessa Specialized Hospital (TASH), Addis Ababa, Ethiopia.

Methods: Wound and corresponding nasal swabs from patients with surgical site infection from general surgery ward ($n = 14$), orthopedic ward ($n = 21$) and those with otitis media ($n = 59$) from Ear Nose and Throat (ENT) ward were cultured for *S. aureus* isolation according to standard procedures from December 2013 to June 2014. Isolates were investigated for susceptibility to panel of 17 antimicrobials using Kirby Bauer disc diffusion assay. Susceptibility to methicillin was phenotypically determined based on sensitivity of isolates to cefoxitin and oxacillin.

Results: A total of 79 *S. aureus* isolates were recovered from 54(57.4%) of patients. The isolates were resistant to ampicillin (100%), oxacillin and cefoxitin (68.4%, each), clindamycin (63.3%), cephalothin (59.5%), tetracycline (57%), sulfamethoxazole + trimethoprim and bacitracin (53.2%, each), and erythromycin (51.9%). Resistance to two or more antimicrobials was recorded in 74 (95%) of the isolates, while resistance to 3 or more antimicrobials was detected in 65(82.3%) of the isolates. Fifty-four (68.4%) of the isolates were methicillin resistant *S. aureus* (MRSA). Rate of occurrence of MRSA was more common among isolates from surgical wards ($p < 0.001$) compared to those from ENT ward. High level of multi-drug resistance (MDR) was detected more commonly among isolates from orthopedic ward than those from general surgical ward and patients with ear infection ($p < 0.001$). One of the isolate cultured from wound swab of a patient with surgical site infection from orthopedic ward was resistant to all of the 17 antimicrobials tested.

Conclusion: *S. aureus* isolates from patients in TASH exhibited resistance to majority of antimicrobials commonly employed for the treatment of staphylococcal infections which calls for urgent need of prudent use of antimicrobials and the need for implementation of effective infection control practices to hamper spread of MDR *S. aureus*.

Keywords: *Staphylococcus aureus*, Methicillin resistant *Staphylococcus aureus*, Surgical site infection, Drug resistance, Otitis media

* Correspondence: tadesse.eguale@aau.edu.et
[2]Aklilu Lemma Institute of Pathobiology, Addis Ababa University, P.O. Box 1176, Addis Ababa, Ethiopia
Full list of author information is available at the end of the article

Background

Staphylococcus aureus is a normal flora associated with skin, skin glands and mucous membrane of almost all warm blooded animals and about 30% of the human population is colonized by *S. aureus* [1]. It is also a leading cause of life- threatening blood stream infection, osteoarticular, skin, soft tissue, respiratory tract, device-associated and surgical site infections particularly in immunocompromised, young and elderly patients [2]. The ability of *S. aureus* to invade the host immune system through various virulence factors and its rapid acquisition of multi-drug resistance phenotype, makes it one of the most notorious organism among gram positive bacterial pathogens [3].

The burden of infection with antimicrobial resistant strains of pathogens involves increased risk of mortality, increased hospital stay, and related attributable costs compared to infection with antimicrobial susceptible pathogens [4]. *S. aureus* is reported to be the most common cause of nosocomial infections and is particularly responsible for majority of surgical site infections [5]. In a previous study in northern Ethiopia, the rate of surgical site infection accounted for 10.2% and *S. aureus* was shown to be the leading bacterial pathogen responsible for surgical site infection [6]. Similarly, *S. aureus* was the most frequently isolated pathogen among patients with otitis media at Bahir Dar, northwest Ethiopia [7], Ayder teaching and Referral Hospital, Mekelle, northern Ethiopia [8] and isolates were resistant to several antimicrobials.

Multidrug resistant (MDR) strains of *S. aureus*, particularly methicillin resistant *Staphylococcus aureus* (MRSA) have potential of rapid spread in a given health facility through colonized or infected patients or health personnel as well as contaminated environments in the facilities, unless there is strict infection control strategy [9]. Recent study showed that infection with MDR strains of *S. aureus* is associated with prolonged length of hospital stay and increased mortality [10]. MRSA is one of the major public health threats globally. Antimicrobial resistance in MRSA is associated with acquisition of large mobile genetic element called staphylococcal cassette chromosome (SCCmec) which carries the central determinant for a broad spectrum beta-lactam resistance encoded by *mec*A or *mec*C genes [11, 12]. Studies showed widespread distribution of MRSA in various countries particularly in hospital environments [13–15] as well as occurrence of community and livestock associated MRSA [16–18]. In addition to *mec*A and *mec*C genes, SCC was reported to carry several other drug resistance genes which confer resistance to mercury, kanamycin, erythromycin, spectinomycin and fusidic acid [19]. Moreover, recent studies showed dramatic increase in the development of resistance to vancomycin, the other alternative drug for the treatment of infections caused by gram positive organisms [20].

It has been shown that overall epidemiology, pathophysiology and clinical manifestations of *S. aureus* vary significantly among different countries and different regions of the same country [2]. In most developing countries like Ethiopia, the potential public health threat due to antimicrobial resistance is high because of the fact that antimicrobial agents can easily be purchased without prescription [21], lack of coordinated routine surveillance of antimicrobial resistance, poor laboratory capacity, and poor infection control mechanisms by health facilities [22]; contributing to the emergence and spread of antimicrobial resistance [23]. Knowledge on the antimicrobial susceptibility status of circulating pathogens in a given health facility is important for better management of infectious pathogens particularly where routine culture and sensitivity testing is not practiced. Recent study at Yekatit 12 Hospital, Addis Ababa, showed isolation rate of *S. aureus* from 14.3% of clinical specimens, of which over 50% of the isolates were MDR and 17.5% were MRSA [24]. Scant information is available on the occurrence and antimicrobial susceptibility of *S. aureus* in patients with surgical site infection and those with otitis media in Ethiopia. Thus, the present study reports occurrence and antimicrobial resistance profile of *S. aureus* among patients with surgical site infection and ear infection and corresponding nasal swab at Tikur Anbessa Specialized Hospital (TASH), Addis Ababa, Ethiopia.

Methods

Study setting, study design and subjects

The study was conducted at Tikur Anbessa Specialized Hospital, a tertiary teaching hospital of Addis Ababa University, from December 2013 to June, 2014. The hospital provides diverse services for patients from different parts of the country. The study design was a hospital based cross-sectional study in which hospitalized patients from general surgical ward and orthopedic ward as well as outpatients from ear, nose, and throat (ENT) ward were involved. Patients with clinical evidence of surgical site infection having surgical wound with pus discharge, serous or seropurulent discharge, signs of sepsis and diagnosed for surgical site infection from general surgical and orthopedic wards were enrolled. These patients were hospitalized for various period and 25(71%) of them were treated with ceftriaxone and others were treated with antimicrobials such as metronidazole, vancomycin, ceftazidime, cloxacillin and gentamicin whereas there was no information on recent history of antimicrobial therapy for 5(14.3%) of the patients. In addition, patients with acute and chronic otitis media with clinically proven discharge from ENT outpatient ward were randomly recruited. Majority of these patients 34(61%) had history of recent treatment with ciprofloxacin and hydrogen peroxide, 4(6.8%) with amoxicillin+clavulanic acid while the rest 19(32.2%) had no history of recent antimicrobial therapy. Only patients who were willing to give their consent to participate in the study were involved.

Sample collection and isolation of *S. aureus*

A total of paired swab samples from 94 patients; wound swab from those with surgical site infection ($n = 14$ from general surgical ward; $n = 21$ from orthopedic ward) and ear swab from patients with otitis media having clinical symptom of ear discharge ($n = 59$) and corresponding nasal swabs from all patients ($n = 94$) were collected. The wound site and ear were first cleaned with sterile saline to remove any purulent debris. Sterile cotton swab was moistened with normal saline and rotated three times on the wound surface and ear opening and placed in test tubes containing 10 ml of sterile Trypton Soya Broth(TSB), (BD, Diagnostic Systems, Heidelberg, Germany). Samples were transported in the ice box to the Microbiology Laboratory of Aklilu Lemma Institute of Pathobiology, Addis Ababa University within 3–4 h of collection and were immediately incubated at 37 °C overnight.

After overnight growth in TSB, loopful of the suspension was streaked into mannitol salt agar (Oxoid, Basingstoke, Hampshire, England). Then the plates were incubated at 37 °C for 24 h and bacterial colonies with typical characteristics of *S. aureus* (i.e. colonies with golden yellow pigmentation on mannitol salt agar) were subjected to subsequent biochemical tests involving Gram stain, catalase, and coagulase tests for confirmation. *Staphylococcus aureus* ATCC25923 was used as a reference strain.

Antimicrobial susceptibility testing

Antimicrobial susceptibility test for *S. aureus* was carried out against a panel of 17 antimicrobials using Kirby Bauer disc diffusion method according to Clinical and Laboratory Standards Institute guidelines [25] on Mueller Hinton agar (MHA) (Oxoid, Basingstoke, England). The bacterial culture was grown in TSB for 4–5 h at 37 °C and the inoculum density was adjusted with 0.5 McFarland standard. A sterile cotton swab was dipped into the suspension and it was pressed against the sides of the tube to avoid excess inoculum. The inoculum was evenly spread on MHA plate and kept for 15 min before antimicrobial discs were dispensed. The plates were then incubated at 37 °C for 24 h and the diameter of zone of inhibition was measured using plastic transparent ruler. The interpretation of the categories of susceptible, intermediate or resistant was based on the CLSI guidelines [25]. Reference strain of *S. aureus* ATCC25923 was used as a quality control organism. The following

antimicrobials with disk potencies (µg) were used (Sensi-Discs, Becton, Dickinson and Company, sparks, MD): oxacillin (Ox; 1), cefoxitin (Fox;30), cephalothin (Cf; 30), bacitracin (B;10 IU), clindamycin (Da; 2), ampicillin (Amp; 10 µg), amoxicillin-clavulanic acid (Amc; 30), ceftriaxone (Cro; 30), chloramphenicol (C) (30 µg), ciprofloxacin (Cip;5), erythromycin (E;15), gentamicin (Gm; 10), amikacin (An; 30), sulphamethoxazole-trimethoprim (Sxt;25), doxycycline (Do,30), tetracycline (Te; 30), and nitrofurantoin(Nitro;300).

Data analysis

The chi-square test was employed to investigate association of sex and age of patients with carriage rate of *S. aureus* and MRSA. One way analysis of variance and student t-test were used to compare the difference in the level of multidrug resistance in *S. aureus* originating from various wards and specimens. The difference between the means was considered significant at $p < 0.05$.

Results

Staphylococcus aureus infection rate

Of all 188 specimens cultured for *S. aureus*, 79 (42.02%) were positive. *S. aureus* was detected from 54 (57.4%) of the 94 patients examined either from wound/ear discharge swab or nasal swab. Rate of recovery of *S. aureus* was higher among specimens obtained from patients with otitis media (44.1% from ear discharge and 50.9% from nasal swab) compared to wound and nasal swab of patients with surgical site infection which ranged from 28 to 38%. However, overall *S. aureus* carriage rate per patient was almost similar among patients from various wards (Table 1). There was no statistically significant difference in occurrence of *S. aureus* among different age group and sex (Table 2).

Antimicrobial resistance profile of *S. aureus*

All *S. aureus* isolates examined in the current study were resistant to at least one of the 17 antimicrobials. All (100%) of the isolates were resistant to ampicillin, 54(68.4%) were resistant to oxacillin and cefoxitin, 50(63.3%) to clindamycin, 47(59.5%) to cephalothin, 45(57%) to tetracycline, 42(53.2%) to sulphamethoxazole+trimethoprim, and bacitracin, 41(51.9%) (Fig. 1).

Based on the sensitivity of isolates to cefoxitin and oxacillin, 54 (68.4%) of the isolates were MRSA. There was no difference in the level of detection of MRSA among *S. aureus* isolates cultured from patients in different age group and from both sexes. Among isolates from various sources, MRSA was detected more frequently in isolates obtained from patients with surgical site infection ($p = 0.001$). Interestingly, all of the 23(100%) of isolates from general surgical and orthopedic wards were

Table 1 Relative isolation rate of S. aureus from wound and nasal swab of patients with surgical site infection and ear discharge swab and nasal swab of patients with otitis media

Patient category	No. of patients	No. of patients positive from one or more specimen (%)	Specimen	No. examined	No. (%) positive	Total no. of isolates
General surgical ward	14	8(57.1)	Wound swab	14	4(28.6)	8
			Nasal swab	14	4(28.6)	
Orthopedic ward	21	10(47.6)	Wound swab	21	8(38.1)	15
			Nasal swab	21	7(33.3)	
ENT ward	59	36(61)	Ear discharge	59	26(44.1)	56
			Nasal swab	59	30(50.9)	
Total	94	54(57.5)		188	79(42.02)	79

MRSA whereas only 31(54.4%) of isolates obtained from patients with ear infection were MRSA (Table 3).

Resistance to two or more antimicrobials was recorded in 74(95%) of the isolates, while resistance to 3 or more antimicrobials was detected in 65(82.3%) of the isolates. Multidrug resistance to 7 or more antimicrobials was detected in 51(64.6%) of the isolates. Majority of isolates cultured from surgical site infection were resistant to several drugs. One of the isolate cultured from a wound swab of patient with surgical site infection from orthopedic ward was found to be resistant to all of the 17 antimicrobials tested (Table 4).

The mean (± SEM) number of drugs to which S. aureus isolates obtained from patients from ENT, general surgical ward and orthopedic ward were 7.1 ± 0.6, 10.63 ± 1.2, 13.3 ± 0.7, respectively (Fig. 2a). The level of MDR was significantly higher in S. aureus isolates obtained from patients in orthopedic ward compared to those obtained from general surgical ward as well as ENT wards ($p < 0.0001$) while no significant difference was observed among isolates obtained from other two wards. Similarly, comparison of level of MDR among S. aureus strains isolated from various specimens revealed that strains isolated from wound swab were resistant to significantly

larger number of antimicrobials compared to those isolated from nasal swab as well as ear swab ($p < 0.001$) (Fig. 2b).

Discussion

The objective of the current study was to assess occurrence and antimicrobial resistance profile of S. aureus among patients with surgical site infection and ear infection and corresponding nasal swab at Tikur Anbessa Specialized Hospital. The overall rate of recovery of S. aureus among patients with surgical site infection in the current study (47.6–57.1%) is in line with previous studies in which S. aureus was shown to be the predominant pathogen responsible for surgical site infection in Ethiopia [6]. Similarly high rate of isolation of S. aureus was reported from patients with pus/wound discharge at Gondar University hospital in north Ethiopia [26], and from ear discharges from Hawassa Hospital, southern Ethiopia [27]. In some of the patients with surgical site infection in the current study, S. aureus was not detected whereas the same patients were positive from nasal swab. Such heterogeneity could be due to direct topical application of antimicrobials to the infection site which might have affected growth of bacteria from this site. The other possible reason could be the real absence of S. aureus from infection site and detection from nasal swab might be due to natural colonization [1]. On the other hand, the absence of S. aureus from nasal swab and detection from wound swab and ear discharge could be due to localized infection in the specific infected sites.

Detection of S. aureus from ear discharge of 44.1% of patients with otitis media in the current study shows that S. aureus is one of the major causes of ear infection in the study population. In previous studies in Ethiopia, S. aureus was the dominant bacterial pathogen isolated from patients with otitis media in Mekelle, north Ethiopia [8] and the 2nd predominantly isolated pathogen in northeastern Ethiopia [28]. Unlike previous studies where recovery of bacterial pathogens including S. aureus varied among patients with different age group [8, 28], in the current study there was no significant

Table 2 Sociodemographic characteristics of patients with surgical site infection, ear infection and carriage rate of S. aureus at Tikur Anbessa Specialized Hospital

Characteristics	No. (%) tested	No. (%) S. aureus culture positive	χ^2	p-value
Sex				
Male	54	28(51.8)	1.6	0.29
Female	40	26(65)		
Age in years				
< 11	18	9(50)		
11–20	26	19(73.1)	3.87	0.42
21–30	20	11(55)		
31–40	15	8(53.3)		
≥ 41	15	7(46.7)		

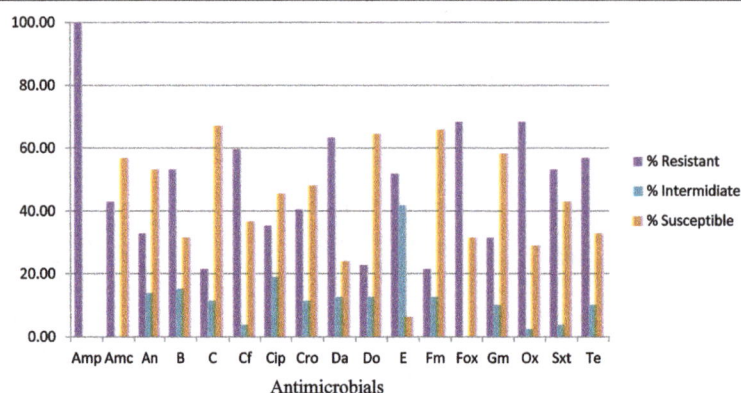

Fig. 1 Proportion of susceptible, intermediately resistant and resistant *S. aureus* isolates (*n* = 79) to 17 antimicrobials examined (Amp = ampicillin; Amc = amoxicillin+clavulanic acid; An = amikacin; B = bacitracin; C = chloramphenicol; Cf = cephalothin; Cip = ciprofloxacin; Cro = ceftriaxone; Fox = cefoxitin; Da = clindamycin Do = doxycycline; E = erythromycin; Gm = gentamicin; Fm = nitrofurantoin; Ox = oxacillin, Sxt = sulfamethoxazole + trimethoprim; Te = tetracycline)

difference in isolation rate of *S. aureus* among age groups, which could be due to small sample size in the current study and due to difference in composition of patient category.

The current study also revealed high rate of resistance to most of the antimicrobials by strains of *S. aureus* isolated from patients with surgical site infection and those with otitis media. Of particular concern is that all strains in this study were resistant to ampicillin unlike previous studies where resistance to ampicillin was observed in 82.2 and 88.5% of *S. aureus* isolates from patients with surgical site infection at Debre Markos Referral Hospital, northwest Ethiopia [29], and patients with otitis media in northeast Ethiopia [28], respectively. On the other hand, it is in agreement with the finding where 100% resistance to ampicillin was recorded in *S. aureus* strains

Table 3 Relative distribution of MRSA among *S. aureus* isolates from patients of different sex, age group and ward type

Characteristics of source of isolates	No. *S. aureus*	No. MRSA (%)	X^2	*p* = value
Sex				
Male	42	28(66.7)	0.12	0.87
Female	37	26(70.3)		
Age in years				
< 11	16	12(75)		
11–20	25	16(64)	2.5	0.65
21–30	18	12(66.7)		
31–40	12	7(58.3)		
≥ 41	8	7(87.5)		
Ward type				
General surgical	8	8(100)	15.02	0.001
Orthopedic	15	15(100)		
ENT	56	31(54.4)		

isolated from patients admitted to Felege Hiwot referral Hospital, North Ethiopia [6]. Such difference could be attributed to variation in patient hospital stay, level of infection control practices by health facilities, and previous exposure of patient to antimicrobials [30]. Some isolates from nasal swab and respective wound or ear discharge swab from a single patient had different antimicrobial susceptibility profile. The possible reason for this could be due to localized infection with different strain of *S. aureus* at the wound site while the one from nasal swab could be due to natural colonization.

Rate of occurrence of MRSA (68.4%) out of total *S. aureus* infection in the current study is higher than study reported by Kahsay et al. [29] from patients with surgical site infection at Debre Markos Referral Hospital, northern Ethiopia (49.7%), various clinical specimens from Yekatit 12 Hospital, in Addis Ababa which was 17.5% [24] as well as reports from HIV infected pediatric patients in northwest Ethiopia [31]. It is also higher than a study in Philippines where *S. aureus* isolated from clinical specimens showed 40% MRSA [32]. This could be attributed to difference in composition of patients from whom samples were collected including patients being outpatients, hospitalized, duration of hospital stay and previous antimicrobial use. Majority of MRSA strains in the current study were isolated from hospitalized patients with surgical site infections and those with chronic otitis media who received antimicrobials. Interestingly, all isolates obtained from patients from general surgical and orthopedic wards were MRSA strains, unlike those from ENT ward where only 54% were MRSA suggesting higher rate of infection of patients with MDR strains from the hospital environment in hospitalized patients either during surgical procedure or during postoperative care. Previous study indicated that most of surgical site infections occur during surgery

Table 4 Resistance pattern of *S. aureus* strains isolated from patients from different wards and specimens

Resistance pattern	No. of drugs to which R is observed	No. (%) isolates	Ward type	Specimen
Amp	1	4(5.1)	ENT	Nasal swab(2)Ear swab(2)
AmpSxt(2),AmpDa,AmpDo, AmpE(2), AmpFox(2), AmpTe(2)	2	10(12.7)	ENT	Ear swab(5), Nasal swab(5)
AmpBSxt, AmpDaOx, AmpTeSxt	3	3(3.8)	ENT	Ear swab(1), Nasal swab(2)
AmpCfFoxOx, AmpDaDoTe,AmpFoxOxSxt, AmpBCfDa	4	4(5.1)	ENT	Ear swab(2) nasal swab(2)
AmpBDoFoxTe, AmpBEOxSxt, AmpDaESxtTe, AmpDoFoxTeOx, AmpBDaETe	5	5(6.3)	ENT(4), Surgical(1)	Ear swab(2), nasal swab(3)
AmpBDaFoxSxtTe, AmpCEFoxOxTe	6	2(2.5)	ENT	Ear swab(1), nasal swab(1)
AmpAnCDaEFoxTe, AmpAnDaFoxOxSxtTe, AmpBCfDaFmFoxOx, AmpBCfCroDaFoxOx, AmpBCfDaFmFoxSxt	7	5(6.3)	ENT(4), Surgical(1)	Ear swab(2), nasal swab(3)
AmpAnCfCroFoxGmOxTe, AmpAnDaDoFoxGmOxTe, AmpBCfDaDoFoxOxTe, AmpBCfDaEOxSxtTe, AmpBCipCroFmGmOxSxt	8	5(6.3)	ENT(2), Surgical(1), Ortho(2),	Nasal swab(1), wound swab(2), ear swab(2),
AmpAnCfDaFoxGmOxSxtTe AmpCCfCipCroDaFoxETe, AmpCCfCipCroFoxGmOx AmpAnBCipDaFoxOxSxtTe, AmpBCCfCroDaFoxGmOx, AmpBCCfCroFoxOxSxtTe	9	6(7.6)	ENT (5), Ortho(1)	Nasal swab(5), ear swab (1)
AmpBCCfCipDaEFmFoxOx, AmpBCCfCipDaEOxSxtTe AmpBCCfCroDaFmFoxOxSxt, AmpBCCfDaDoEFmOxTe	10	4(5.1)	ENT(3), Surgical(1)	Ear swab(3), Wound swab(1)
AmpAnBCfCipDaDoEFoxOxTe, AmpAnBCCfCroDaDoFoxOxTe, AmpAnCCipCroDaEFoxOxSxtTe, AmpAnCCipCroDaEFoxOxSxtTe, AmpAnCCfCipCroDaEFoxGmOx, AmpAmcAnCCfCipEFoxOxSxtTe, AmpAmcBCfCroDaEFmFoxOxSxt, AmpAmcAnBCfCroDaEFmFoxOx, AmpAmcBCfCipCroEFoxOxSxtTe, AmpAnBCfCroDaEFoxGmOxTe	11	9 (11.4)	ENT(6), Ortho(2), Surgical(1)	Ear swab(2), nasal swab(6), wound swab(1)
AmpAnBCfDaDoEFoxGmOxSxtTe, AmpAmcAnBCfDaEFmFoxOxSxtOx, AmpAmcAnBCCfCroDaEFoxOxTe, AmpAmcBCfCipCroEFoxGmOxSxtTe, AmpAmcBCfCipDaDoEFmOxSxtTe	12	5(6.3)	ENT(3), Ortho(2)	Ear swab(2), nasal swab(1), Wound swab(2)
AmpAmcAnCCfCipCroDaEFoxGmOxSxt, AmpAmcBCfCipCroDaEFoxGmOxSxtTe, AmpAmcAnBCfCipCroEFmFoxGmOxSxt, AmpCCfCipCroDaDoEFoxGmOxSxtTe, AmpAnCCfCipCroDaDoFoxGmOxSxtTe, AmpAmcBCCfCipCroDaFoxGmOxSxtTe, AmpAmcBCfCipCroDaFmFoxGmOxSxtTe	13	7(8.9)	ENT(2), Surgical(2), Ortho(3)	Ear swab(2), wound swab(2), nasal swab(3)
AmpAmcAnCCfCipCroDaEFoxGmOxSxtTe, AmpAmcAnBCfCipCroDaEFoxGmOxSxtTe, AmpAmcAnCfCipCroDaDoEFoxGmOxSxtTe, AmpAmcAnBCfCipCroDaEFoxGmOxSxtTe, AmpAmcAnBCCfCipCroDaEFoxOxSxtTe,	14	5(6.3)	Ortho(3), ENT(2)	Nasal swab(4), wound swab(1)
AmpAmcBCCfCipCroDaEFmFoxGmOxSxtTe, AmpAmcAnBCCfCipCroDaEFoxGmOxSxtTe, AmpAmcBCCfCipCroDaDoEFoxGmOxSxtTe	15	3(3.8)	Surgical(1) Ortho(2)	Wound swab (2), nasal swab(1)
AmpAmcAnBCCfCipCroDaDoEFoxGmOxSxtIe	16	1(1.3)	EVNT(1)	Ear swab(1)
AmpAmcAnBCCfCipCroDaDoEFmFoxGmOxSxtTe	17	1(1.3)	Ortho	Wound swab(1)

Amp ampicillin, *Amc* amoxicillin+clavulanic acid, *An* amikacin, *B* bacitracin, *Cf* cephalothin, *C* chloramphenicol, *Cip* ciprofloxacin, *Cro* ceftriaxone, *Fox* cefoxitin, *Da* clindamycin, *Do* doxycycline, *E* erythromycin, *Gm* gentamicin, *Nitro* nitrofurantoin, *Ox* oxacillin, *Sxt* sulfamethoxazole + trimethoprim, *Te* tetracycline, *R* resistant

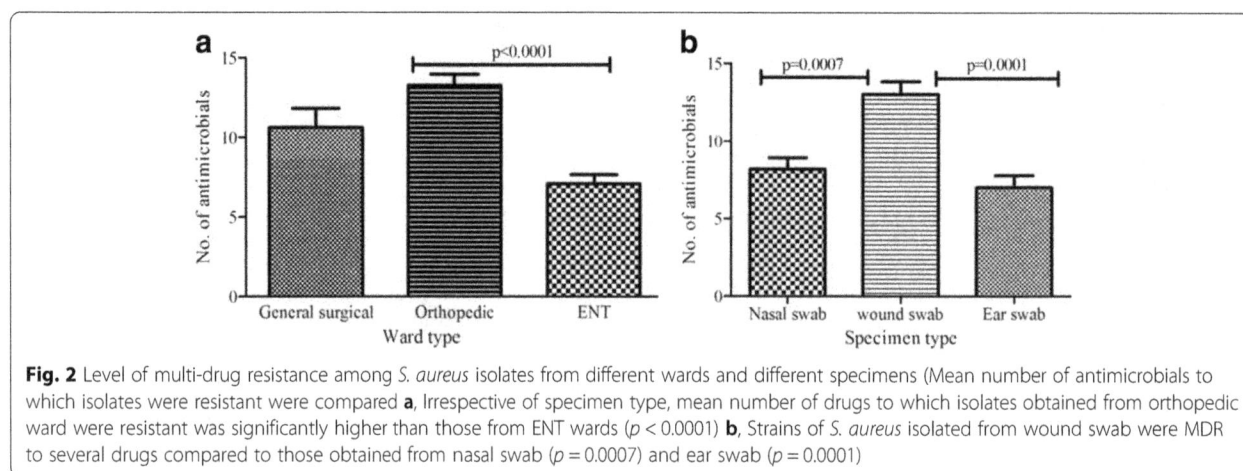

Fig. 2 Level of multi-drug resistance among *S. aureus* isolates from different wards and different specimens (Mean number of antimicrobials to which isolates were resistant were compared **a**, Irrespective of specimen type, mean number of drugs to which isolates obtained from orthopedic ward were resistant was significantly higher than those from ENT wards ($p < 0.0001$) **b**, Strains of *S. aureus* isolated from wound swab were MDR to several drugs compared to those obtained from nasal swab ($p = 0.0007$) and ear swab ($p = 0.0001$)

demonstrated by matching of strains of pathogens from surgeon's fingers and post-operative infection [33].

The probable reason for high rate of overall MDR in *S. aureus* isolates obtained from orthopedic surgery ward compared to those from other wards could be due to high contamination of this specific ward with MDR strains of *S. aureus*. The reason why isolates cultured from nasal swab and ear swab were resistant to less number of drugs compared to those obtained from surgical wound could possibly because the level of previous exposure to antimicrobial agents might not be as high as those from surgical ward who were hospitalized. All isolates from ear discharge and most of the isolates from nasal swab were obtained from outpatients in ENT ward who had less exposure to antimicrobials. MRSA and other MDR nosocomial pathogens can be transmitted through skin contact among patients, from health personnel and hospital environment and surfaces unless proper infection control measures are practiced [34]. The poor sanitary conditions of the hospital and lack of routine surveillance of antimicrobial susceptibility of circulating bacterial strains might have contributed to spread of resistant bacteria in the hospital.

Conclusion
In general, this study revealed high rate of MDR strains of *S. aureus* in TASH, majority of which being MRSA. As this study involved limited wards in a single hospital and small sample size, it may not represent the whole hospital situation and the country as well. Despite this limitation, the finding warrants implementation of measures to control spread of MDR strains in the hospital and the community. Some of the measures to be undertaken include, improving antimicrobial stewardship through routine monitoring of antimicrobial susceptibility of circulating strains and avoiding or reducing empirical therapy, effective infection control practices, training

of health personnel and patients on the risk of antimicrobial resistance.

Abbreviations
CLSI: Clinical and Laboratory Standards Institute; ENT: Ear nose and throat; MDR: multidrug resistance; MHA: Mueller Hinton agar; MRSA: Methicillin resistant *Staphylococcus aureus*; TASH: Tikur Anbessa Specialized Hospital; TSB: Trypton Soya Broth

Acknowledgements
The authors would like to thank staff of ENT, surgical and orthopedic wards of TASH for their technical support during sample collection and all study participants.

Funding
This study was financially supported by Addis Ababa University.

Authors' contributions
ST, TE, AT, GT, TS and WS participated in conception of the study. ST was involved in sample collection, laboratory work and preparation of draft manuscript. TE supervised data collection and participated in preparation of draft manuscript. HA participated in laboratory investigation. All authors read and approved the final manuscript.

Author details
¹Yekatit 12 Hospital Medical College, P.O. Box157, Addis Ababa, Ethiopia. ²Aklilu Lemma Institute of Pathobiology, Addis Ababa University, P.O. Box 1176, Addis Ababa, Ethiopia. ³Department of Internal Medicine, School of Medicine, College of Health Sciences, Addis Ababa University, Churchill Avenue, P.O.Box 9086, Addis Ababa, Ethiopia. ⁴Department of Biomedical Sciences, College of Veterinary medicine and Agriculture, Addis Ababa

University, P.O. Box 34, Debrezeit, Ethiopia. [5]Institute of Biotechnology, College of natural and Computational sciences, Addis Ababa University, P.O. Box, 1176, Addis Ababa, Ethiopia. [6]Department of Pharmacology and Clinical Pharmacy, School of Pharmacy, College of Health Sciences, Addis Ababa University, Churchill Avenue, P.O. Box 9086, Addis Ababa, Ethiopia.

References

1. Wertheim HF, Melles DC, Vos MC, van Leeuwen W, van Belkum A, Verbrugh HA, Nouwen JL. The role of nasal carriage in Staphylococcus aureus infections. Lancet Infect Dis. 2005;5(12):751–62.

2. Tong SY, Davis JS, Eichenberger E, Holland TL, Fowler VG Jr. Staphylococcus aureus infections: epidemiology, pathophysiology, clinical manifestations, and management. Clin Microbiol Rev. 2015;28(3):603–61.

3. Davies J, Davies D. Origins and evolution of antibiotic resistance. Microbiol Mol Biol Rev. 2010;74(3):417–33.

4. Mulvey MR, Simor AE. Antimicrobial resistance in hospitals: how concerned should we be? CMAJ. 2009;180(4):408–15.

5. Cheadle WG. Risk factors for surgical site infection. Surg Infect. 2006;7(Suppl 1):S7–11.

6. Mulu W, Kibru G, Beyene G, Damtie M. Postoperative nosocomial infections and antimicrobial resistance pattern of Bacteria isolates among patients admitted at Felege Hiwot referral hospital, Bahirdar, Ethiopia. Ethiop J Health Sci. 2012;22(1):7–18.

7. Abera B, Biadeglegne F. Antimicrobial resistance patterns of Staphylococcus aureus and Proteus spp. isolated from otitis media at Bahir Dar regional laboratory, north West Ethiopia. Ethiop Med J. 2009;47(4):271–6.

8. Wasihun AG, Zemene Y. Bacterial profile and antimicrobial susceptibility patterns of otitis media in Ayder Teaching and Referral Hospital, Mekelle University, Northern Ethiopia. Springerplus. 2015;4:701. https://doi.org/10.1186/s40064-015-1471-z.

9. Kesah C, Ben Redjeb S, Odugbemi TO, Boye CS, Dosso M, Ndinya Achola JO, Koulla-Shiro S, Benbachir M, Rahal K, Borg M. Prevalence of methicillin-resistant Staphylococcus aureus in eight African hospitals and Malta. Clin Microbiol Infect. 2003;9(2):153–6.

10. Rauber JM, Carneiro M, Arnhold GH, Zanotto MB, Wappler PR, Baggiotto B, Valim AR, d'Azevedo PA. Multidrug-resistant Staphylococcus spp and its impact on patient outcome. Am J Infect Control. 2016;44(11):e261–3.

11. Katayama Y, Ito T, Hiramatsu K. A new class of genetic element, staphylococcus cassette chromosome mec, encodes methicillin resistance in Staphylococcus aureus. Antimicrob Agents Chemother. 2000;44(6):1549–55.

12. Garcia-Alvarez L, Holden MT, Lindsay H, Webb CR, Brown DF, Curran MD, Walpole E, Brooks K, Pickard DJ, Teale C, et al. Meticillin-resistant Staphylococcus aureus with a novel mecA homologue in human and bovine populations in the UK and Denmark: a descriptive study. Lancet Infect Dis. 2011;11(8):595–603.

13. Bhattacharya S, Pal K, Jain S, Chatterjee SS, Konar J. Surgical site infection by methicillin resistant Staphylococcus aureus- on decline? J Clin Diagn Res. 2016;10(9):DC32–6.

14. Stefani S, Chung DR, Lindsay JA, Friedrich AW, Kearns AM, Westh H, Mackenzie FM. Meticillin-resistant Staphylococcus aureus (MRSA): global epidemiology and harmonisation of typing methods. Int J Antimicrob Agents. 2012;39(4):273–82.

15. Nwankwo EO, Nasiru MS. Antibiotic sensitivity pattern of Staphylococcus aureus from clinical isolates in a tertiary health institution in Kano, Northwestern Nigeria. Pan Afr Med J. 2011;8:4.

16. Takano T, Higuchi W, Zaraket H, Otsuka T, Baranovich T, Enany S, Saito K, Isobe H, Dohmae S, Ozaki K, et al. Novel characteristics of community-acquired methicillin-resistant Staphylococcus aureus strains belonging to multilocus sequence type 59 in Taiwan. Antimicrob Agents Chemother. 2008;52(3):837–45.

17. Aires-de-Sousa M. Methicillin resistant Staphylococcus aureus among animals:current overview. Clin Microbiol Infect. 2016;23(6):373–80.

18. Guimares FF, Manzi MP, Joaquim SF, Richini-Pereira VB, Langoni H. Outbreak of methicillin-resistant Staphylococcus aureus (MRSA)-associated mastitis in a closed dairy herd. J Dairy Sci. 2017;100(1):726–30.

19. Holden MT, Feil EJ, Lindsay JA, Peacock SJ, Day NP, Enright MC, Foster TJ, Moore CE, Hurst L, Atkin R, et al. Complete genomes of two clinical

20. Cameron DR, Howden BP, Peleg AY. The interface between antibiotic resistance and virulence in Staphylococcus aureus and its impact upon clinical outcomes. Clin Infect Dis. 2011;53(6):576–82.

21. Morgan DJ, Okeke IN, Laxminarayan R, Perencevich EN, Weisenberg S. Non-prescription antimicrobial use worldwide: a systematic review. Lancet Infect Dis. 2011;11(9):692–701.

22. Vernet G, Mary C, Altmann DM, Doumbo O, Morpeth S, Bhutta ZA, Klugman KP. Surveillance for antimicrobial drug resistance in under-resourced countries. Emerg Infect Dis. 2014;20(3):434–41.

23. Okeke IN, Lamikanra A, Edelman R. Socioeconomic and behavioral factors leading to acquired bacterial resistance to antibiotics in developing countries. Emerg Infect Dis. 1999;5(1):18–27.

24. Dilnessa T, Bitew A. Prevalence and antimicrobial susceptibility pattern of methicillin resistant Staphylococcus aureus isolated from clinical samples at Yekatit 12 hospital medical college, Addis Ababa, Ethiopia. BMC Infect Dis. 2016;16:398.

25. CLSI. Performance standards for antimicrobial susceptibility testing; twenty-third informational SupplementM100-S23, vol. 33; 2013.

26. Muluye D, Wondimeneh Y, Ferede G, Nega T, Adane K, Biadgo B, Tesfa H, Moges F. Bacterial isolates and their antibiotic susceptibility patterns among patients with pus and/or wound discharge at Gondar university hospital. BMC Res Notes. 2014;7:619.

27. Deyno S, Toma A, Worku M, Bekele M. Antimicrobial resistance profile of staphylococcus aureus isolates isolated from ear discharges of patients at University of Hawassa comprehensive specialized hospital. BMC Pharmacol Toxicol. 2017;18(1):35.

28. Argaw-Denboba A, Abejew AA, Mekonnen AG. Antibiotic-resistant Bacteria are major threats of otitis Media in Wollo Area, northeastern Ethiopia: a ten-year retrospective analysis. Int J Microbiol. 2016;2016:8724671.

29. Kahsay A, Mihret A, Abebe T, Andualem T. Isolation and antimicrobial susceptibility pattern of Staphylococcus aureus in patients with surgical site infection at Debre Markos referral hospital, Amhara region, Ethiopia. Arch Public Health. 2014;72(1):16.

30. Harrop JS, Styliaras JC, Ooi YC, Radcliff KE, Vaccaro AR, Wu C. Contributing factors to surgical site infections. J Am Acad Orthop Surg. 2012;20(2):94–101.

31. Lemma MT, Zenebe Y, Tulu B, Mekonnen D, Mekonnen Z. Methicillin resistant Staphylococcus aureus among HIV infected pediatric patients in Northwest Ethiopia: carriage rates and antibiotic co-resistance profiles. PLoS One. 2015;10(9):e0137254.

32. Juayang AC, de Los Reyes GB, de la Rama AJ, Gallega CT. Antibiotic resistance profiling of Staphylococcus aureus isolated from clinical specimens in a tertiary hospital from 2010 to 2012. Interdiscip Perspect Infect Dis. 2014;2014:898457.

33. Uckay I, Hoffmeyer P, Lew D, Pittet D. Prevention of surgical site infections in orthopaedic surgery and bone trauma: state-of-the-art update. J Hosp Infect. 2013;84(1):5–12.

34. Wang X, Xiao Y, Wang J, Lu X. A mathematical model of effects of environmental contamination and presence of volunteers on hospital infections in China. J Theor Biol. 2012;293:161–73.

5

The use of clonidine in elderly patients with delirium; pharmacokinetics and hemodynamic responses

Karen Roksund Hov[1,2*†], Bjørn Erik Neerland[1,2†], Anders Mikal Andersen[3], Øystein Undseth[4], Vegard Bruun Wyller[2,5], Alasdair M. J. MacLullich[6], Eva Skovlund[7], Eirik Qvigstad[8] and Torgeir Bruun Wyller[1,2]

Abstract

Background: The Oslo Study of Clonidine in Elderly Patients with Delirium (LUCID) is an RCT investigating the effect of clonidine in medical patients > 65 years with delirium. To assess the dosage regimen and safety measures of this study protocol, we measured the plasma concentrations and hemodynamic effects of clonidine in the first 20 patients.

Methods: Patients were randomised to clonidine ($n = 10$) or placebo ($n = 10$). The treatment group was given a loading dose (75μg every 3rd hour up to a maximum of 4 doses) to reach steady state, and further 75μg twice daily until delirium free for 2 days, discharge or a maximum of 7 days. Blood pressure (BP) and heart rate (HR) were measured just before every dose. If the systolic BP was < 100 mmHg or HR < 50 beats per minute the next dose was omitted. Plasma concentrations of clonidine were measured 3 h after each drug intake on day 1, just before intake (day 2 and at steady state day 4–6) and 3 h after intake at steady state (C_{max}). Our estimated pre-specified plasma concentration target range was 0.3–0.7μg/L.

Results: 3 h after the first dose of 75μg clonidine, plasma concentration levels rose to median 0.35 (range 0.24–0.40) μg/L. Median trough concentration (C_0) at day 2 was 0.70 (0.47–0.96)μg/L. At steady state, median C_0 was 0.47 (0.36–0.76)μg/L, rising to C_{max} 0.74 (0.56–0.95)μg/L 3 h post dose. A significant haemodynamic change from baseline was only found at a few time-points during the loading doses within the clonidine group. There was however extensive individual BP and HR variation in both the clonidine and placebo groups, and when comparing the change scores (delta values) between the clonidine and the placebo groups, there were no significant differences.

Conclusions: The plasma concentration of clonidine was at the higher end of the estimated therapeutic range. Hemodynamic changes during clonidine treatment were as expected, with trends towards lower blood pressure and heart rate in patients treated with clonidine, but with dose adjustments based on SBP this protocol appears safe.

Keywords: Delirium, Clonidine, RCT, Pharmacokinetic

* Correspondence: karenroksundhov@gmail.com
†Karen Roksund Hov and Bjørn Erik Neerland contributed equally to this work.
[1]Oslo Delirium Research Group, Department of Geriatric Medicine, Oslo University Hospital, Oslo, Norway
[2]Institute of Clinical Medicine, University of Oslo, Oslo, Norway
Full list of author information is available at the end of the article

Background

Despite their dominance in the clinical practice of medicine, older people are poorly represented in drug trials [1]. There are many potential reasons for this, including heterogeneity due to variations in biological aging, the wide range of comorbidities and polypharmacy. For informed decisions to be made in older people, however, it is important that drug trials overcome these challenges.

Delirium is a disturbance in attention, awareness and cognition with acute onset resulting from medical illness, trauma, surgery or drugs. Delirium affects 20% of hospitalised patients [2] and is associated with poor outcomes [3]. Drugs are widely used in the treatment of delirium [4, 5], despite the lack of positive evidence of their effectiveness [6, 7]. The pathogenesis is not well understood, but one prominent hypothesis is that delirium may in part result from exaggerated and/or prolonged stress responses [8].

Dexmedetomidine, a parenterally administered alpha2-adrenergic receptor agonist which attenuates sympathetic nervous system activity [9], shows promise as treatment for delirium in intensive care units (ICU) [10–16]. A recently published RCT showed that prophylactic low-dose dexmedetomidine significantly decreased occurrence of post-operative delirium [17]. Indeed, it is now in clinical use in the USA and Europe [18]. However, most patients with delirium are outside of ICUs, where intravenous use of dexmedetomidine is not feasible. An alternative agent is orally administered clonidine, which has very similar pharmacological properties to dexmedetomidine [19], even though its alpha-2-adrenergic selectivity is lower [20]. Clonidine in delirium is poorly studied, but a pilot study showed that the use of clonidine infusion during the weaning period after surgery for type-A aortic dissection might reduce the severity of delirium [21].

The Oslo Study of Clonidine in Elderly Patients with Delirium (LUCID) is an RCT designed to investigate the effectiveness of clonidine as a treatment for delirium in geriatric medical patients [22]. The properties of clonidine make it challenging to anticipate the right dosage to achieve an appropriate balance between efficacy and safety in older patients. Most pharmacological studies of clonidine have been conducted in younger adults [23–25] or in children [26, 27]. Concentrations of clonidine known to have clinical effects in adults range from 0.2 to 2.0 µg/L [24, 25, 27]. After oral administration the maximum plasma concentration (C_{max}) occurs after 1–3 h [23]; higher doses yield proportionately higher concentrations [25]. The metabolism of clonidine is hepatic, mainly through CYP2D6 [28], but varying amounts of unmetabolised clonidine are excreted by the kidneys. The reduction in mean arterial pressure (MAP), as well as the risk of side effects like sedation and dry mouth, is highest when the plasma concentration of clonidine peaks (i.e. between 2 and 3 h after administration), even though only the hemodynamic effects (i.e. blood pressure and heart rate) correlate with the concentration levels [25].

To the best of our knowledge, there are no studies on the safety of clonidine and its hemodynamic effects in geriatric hospitalized patients with delirium. This study aims to investigate in detail the dosage regimen of clonidine in the LUCID protocol through measuring both plasma concentrations and hemodynamic effects. We aimed for the intermediate to low levels, that is, between 0.3 and 0.7 µg/L, because higher plasma concentration levels may increase the risk of adverse events, including hypotension, whereas plasma concentration levels lower than 0.3 µg/L might be insufficient to give a significant clinical effect.

Methods

LUCID is a randomised, placebo-controlled, double-blind, parallel group study with 4-month prospective follow-up [22]. Acutely admitted medical patients > 65 years with delirium or subsyndromal delirium are eligible for inclusion. The selection criteria are presented in Table 1. Included patients were randomised to treatment with oral clonidine or placebo for a maximum of 7 days. The goal is to include 100 patients and the primary endpoint is the trajectory of delirium including measurements of attention, awareness and cognitive function. However, according to the pre-specified protocol, pharmacological analysis of clonidine and safety of the treatment will be assessed in the first 20 patients, before the final protocol for dosage regimen and safety assessments in the final 80 patients are decided. Our pre-specified target values were plasma-concentrations 0.3–0.7 µg/L, but a small number of measurements outside this range would be considered acceptable.

Study medication

Each capsule (CAPSUGEL) contained either 75 µg Catapresan (clonidine hydrochloride) or 75 µg placebo, and was produced and labelled by "Kragerø tablettproduksjon A/S".

Dosage plan and safety

A loading dose (one capsule every 3rd hour up to a maximum of 4 doses on day 1) was given to achieve steady state. Further dosage was one capsule twice daily (8 am and 8 pm) until delirium free for 2 days, discharge or a maximum of 7 days treatment, whichever came first (see Table 2). Blood pressure (BP) and heart rate (HR) was measured just before every dose. The capsule was

Table 1 Eligibility criteria

Inclusion criteria

- Patient > 65 years old admitted to an acute medical ward
- Delirium or subsyndromal delirium within the last 48 h
- Signed informed consent from patient or relatives including advance consent for on-going treatment and follow up

Exclusion criteria

- Symptomatic bradycardia, bradycardia due to sick sinus syndrome, second- or third- degree AV-block (if not treated with pacemaker) or any other reason causing HR[a] < 50 bpm[b] at time of inclusion
- Symptomatic hypotension or orthostatic hypotension, or a systolic BP[c] < 120 at the time of inclusion
- Ischemic stroke within the last 3 months or critical peripheral ischemia
- Acute coronary syndrome, unstable or severe coronary heart disease (symptoms at minimal physical activity; NYHA[d] 3 and 4) and moderate to severe heart failure (NYHA 3 and 4). (Acute coronary syndrome is defined according to international guidelines)
- A diagnosis of polyneuropathy, phaeochromocytoma or renal insufficiency (estimated GFR[e] < 30 ml/min according to the MDRD[f] formula)
- Body weight < 45 kg
- Considered as moribund on admission
- Unable to take oral medications
- Current use of tricyclic antidepressants, monoamine reuptake inhibitors or cyclosporine
- Previously included in this study
- Adverse reactions to clonidine or excipients (lactose, saccharose)
- Not speaking or reading Norwegian
- Any other condition as evaluated by the treating physician
- Admitted to the intensive care unit

[a]HR = heart rate
[b]bpm = beats per minute
[c]BP = blood pressure
[d]NYHA = New York Heart Association Functional Classification
[e]GFR = glomerular filtration rate
[f]MDRD = Modification of Diet in Renal Disease formula for estimated GFR

not given if the systolic BP (SBP) was < 100 mmHg or HR < 50 beats per minute (bpm). Serum creatinine, blood glucose, ECG, a clinical assessment of hydration and the Richmond Agitation Sedation Scale [29] were scheduled for daily assessments for safety reasons. Orthostatic BP tests were planned at day 5, 6 or 7 at 11.00 (approximately 3 h after drug intake), but occasionally done on day 4 if study drug was planned halted following protocol. All adverse events were recorded.

Measurements and procedures

Venous puncture for collection of plasma was scheduled 3 h after each drug intake on day 1, just before drug intake (between 8 am and 9 am on day 2 and day 5, 6 or 7) and 3 h after intake (C_{max}) at day (4), 5, 6 or 7. Heparin tubes (4 ml) with blood were collected by venous puncture and centrifuged (2000G) for 10 min and two aliquots of at least 250 µl were stored in polypropylene tubes at − 80 °C pending analyses. Clonidine in plasma was determined by the method of Muller et al. [30] with modifications as described by Sulheim et al. [31]. The Data Monitoring Committee (represented by Leiv Otto Watne) was un-blinded to the randomisation, and identified the samples from the 10 patients that had received clonidine for plasma analyses.

Statistical methods

Statistical analyses were performed in SPSS Statistics version 21 (IBM, Armonk NY) and Prism v7 (Graph Pad Software Inc., La Jolla, CA, USA).

Due to non-normally distributed data, non-parametric tests were used to compare continuous variables between the groups (Mann-Whitney tests) and to compare paired samples (Wilcoxon signed rank tests). To compare change from baseline to given time points between the groups, delta values were calculated and compared with Mann-Whitney U tests. A p-value of < 0.05 was considered statistically significant.

Results

Between April 2014 and February 2017, of 407 inpatients considered to probably have delirium, 20 patients fulfilled the selection criteria and were included in LUCID and randomised to either clonidine ($n = 10$) or placebo ($n = 10$). Median age was 86 years (range 66–95), and 13 (65%) were women. Polypharmacy and use of other antihypertensive drugs were common (see Table 3), but none of the patients were using any known strong CYP2D6 inhibitors (i.e. fluoxetine/paroxetine [32], bupropion [33], quinidine [34], cinacalcet [35] or ritonavir [36]). See Table 3 for baseline characteristics.

Table 2 Dosage plan for clonidine

Time	Safety	Dosage
Day 1 Loading doses	Systolic BP[a] must be > 120 mmHg at inclusion (i.e. before the first loading dose). For any of the subsequent loading doses: If systolic BP is < 100 mmHg, HR[b] < 50 beats/min, or if RASS[c] is − 3 or less no more study medication will be given until the planned maintenance dose the next morning. If RASS is − 2, the treating physician has to assess if study medication will be given or not	75 µg every 3rd hour until maximum 4 doses, (e.g.: at 2, 5, 8 and 11 pm)
Day 2–7 Maintenance doses	If systolic BP is < 100 mmHg, HR < 50 beats/min, or if RASS is − 3 or less just before a planned dose, no study medication will be given until the next planned dose 12 h later. If RASS is − 2, the treating physician has to assess if study medication will be given or not	75 µg BID[d], at 8–9 am and 8–9 pm

[a]BP = blood pressure
[b]HR = heart rate
[c]RASS = Richmond Agitation Sedation Scale
[d]BID = bis in die (i.e. twice a day)

Table 3 Baseline characteristics of study participants, $n = 20$

Variable	Clonidine, $n = 10$	Placebo, $n = 10$
Age, years, median (range)	85 (73–94)	88 (66–95)
Female, n/N (%)	6/10 (60)	7/10 (70)
Body mass index, kg/m^2, median (range)	23 (19–29)	24 (17–28)
Creatinine at baseline, median (range)	78 (34–128)	88 (32–140)
Number of patients using other antihypertensive drugs[a], n/N (%)	8/10 (80)	7/10 (70)

[a]Antihypertensive drugs used in the clonidine group (patients using the drug, n); metoprolol (5), furosemide (2), nifedipine (2), amlodipine (1), atenolol (1), bisoprolol (1), candesartan/hydrochlorthiazide (1), nitroglycerin (1) and tamsulosin (1)

Plasma concentrations

The plasma concentrations in relation to time of drug administration are shown in Table 4. Three hours after the first dose of 75 µg clonidine, plasma concentration rose to median 0.35 µg/L (range 0.24–0.46). Median trough concentration before drug administration at day 2 was 0.70 (0.47–0.96) µg/L. After 4–6 days of clonidine treatment, median trough concentration (C_0) was 0.47 (0.36–0.76) µg/L, rising to a level of 0.74 (0.56–0.95) µg/L (C_{max}) 3 h after administration of the regular dose of 75 µg clonidine.

Hemodynamic changes during treatment

Hemodynamic variables before and during clonidine treatment are presented in Table 5 and Fig. 1a and b for the clonidine and placebo groups, respectively. There was extensive individual BP variation in both treatment groups. The change in SBP from baseline to day 2 (delta values) was median – 16 (range – 61–40) in the clonidine group and median 7 (range – 40–47) in the placebo groups, but this difference was not statistically significant (median difference 21 mmHg (95%CI -12–44), $p = 0.17$).

Time points with a significant change from baseline were only found during the loading dosage regimen at day 1 within the clonidine group. A reduction in SBP from median 141 (range 124–190) mmHg at baseline to 135 (81–170) mmHg at day 2 in the intervention group was also noted, while no reduction was observed in the placebo group (Table 5). No adverse events were reported related to changes in BP and HR.

A test for orthostatic hypotension was performed in 11/20 patients. In the clonidine group, 1 of 6 patients had a fall in SBP > 20 mmHg, versus 1 of 5 patients in the placebo group. During the whole treatment period, a SBP < 100 mmHg was measured 3 times in the clonidine group (after the 4th loading dose and in the morning day 2 in patient no. 10, and in the morning day 2 in patient no. 5). SBP was also measured < 100 mmHg once

Table 4 Clonidine concentrations (µg/L) measured at day 1, day 2 and at steady state

Patient	Day 1				Day 2	Steady state Day 4,5 or 6 [a]	
	Dose 1 C_{max}	Dose 2 C_{max}	Dose 3 C_{max}	Dose 4 C_{max}	C_0	C_0	C_{max}
1	0.32	0.74	0.76		0.65	0.76	0.95
2	0.24	0.43			0.67	[b]	[b]
3				[c]	0.63		0.56
4	0.34	0.59	0.74	0.91	0.71	0.36	
5	0.39				0.77		0.61
6	0.27	0.41		[c]	0.47	0.41	
7	0.46	0.45	0.63		0.74	0.47	0.71
8		0.71		[c]	0.69		0.92
9	0.40	0.41	0.52		0.82	0.67	[b]
10	0.35	0.85	1.00		0.96		0.77
Median, µg/L	0.35	0.52	0.74	0.91	0.70	0.47	0.74
Range, µg/L	0.24–0.46	0.41–0.85	0.52–1.00		0.47–0.96	0.36–0.76	0.56–0.95
Missing, n	2	2	5	9	0	5	4

All samples were taken 3 h after administration of clonidine, except for C_0 at day 2 and at steady state, taken just before administration of clonidine
[a]The samples at steady state were taken at day 4 (patients 5 and 10), day 5 (patients 3, 8 and 9), and day 6 (patients 1, 4, 6 and 7)
[b]The treatment was halted early (according to the protocol) and complete steady state measurements were not available
[c]4th dose not given (according to the protocol as patients were asleep)

Table 5 Hemodynamic variables before and during clonidine treatment

		Baseline	Day 1, 3 h after dose 1	Day 1, 3 h after dose 2	Day 1, 3 h after dose 3	Day 1, 3 h after dose 4	Day 2, before morning dose	Last measurement during treatment	Delta 1[a]	Delta 2[b]
Clonidine										
SBP[c], mmHg	Median	141	138	**130**	133	**128**[d]	135	137	−16	−10
	Range	124–190	121–182	106–184	125–160	98 – 153[d]	81–170	102 – 238[e]	− 61 - 40	−46 - 98
DBP[f], mmHg	Median	74	78	**67**	72	65[d]	78	75	−5	−9
	Range	62–105	64–93	59–84	62–87	58–77[d]	49–97	56–109	− 24 - 28	− 23 - 40
HR[g], bpm[h]	Median	89	85	79	**66**	67[d]	84	76	−6	−12
	Range	71–106	64–92	63–101	62–92	60–89[4d]	72–90	62–146	−41 - 18	− 32 - 61
Placebo										
SBP, mmHg	Median	130	132	134	118	170[i]	140	136	7	8
	Range	122–181	94–163	110–152	113–149	–	119–170	110–149	− 40 - 47	− 56 - 19
DBP, mmHg	Median	72	76	72	70	85[i]	77	62	5	1
	Range	54–105	58–103	56–105	56–85	–	61–103	58–96	− 27 - 19	−31 - 22
HR, bpm	Median	87	85	84	75	75[i]	84	80	1	1
	Range	53–123	58–105	64–106	58–88	–	65–140	64–130	− 34 - 30	− 36 - 36

Bold characters mark time points with a significant change in value from baseline (for SBP at 3 h after dose 2 and 4 (respectively p = 0.047 and p = 0.043), for DBP 3 h after dose 2 (p = 0.047) and for HR 3 h after dose 3 (p = 0.028)). The within group differences were otherwise not statistically significant

[a] baseline to day 2, before morning dose
[b] from baseline to last measurement during treatment
[c] SBP = systolic blood pressure
[d] Measurements from 5 of 7 patients that received the 4th loading dose
[e] One patient had SBP 238 mmHg at the last measurement during treatment, as a part of a hypertensive pulmonary oedema
[f] DBP = diastolic blood pressure
[g] HR = heart rate
[h] bpm = beats per minute
[i] Measurements only from one patient

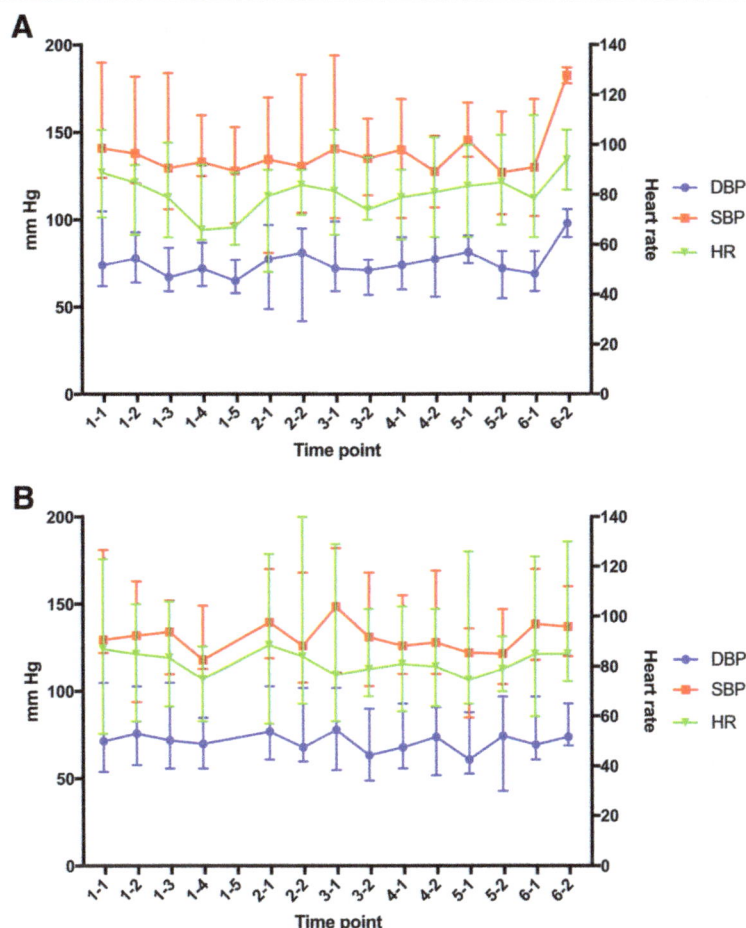

Fig. 1 Panel **a** shows hemodynamic variables in the clonidine group and Panel **b** shows variables in the placebo group. Time points: First digit= day number, second digit = measurement at that day. At day two 2–1 is before morning dose and 2–2 is before evening dose. For panel **b**, time point 1–5 is not included in the figure as there were only measurements available from one patient. Median (range) values are displayed. DBP= Diastolic Blood Pressure SBP= Systolic Blood Pressure HR= Heart rate

in the placebo group. One patient (patient no. 10, morning day 2) had one measurement of HR 49, all other HR measurements were > 50 at all times and no patients had any relevant ECG changes.

Patient no. 10 had a large drop in SBP from baseline to day 2 (from 142 to 81 mmHg). This patient also had the highest plasma concentration level after the third loading dose (1.0 µg/L), and before the drug administration on day 2 (0.96 µg/L), but kidney function and body mass index were within the normal range. However, as per the protocol, the patient did not receive the next dose, and the SBP and HR was within the accepted range during the rest of the treatment (4 days). Considering all 10 intervention patients, there was no correlation between the clonidine concentrations and the level of drop of SBP from baseline to the morning at day 2 (Pearson coefficient 0.271, $p = 0.448$ (Fig. 2)).

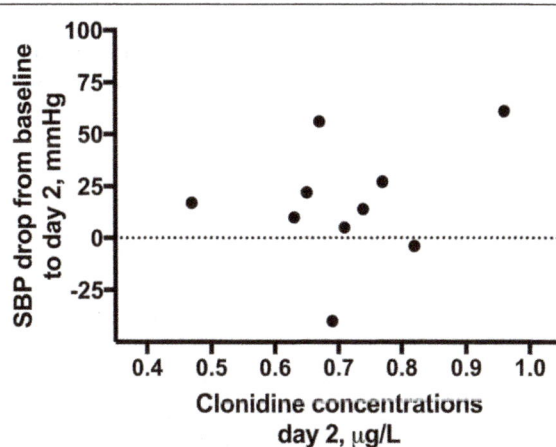

Fig. 2 Scatterplot of clonidine concentrations and drop in SBP from baseline to day 2. There was no significant correlation between the clonidine concentrations and the level of drop of SBP from baseline to the morning at day 2. Pearson coefficient 0.271, $p = 0.448$

Other adverse events

On the 5th day of treatment one patient in the clonidine group developed hypertensive pulmonary oedema (SBP 238 mmHg). According to the study protocol the study drug was halted. The Principal Investigator chose to report this to The Norwegian Medicines Agency as a Serious Unexpected Serious Adverse Reaction as causality may have been possible, although considering the known pharmacological effects of clonidine, hypertension caused by the treatment would not be expected. The patient died 2 weeks later and a follow up report was filed. In the placebo group two patients died during the hospital stay or shortly after discharge.

Regarding minor adverse events, two patients in both the clonidine and the placebo group reported dry mouth. One patient in the clonidine group experienced a fall during the treatment, but it was not considered related to hypotension and there was no orthostatic hypotension measured in this patient. There were no significant alterations in blood-glucose or significant episodes of sedation (RASS -3 or less) in either treatment group.

Missing samples

27 of 70 (39%) scheduled blood samples were missing. For the planned sample after loading dose 4, 9 of 10 samples were missing (including 3 cases in which the patients never received the 4th dose). The other reasons for missing samples were: not all patients were willing to give repeated blood samples; some patients had veins that were difficult to puncture, making repeated punctures too uncomfortable; if the patients were asleep at midnight, we did not wake them up because it could worsen the delirium. Additionally, one patient (patient no. 2) was treated only for 3 days and gave no sample in steady state. No blood samples were lost after collection.

Of the 7 patients that received the 4th loading dose of clonidine, a control BP 3 h after this last dose was missing in 2 patients as they were asleep and waking them up might worsen the delirium.

Discussion

The main findings of this study is that the dosage regimen described in the LUCID protocol, with a loading dose of 75 µg clonidine every 3rd hour up to a maximum of 4 doses on day 1 and further 75 µg twice daily, is generally adequate for target concentration of 0.3–0.7 µg/L. However, as the trough concentrations on day 2 were slightly high, a loading dose seems unnecessary and we propose that a revised dosage regimen of 75 µg twice daily from day 1 is both adequate and easier to administer. There was a trend that clonidine had an effect on BP and HR also in these geriatric medical patients, and these effects might relate to concentration levels.

Our safety protocol with measurements of BP and HR before administering clonidine to this patient group thus proved both necessary and adequate.

The step-wise regimen with repeated doses of 75 µg every 3rd hour, up to a maximum of 300 µg the first day, was effective and resulted in plasma concentration levels at the higher end of the expected therapeutic range. We aimed for plasma concentration levels between 0.3 and 0.7 µg/L, and calculated theoretically that C_{max} at day one should be lower than 1.2 µg/L [22]. No measurements showed higher values than 1.0 µg/L, but many samples are missing after the last dose at day 1, and so we cannot rule out that some patients had concentrations above 1.2 µg/L. Also, the trough concentration at day 2 was at the higher end of our pre-specified target concentration, and would rise further after the next dose (even though this was not measured in this study). The three patients that only received 3 loading doses had among the lower values at day 2 as expected. A few patients had some measurements higher than 0.7 µg/L, and no patients had lower levels than 0.3 µg/L on day 2. Based on our findings of some concentration levels higher than expected and trough concentrations in the higher end at day 2, we suggest a loading dose is unnecessary and a dosage regimen of 75 µg twice daily from day 1 is both adequate and easier to administer.

Examining the response from the very first dose of 75 µg clonidine, the median plasma concentration level (0.35 µg/L) was already within our pre-specified expected range. This finding is in line with previously published studies of plasma concentrations of clonidine in younger adults [23] where it was shown that a single dose of 75 µg clonidine gave concentration max of 0.285 (+/− 0.001) ng/ml. That study seemingly had a lower inter-patient variability than we found, possibly due to a healthier, younger population. We chose a single time-point for C_{max} concentration measures (3 h post dose). As the time (T_{max}) from intake to C_{max} varies inter-individually, our variability might simply be a reflection of this. Several repeated samples (e.g. from in-dwelling cannulas) could have given more accurate measures of T_{max} and thus C_{max} for every patient. However, in our population of frail, elderly patients even more blood samples, or the use of in-dwelling cannulas, would raise both practical and ethical issues. Also, we assume that by collecting samples at a time corresponding with a late T_{max} (i.e. 3 h) we will still be relatively close to C_{max} even in patients who may have a shorter T_{max}, given the relatively long half-life of clonidine (between 5 to 25.5 h).

The clonidine concentration levels measured at steady state (day 4–6) were also within the target range. After the initial loading doses, clonidine 75 µg twice daily was sufficient to reach trough concentrations (C_0) at median

0.47 µg/L, rising to a median level of 0.74 µg/L (C_{max}) after intake of another 75 µg clonidine. These results are also in line with previous studies. In a study of adolescents with chronic fatigue syndrome, a dosage of 50 µg twice per day for 14 days resulted in median C_0 at 0.21 µg/L, rising to median 0.41 µg/L (C_{max}) 2 h after administration of one regular dose of 50 µg [26]. In subjects receiving oral clonidine 100 µg twice per day for 6 weeks, plasma concentration ranged between 0.4 and 0.7 µg/L (2 h after intake of 100 µg) [25]. Another study found that a single dose of 75 µg gave a C_{max} of 0.66 µg/L after achieving steady state with two 75 µg doses [37].

Clonidine has well known antihypertensive effects and it also lowers the heart rate [37]. The maximum hypotensive effect and degree of bradycardia are related to dose and peak plasma concentrations [23]. Therefore, the hemodynamic changes with a trend of lower BP and HR during clonidine treatment were as expected as we reached the assumed therapeutic concentrations. The changes in BP and HR in patients treated with clonidine were not significantly larger than in the placebo group. Wide 95% confidence intervals indicate that this is likely due to the low number of participants as the trend was clearly present in the clonidine group and not in the placebo group. Our main goal was, however, not to formally establish differences in BP between the clonidine and the placebo group. In order to ensure sufficient statistical power for this comparison, a much larger study would have been necessary. It has previously been shown that there is a correlation between plasma concentration levels and drop in SBP [25]. In this group as a whole we could not statistically confirm this, but again this might be due to the small sample size.

Also, a great variability in blood pressure and heart rate values would be expected in a geriatric hospital population due to the natural course of the illnesses and other treatment received. Notably, even if the median blood pressure and heart rate values were lower in the patients that received clonidine, the values were not below that what would be generally considered safe and adverse symptoms were not reported related to changes in BP and HR. So, even if the plasma concentration levels of clonidine occasionally were higher than 0.7 µg/ L, this dosage regimen did not have any hemodynamic effects considered unsafe.

Large variability in the half-life of clonidine has previously been reported, and for elderly patients who tend to have an increase in volume of distribution of lipid soluble drugs [38] (like clonidine) such an increase of half-life would be expected to be more frequent. Half-life was however not estimated in this study. Effects of polypharmacy and interactions related to metabolizing enzymes are another source of variability and heterogeneity. To avoid known interactions, a few

drugs were listed as exclusion criteria and to our knowledge; none of the medications used in our patients are strong CYP2D6 inhibitors. However, several other antihypertensive medications were in use affecting the BP variation. Also, in this elderly population a varying degree of reduction of renal and hepatic clearance must be expected. Dose adjustments based on renal function is recommended, and thus an eligibility criterion of eGFR > 30 was chosen as it was not feasible to include individual dose adjustments in our protocol. For hepatic function, the manufacturer suggests no dose adjustments. Accordingly, no dose adjustments or safety measures of liver function were included.

Patient no. 10 illustrates the difficulties in predicting individual effects on BP. The patient had a large reduction in SBP during the first day of treatment, but both the kidney function and the body mass index were within the normal range, and the patient did not otherwise differ from the other patients receiving clonidine. Many of these issues are not unique to clonidine, but illustrate some of the challenges in administering drugs in the geriatric population. This emphasizes the importance of clinical efficacy measurements for safety assessments.

The reasons for missing samples illustrate some of the feasibility issues with intensive follow-up studies in this population. Despite signalising a positive attitude at inclusion, not all patients were willing to give repeated blood samples. In other cases, we had to consider what was best for the patients (i.e. veins that were difficult to puncture, making repeated punctures too uncomfortable; and the risk of worsening delirium if the patient was asleep). Pharmacological studies are rarely performed in elderly patients, and in future studies these challenges must be taken into account in the study design both regarding sample schedules (e.g. timing of samples; which are the most crucial and which can be 'optional') and sample size (anticipating the proportion of samples likely to be missed).

This study is part of a well-designed RCT with a pre-published protocol. The study included a real-life, placebo-treated control group in the assessment of hemodynamic changes. There was a clear pre-defined prediction of plasma concentration levels, based on theoretical calculations. The patients were monitored very closely; safety and optimal clinical care of the patients was the priority. Some limitations of the study need to be acknowledged. Some planned plasma concentration samples are missing. The sample size was small. Additionally, because of the strict exclusion criteria, the external validity of our findings might be limited, at least regarding the pharmacodynamic effects of clonidine.

Conclusion

The main finding of this study is that a dosage regimen, as described in the LUCID protocol, with a loading dose of 75 μg every 3rd hour up to a maximum of 4 doses on day 1 and further 75 μg twice daily, seems safe, with the limitation that this is based on a small sample size. For a target concentration of 0.3–0.7 μg/L, a loading dose is unnecessary and we propose that a dosage regimen of 75 μg twice daily from day 1 is both adequate and easier to administer. There was a clear trend that clonidine has an effect on BP and HR, which might relate to concentration levels, and we believe a safety protocol with measurements of BP and HR before administering clonidine to this patient group is both a necessary and a sufficient precaution. We also found that this geriatric population does have a higher inter-patient variability of plasma concentration levels compared to previous studies done in healthier, younger populations, which illustrates the difficulties of geriatric pharmacological treatment and supports the need for clinical efficacy measurements for these patients.

Abbreviations

BP: Blood pressure; bpm: Beats per minute; C_0: Trough concentration; C_{max}: Maximum plasma concentration; DBP: Diastolic blood pressure; HR: Heart rate; ICU: Intensive care unit; LUCID: The Oslo Study of Clonidine in Elderly Patients with Delirium; MAP: Mean arterial pressure; RCT: Randomised controlled trial; SBP: Systolic blood pressure; T_{max}: Time from intake to C_{max}

Acknowledgments

The authors wish to thank the patients and staff at the Department of Geriatric Medicine and Department of Acute Medicine at Oslo University Hospital, Ullevål. They also thank research assistants Helene Halsteinli Unsvåg and Therese Omland for assisting in data collection and Leiv Otto Watne for work with Data Monitor Committee.

Funding

LUCID was mainly funded by South-Eastern Norway Regional Health Authority and the University of Oslo. The sponsors had no role in the design, collection, analysis and interpretation of the data or in writing the manuscript.

Authors' contributions

TBW initiated the study. The study was designed by TBW, EQ, VBW, ES, KRH and BEN. KRH and BEN were the daily responsible of running the study and collecting the data, ØU also made substantial contributions in acquisition of data. AMA had particular responsibility for planning and performing the analyses of clonidine in plasma samples. EQ and VBW had particular responsibility for analysis and interpreting of pharmacological data and have contributed to the design of the pharmacological part of intervention. AM participated in all aspects of the project planning. ES carried out the randomisation procedure and has participated in planning of the statistical analyses. All authors made substantive intellectual contributions to the manuscript and all authors read and approved the final manuscript. KRH and BEN contributed equally and are both primary authors to this manuscript.

Competing interests

The authors declare that they have no competing interests.

Author details

[1]Oslo Delirium Research Group, Department of Geriatric Medicine, Oslo University Hospital, Oslo, Norway. [2]Institute of Clinical Medicine, University of Oslo, Oslo, Norway. [3]Department of Pharmacology, Oslo University Hospital, Oslo, Norway. [4]Department of Acute Medicine, Oslo University Hospital, Oslo, Norway. [5]Department of Paediatrics, Akershus University Hospital, Lørenskog, Norway. [6]Edinburgh Delirium Research Group, Geriatric Medicine, University of Edinburgh, Edinburgh, UK. [7]Department of Public Health and Nursing, Norwegian University of Science and Technology, Trondheim, Norway. [8]Department of Cardiology, Oslo University Hospital, Oslo, Norway.

References

1. Briggs R, Robinson S, O'Neill D. Ageism and clinical research. Ir Med J. 2012; 105(9):311–2.
2. Ryan DJ, O'Regan NA, Caoimh RO, Clare J, O'Connor M, Leonard M, McFarland J, Tighe S, O'Sullivan K, Trzepacz PT, et al. Delirium in an adult acute hospital population: predictors, prevalence and detection. BMJ Open. 2013;3(1). https://doi.org/10.1136/bmjopen-2012-001772.
3. Witlox J, Eurelings LS, de Jonghe JF, Kalisvaart KJ, Eikelenboom P, van Gool WA. Delirium in elderly patients and the risk of postdischarge mortality, institutionalization, and dementia: a meta-analysis. JAMA. 2010;304(4):443–51.
4. Carnes M, Howell T, Rosenberg M, Francis J, Hildebrand C, Knuppel J. Physicians vary in approaches to the clinical management of delirium. J Am Geriatr Soc. 2003;51(2):234–9.
5. Morandi A, Davis D, Taylor JK, Bellelli G, Olofsson B, Kreisel S, Teodorczuk A, Kamholz B, Hasemann W, Young J, et al. Consensus and variations in opinions on delirium care: a survey of European delirium specialists. Int Psychogeriatrics. 2013;25(12):2067–75.
6. Neufeld KJ, Yue J, Robinson TN, Inouye SK, Needham DM. Antipsychotic medication for prevention and treatment of delirium in hospitalized adults: a systematic review and meta-analysis. J Am Geriatr Soc. 2016;64(4):705–14.
7. Inouye SK, Westendorp RG, Saczynski JS. Delirium in elderly people. Lancet. 2014;383(9920):911–22.
8. Maclullich AM, Ferguson KJ, Miller T, de Rooij SE, Cunningham C. Unravelling the pathophysiology of delirium: a focus on the role of aberrant stress responses. J Psychosom Res. 2008;65(3):229–38.
9. Smith H, Elliott J. Alpha(2) receptors and agonists in pain management. Curr Opin Anaesthesiol. 2001;14(5):513–8.
10. Pandharipande PP, Pun BT, Herr DL, Maze M, Girard TD, Miller RR, Shintani AK, Thompson JL, Jackson JC, Deppen SA, et al. Effect of sedation with dexmedetomidine vs lorazepam on acute brain dysfunction in mechanically ventilated patients: the MENDS randomized controlled trial. JAMA. 2007; 298(22):2644–53.
11. Riker RR, Shehabi Y, Bokesch PM, Ceraso D, Wisemandle W, Koura F, Whitten P, Margolis BD, Byrne DW, Ely EW, et al. Dexmedetomidine vs midazolam for sedation of critically ill patients: a randomized trial. JAMA. 2009;301(5):489–99.
12. Maldonado JR, Wysong A, van der Starre PJ, Block T, Miller C, Reitz BA. Dexmedetomidine and the reduction of postoperative delirium after cardiac surgery. Psychosomatics. 2009;50(3):206–17.
13. Shehabi Y, Grant P, Wolfenden H, Hammond N, Bass F, Campbell M, Chen J. Prevalence of delirium with dexmedetomidine compared with morphine based therapy after cardiac surgery: a randomized controlled trial (DEXmedetomidine COmpared to morphine-DEXCOM study). Anesthesiology. 2009;111(5):1075–84.
14. Mo Y, Zimmermann AE. Role of dexmedetomidine for the prevention and treatment of delirium in intensive care unit patients. Ann Pharmacother. 2013;47(6):869–76.
15. Zhang H, Lu Y, Liu M, Zou Z, Wang L, Xu FY, Shi XY. Strategies for prevention of postoperative delirium: a systematic review and meta-analysis of randomized trials. Crit Care. 2013;17(2):R47.
16. Reade MC, O'Sullivan K, Bates S, Goldsmith D, Ainslie WR, Bellomo R. Dexmedetomidine vs. haloperidol in delirious, agitated, intubated patients:

a randomised open-label trial. Crit Care. 2009;13(3):R75.

17. Su X, Meng ZT, Wu XH, Cui F, Li HL, Wang DX, Zhu X, Zhu SN, Maze M, Ma D. Dexmedetomidine for prevention of delirium in elderly patients after non-cardiac surgery: a randomised, double-blind, placebo-controlled trial. Lancet. 2016;388(10054):1893–902.

18. Bajwa S, Kulshrestha A. Dexmedetomidine: an adjuvant making large inroads into clinical practice. Ann Med Health Sci Res. 2013;3(4):475–83.

19. Pichot C, Ghignone M, Quintin L. Dexmedetomidine and clonidine: from second- to first-line sedative agents in the critical care setting? J Intensive Care Med. 2012;27(4):219–37.

20. Khan ZP, Ferguson CN, Jones RM. Alpha-2 and imidazoline receptor agonists. Their pharmacology and therapeutic role. Anaesthesia. 1999; 54(2):146–65.

21. Rubino AS, Onorati F, Caroleo S, Galato E, Nucera S, Amantea B, Santini F, Renzulli A. Impact of clonidine administration on delirium and related respiratory weaning after surgical correction of acute type-a aortic dissection: results of a pilot study. Interact Cardiovasc Thorac Surg. 2010; 10(1):58–62.

22. Neerland BE, Hov KR, Bruun Wyller V, Qvigstad E, Skovlund E, MacLullich AM, Bruun Wyller T. The protocol of the Oslo study of clonidine in elderly patients with delirium; LUCID: a randomised placebo-controlled trial. BMC Geriatr. 2015;15:7.

23. Anavekar SN, Jarrott B, Toscano M, Louis WJ. Pharmacokinetic and pharmacodynamic studies of oral clonidine in normotensive subjects. Eur J Clin Pharmacol. 1982;23(1):1–5.

24. Keranen A, Nykanen S, Taskinen J. Pharmacokinetics and side-effects of clonidine. Eur J Clin Pharmacol. 1978;13(2):97–101.

25. Hogan MJ, Wallin JD, Chu LC. Plasma clonidine concentration and pharmacologic effect. Clin Pharmacol Ther. 1981;30(6):729–34.

26. Fagermoen E, Sulheim D, Winger A, Andersen AM, Vethe NT, Saul JP, Thaulow E, Wyller VB. Clonidine in the treatment of adolescent chronic fatigue syndrome: a pilot study for the NorCAPITAL trial. BMC Res Notes. 2012;5:418.

27. Almenrader N, Larsson P, Passariello M, Haiberger R, Pietropaoli P, Lonnqvist PA, Eksborg S. Absorption pharmacokinetics of clonidine nasal drops in children. Paediatr Anaesth. 2009;19(3):257–61.

28. Claessens AJ, Risler LJ, Eyal S, Shen DD, Easterling TR, Hebert MF. CYP2D6 mediates 4-hydroxylation of clonidine in vitro: implication for pregnancy-induced changes in clonidine clearance. Drug Metab Dispos. 2010;38(9):1393–6.

29. Sessler CN, Gosnell MS, Grap MJ, Brophy GM, O'Neal PV, Keane KA, Tesoro EP, Elswick RK. The Richmond agitation-sedation scale: validity and reliability in adult intensive care unit patients. Am J Respir Crit Care Med. 2002; 166(10):1338–44.

30. Muller C, Ramic M, Harlfinger S, Hunseler C, Theisohn M, Roth B. Sensitive and convenient method for the quantification of clonidine in serum of pediatric patients using liquid chromatography/tandem mass spectrometry. J Chromatogr A. 2007;1139(2):221–7.

31. Sulheim D, Fagermoen E, Winger A, Andersen AM, Godang K, Muller F, Rowe PC, Saul JP, Skovlund E, Oie MG, et al. Disease mechanisms and clonidine treatment in adolescent chronic fatigue syndrome: a combined cross-sectional and randomized clinical trial. JAMA Pediatr. 2014;168(4):351–60.

32. Alfaro CL, Lam YW, Simpson J, Ereshefsky L. CYP2D6 inhibition by fluoxetine, paroxetine, sertraline, and venlafaxine in a crossover study: intraindividual variability and plasma concentration correlations. J Clin Pharmacol. 2000; 40(1):58–66.

33. Sager JE, Tripathy S, Price LS, Nath A, Chang J, Stephenson-Famy A, Isoherranen N. In vitro to in vivo extrapolation of the complex drug-drug interaction of bupropion and its metabolites with CYP2D6; simultaneous reversible inhibition and CYP2D6 downregulation. Biochem Pharmacol. 2017;123:85–96.

34. Bramer SL, Suri A. Inhibition of CYP2D6 by quinidine and its effects on the metabolism of cilostazol. Clin Pharmacokinet. 1999;37(Suppl 2):41–51.

35. Padhi D, Harris R. Clinical pharmacokinetic and pharmacodynamic profile of cinacalcet hydrochloride. Clin Pharmacokinet. 2009;48(5):303–11.

36. Foisy MM, Yakiwchuk EM, Hughes CA. Induction effects of ritonavir: implications for drug interactions. Ann Pharmacother. 2008;42(7):1048–59.

37. Anavekar SN, Howes LG, Jarrott B, Syrjanen M, Conway EL, Louis WJ. Pharmacokinetics and antihypertensive effects of low dose clonidine during chronic therapy. J Clin Pharmacol. 1989;29(4):321–6.

38. Mangoni AA, Jackson SH. Age-related changes in pharmacokinetics and pharmacodynamics: basic principles and practical applications. Br J Clin Pharmacol. 2004;57(1):6–14.

6

Involvement of methylation of MicroRNA- 122, −125b and -106b in regulation of Cyclin G1, CAT-1 and STAT3 target genes in isoniazid-induced liver injury

Yuhong Li[1], Qi Ren[1], Lingyan Zhu[1], Yingshu Li[1], Jinfeng Li[1], Yiyang Zhang[1], Guoying Zheng[1], Tiesheng Han[1], Shufeng Sun[2] and Fumin Feng[1]*

Abstract

Background: This investigation aimed to evaluate the role of methylation in the regulation of microRNA (miR)-122, miR-125b and miR-106b gene expression and the expression of their target genes during isoniazid (INH)-induced liver injury.

Methods: Rats were given INH 50 mg kg^{-1}·d^{-1} once per day for 3, 7, 10, 14, 21 and 28 days and were sacrificed. Samples of blood and liver were obtained.

Results: We analysed the methylation and expression levels of miR-122, miR-125b and miR-106b and their potential gene targets in livers. Liver tissue pathologies, histological scores and alanine aminotransferase (ALT) and aspartate aminotransferase (AST) activities changed, indicating the occurrence of liver injury. Relative expression levels of miR-122, miR-125b and miR-106b genes in the liver decreased after INH administration and correlated with the scores of liver pathology and serum AST and ALT activities, suggesting that miR-122, miR-125b and miR-106b are associated with INH-induced liver injury. The amount of methylated miR-122, miR-125b and miR-106b in the liver increased after INH administration and correlated with their expression levels, suggesting the role of methylation in regulating miRNA gene expression. Two miR-122 gene targets, cell cycle protein G1 (Cyclin G1) and cationic amino acid transporter-1 (CAT-1), also increased at the mRNA and protein levels, which suggests that lower levels of miR-122 contribute to the upregulation of Cyclin G1 and CAT-1 and might play a role in INH-induced liver injury. Signal transducer and activator of transcription 3 (STAT3) was a common target gene of miR-125b and miR-106b, and its expression levels of mRNA and protein increased after INH administration. The protein expression of phosphorylated (p)-STAT3 and the mRNA expression of RAR-related orphan receptor gamma (RORγt) regulated by p-STAT3 also increased. Meanwhile, the mRNA and protein expression of interleukin (IL)-17 regulated by RORγt, and the mRNA and protein expression of CXCL1 and MIP-2 regulated by IL-17 increased after INH administration. These results demonstrate that lower levels of hepatic miR-125b and miR-106b contribute to the upregulation of STAT3 in stimulating the secretion of inflammatory factors during INH-induced liver injury.

Conclusions: Our results suggested that DNA methylation probably regulates the expression of miRNA genes (miR-122, miR-125b, and miR-106b), affecting the expression of their gene targets (Cyclin G1, CAT-1, and STAT3) and participating in the process of INH-induced liver injury.

* Correspondence: fm_feng@sina.com
[1]Hebei Province Key Laboratory of Occupational Health and Safety for Coal Industry, School of Public Health, North China University of Science and Technology, No.21 Bohai Road, Tangshan 063210, People's Republic of China
Full list of author information is available at the end of the article

Background

Isoniazid (INH) is the preferred drug in the treatment of tuberculosis, but the major side-effect in clinical practice is drug-induced liver injury (DILI) [1]. A previous study has shown that the morbidity of hepatotoxicity is 7% from INH and 23% from the administration of anti-tuberculosis drugs rifampicin and pyrazinamide [2]. INH-induced liver injury is related to toxic metabolites [3], immune response [4] and genetic polymorphisms of drug-metabolising enzymes [5]. However, the mechanism of the INH-induced liver injury is not yet fully understood.

MicroRNAs (miRNAs/miRs) are endogenous small non-coding RNAs (19–24 nucleotides) involved in several biological processes, such as lipid metabolism, apoptosis and cancer. Many liver diseases, including fatty liver [6], viral hepatitis [7] and obstructive cholestasis [8], are related to the abnormal changes of miRNAs. The mechanism of miRNA action has been unravelled recently. Most miRNAs can bind with the 3′ untranslated region (UTR) of their mRNA targets for complete or incomplete complementary pairing, resulting in the degradation or translational repression of mRNAs [9]. However, some studies have also shown that miRNAs could bind with other parts of the 3′UTR of their mRNA targets to increase mRNA stability [10, 11]. MiRNAs and their target genes constitute a complex regulatory network, which brings the regulation of mRNA expression and miRNA function to a new level.

More recently, it has been suggested that miRNAs are involved in the incidence and progression of DILI. MiR-122 is a highly abundant and liver-specific miRNA that accounts for 72% of the total liver miRNA population [12]. There was evidence of high miR-122 expression levels in plasma after acetaminophen (APAP) treatment, but their expression levels decreased in the liver [13]. One study also demonstrated that inflammatory miR-125b is dysregulated in APAP-induced liver injury, and this miRNA could potentially represent a biomarker of DILI. Another inflammatory miR-106b has been shown to be associated with halothane-induced liver injury [14]. Although this evidence indicates that these three miRNAs are involved in the occurrence and development of DILI, their detailed effects on INH-induced liver injury remain unknown.

Epigenetic modification, especially DNA methylation, may also influence miRNA genes in regulating miRNA expression. DNA methylation occurs at the C-5 position of the cytosine in CpG dinucleotide sequences, which are mainly concentrated in regions known as CpG islands. Methylation in CpG islands within gene promoters strongly correlates with gene expression [15]. For instance, lower expression levels of miR-200b, miR-152 and miR-10a were associated with increased DNA methylation in

bladder cancer [16], and miR-10a was silenced by aberrant DNA methylation in gastric cancer [17]. Because different diseases have unique characteristics, the methylation statuses of different diseases have commonness and personality characteristics. Unfortunately, research on CpG island methylation status of miRNA genes in INH-induced liver injury remains lacking.

Therefore, we first analysed the expression levels of hepatic miR-122, miR-125b and miR-106b after INH administration and explored their correlation with INH-induced liver injury. Following this, we measured the methylation levels of these miRNAs after INH administration and tested whether the methylation levels correlated with their expression levels. Finally, we detected the expression levels of their target genes cell cycle protein G1 (Cyclin G1), cationic amino acid transporter-1 (CAT-1) and signal transducer and activator of transcription 3 (STAT3)) and explored the possible regulation mechanisms of miR-122, miR-125b and miR-106b during INH-induced liver injury.

Methods

Animals

Male Sprague-Dawley rats, aged 8–9 weeks old, were purchased from Hua-Fu-Kang Animal Company (Beijing, China). All rats were maintained at 22–23 °C under 65%–69% relative humidity and a 12 h/12 h light/dark cycle with free access to food and water. All rats were acclimatised for one week before the experiment. The experimental protocol was approved by the Institutional Animal Care Committee of North China University of Science and Technology (Permit Number: 14–016).

Experimental design

After acclimatisation for one week, a total of 56 rats were divided into a control group ($n = 8$) and experimental groups ($n = 48$). The experimental groups were subdivided to 3-, 7-, 10-, 14-, 21- and 28-day groups, which were given INH orally at 50 mg·kg^{-1}·d^{-1} for each time point. Rats were fasted overnight and sacrificed the following morning by light ether anaesthesia. Plasma and liver tissue samples were collected at the time of animal sacrifice. Blood was drawn by cardiac puncture and collected into silicon disposable glass tubes with ethylenediaminetetraacetic acid (EDTA) as an anticoagulant. Tubes were centrifuged at 4000 g for 15 min at 4 °C. Plasma samples were stored at − 80 °C for later determination of alanine aminotransferase (ALT) and aspartate aminotransferase (AST) activities. Liver tissues were excised immediately and washed with an ice-cold physiologic saline solution (0.9%, w/v) and blotted dry with filter paper. Liver tissues were split equally into two portions. A portion of liver tissue was fixed in phosphate-buffered formalin and used for histological analysis, while another portion of the liver tissue was stored under refrigeration for subsequent RNA/DNA extraction and polymerase chain reaction (PCR) analysis.

Histological examination and liver injury scoring
Rat liver specimens, fixed in 10% formaldehyde, went through conventional dehydration, wax-dipping, embedding and slicing. The slices were stained with haematoxylin and eosin (HE) for histopathological examination and scoring. Pathological changes were observed in an optical microscope under 20× magnification [18].

Biochemical assays
Plasma ALT and AST levels were assessed using an automatic biochemical analyzer (Hitachi, Japan).

Quantitative real-time PCR (qRT-PCR)
Expression levels of the selected miRNAs (U6, miR-122, miR-125b and miR-106b) and selected mRNAs (β-actin, Cyclin G1, CAT-1, mitogen-activated protein kinase 14 MAPK14, STAT3, RAR-related orphan receptor gamma (RORγt), IL-17, IL-6, TNF-α, CXCL1 and MIP-2) were quantified using real-time RT-PCR analysis. Table 1 lists the primers used in this study. According to the manufacturer's instructions, rat liver RNA was isolated using TRI reagent (Invitrogen, Carlsbad, CA, USA) and was reverse-transcribed into cDNA. Reverse transcription and real-time RT-PCR were performed as previously described [19]. Relative differences in expression between groups were indicated in terms of cycle time (*Ct*) values, which were generated under the ABI StepOne™ Real-Time PCR System (Applied Biosystems, Carlsbad, CA). Calculations were measured using the $2^{-\Delta\Delta Ct}$ method.

Quantitative methylation-specific-PCR (qMSP)
Genomic DNA was extracted from the liver tissue of rats using a DNA Extraction Kit (Aidlab, BJ, China). Extracted DNA was treated with sodium bisulphite using the EZ DNA Methylation-Gold kit (ZYMO Research Corporation, Irvine, CA, USA) according to the manufacturer's protocols. The CpG island methylation of miR-122, miR-125b and miR-106b was analysed using SYBR Green-based quantitative methylation-specific PCR (qMSP). The UCSC Genome Browser (http://genome.ucsc.edu/) was used to obtain a 2000 bp promoter sequence in the upstream of miR-122, miR-125b and miR-106b genes. Then, we copied the 5′ sequence and fed it into MethPrimer (http://www.urogene.org/methprimer) to predict CpG islands. PCR primers were also designed using the online bioinformatics tool MethPrimer (www.urogene.org/methprimer), which are shown in Table 2. The PCR mixture (20 μL) contained a bisulphite-treated DNA template (2 μL), 2× Power SYBR Green PCR Master Mix (10 μL, Invitrogen, USA) and the forward (1 μL) and reverse (1 μL) primers. PCR conditions

Table 1 Sequences of primers used for real-time RT-PCR analyses

Primer Name	Primer sequence
U6	RT: 5′-AACGCTTCACGAATTTGCGTG-3′
	F: 5′-GCTCGCTTCGGCAGCACA-3′
	R: 5′-GAGGTATTCGCACCAGAGGA-3′
miR-122	RT: 5′-GTCGTATCCAGTGCAGGGTCCGAG
	GTATTCGCACTGGATACGACCAAACA-3′
	F: 5′-GGAAAATCGCCATAGCCAGG-3′
	R: 5′-AGATCAGGGTGGCCCCATTT-3′
miR-125b	RT: 5′-GTCGTATCCAGTGCAGGGTCCG
	AGGTATTCGCACTGGAACGACTTCACAA-3′
	F: 5′-CATGGCACTTCCAAGGTTGC-3′
	R: 5′-GCAGACTGACAGACCACACA-3′
miR-106b	RT: 5′-GTCGTATCCAGTGCAGGGTCCGA
	GGTATTCGCACTGGATACGACATCTGC-3′
	F: 5′-CGCCCAGGAAAACATCAAGC-3′
	R: 5′-GGAACTGGCTTTGTTCTGCG-3′
β-actin	F: 5′-GTGGACTAGCAAGCAGGAGT-3′
	R: 5′-CGCAGCTCAGTAACAGTCCG-3′
Cyclin G1	F: 5′-CTGCACGACAACTGAAGCAC-3′
	R: 5′-CTGCGGTACACAGTGAATGC-3′
CAT-1	F: 5′-GCTCCGCAATCCTACACCAT-3′
	R: 5′-GTGGTCAGGACATCGGGTTT-3′
MAPK14	F: 5′-TGCCGTCTCCTTAGGGATGT-3′
	R: 5′-CGCGCCCTTCTCTCCTTTTA-3′
STAT3	F: 5′-TCTGTGTGACACCAACGACC-3′
	R: 5′-AGGCGGACAGAACATAGGTG-3′
RORγt	F: 5′-ACTGACGGCCAGCTTACTCT-3′
	R: 5′-CTGGCACGTCTCTCGGTAG-3′
IL-6	F: 5′-ACAGCGATGATGCACTGTCA-3′
	R: 5′-AGCACACTAGGTTTGCCGAG-3′
TNFα	F: 5′-CTCAAGCCCTGGTATGAGCC-3′
	R: 5′-GGCTGGGTAGAGAACGGATG-3′
IL-17	F: 5′-TCAACCGTTCCACTTCACCC-3′
	R: 5′-CTCCACCCGGAAAGTGAAGG-3′
CXCL1	F: 5′-ACTCAAGAATGGTCGCGAGG-3′
	R: 5′-TTCACCAGACAGACGCCATC-3′
MIP-2	F: 5′-ACCATCAGGGTACAGGGGTT-3′
	R: 5′-CACCGTCAAGCTCTGGATGT-3′

RT Reverse-transcription primer, *R* Reverse primer, *F* Forward primer, *Cyclin G1* Cell cycle protein G1, *CAT-1* Cationic amino acid transporter-1, *MAPK14* Mitogen activated protein kinase 14, *STAT3* Signal Transducer and Activator of Transcription 3, *RORγt* Retinoid-related orphan receptoryt, *IL-17* Interleukin-17, *IL-6* Interleukin-6, *TNFα* Tumor necrosis factor alpha, *CXCL1* Cytokineinduced neutrophil chemoattractant 1, *MIP-2* Crophage Inflammatory Protein 2

Table 2 Primers sequences used in direct qMSP

MiRNA gene	Methylated primers	Unmethylated primers	Temperature (°C) M	U	Amplicon size (bp) M	U
miRNA-122	F:5'-TTGTTTTGAAAATTATTTTTTTGTTC-3'	F:5'-TTTTGAAAATTATTTTTTTGTTTGA-3'	57.2	57.3	122	120
	R:5'-CATCTACTCACCTAATCCACGAT-3'	R:5'-CCATCTACTCACCTAATCCACAAT-3'	56.5	58.5		
miRNA-125b	F:5'-CGGTTAAAGTATAAATTATAGAGTTACGG-3'	F:5'-TGGTTAAAGTATAAATTATAGAGTTATGG-3'	57.8	57.3	181	179
	R:5'-ACTAACTACAAAACTTCCAAAAACG-3'	R:5'-TAACTACAAAACTTCCAAAAACACC-3'	54.7	56.9		
miRNA-106b	F:5'-TCGGAAATTTATTTGGAAGTTTATC-3'	F:5'-TGGAAATTTATTTGGAAGTTTATTG-3'	59.2	53.9	105	105
	R:5'-GACAATCTACTTCAACTCCTCGAC-3'	R:5'-CAACAATCTACTTCAACTCCTCAAC-3'	57.2	57.7		

included initial incubation at 95 °C for 10 min, 45 cycles of 95 °C for 15 s and 45 cycles of annealing at the temperatures specified in Table 2 for 60 s. PCR products were analysed in 2% agarose gel, stained with ethidium bromide and visualised under ultraviolet (UV) illumination. The CpG methylation percentage in a sample was estimated as previously described [20].

$$\text{Methylation rate}(\%) = \frac{M}{M+U} \times 100\%$$
$$= \frac{1}{1+\dfrac{U}{M}} \times 100\%$$
$$= \frac{1}{1+2^{-\Delta Ct}} \times 100\%$$

where M is the copy number of methylated miR-122, miR-125b and miR-106b; U is the copy number of unmethylated miR-122, miR-125b and miR-106b, and $\Delta Ct = Ct_U - Ct_M$.

Enzyme-linked immunosorbent assays (ELISA)

Protein contents of Cyclin G1, CAT-1, (MAPK14, p38a), STAT3, IL-17, IL-6, tumor necrosis factor (TNF)-α, chemokine ligand 1(CXCL1), and MIP-2 (MIP-2) in the livers were measured with ELISA Kits (Beijing, Winter Song Boye Biotechnology Co., Ltd., BJ, Beijing, China) according to the manufacturer's protocols. Intra- and interassay CVs were both less than 15%.

Statistical analysis

Statistical analysis was performed using SPSS 17.0 software (SPSS, Inc., Chicago, IL, USA). Data were expressed as mean ± SD. Normality and homogeneity-of-variance tests were sequentially conducted on the data. Comparison of variance among groups was performed using one-way analysis of variance (ANOVA). The Student-Newman-Keuls method was used to analyse the differences among the groups. Pearson correlation analyses were used to determine the degree of correlation between different parameters. Differences were considered statistically significant at $p < 0.05$.

Results

INH administration caused extensive hepatic damage

Liver histopathology, histological scoring, and ALT and AST activities in serum were evaluated to show the effect of INH on liver injury. Histopathological analysis of liver sections obtained from control rats showed normal architecture of the liver. The structure of liver lobules was intact in the normal control group (Fig. 1a). INH treatment in rats changed the function and structure of liver. The difference in the pathological changes between INH-treated 3-day and 7-day groups was not significant, although a small amount of inflammatory cell infiltration was present (Fig. 1b, c). After 10-day treatment with INH, the hepatocytes were swollen, and necrosis was occasionally visible (Fig. 1d). Ballooning degeneration of liver cells and diffusion were observable at 14 d (Fig. 1e). The liver cells had a more visibly dissolved putrescent state at 21 d (Fig. 1f). The structure of the hepatic cord was heavily destroyed, and many large hepatic cells had necrotised at 28 d (Fig. 1g, h).

In comparison with the control group, all liver pathology scores dramatically increased at 7, 10, 14, 21 and 28 days after INH administration (Fig. 2 and see Additional file 1, $p < 0.05$ versus control). This result indicates worsening liver damage.

ALT and AST are the most sensitive liver enzymes and were widely used as indicators of liver injury. As shown in Fig. 3, the activities of serum AST and ALT after INH administration were significantly higher in the experimental group (Fig. 3 and see Additional file 2, $p < 0.05$ versus control) than in the control group. Both ALT and AST significantly increased after administering INH for 10 days, which proved the occurrence of liver injury.

Involvement of IL-6 and TNF-α in the pathogenesis of INH-induced liver injury

To explore the involvement of inflammation-related factors in INH-induced liver injury, the hepatic mRNA and protein expression levels of the cytokines, including IL-6 and TNF-α were measured. INH-administered rats showed increased mRNA and protein levels of IL-6 and TNF-α compared to the control rats (Figs. 4a, b and see Additional file 3, $p < 0.05$

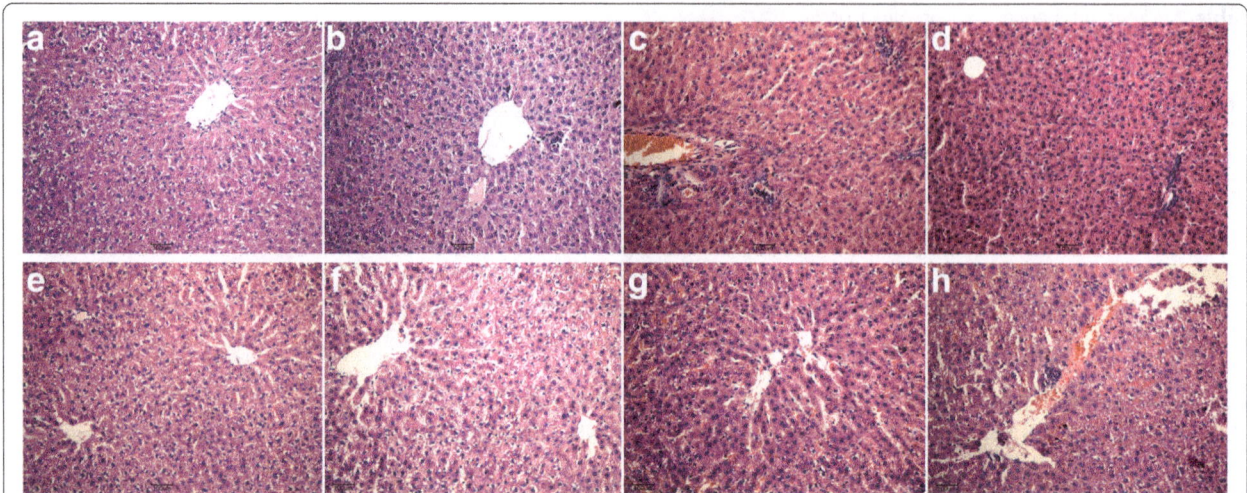

Fig. 1 Effect of INH on liver histopathological changes in rats. Rats were administered with 55 mg·kg^{-1} d^{-1} INH. At 3, 7, 10, 14, 21 and 28 d after administration, the livers were collected to observe for histopathological changes in HE staining of livers (original magnification, × 20). Representative microphotographs taken from the control (**a**) group or INH-treated for 3 (**b**), 7 (**c**), 10 (**d**), 14 (**e**), 21 (**f**), 28 (**g**) and 28 (**h**) days groups, respectively

versus control). These results suggested that inflammation response participated in INH-induced liver injury.

Downregulation of miRNA levels were associated with INH-induced liver injury

To evaluate the relationship of miR-122, miR-125b and miR-106b expression levels with INH-induced liver injury, we examined the expression levels of miR-122, miR-125b and miR-106b using RT-PCR. Compared with the control group, all hepatic miR-122, miR-125b and miR-106b levels dramatically decreased after 3-, 7-, and 7-day INH administration, respectively (Fig. 5 and see Additional file 4, $p < 0.05$ versus control). Moreover,

expression levels of miR-122, miR-125b and miR-106b reached a nadir after 14-, 21-, and 21-day administration. These results occurred earlier than the changes of the serum ALT and AST, and histological examination.

The analysis of Pearson correlation coefficients demonstrated that the expression levels of miR-122, miR-125b and miR-106b were negatively correlated with liver scores ($r = -0.591$, -0.654 and -0.701, $p < 0.001$, see Additional file 5: Figure S3) and serum ALT and AST activities (ALT, $r = -0.672$, -0.771 and -0.695, $p < 0.001$, see Additional file 5: Figure S1; AST, $r = -0.462$, -0.584 and -0.606, $p < 0.001$, see Additional file 5: Figure S2). These results suggested that miR-122, miR-125b and miR-106b participated during the early phases of INH-induced liver injury.

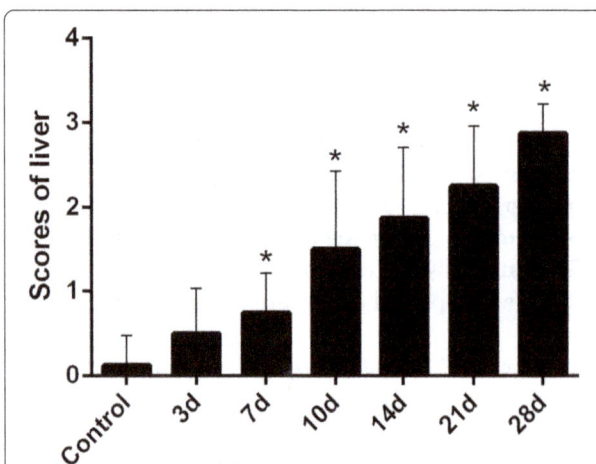

Fig. 2 Quantification of histological scoring. Liver pathology scores after 7-, 10-, 14-, 21- and 28-day INH administration were significantly higher compared with that in the normal control group (*$p < 0.05$ versus control group)

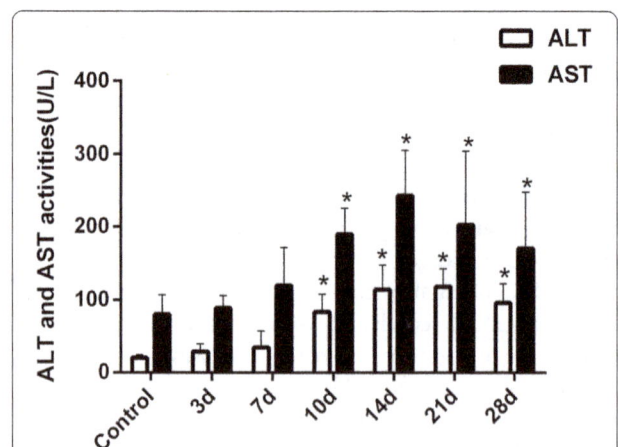

Fig. 3 Serum ALT and AST levels of different groups. ALT and AST were significantly higher after 10-day INH administration than the control group (*$p < 0.05$ versus control group)

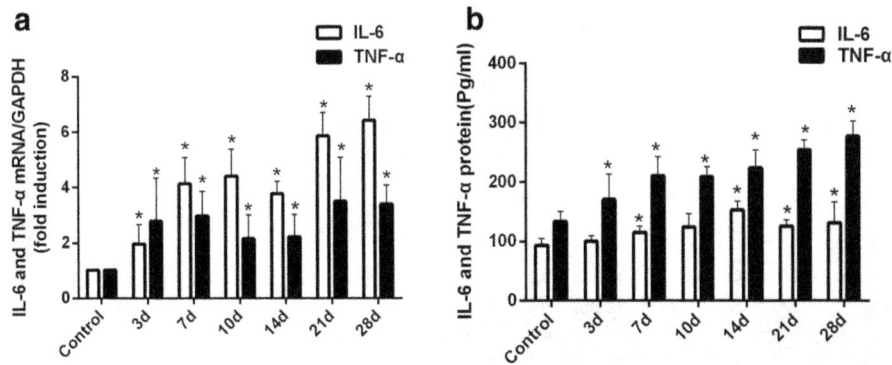

Fig. 4 MRNA and protein expression levels of IL-6 and TNF-α in the liver tissue of the different groups. (**a**) IL-6 and TNF-α mRNA expression levels significantly increased in the livers of INH-administered rats compared with the controls. (**b**) IL-6 and TNF-α protein expression levels were significantly higher in the livers of INH-administered rats compared with the controls (*$p < 0.05$ versus control group)

Downregulation of MiRNAs were due to the Hypermethylation of MiRNAs gene promoter region in INH-induced liver injury

Previous studies have demonstrated that hypermethylation of CpG islands in the promoter region of miRNA genes is one of the most important mechanisms that leads to the downregulation of miRNA expression [21]. The analysis of the promoter region revealed that miR-122, miR-125b and miR-106b had CpG islands within the 2000 bp upstream of the transcriptional start site (Fig. 6a–e), providing the structural basis of DNA methylation. Thus, we hypothesised that hypermethylation is responsible for the downregulation of these three miRNAs. To test this hypothesis, we performed quantitative methylation-specific PCR (qMSP) analysis to detect the methylation levels of the promoter regions of these three miRNAs. Results demonstrated that the methylation levels of miR-122, miR-125b and miR-106b in rat liver tissues treated with INH were significantly

higher than those in the control group (Figs. 6c–i and see Additional file 6, $p < 0.05$ versus control). In addition, hepatic miR-122, miR-125b and miR-106b methylation levels significantly increased at 7 days after INH administration. Products from methylated and unmethylated miR-122 primers were 122 and 120 bp in size, respectively (Fig. 6b). Products of the methylated and unmethylated miR-125b primers were 181 and 179 bp in size, respectively (Fig. 6e). Both products of the methylated and unmethylated miR-106b primers were 105 bp in size (Fig. 6h).

We also analysed the correlation between methylation levels and the gene expression of miR-122, miR-125b and miR-106b. The results showed the negative correlation between methylation and expression levels of miR-122, miR-125b and miR-106b (miRNA-122, $r = -0.587$, $p < 0.001$; miRNA-125b, $r = -0.536$, $p < 0.001$; miRNA-106b, $r = -0.568$, $p < 0.001$, see Additional file 5: Figure S4). Thus, the correlation between the expression levels and methylation of CpG islands of the miR-122, miR-125b and miR-106b genes have been revealed, indicating the possibility of epigenetic regulation of these genes during INH-induced liver injury.

MiRNA-122 regulated Cyclin G1 and CAT-1 in INH-induced liver injury

Our results indicated that the expression level of miR-122 decreased at 3 days after INH administration and declined to a minimum at 14 days, before rising rapidly (Fig. 5). This phenomenon raised the question of what the role miR-122 played during INH-induced liver injury. The biological target genes of miR-122 should be taken into consideration. We search for putative miR-122 target genes that may participate in the regulation of liver injury. Previous studies identified cell cycle protein G1 (Cyclin G1) and the cationic amino acid transporter-1 (CAT-1) were targets of miR-122 [22, 23]. Cyclin G1 and CAT-1 played a crucial role in cell survival and

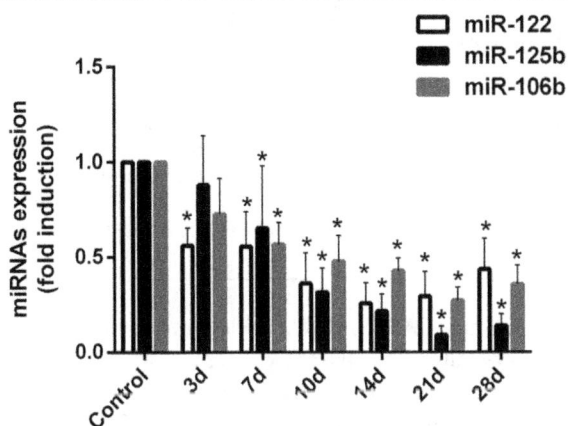

Fig. 5 Expression levels of miR-122, miR-125b and miR-106b in the liver tissue of different groups. Hepatic miR-122, miR-125b and miR-106b expression levels dramatically decreased after INH administration for 3, 7 and 7 days (*$p < 0.05$ versus control group)

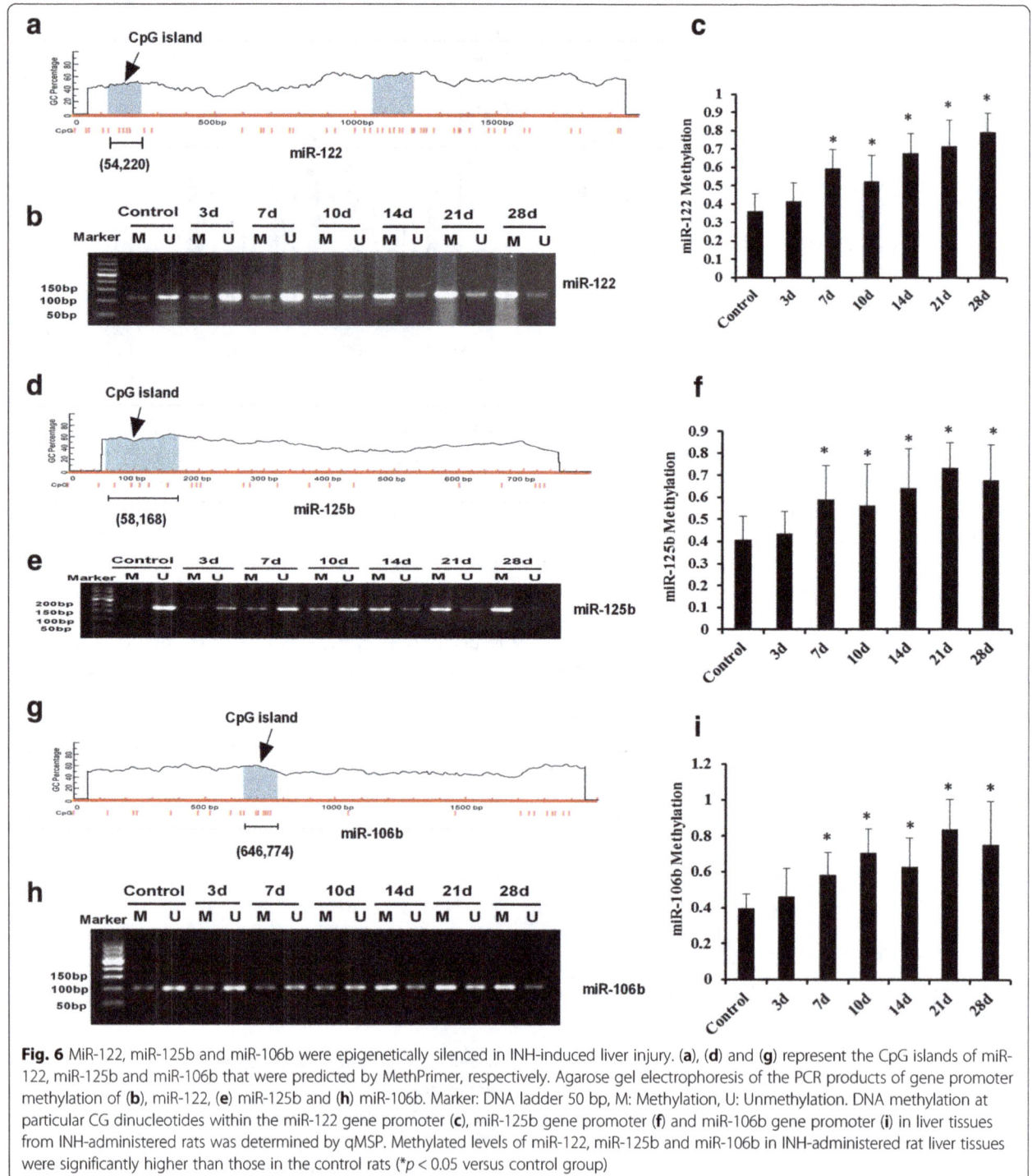

Fig. 6 MiR-122, miR-125b and miR-106b were epigenetically silenced in INH-induced liver injury. (**a**), (**d**) and (**g**) represent the CpG islands of miR-122, miR-125b and miR-106b that were predicted by MethPrimer, respectively. Agarose gel electrophoresis of the PCR products of gene promoter methylation of (**b**), miR-122, (**e**) miR-125b and (**h**) miR-106b. Marker: DNA ladder 50 bp, M: Methylation, U: Unmethylation. DNA methylation at particular CG dinucleotides within the miR-122 gene promoter (**c**), miR-125b gene promoter (**f**) and miR-106b gene promoter (**i**) in liver tissues from INH-administered rats was determined by qMSP. Methylated levels of miR-122, miR-125b and miR-106b in INH-administered rat liver tissues were significantly higher than those in the control rats (*$p < 0.05$ versus control group)

proliferation in the carbon tetrachloride- and thioacetamide-induced liver injury models [24]; however, their role in INH-induced liver injury models has yet to be evaluated under the rationale for testing Cyclin G1 and CAT-1 expression in our INH-induced liver injury model.

Along with lower miR-122 (Fig. 5), we found higher levels of Cyclin G1 and CAT-1 mRNAs in the livers of the experimental group rats compared with the control (Fig. 7a). All

Cyclin G1 and CAT-1 mRNA levels significantly increased at 7 days after the INH treatment (Fig. 7a and see Additional file 7, $p < 0.05$ versus control).

To investigate the role of Cyclin G1 and CAT-1 in INH-induced liver injury, we measured the Cyclin G1 and CAT-1 protein levels. Expectedly, we found a significant increase of Cyclin G1 and CAT-1 proteins in the livers (Fig. 7b and see Additional file 7, $p < 0.05$ versus

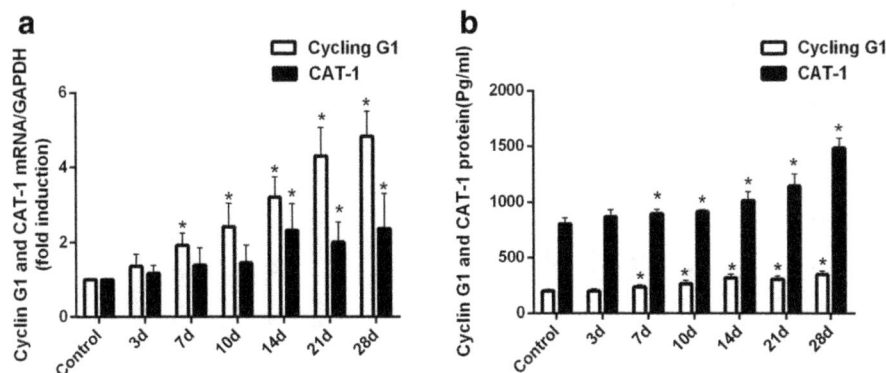

Fig. 7 mRNA and protein expression levels of Cyclin G1 and CAT-1 in the liver tissue of the different groups. (**a**) Cyclin G1 and CAT-1 mRNA expression levels were significantly higher in the livers of INH-administered rats compared with the control group. (**b**) Cyclin G1 and CAT-1 protein expression levels were significantly higher in the livers of INH-administered rats compared with the controls (*$p < 0.05$ versus control group)

control). The higher protein levels might suggest that miRNA-122 could upregulate translation.

Generally, the low expression level of miR-122 and high expression of Cyclin G1 and CAT-1 at both mRNA and protein levels during INH-induced liver injury suggested that miR-122 could upregulate translation.

MiR-125b and MiR-106b regulated STAT3 in INH-induced liver injury

Previous studies have confirmed that miR-125b and miR-106b were two important indicators that reflect inflammatory response. Our results also confirmed that both miR-125b and miR-106b expression levels dramatically decreased during INH-induced liver injury. The time of significant changes and the changing trends of miR-125b and miR-106b were all consistent. We also found a higher degree of inflammatory cell infiltration in liver histopathology (Fig. 1b) and significantly increased mRNA and protein levels of IL-6 and TNF-α in the livers (Fig. 4a, b) after 3 days of INH administration. Altogether, this discovery raised the question of whether miR-125b and miR-106b were related to the inflammatory immune response in INH-induced liver injury.

First, we searched for putative miR-125b and miR-106b targets that might regulate inflammatory immune response. These gene targets are identified as MAPK14 and STAT3. Previous studies confirmed that MAPK14 and STAT3 were common gene targets of miR-125b and miR-106b [25–27]. Considering the fact that one miRNA can regulate multiple target genes, and several miRNAs can regulate the single gene to exert its effect, the modulation of MAPK14 and STAT3 during INH-induced liver injury may be conceivable. In this study, we found significant elevation of STAT3 in both mRNA and protein levels after administering INH for 10 days (Fig. 8a, b and see Additional file 8, $p < 0.05$ versus control). MAPK14 mRNA levels were higher (Fig. 8a), but the protein levels

were lower (Fig. 8b), indicating the absence of correlation between these expression levels. These results suggested the possible activation of STAT3 during INH-induced liver injury.

To explore the activation of STAT3, we detected the protein content of its activated form, p-STAT3. We found that the protein content of p-STAT3 was significantly higher in the livers of the experimental group rats after 10-day INH administration than those of the control group (Fig. 9a and see Additional file 8, $p < 0.05$ versus control). The time of significant change in p-STAT3 was consistent with STAT3. These results showed that STAT3 was activated during INH-induced liver injury.

Some studies confirmed that STAT3 further regulated its downstream RORγt gene to induce inflammatory cytokine IL-17 [28]. We detected mRNA levels of RORγt, and found that RORγt mRNA levels significantly increased in the livers of experimental group rats compared with those of the control group after 10-day administration of INH in the former (Fig. 9b and see Additional file 9, $p < 0.05$ versus control). In addition, IL-17, a newly discovered pro-inflammatory cytokine, is highly abundant in drug-induced liver injury [29] and produces the chemokines CXCL1 and MIP-2 [30]. The mRNA and protein levels of IL-17, CXCL1 and MIP-2 also significantly increased in INH-administered rats (Figs. 9c–f and see Additional file 9, $p < 0.05$ versus control). The above results suggested that the aberrantly downregulated miR-125b and miR-106b upregulated the STAT3 expression to stimulate the secretion of inflammatory factors during INH-induced liver injury.

Discussion

In the present study, the expression levels of hepatic miR-122, miR-106b and miR-125b were downregulated and correlated with liver pathology scores and serum AST and ALT activities, suggesting that the dynamic

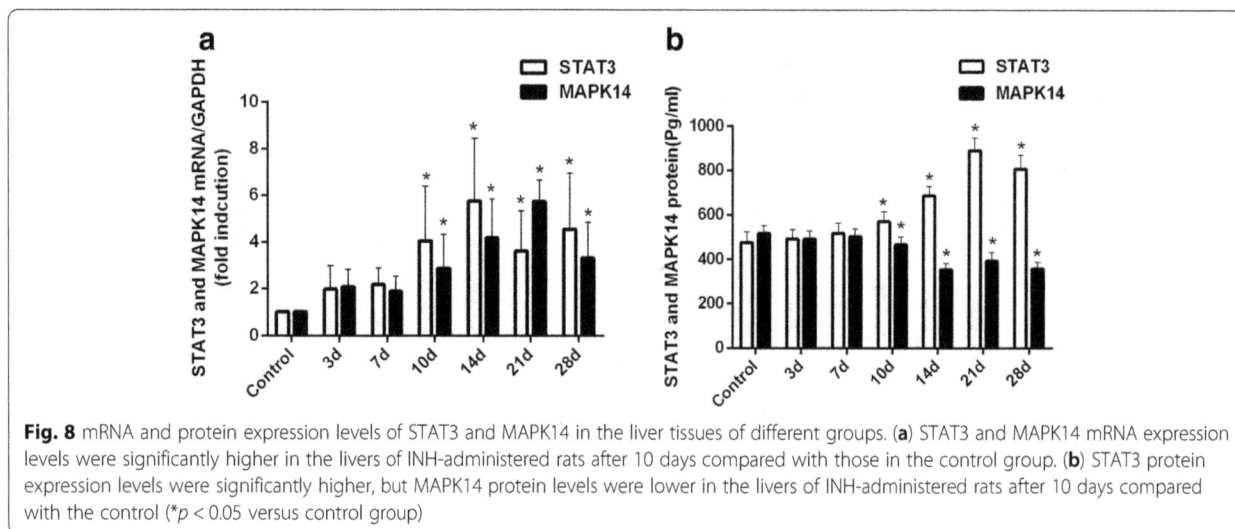

Fig. 8 mRNA and protein expression levels of STAT3 and MAPK14 in the liver tissues of different groups. (**a**) STAT3 and MAPK14 mRNA expression levels were significantly higher in the livers of INH-administered rats after 10 days compared with those in the control group. (**b**) STAT3 protein expression levels were significantly higher, but MAPK14 protein levels were lower in the livers of INH-administered rats after 10 days compared with the control (*$p < 0.05$ versus control group)

change in the expression levels of miR-122, miR-106b and miR-125b were related to INH-induced liver injury. Methylated levels of miR-122, miR-106b and miR-125b were upregulated in INH-induced liver injury and correlated with their expression levels. These results suggested that methylation was responsible for the downregulation of miR-122, miR-106b and miR-125b expression during INH-induced liver injury. INH also decreased the expression of miR-122, which corresponded to the increase of two gene targets: Cyclin G1 and CAT-1. Finally, the aberrant downregulation of miR-125b and miR-106b upregulated the STAT3 expression to stimulate the secretion of inflammatory factors during INH-induced liver injury.

MiRNAs have emerged as an important mechanism in drug-induced liver injury. Mitsugi et al. [31] implicated miR-877-5p-induced PEPCK as a trigger involved in the development of trovafloxacin-induced liver injury. Uematsu et al. [32] reported that regulating the expression of SRY-box 4 (SOX4) and lymphoid enhancer-binding factor 1 (LEF1) by miR-29b-1-5p and miR-449a-5p are important in the development of Th2 bias in methimazole-induced liver injury. These studies suggest the importance of miRNAs in the regulation of drug-induced liver injury. Changes in miRNA profiles, including lower miR-122, miR-106b and miR-125b levels, have been reported in animal model studies on drug-induced liver injury. However, the expression of miRNAs in INH-induced liver injury remains largely unexplored. To our knowledge, this study shows for the first time that hepatic miR-122, miR-125b and miR-106b expression levels gradually decreased during a model of INH-induced liver injury. Moreover, we clearly found that the expression of miR-122, miR-125b and miR-106b were significantly lower at different times. The miR-122 expression was significantly lower after 3 days, while both miR-125b and miR-106b significantly decreased after 7 days. The reason for this change

might be related to the tissue specificity of miRNA expression. miR-122 was one of the most abundant miRNAs in the liver, accounting for up to 72% of all hepatic miRNAs [12], while the expressions of miR-106b and miR-125b not only occur in the liver, but also in many other tissues, including the uterus, ovaries and lungs. A common characteristic of these miRNAs in the expression was that they initially decreased before gradually increasing through time. The occurrence of drug-induced liver injury can explain this phenomenon. Unlike other organs, the liver has an amazing regenerative ability, as evidenced by its recovery after toxic and drug-induced liver injury [33–35]. We further analysed whether the expression levels of miR-122, miR-106b and miR-125b are correlated with the ongoing liver damage according to liver histopathology and serum ALT and AST activities. miR-122, miR-106b and miR-125b expression levels are correlated with liver pathology scores and AST and ALT levels, supporting the correlation of these three miRNAs with INH-induced liver injury.

Previous studies have shown that aberrant hypermethylation of CpG islands in miRNA promoter sequences occurred in some cancer types, such as gastric, oral and hepatocellular cancer, leading to the downregulation of miRNA expression [36–38]. Another study found that the expression of miR-34a during alcoholic liver injury might be regulated by methylation [39]. These publications demonstrated that methylation of CpG-islands affects miRNA gene expression. Thus, we hypothesise that methylation is responsible for the downregulation of miR-122, miR-125b and miR-106b in INH-induced liver injury. To verify this hypothesis, we used qMSP analysis to detect the methylation level of hepatic miR-122, miR-125b and miR-106b. As a result, the methylation of CpG islands in these three miRNA genes was detected. For the first time, we have detected the frequent methylation of miR-122, miR-125b and miR-106b. In our work,

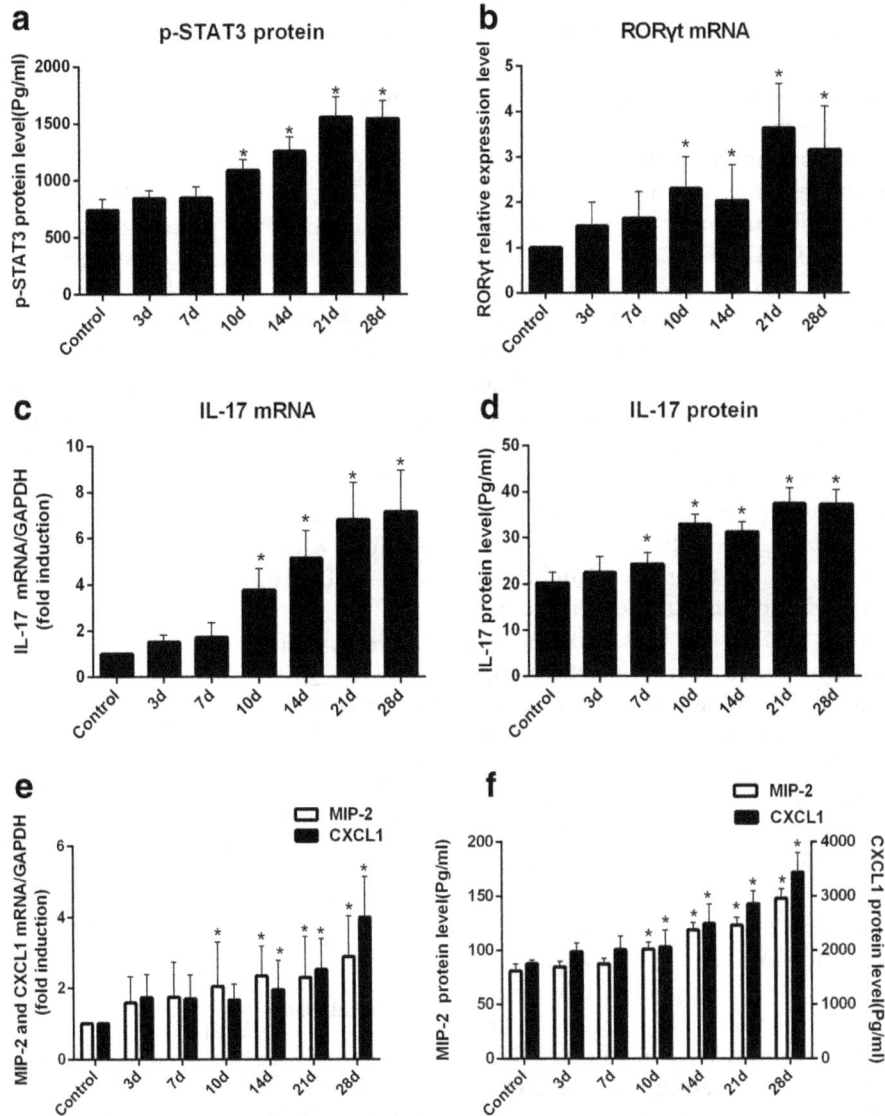

Fig. 9 INH administration causes alterations in RORγt (**b**), IL-17 (**c**), MIP-2, and CXCL1 (**e**) mRNA expression levels and p-STAT3 (**a**), IL-17 (**d**), MIP-2 and CXCL1 (**f**) protein levels in the liver

statistically significant correlation was detected between the expression level of miRNA genes and the methylation status of CpG islands of these genes in the liver tissue, indicating the possibility of the epigenetic regulation of these genes during INH-induced liver injury.

To develop a deeper understanding of the molecular mechanism of miRNA genes involved in INH-induced liver injury, mRNA and protein expression of the miRNA gene targets were determined. CAT-1 and Cyclin G1 genes are miR-122 targets. We have revealed that INH decreased the expression of miR-122, which corresponded with the increase of Cyclin G1 and CAT-1. However, we revealed a situation in which the expression level of miR-122 did not continuously decrease after INH administration. Instead, miR-122 levels initially

declined before rising. We also found that ALT and AST activities were not always higher after INH administration, as both reached a maximum at 21 and 14 days, respectively, before decreasing. These phenomena can be partially explained by liver regeneration. CAT-1 is responsible for cationic amino acid transport, and this intake stimulates DNA synthesis for cell replication [40]. Cyclin G1, a cell-cycle-regulatory protein, participates in G2/M arrest of cells in response to DNA damage, promotes DNA damage repair, and induces apoptosis [41]. Previous studies have also discovered that Cyclin G1 is important for cell proliferation [42]. Therefore, the reduction of miR-122 levels may regulate the target genes, Cyclin G1 and CAT-1, to activate cell proliferation and to repair the damaged liver tissue caused by

INH. However, the specific biological role of Cyclin G1 and CAT-1 in INH-induced liver injury deserves further investigation.

DILI pathogenesis usually involves parent compounds that become hepatotoxic through metabolism, oxidative stress, lipid peroxidation, mitochondrial dysfunction, apoptosis and immune response [43]. A growing body of research suggests that inflammation is an important factor that contributes to DILI. miR-125b and miR-106b are two miRNAs identified to be associated with inflammation. We attempted to elucidate the underlying mechanism of miR-125b and miR-106b involved in INH-induced liver injury. TNF-a and IL-6 are key pro-inflammatory cytokines that initiate the inflammatory response and induce massive hepatocyte apoptosis. Previous studies have demonstrated that the liver can activate Kupffer cells to release inflammatory cytokines (IL-6 and TNF-α) and to aggravate hepatic cell death when stimulated by toxic substances [28, 30]. In the present study, analysis of inflammatory indicators in rats after INH administration showed that TNF-a and IL-6 mRNA and protein levels in the liver tissue of experimental groups were significantly higher than those of the control group. At the same time, a large number of capillaries and inflammatory cell infiltration was also present in liver pathology. Therefore, INH can activate inflammation during liver injury. We also found that STAT3, an important signal transduction pathway, was predicted and experimentally proven as the common gene target of miR-125b and miR-106b [25–27]. STAT3 can be activated in hepatocytes following TNF-α and IL-6 stimulation. STAT3 activation plays an important role in cell survival, differentiation, transformation, apoptosis and inflammation [44]. In this study, we showed that STAT3 in mRNA and protein levels increased, and the protein content of p-STAT3 was significantly higher after INH administration. These results suggested the possible activation of STAT3 during INH-induced liver injury. STAT3 is an important determinant in the differentiation of T-helper 17 (Th17) cells and regulates the transcription of inflammatory genes [45]. Th17 cells mainly secrete pro-inflammatory cytokine IL-17 [46], which stimulate the activation of various pro-inflammatory cytokines and chemokines and participate in drug-induced liver injury [47]. Given this information, we speculate that STAT3 activation induces IL-17 to produce chemokines, such as MIP-2 and CXCL1, and exacerbates INH-induced liver injury. To confirm this hypothesis, we examined the expression of IL-17, MIP-2 and CXCL1 in both mRNA and protein levels after INH treatment and found their enhanced levels under such conditions. Taking these experimental data into consideration, we can conclude that aberrant downregulation of miR-125b and miR-106b can upregulate STAT3 expression to stimulate

the secretion of inflammatory factors involved in INH-induced liver injury.

Conclusion

In this study, lower hepatic levels of miR-122, miR-125b and miR-106b are associated with INH-induced liver injury. CpG island hypermethylation of miR-122, miR-125b and miR-106b genes correlate with their expression levels. Furthermore, the expression level of miR-122 has a causal role in higher levels of Cyclin G1 and CAT-1 mRNA and protein expression. Furthermore, the expression of miR-125b and miR-106b has a causal role in enhanced STAT3 mRNA and protein expression during INH-induced liver injury. Our results suggested that DNA methylation likely regulated the expression of miRNA genes (miR-122, miR-125b and miR-106b), thereby affecting the expression of their target genes (Cyclin G1, CAT-1 and STAT3) and participating in the process of INH-induced liver injury.

Additional files

Additional file 1: Quantification of histological scoring. Supplementary data and statistical analysis for **Figure S3**. (XLSX 16 kb)

Additional file 2: Serum ALT and AST levels of different groups. Supplementary data and statistical analysis for **Figure S4**. (XLSX 19 kb)

Additional file 3: mRNA and protein expression levels of IL-6 and TNF-α in the liver tissue of the different groups. Supplementary data and statistical analysis for **Figure S5**. (XLSX 27 kb)

Additional file 4: Expression levels of miR-122, miR-125b, and miR-106b in the liver tissue of different groups. Supplementary data and statistical analysis for **Figure S6**. (XLSX 24 kb)

Additional file 5: Figures of pearson correlation analysis. (DOC 917 kb)

Additional file 6: DNA methylation at particular CG dinucleotides within the gene promoter of miR-122, miR-125b, and miR-106b in liver tissues from INH-administered rats . Supplementary data and statistical analysis for **Figure S7**. (XLSX 25 kb)

Additional file 7: mRNA and protein expression levels of Cycling G1 and CAT-1 in the liver tissue of the different groups. Supplementary data and statistical analysis for **Figure S8**. (XLSX 27 kb)

Additional file 8: mRNA and protein expression levels of STAT3 and MAPK14 in the liver tissue of different groups. Supplementary data and statistical analysis for **Figure S9**. (XLSX 28 kb)

Additional file 9: INH administration causes alterations in RORγt, IL-17, MIP-2, and CXCL1 mRNA expression levels and p-STAT3, IL-17, MIP-2, and CXCL1 protein levels in the liver. Supplementary data and statistical analysis for **Figure S10**. (XLSX 51 kb)

Abbreviations

ALT: Alanine aminotransferase; ANOVA: Analysis of variance; AST: Aspartate aminotransferase; CAT-1: Cationic amino acid transporter-1; CXCL1: Cytokineinduced neutrophil chemoattractant 1; Cyclin G1: Cell cycle protein G1; DILI: Drug-induced liver injury; ELISA: Enzyme Linked Immunoasorbent Assays; F: Forward primer; HE: Hematoxylin and eosin; IL-17: Interleukin-17; IL-6: Interleukin-6; INH: Isoniazid; MAP K14: Mitogen activated protein kinase 14; MIP-2: Crophage inflammatory protein 2; qMSP: Quantitative Methylation-Specific-PCR; qRT-PCR: Quantitative Real-Time Polymerase Chain Reaction; R: Reverse primer; RORγt: Retinoid-related orphan receptoryt; RT: Reverse-transcription primer; SD: Standard deviation; STAT3: Signal Transducer and Activator of Transcription 3; TNF-α: Tumor necrosis factor alpha

Acknowledgments
Special acknowledgements should be given to the teachers in the Animal Laboratory, School of North China University of Science and Technology.

Funding
This study was supported by National Natural Science Foundation of China (No: 81041096).

Authors' contributions
YH Li, SFS and FMF designed the research. YH Li, LYZ and QR performed the experiments. GYZ, YSL, JFL, YYZ analyzed these data and participated in interpretation of the results. YH Li organized the data and wrote the manuscript. TSH revised the manuscript and gave valuable advice for the modification of this paper. All the authors read and approved the paper.

Competing interests
The authors declare that they have no competing interests.

Author details
[1]Hebei Province Key Laboratory of Occupational Health and Safety for Coal Industry, School of Public Health, North China University of Science and Technology, No.21 Bohai Road, Tangshan 063210, People's Republic of China. [2]College of Nursing and Rehabilitation, North China University of Science and Technology, Tangshan 063210, China.

References
1. Ramappa V, Aithal GP. Hepatotoxicity related to anti-tuberculosis drugs: mechanisms and management. J Clin Exp Hepatol. 2013;3(1):37–49.
2. Schaberg T, Rebhan K, Lode H. Risk factors for side-effects of isoniazid, rifampin and pyrazinamide in patients hospitalized for pulmonary tuberculosis. Eur Respir J. 1996;9(10):2026–30.
3. Meng X, Maggs JL, Usui T, Whitaker P, French NS, Naisbitt DJ, Park BK. Auto-oxidation of isoniazid leads to Isonicotinic-lysine adducts on human serum albumin. Chem Res Toxicol. 2015;28(1):51–8.
4. Metushi IG, Uetrecht J. Isoniazid-induced liver injury and immune response in mice. J Immunotoxicol. 2014;11(4):383–92.
5. Leiro V, Fernandez-Villar A, Valverde D, Constenla L, Vazquez R, Pineiro L, Gonzalez-Quintela A. Influence of glutathione S-transferase M1 and T1 homozygous null mutations on the risk of antituberculosis drug-induced hepatotoxicity in a Caucasian population. Liver Int. 2008;28(6):835–9.
6. Sobolewski C, Calo N, Portius D, Foti M. MicroRNAs in fatty liver disease. Semin Liver Dis. 2015;35(1):12–25.
7. Fan HX, Tang H. Complex interactions between microRNAs and hepatitis B/C viruses. World J Gastroenterol. 2014;20(37):13477–92.
8. Dai BH, Geng L, Wang Y, Sui CJ, Xie F, Shen RX, Shen WF, Yang JM. microRNA-199a-5p protects hepatocytes from bile acid-induced sustained endoplasmic reticulum stress. Cell Death Dis. 2013;4:e604.
9. Bartel DP. MicroRNAs: genomics, biogenesis, mechanism, and function. Cell. 2004;116(2):281–97.
10. Vasudevan S, Tong Y, Steitz JA. Switching from repression to activation: microRNAs can up-regulate translation. Science. 2007;318(5858):1931–4.
11. Masaki T, Arend KC, Li Y, Yamane D, McGivern DR, Kato T, Wakita T, Moorman NJ, Lemon SM. miR-122 stimulates hepatitis C virus RNA synthesis by altering the balance of viral RNAs engaged in replication versus translation. Cell Host Microbe. 2015;17(2):217–28.
12. Shi Q, Yang X, Mendrick DL. Hopes and challenges in using miRNAs as translational biomarkers for drug-induced liver injury. Biomark Med. 2013;7(2):307–15.
13. Wang K, Zhang S, Marzolf B, Troisch P, Brightman A, Hu Z, Hood LE, Galas DJ. Circulating microRNAs, potential biomarkers for drug-induced liver injury. Proc Natl Acad Sci U S A. 2009;106(11):4402–7.
14. Endo S, Yano A, Fukami T, Nakajima M, Yokoi T. Involvement of miRNAs in the early phase of halothane-induced liver injury. Toxicology. 2014;319:75–84.
15. Irizarry RA, Ladd-Acosta C, Wen B, Wu Z, Montano C, Onyango P, Cui H, Gabo K, Rongione M, Webster M, Ji H, Potash JB, Sabunciyan S, Feinberg AP. The human colon cancer methylome shows similar hypo- and hypermethylation at conserved tissue-specific CpG island shores. Nat Genet. 2009;41(2):178–86.
16. Kohler CU, Bryk O, Meier S, Lang K, Rozynek P, Bruning T, Kafferlein HU. Analyses in human urothelial cells identify methylation of miR-152, miR-200b and miR-10a genes as candidate bladder cancer biomarkers. Biochem Biophys Res Commun. 2013;438(1):48–53.
17. Jia H, Zhang Z, Zou D, Wang B, Yan Y, Luo M, Dong L, Yin H, Gong B, Li Z, Wang F, Song W, Liu C, Ma Y, Zhang J, Zhao H, Li J, Yu J. MicroRNA-10a is down-regulated by DNA methylation and functions as a tumor suppressor in gastric cancer cells. PLoS One. 2014;9(1):e88057.
18. Eckhoff DE, Bilbao G, Frenette L, Thompson JA, Contreras JL. 17-Beta-estradiol protects the liver against warm ischemia/reperfusion injury and is associated with increased serum nitric oxide and decreased tumor necrosis factor-alpha. Surgery. 2002;132(2):302–9.
19. Jiang CB, Wei MG, Tu Y, Zhu H, Li CQ, Jing WM, Sun W. Triptolide attenuates podocyte injury by regulating expression of miRNA-344b-3p and miRNA-30b-3p in rats with Adriamycin-induced nephropathy. Evid Based Complement Alternat Med. 2015;2015:107814.
20. Lu L, Katsaros D, de la Longrais IA, Sochirca O, Yu H. Hypermethylation of let-7a-3 in epithelial ovarian cancer is associated with low insulin-like growth factor-II expression and favorable prognosis. Cancer Res. 2007;67(21):10117–22.
21. Lynch SM, O'Neill KM, McKenna MM, Walsh CP, McKenna DJ. Regulation of miR-200c and miR-141 by methylation in prostate Cancer. Prostate. 2016; 76(13):1146–59.
22. Gramantieri L, Ferracin M, Fornari F, Veronese A, Sabbioni S, Liu CG, Calin GA, Giovannini C, Ferrazzi E, Grazi GL, Croce CM, Bolondi L, Negrini M. Cyclin G1 is a target of miR-122a, a microRNA frequently down-regulated in human hepatocellular carcinoma. Cancer Res. 2007;67(13):6092–9.
23. Chang J, Nicolas E, Marks D, Sander C, Lerro A, Buendia MA, Xu C, Mason WS, Moloshok T, Bort R, Zaret KS, Taylor JM. miR-122, a mammalian liver-specific microRNA, is processed from hcr mRNA and may downregulate the high affinity cationic amino acid transporter CAT-1. RNA Biol. 2004;1(2):106–13.
24. Lardizabal MN, Rodriguez RE, Nocito AL, Daniele SM, Palatnik JF, Veggi LM. Alteration of the microRNA-122 regulatory network in rat models of hepatotoxicity. Environ Toxicol Pharmacol. 2014;37(1):354–64.
25. Carraro G, El-Hashash A, Guidolin D, Tiozzo C, Turcatel G, Young BM, De Langhe SP, Bellusci S, Shi W, Parnigotto PP, Warburton D. miR-17 family of microRNAs controls FGF10-mediated embryonic lung epithelial branching morphogenesis through MAPK14 and STAT3 regulation of E-cadherin distribution. Dev Biol. 2009;333(2):238–50.
26. Surdziel E, Cabanski M, Dallmann I, Lyszkiewicz M, Krueger A, Ganser A, Scherr M, Eder M. Enforced expression of miR-125b affects myelopoiesis by targeting multiple signaling pathways. Blood. 2011;117(16):4338–48.
27. Tan G, Niu J, Shi Y, Ouyang H, Wu ZH. NF-kappaB-dependent microRNA-125b up-regulation promotes cell survival by targeting p38alpha upon ultraviolet radiation. J Biol Chem. 2012;287(39):33036–47.
28. Yano A, Higuchi S, Tsuneyama K, Fukami T, Nakajima M, Yokoi T. Involvement of immune-related factors in diclofenac-induced acute liver injury in mice. Toxicology. 2012;293(1–3):107–14.
29. Kobayashi E, Kobayashi M, Tsuneyama K, Fukami T, Nakajima M, Yokoi T. Halothane-induced liver injury is mediated by interleukin-17 in mice. Toxicol Sci. 2009;111(2):302–10.
30. Takai S, Higuchi S, Yano A, Tsuneyama K, Fukami T, Nakajima M, Yokoi T. Involvement of immune- and inflammatory-related factors in flucloxacillin-induced liver injury in mice. Appl Toxicol. 2015;35(2):142–51.
31. Mitsugi R, Itoh T, Fujiwara R. MicroRNA-877-5p is involved in the trovafloxacin-induced liver injury. Toxicol Lett. 2016;263:34–43.
32. Uematsu Y, Akai S, Tochitani T, Oda S, Yamada T, Yokoi T. MicroRNA-mediated Th2 bias in methimazole-induced acute liver injury in mice. Toxicol Appl Pharmacol. 2016;307:1–9.
33. Riehle KJ, Dan YY, Campbell JS, Fausto N. New concepts in liver regeneration. J Gastroenterol Hepatol. 2011;26(Suppl 1):203–12.
34. Lei YC, Li W, Luo P. Liuweiwuling tablets attenuate acetaminophen-induced acute liver injury and promote liver regeneration in mice. World J Gastroenterol. 2015;21(26):8089–95.
35. Tan CY, Lai RC, Wong W, Dan YY, Lim SK, Ho HK. Mesenchymal stem cell-derived exosomes promote hepatic regeneration in drug-induced liver injury models. Stem Cell Res Ther. 2014;5(3):76.

36. Yin H, Song P, Su R, Yang G, Dong L, Luo M, Wang B, Gong B, Liu C, Song W, Wang F, Ma Y, Zhang J, Wang W, Yu J. DNA methylation mediated down-regulating of MicroRNA-33b and its role in gastric cancer. Sci Rep. 2016;6:18824.

37. Hou YY, You JJ, Yang CM, Pan HW, Chen HC, Lee JH, Lin YS, Liou HH, Liu PF, Chi CC, Ger LP, Tsai KW. Aberrant DNA hypomethylation of miR-196b contributes to migration and invasion of oral cancer. Oncol Lett. 2016; 11(6):4013–21.

38. Long XR, He Y, Huang C, Li J. MicroRNA-148a is silenced by hypermethylation and interacts with DNA methyltransferase 1 in hepatocellular carcinogenesis. Int J Oncol. 2014;44(6):1915–22.

39. Meng F, Glaser SS, Francis H, Yang F, Han Y, Stokes A, Staloch D, McCarra J, Liu J, Venter J, Zhao H, Liu X, Francis T, Swendsen S, Liu CG, Tsukamoto H, Alpini G. Epigenetic regulation of miR-34a expression in alcoholic liver injury. Am J Pathol. 2012;181(3):804–17.

40. Hatzoglou M, Fernandez J, Yaman I, Closs E. Regulation of cationic amino acid transport: the story of the CAT-1 transporter. Annu Rev Nutr. 2004;24:377–99.

41. Kimura SH, Ikawa M, Ito A, Okabe M, Nojima H. Cyclin G1 is involved in G2/M arrest in response to DNA damage and in growth control after damage recovery. Oncogene. 2001;20(25):3290–300.

42. Jiang L, Liu R, Wang Y, Li C, Xi Q, Zhong J, Liu J, Yang S, Wang J, Huang M, Tang C, Fang Z. The role of cyclin G1 in cellular proliferation and apoptosis of human epithelial ovarian cancer. J Mol Histol. 2015;46(3):291–302.

43. Tarantino G, Di Minno MN, Capone D. Drug-induced liver injury: is it somehow foreseeable? World J Gastroenterolo. 2009;15(23):2817–33.

44. Bromberg J, Darnell JE Jr. The role of STATs in transcriptional control and their impact on cellular function. Oncogene. 2000;19(21):2468–73.

45. Harris TJ, Grosso JF, Yen HR, Xin H, Kortylewski M, Albesiano E, Hipkiss EL, Getnet D, Goldberg MV, Maris CH, Housseau F, Yu H, Pardoll DM, Drake CG. Cutting edge: an in vivo requirement for STAT3 signaling in TH17 development and TH17-dependent autoimmunity. J Immunol. 2007; 179(7):4313–7.

46. McGeachy MJ, Cua DJ. Th17 cell differentiation: the long and winding road. Immunity. 2008;28(4):445–53.

47. Wang X, Jiang Z, Xing M, Fu J, Su Y, Sun L, Zhang L. Interleukin-17 mediates triptolide-induced liver injury in mice. Food Chem Toxicol. 2014;71:33–41.

7

Effect of β-Eudesmol on NQO1 suppression-enhanced sensitivity of cholangiocarcinoma cells to chemotherapeutic agents

Pimradasiri Srijiwangsa[1], Saranyoo Ponnikorn[1] and Kesara Na-Bangchang[1,2*]

Abstract

Background: Cholangiocarcinoma (CCA), an epithelial malignancy of the biliary tree, is one of the aggressive cancers with poor prognosis and unsatisfactory response to chemotherapy with acquired resistance. NAD(P)H-quinone oxidoreductase 1 (NQO1), an antioxidant/detoxifying enzyme, plays important roles in chemo-resistance and proliferation in several cancer cells. The study aimed to investigate the inhibitory effect of β-eudesmol on NQO1 enhanced chemotherapeutic effects of 5-fluorouracil (5-FU) and doxorubicin (DOX) in the high NQO1-expressing human CCA cell line, NQO1-KKU-100. In addition, the molecular events associated with the inhibition of the cell proliferation, cell migration, and induction of apoptosis were investigated.

Methods: Human CCA KKU-100 cells were exposed to β-eudesmol at various concentrations. NQO1 enzyme activity and protein expression were measured by enzymatic assay and Western blot analysis, respectively. Sulforhodamine B (SRB) assay and wound healing assay were performed to detect the inhibitory effect of β-eudesmol on cell proliferation, cell migration, and sensitivity to 5-FU and DOX. Apoptotic induction was detected by flow cytometry with annexin V/PI and DAPI nuclear staining. Caspase 3/7 activation was determined by fluorescence microscopy. The mechanism of enhanced chemo-sensitivity was evaluated by Western blot analysis.

Results: β-Eudesmol significantly suppressed NQO1 enzyme activity (both in KKU-100 cells and cell lysates) and protein expression in KKU-100 cells in a concentration-dependent manner. β-Eudesmol exhibited potent cytotoxicity on KKU-100 cells with mean ± SD IC_{50} values of 47.62 ± 9.54 and 37.46 ± 12.58 μM at 24 and 48 h, respectively. In addition, it also potentiated the cytotoxic activities and inhibitory activities of 5-FU and DOX on cell migration through induction of cell apoptosis and activation of caspase 3/7. Western blot analysis suggested that β-eudesmol enhanced chemosensitivity was associated with the suppression of NQO1 protein and activation of Bax/Bcl-2 protein expression ratio in CCA cells.

Conclusions: β-Eudesmol may serve as a potential anti-CCA candidate particularly when used in combination with conventional chemotherapeutics. The mechanisms involved may be mediated via NQO1 suppression-related apoptosis pathway.

Keywords: Cholangiocarcinoma, NAD(P)H-quinone oxidoreductase 1, β-Eudesmol, 5-Fluorouracil, Doxorubicin, Apoptosis, Migration

* Correspondence: kesaratmu@yahoo.com
[1]Chulabhorn International College of Medicine, Thammasat University, (Rangsit Campus), Pathum Thani 12121, Thailand
[2]Center of Excellence in Pharmacology and Molecular Biology of Malaria and Cholangiocarcinoma, Chulabhorn International College of Medicine, Thammasat University, Pathum Thani, Thailand

Background

Cholangiocarcinoma (CCA) is an extremely aggressive malignant tumor of the bile duct that becomes one of the major health problems worldwide. It is originating from the epithelial cells of the extrahepatic or intrahepatic bile ducts [1]. The northeastern region of Thailand including countries around Mekong basin are documented as areas with highest CCA incidence in the world [2, 3]. Epidemiological and experimental studies provide evidence that chronic inflammation and cell injury as a consequence of infection with the liver flukes *Opisthorchis viverrini* or *Chlonorchis sinensis* is the main risk factor of CCA [4]. The diagnosis of CCA is challenging because most patients are present with progressive and advanced stages resulting in disease poor prognosis [5]. Currently, management of CCA remains a challenge because the only occasional therapy is surgical resection. Chemoresistance is the major obstacle in the treatment of CCA particularly in unresectable tumors [6]. Multiple mechanisms involved in resistance of CCA to chemotherapeutic agents have been proposed. These include alteration of drug metabolizing enzymes, efflux transporters, cytoprotective enzymes, or derangement of intracellular signaling system [7, 8]. Novel effective therapy to overcome the chemoresistance of CCA is urgently needed.

NAD(P)H-quinone oxidoreductase 1 (NQO1; EC 1.6.5.2) is mainly a cytosolic phase II detoxification enzyme that reduces quinones to hydroquinones and thus bypassing the toxic semiquinone intermediates. The resultant hydroquinones undergo further conjugation and excretion [9]. NQO1 is ubiquitously expressed at low basal levels in all types of normal human tissues except liver through Nrf2 dependent pathway and proteasome degradation [10, 11]. The enzyme is induced along with a battery of defensive enzymes in response to cellular stress to prevent carcinogenesis process in body tissues through its free radical scavenging activity [9, 12, 13]. Conversely, the expression of NQO1 has been found to be increased in cancers of lung [14], pancreas [15], breast [16], thyroid [17], stomach [18], and bile duct (CCA) [19]. It is hypothesized that high level of NQO1 expression promotes carcinogenesis and cancer progression while also making cells more resistant to anticancer drugs particularly oxidative stress inducers. The critical role of NQO1 as a promising target for cancer chemotherapy has been demonstrated in various studies. Inhibition of NQO1 activity by dicoumarol, the pharmacological NQO1 inhibitor, was shown to suppress urogenital cancer cell growth and potentiate cytotoxicity of doxorubicin and cisplatin [20, 21]. In CCA, dicoumarol was shown to potentiate gemcitabine-induced cytotoxicity in the high NQO1-expressing CCA [22]. Furthermore, knocking down of NQO1 gene expression by small

interfering RNA (siRNA) in the high NQO1-expressing CCA cells was shown to enhance the cytotoxic effect of 5-fluorouracil, doxorubicin, and gemcitabine [23]. Searching for specific NQO1 inhibitors would therefore be one of the promising approaches for discovery and development of new chemotherapeutics for CCA. A large number of moderate to potent NQO1 inhibitors from natural and synthetic sources have been reported including flavonoids, coumarins, curcumin, and ES936, of which the most demonstrative inhibitors are dicoumarol and ES936 [24–26]. Dicoumarol acts by completing with NAD(P)H and thereby preventing the reduction of FAD in cells. The compound is commonly used to investigate the inhibitory effect on NQO1 activity and its consequences in several cell types. Based on X-crystallography, the conformational change of the amino acid residues Tyr128 and Phe232 located in the catalytic pocket of NQO1 have been demonstrated upon binding of dicoumarol [27]. Unlike dicoumarol, flavonoids have been identified as strong NQO1 inhibitors through competitive inhibition of NAD(P)H [27]. Preliminary molecular dynamic studies suggested that flavonoids bind to different active site of NQO1 from that of dicoumarol; the 7-hydroxyl moiety of the flavonoids interacts with His161 residue in the active site [28]. The inhibition of NQO1 by flavonoids is pointing at a mechanism contradicting the proven beneficial properties of these phytochemicals. Novel NQO1 inhibitors are being identified by a structure-based or mechanism-based approach using reference NQO1 inhibitors.

β-Eudesmol is a one of the major constituents of the rhizome of *Atractylodes lancea* (Thunb) DC. (AL: Khod-Kha-Mao or Cang Zhu) of the Compositae family. It is the common medical plant used in Thai and Chinese traditional medicine for treatment of fever, colds, flu, sore throat, rheumatic diseases, digestive disorders, night blindness, and influenza [29, 30]. Various pharmacological activities of AL as well as its active compounds β-eudesmol, atracylodin, hinesol and atracylon have been demonstrated [26]. With regard to anticancer activity, inhibitory effect of AL on gastric and colon cancer cells were demonstrated [31, 32]. In addition, the potential role of AL and β-eudesmol in CCA has previously been demonstrated both in vitro and in vivo models [33–35]. Both exhibited promising inhibitory activity in CCA-xenografted nude mice with a marked reduction of tumor size and lung metastasis, as well as prolongation of survival time [34]. β-Eudesmol is a member of the class of compounds known as eudesmane, isoeudesmane or cycloeudesmane sesquiterpenoids [36]. Sesquiterpenoids were shown to inhibit phase II detoxification enzymes including superoxide dismutase (SOD), and UDP-glucuronosyltransferase (UGT). The cytotoxic and apoptotic activities on HL-60 cells of sesquiterpenolides (atractylenolide I, AT-I) from the dried rhizome of

Effect of β-Eudesmol on NQO1 suppression-enhanced sensitivity of cholangiocarcinoma cells...

69

Atractylodes ovata were shown to be through inhibition of Cu-Zn-SOD activity [37]. In addition, the inhibitory effect on UGT activity of the sesquiterpenoid xanthorrhizol, a major component of the essential oil of *Curcuma xanthorrhiza* was demonstrated in an in vivo study [38]. Nevertheless, the cytotoxic activity of sesquiterpenoids through modulation of NQO1 or other detoxifying enzymes has not been fully investigated. We have previously reported that β-eudesmol exerts potent growth inhibitory activity on CCA cells which might be linked to its suppressive effect on heme oxygenase-1 (HO-1) production, STAT1/3 activation, and NF-κB downregulation [39]. Based on this information together with the complex multidirectional biological activity of β-eudesmol, it is also worth investigating its activity on the NQO1 target which is highly expressed in CCA. In the present study, the effect of β-eudesmol on NQO1 suppression-enhanced chemotherapeutic effects of 5-fluorouracil (5-FU) and doxorubicin (DOX) was observed in the human CCA cell line, KKU-100. In addition, the molecular events associated with the inhibition of cell proliferation, cell migration, and induction of apoptosis were investigated.

Methods

Chemical and reagents

The cell culture medium Ham's F12, fetal bovine serum, 0.25% trypsin-EDTA, and penicillin-streptomycin solution were purchased from Gibco BRL Life Technologies (Grand Island, NY, USA). β-Eudesmol and 5-fluorouracil (5-FU) were purchased from Wako Pure Chemical Industries Ltd. (Osaka, Japan). Doxorubicin hydrochloride (DOX) was obtained from Boryung Pharm (Seoul, South Korea). Dimethyl sulfoxide (DMSO) was purchased from Lab-Scan Analytical Science (Dublin, Ireland). β-Eudesmol was dissolved in 100% ethanol. 5-FU and DOX were dissolved in 100% DMSO. Concentrations of both solvents used in all experiments were less than 1% (*v/v*).

All reagents used for NQO1 activity assay and sulforhodamine B (SRB) assay were obtained from Sigma Chemical Co. Ltd. (St. Louis, MO, USA). The primary rabbit polyclonal IgG NQO1 antibody (1:2500) (ab34173) was purchased from Abcam (Cambridge, MA, USA). The rabbit polyclonal IgG Bax (1:2500) (#sc-493), mouse monoclonal IgG Bcl-2 (1:1000) (#sc-7382) and mouse monoclonal IgG β-actin (1:2500) (#sc-1616), and the secondary horseradish peroxidase (HRP)-linked antibodies (goat anti-rabbit IgG; #sc-2004 and goat anti-mouse IgG; #sc-2005 at 1:5000 dilution) were obtained from Santa Cruz Biotechnology, Inc. (California, USA). The Amersham™ ECL™ Prime Western Blotting Detection Reagent was obtained from Amersham Biosciences Crop. (NJ, USA). Annexin V-FITC apoptosis detection kit (Cat no. 420201) and 4'-6-diamidino-2-phenylindole

(DAPI) (Cat no. 422801) were purchased from BioLegend Inc. (San Diego, CA, USA). CellEvent™ Caspase-3/7 green detection reagent (Cat no. C10723) was obtained from Invitrogen (Thermo Fisher Scientific Inc., Massachusetts, USA).

Cell lines and cell culture

The human CCA cell line, KKU-100, with a high expression level of NQO1 was used in the study [23]. The cell was originally derived from intrahepatic CCA tissue of a patient and was kindly provided by Professor Banchob Sripa, Department of Pathology, Faculty of Medicine, Khon Kean University. The cell was routinely cultured in complete medium consisting of Ham's F12 supplemented with 10% fetal calf serum, 12.5 mM HEPES (pH 7.3), 100 U/mL penicillin G, and 100 μg/mL streptomycin and maintained at 37 °C under an atmosphere of 5% CO_2. Culture medium was renewed every 3 days. Cells were trypsinized with 0.25% trypsin-EDTA and subcultured in the same culture medium.

NAD(P)H-quinone oxidoreductase 1 (NQO1) activity assay

The NQO1 activity assay was performed according to the previously described method [40]. In brief, the KKU-100 cells were cultured overnight at 37 °C in a 96-well microtiter plate (7.5×10^3 cells/well). The cells were exposed to various concentrations of β-eudesmol (0, 1, 10, 30, and 100 μM) and dicoumarol (1 μM), a potent pharmacological NQO1 enzyme inhibitor (37 °C, 24 h). Cells were lysed with 50 μL of 0.8% digitonin in 2 nM EDTA with agitation for 10 min. The assay was performed using menadiol and MTT [3-(4, 5-dimethylthiazol-2-yl)-2,5-diphenyltetrazolium bromide] in the substrate coupling reaction and measured as rate-kinetics at the wavelength of 620 nm. To further investigate the direct effect of β-eudesmol on NQO1 activity, β-eudesmol (1–100 μM) was added to KKU-100 cell lysates. Following incubation (37 °C, 15 min), the NQO1 activity of the lysates was determined. Using the extinction coefficient of MTT formazan of 11,300 M^{-1} cm^{-1} at 620 nm and correction for the light path of the microplate, activity of NQO1 is expressed as nmol/min/mg protein. The assay was performed as three independent experiments, triplicate each.

Western blot analysis

Western blot analysis was performed to determine the expression levels of NQO1 and apoptotic proteins following exposure to various concentrations of β-eudesmol with or without 5-FU or DOX. In brief, KKU-100 cells were washed with PBS and lysed with 1× cell lysis buffer (4 °C) containing 1 mmol/L dithiothreitol (DTT), and 0.1 mmol/L phenylmethylsulfonyl fluoride (PMSF) with vigorous shaking. Following centrifugation at 12,000 g for 30 min, the cell supernatant was collected and stored at − 80 °C until use. The sample was mixed with 5× loading dye buffer and heated at 90 °C for 10 min. Proteins were separated by electrophoresis (in 10% SDS-polyacrylamide gel) and transferred to polyvinylidene difluoride (PVDF) membranes (180 mA, 1 h). The PVDF membranes were blocked with 5% (w/v) skimmed milk powder in PBS and 0.1% Tween-20 (25 °C, 1 h) and incubated overnight at 4 °C with primary antibodies diluted with PBS and 0.1% Tween-20. The antibodies used were as follows: rabbit polyclonal IgG NQO1 (1:2500), rabbit polyclonal IgG Bax (1:2500), mouse monoclonal IgG Bcl-2 (1:1000) and mouse monoclonal IgG β-actin (1:2500). The primary antibody was removed and the blots were extensively washed with PBS/Tween-20 and incubated (25 °C, 2 h) with the secondary antibodies (horseradish peroxidase goat anti-mouse IgG and goat anti-rabbit IgG at 1:5000 dilution in PBS buffer). After removal of the secondary antibody and washing with PBS/Tween-20, the blots were incubated with the ECL substrate solution. Densities of the specific bands of NQO1, Bcl-2, Bax, and β-actin were visualized and captured by Imagequant™ LAS4000.

Cell cytotoxicity assay

Cytotoxicity testing was performed using the sulphorhodamine B (SRB) assay. Briefly, KKU-100 cells were seeded onto a 96-well microtiter plate (7.5×10^3 cells/well) and incubated overnight at 37 °C. Cells were exposed to various concentrations of the test compounds (200 μL) for specified periods as follows: (i) β-eudesmol alone (0, 1, 10, 30, and 100 μM) for 24 and 48 h; (ii) 30 μM β-eudesmol in combination with 5-FU (0, 3, 10, 30, and 100 μM) for 24 and 48 h; and (iii) 30 μM β-eudesmol in combination with DOX (0, 0.1, 0.01, 1, and 10 μM) for 24 and 48 h. The cells were fixed with 100 μL of ice-cold 10% trichloroacetic acid (TCA) at 4 °C for at least 1 h. TCA was removed and the cells were washed 5 times with distilled water. After 10 min of air drying, 50 μL of 0.4% sulforhodamine in 1% acetic acid was added and the cell suspension was incubated at 25 °C for 30 min. Cells were rinsed 3–4 times with 1% acetic acid and air dried at 25 °C for 1 h. Finally, the adhered cells were dissolved in 10 mM Tris base (200 μL) and the plate was shaken for 20 min. The absorbance of cell suspension was measured at the wavelength of 540 nm. Cell growth inhibition was expressed in term of percentage of untreated control absorbance. The IC_{50} (concentration that inhibits cell growth by 50%) was estimated from concentration-response curve analysis using Prism 5 program (GraphPad Software, San Diego, CA, USA).

Cell migration by wound healing assay

Cell migration was assessed using wound healing assay according to the previously described method [41].

Briefly, KKU-100 cells (1.5×10^5 cells/well) were seeded onto a 24-well microtiter plate and allowed to grow overnight at 37 °C in Ham's F12 medium supplemented with 10% fetal calf serum. A scratch wound was made using a sterile 200 μL pipette tip and the scratched cells were washed twice with PBS to remove any detached cells. Cells were exposed to various concentrations of the test compounds (200 μL) for 48 h as follows: (i) β-eudesmol (30 μM) in combination with 5-FU (30 μM); and (ii) β-eudesmol (30 μM) in combination with DOX (0.1 μM). The width of the wound outline was monitored under a phase-contrast microscope. The closing of the scratched wound was determined by capturing the denuded area along the scratch using Image-Pro Plus software (Media Cybernetics, LP, USA).

Cell apoptosis analysis and caspase 3/7 activation

The potentiating effect of β-eudesmol (30 μM) on 5-FU (30 μM) or DOX (0.1 μM)-induced apoptosis in KKU-100 cells was investigated using Annexin V-FITC Apoptosis Detection Kit. Following a 24 h incubation, cells were washed twice with cold BioLegend's cell staining buffer and resuspended in Annexin V binding buffer to obtain the cell density of 5×10^5 cells/mL. FITC Annexin V and propidium iodide solution (5 μL each) were added and the cells were incubated at 25 °C for 15 min in the dark. Apoptotic cells were analyzed by flow cytometry (BD FACSCan to II, BD Biosciences, San Joes, CA, USA). Intact nuclei within apoptotic cells were stained and observed by DAPI method according to the manufacturer's procedure. Following exposure to β-eudesmol in combination with 5-FU or DOX for 24 h, KKU-100 cells (1.5×10^5 cells/well of a 24 well microtiter plate) were washed with PBS, fixed with iced methanol for 10 min, and stained with 1 μg/mL DAPI for 15 min (25 °C in the dark). Results are expressed with complementary nuclear morphological observations gathered using fluorescence microscope (ZOE™ fluorescent Cell imager: BIO-RAD, California, USA).

The effects of β-eudesmol in combination with 5-FU or DOX on stimulation of caspase 3 and caspase 7 of the apoptosis pathway in the KKU-100 cells were investigated using CellEvent™ Caspase 3/7 Green detection assay. Caspase 3/7 Green is a novel fluorogenic substrate that activates caspase 3 and caspase 7 which constitute a hallmark of the apoptotic process. The reagent consists of a four amino acid peptide (DEVD) conjugated to a nucleic acid binding dye. This cell-permeant substrate is intrinsically non-fluorescent because the DEVD peptide inhibits the ability of the dye to bind to DNA. After activation of caspase 3 or caspase 7 in apoptotic cells, the DEVD peptide is cleaved, enabling the dye to bind to DNA and produce a bright, fluorogenic response with an absorption/emission maxima of ~502/530 nm. The KKU-100 cells (1.5×10^5 cells) were mixed with the test compounds as described above and seeded onto each well of a 24-well culture plate. Following incubation (37 °C under 5% CO_2 for 24 h), cells were washed with PBS and fixed with iced methanol (10 min). CellEvent™ caspase 3/7 Green Detection Reagent was added to each well at a final concentration of 10 mM and incubated at 25 °C for 30 min in the dark. Cells were observed under a light and a fluorescence microscope (ZOE™ fluorescent Cell imager: BIO-RAD, California, USA).

Statistical analysis

Statistical analysis was performed using the Prism 5 program (GraphPad Software, San Diego, CA, USA). Quantitative data are expressed as mean ± SD of three independent assays, triplicate each. Comparison of difference in data of two dependent quantitative groups was performed using paired t-test at a statistical significance level of $p < 0.05$.

Results

The sensitivity of NQO1 to β-eudesmol

β-Eudesmol at the concentration range 1–100 μM significantly inhibited NQO1 enzyme activity of the KKU-100 cells in a concentration-dependent manner (Fig. 1a). Dicoumarol was the most potent inhibitor of NQO1 activity (77.96% inhibitory effect at 1 μM). For β-eudesmol, significant inhibitory activity on NQO1 activity was observed at 30 and 100 μM (37.68 and 50.06%, respectively). β-Eudesmol also produced an inhibitory effect on the NQO1 activity of the cell lysates in a concentration-dependent manner (Fig. 1b). The inhibitory effect occurred within 15 min of exposure. At the lowest concentration (1 μM), the enzyme activity was inhibited by 71.86% and almost complete inhibitory effect (95.56%) occurred at the highest concentration (100 μM). Furthermore, Western blot analysis was performed to verify whether the suppressive action of β-eudesmol towards NQO1 activity was due to direct inhibition of the enzyme activity or modulation of its expression. These results showed that the NQO1 protein expression was significantly suppressed only when the cells were exposed to the highest concentration (100 μM) of β-eudesmol (Fig. 1c).

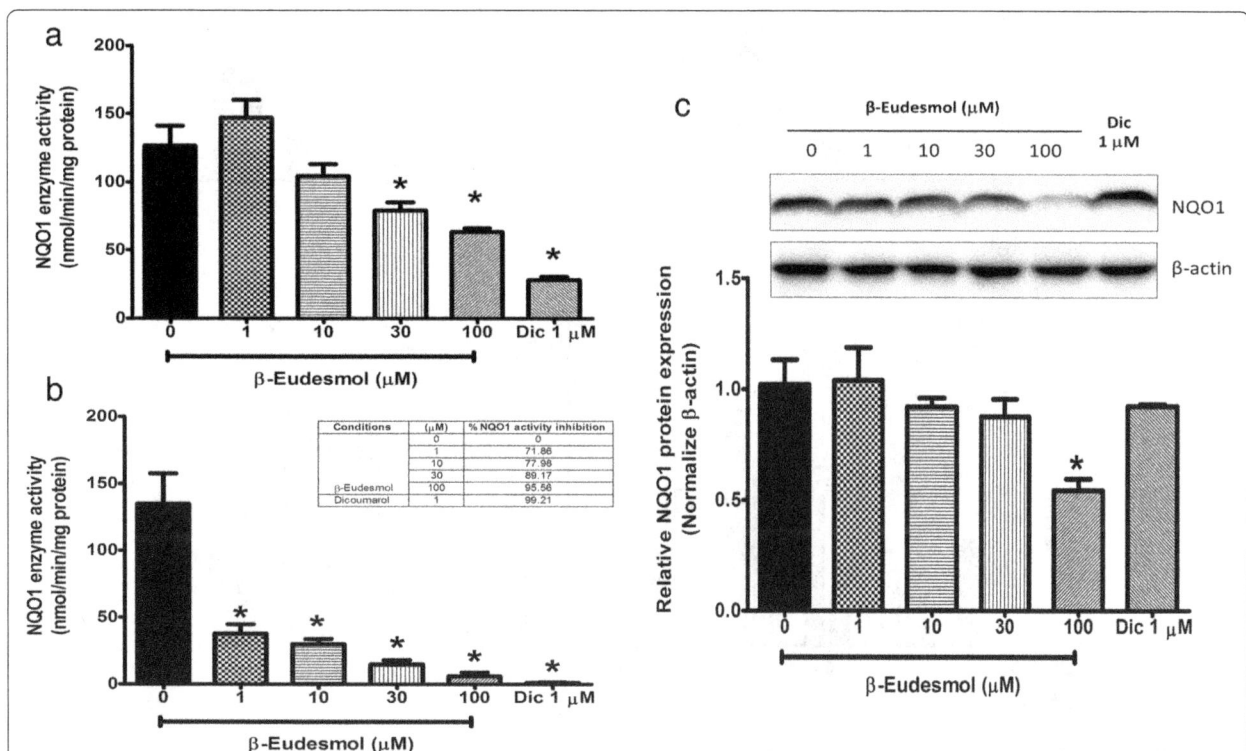

Fig. 1 Concentration responses of NQO1 suppression by β-eudesmolKKU-100 cells were seeded onto a 96-well microtiter plate overnight and cells were exposed to β-eudesmol (1–100 μM) and dicoumarol as a potent positive NQO1 inhibitor (1 μM) for 24 h. **a** The effect of β-eudesmol on NQO1 enzyme activity of KKU-100 cells analyzed by the enzymatic method, **b** The effect of β-eudesmol on NQO1 enzyme activity of cell lysates analyzed by the enzymatic method, and **c** The effect of β-eudesmol on the expression of the NQO1 protein by Western blot analysis using β-actin as an internal control for equal protein loading. The relative bar that was normalized with β-actin of each band is shown below. Each bar represents mean ± SD of three independent experiments, triplicate each. * indicates statistically significant difference with untreated control (paired t-test, $p < 0.05$)

Potentiating effect of β-eudesmol on cytotoxic activities of 5-FU and DOX

To investigate whether the inhibitory activity of β-eudesmol on NQO1 activity and protein expression in the CCA cells resulted in an enhanced sensitivity of the cells to chemotherapeutic agents, the KKU-100 cells were incubated with β-eudesmol in the absence and presence of 5-FU or DOX for 24 or 48 h. β-Eudesmol potently inhibited cell growth with mean (±SD) IC_{50} of 47.62 ± 9.54 and 37.46 ± 12.58 μM following 24 and 48 h exposure (Fig. 2a). The concentration of β-eudesmol below the IC_{50} (30 μM) was therefore used in subsequent

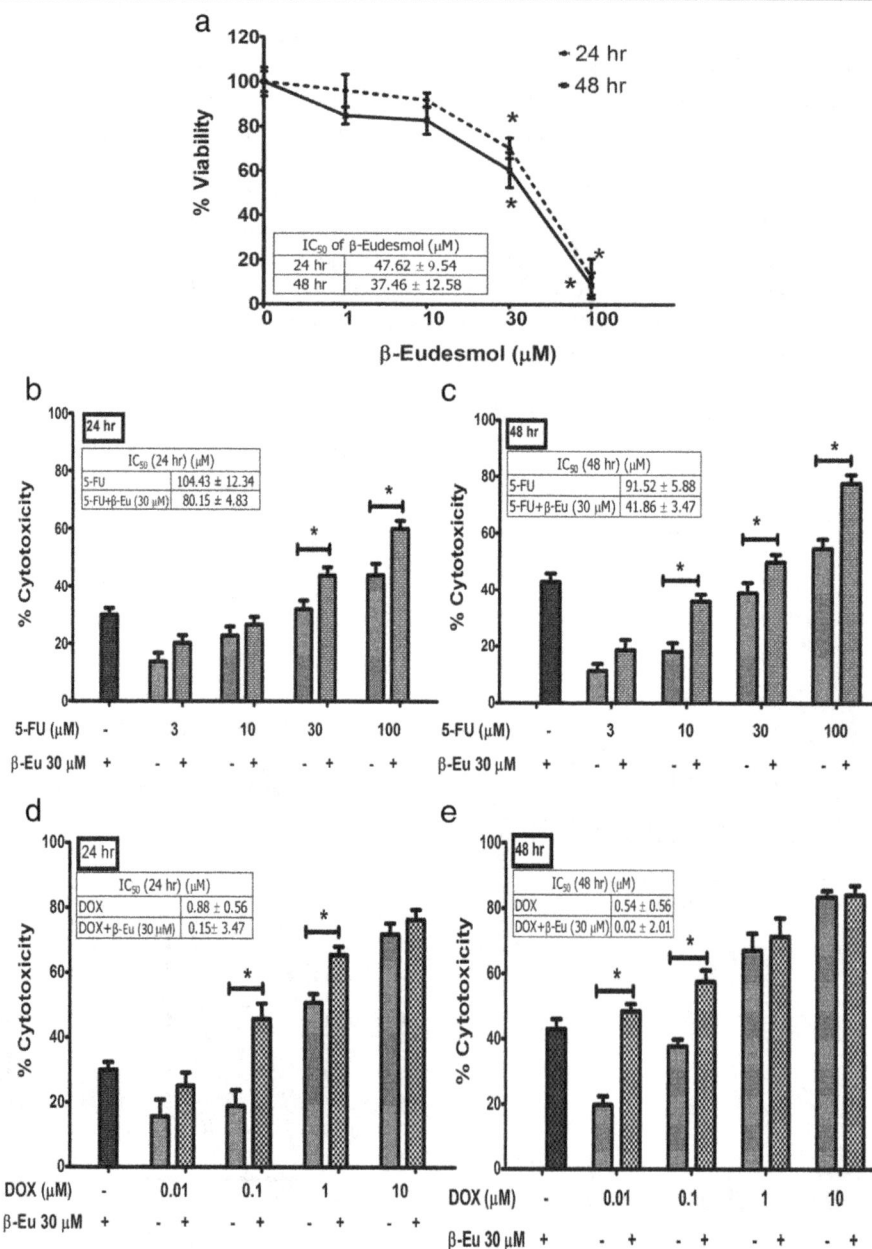

Fig. 2 Potentiating effect of β-eudesmol on cytotoxic activities of 5-FU and DOX. KKU-100 cells were seeded onto a 96-well microtiter plate overnight and cells were treated with β-eudesmol (1, 10, 30 and 100 μM) in the absence and presence of 5-FU or DOX for 24 and 48 h. Cell death was determined using SRB assay. **a** KKU-100 cells were incubated with β-eudesmol (1, 10, 30 and 100 μM) for 24 and 48 h. The results are presented as the percentage of viable cells. **b-e** The cytotoxic effect of β-eudesmol in combination with chemotherapeutic agents was determined. **b-c** KKU-100 cells were treated with β-eudesmol (30 μM) in the absence and presence of 5-FU (3, 10, 30 and 100 μM) for 24 and 48 h. **d-e** KKU-100 cells were treated with β-eudesmol (30 μM) in the absence and presence of DOX (0.01, 0.1, 1 and 10 μM) for 24 and 48 h. Each bar represents mean ± SD of three independent experiments, triplicate each. * indicates statistically significant difference with each drug alone (t-test, $p < 0.05$). β-Eu; β-Eudesmol, 5-FU; 5-Fluorouracil, DOX; Doxorubicin

experiments (potentiating effect on cytotoxic activities, inhibitory effect on cells migration, and enhancing the effect on cell apoptosis) to avoid the complete cytotoxic effect of β-eudesmol. Combination of β-eudesmol with 5-FU or DOX resulted in a markedly enhanced cytotoxic effect of each drug in concentration- and time-dependent manners (Fig. 2b-e). The cytotoxic activity of 5-FU was increased by 24 and 55% at 24 and 48 h of β-eudesmol exposure, respectively. The enhancement effect of β-eudesmol on the cytotoxic activity of DOX by greater than 80% was observed following 24 and 48 h of exposure.

Inhibitory effects of β-eudesmol in combination with 5-FU or DOX on CCA cell migration

Based on the wound closure assay, closure of the scratched wound of the monolayer culture of KKU-100 cells significantly occurred following exposure to β-eudesmol (30 μM) with or without 5-FU (30 μM) or DOX (0.1 μM) for 48 h (Fig. 3a and b).

Enhancing effect of β-eudesmol on apoptotic activities of 5-FU and DOX on CCA cells

Annexin V/PI and DAPI staining assay was used to further examine whether KKU-100 cell death following exposure to β-eudesmol in combination with 5-FU or DOX was associated with cell apoptosis (Fig. 4, 5 and 6). Percentage of annexin V/PI stained cells following

exposure to β-eudesmol in combination with 5-FU or DOX (Fig. 4e, f) was compared with that following exposure to each compound alone (Fig. 4b-d). The calculated percentage of the stained cells is shown in Fig. 4g. The inducing effect of β-eudesmol (30 μM) alone on cell apoptosis was relatively weak but was markedly increased in the presence of 5-FU or DOX. This observation of the enhancing cytotoxic activities of 5-FU or DOX by β-eudesmol through induction of cell apoptosis was supported by the analysis of cell morphology after staining with DAPI (Fig. 5). The number of apoptotic cells, nuclear condensation, and fragmentation were more prominent following exposure to the combination of β-eudesmol and 5-FU or DOX (Fig. 5e, f) compared with 5-FU or DOX alone (Fig. 5b-d).

Enhancing effect of β-eudesmol on caspase activation on CCA cells by 5-FU and DOX

To demonstrate the mechanisms underlying apoptotic induction, activation of caspase 3/7 of the cell apoptosis cascade was investigated following exposing the KKU-100 cells to β-eudesmol in combination with 5-FU or DOX. The caspase 3/7 activity of the cells in the presence of β-eudesmol alone (30 μM) was slightly but significantly increased compared with untreated control cells. However, the activity was markedly increased following exposure to β-eudesmol (30 μM) in combination

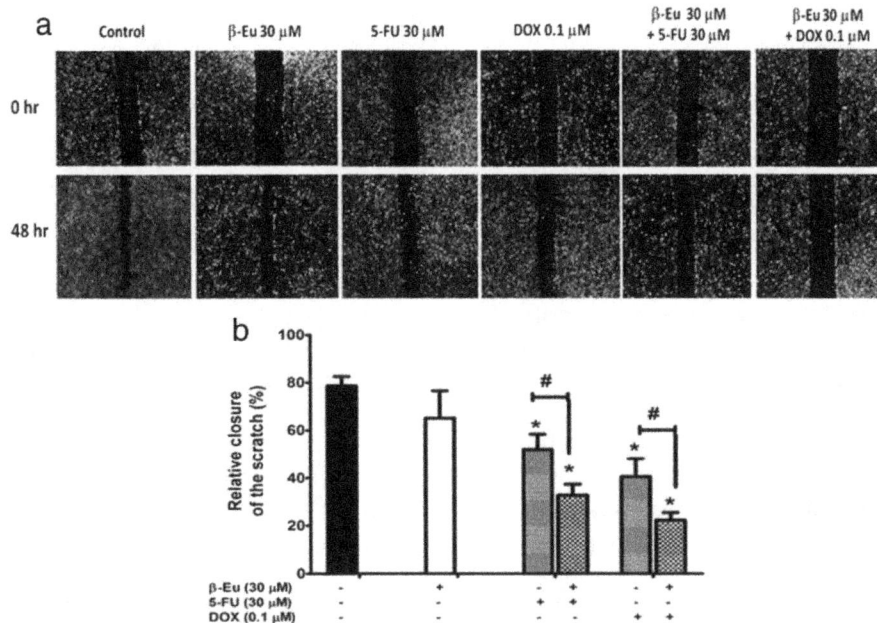

Fig. 3 Inhibitory effects of β-eudesmol in combination with 5-FU or DOX on CCA cells migration. Scratched wounds of monolayer KKU-100 cells were exposed to β-eudesmol (30 μM), 5-FU (30 μM), DOX (0.1 μM), and the combination of β-eudesmol (30 μM) with 5-FU (30 μM) or DOX (0.1 μM). Cell migration was monitored under phase-contrast microscopy (× 4 magnification). Representative images of wound healing were obtained at the time of the scratch and 48 h later (**a**). **b** The graph shows the level of cell migration into the wound scratch quantified as the percentage of wound closure at 48 h. Each bar represents mean ± SD of three independent experiments, triplicate each. * indicates statistically significant difference with each drug alone (paired t-test, $p < 0.05$). β-Eu = β-Eudesmol, 5-FU = 5-Fluorouracil, DOX = Doxorubicin

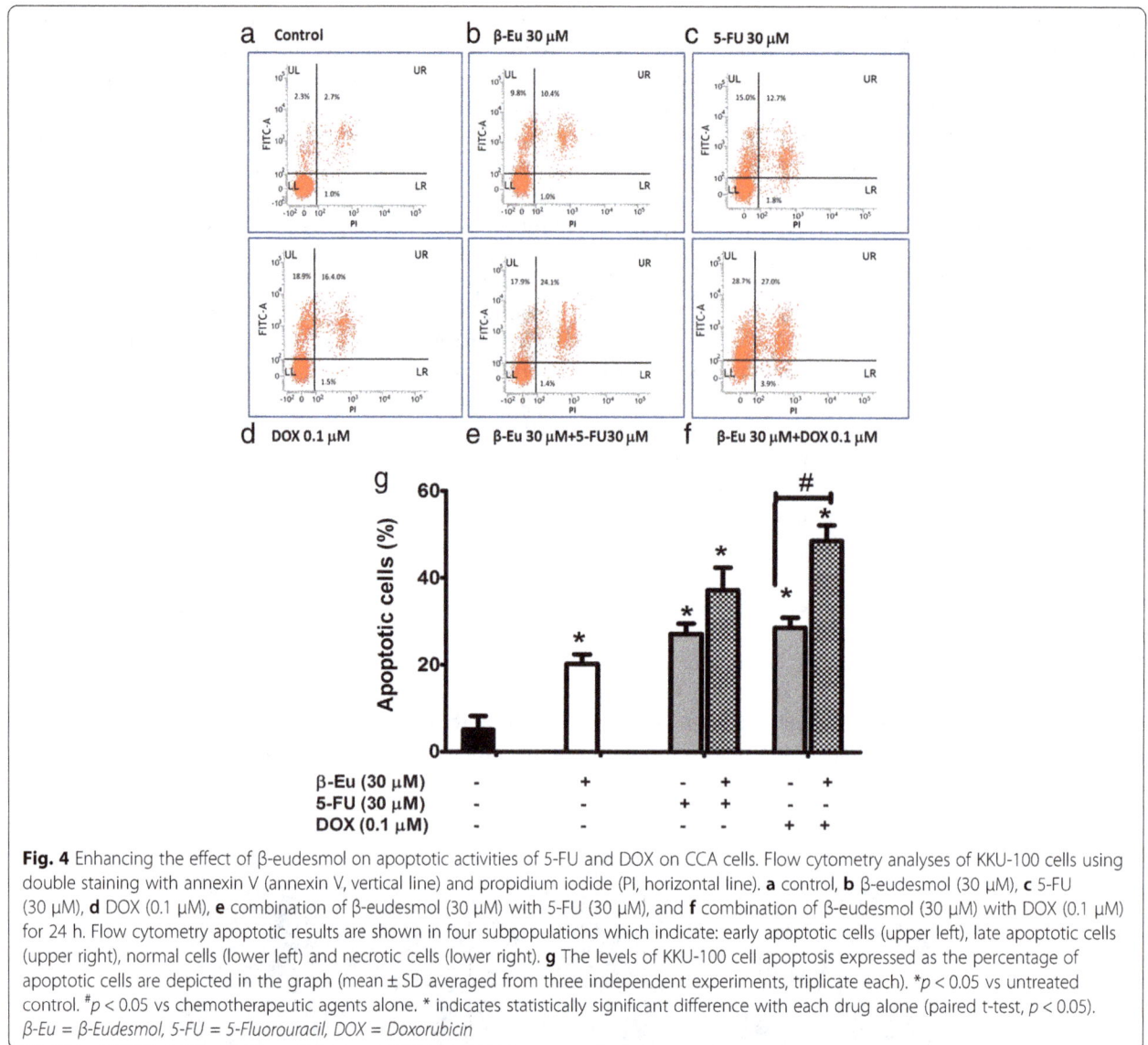

Fig. 4 Enhancing the effect of β-eudesmol on apoptotic activities of 5-FU and DOX on CCA cells. Flow cytometry analyses of KKU-100 cells using double staining with annexin V (annexin V, vertical line) and propidium iodide (PI, horizontal line). **a** control, **b** β-eudesmol (30 μM), **c** 5-FU (30 μM), **d** DOX (0.1 μM), **e** combination of β-eudesmol (30 μM) with 5-FU (30 μM), and **f** combination of β-eudesmol (30 μM) with DOX (0.1 μM) for 24 h. Flow cytometry apoptotic results are shown in four subpopulations which indicate: early apoptotic cells (upper left), late apoptotic cells (upper right), normal cells (lower left) and necrotic cells (lower right). **g** The levels of KKU-100 cell apoptosis expressed as the percentage of apoptotic cells are depicted in the graph (mean ± SD averaged from three independent experiments, triplicate each). *$p < 0.05$ vs untreated control. #$p < 0.05$ vs chemotherapeutic agents alone. * indicates statistically significant difference with each drug alone (paired t-test, $p < 0.05$). β-Eu = β-Eudesmol, 5-FU = 5-Fluorouracil, DOX = Doxorubicin

with 5-FU (30 μM) or DOX (0.1 μM) for 24 h (Fig. 6). These results suggested that combination of β-eudesmol and 5-FU or DOX enhanced KKU-100 cell apoptosis through caspase 3/7 activation.

Potentiating effect of β-eudesmol on suppression Bcl-2 and Bax protein expression of CCA cells by 5-FU and DOX and the involvement of mitochondrial pathway

The NQO1 enzyme activity and protein expression in KKU-100 cells were determined to examine whether the potentiating effect of β-eudesmol on cytotoxic activities of 5-FU or DOX was mediated through suppression of oxidative stress produced by NQO1. Cells were treated with β-eudesmol with or without 5-FU (30 μM) or DOX (0.1 μM) for 24 h. 5-FU and DOX alone significantly enhanced NQO1 activity and protein expression in KKU-100 cells. In the presence of β-eudesmol however,

enzyme activity and protein expression were markedly decreased (Fig. 7a and b).

In order to further confirm the involvement of the mitochondrial pathway in β-eudesmol enhanced chemosensitivity of KKU-100 cells through the induction of cell apoptosis, the expression levels of Bcl-2 family proteins Bcl-2 and Bax were investigated by Western blot analysis. β-Eudesmol (30 μM) alone did not alter Bax and Bcl-2 protein expression. On the other hand, the combination of β-eudesmol with 5-FU (30 μM) or DOX (0.1 μM) significantly increased the Bax/Bcl-2 expression ratios (1.23 vs. 2.81 and 1.84 vs. 2.98 for 5-FU alone vs. 5-FU + β-eudesmol and DOX alone vs. DOX + β-eudesmol, respectively) (Fig. 7b). These results suggested that β-eudesmol-potentiated cytotoxic activity of 5-FU and DOX was mediated through induction of apoptosis by Bcl-2 protein family in the mitochondrial pathway.

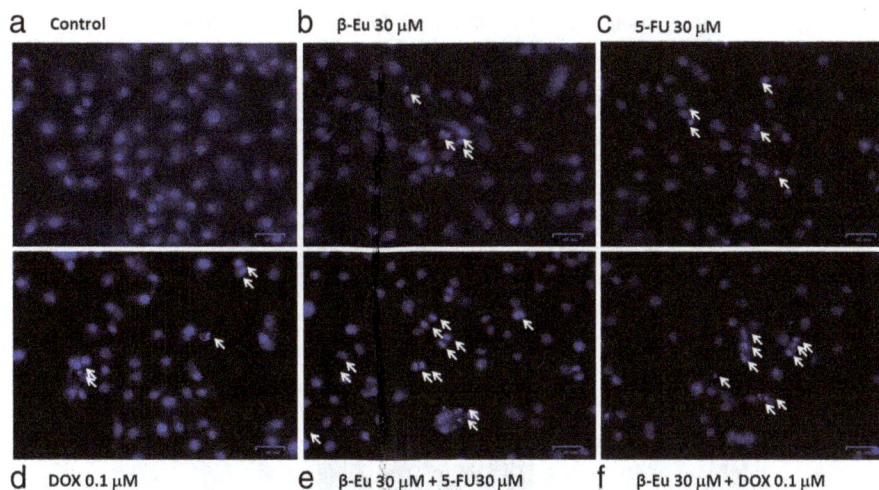

Fig. 5 Apoptotic bodies of KKU-100 CCA cells following treatment with β-eudesmol, 5-FU, and DOX, and the combination of β-eudesmol with 5-FU or DOX by DAPI staining. **a** control, **b** β-eudesmol (30 μM), **c** 5-FU (30 μM), **d** DOX (0.1 μM), **e** combination of β-eudesmol (30 μM) with 5-FU (30 μM), and **f** combination of β-eudesmol (30 μM) with DOX (0.1 μM) for 24 h. Apoptotic bodies were observed under inverted fluorescence microscopy (Scale bars represent 40 μm). *β-Eu= β-Eudesmol, 5-FU= 5-Fluorouracil, DOX= Doxorubicin*

Discussion

Since the up-regulation of NQO1 in certain types of solid tumor including CCA was associated with poor prognosis [14–19], compounds targeting NQO1 would be of therapeutic potential. Previous studies have suggested possible role of NQO1 suppression-enhanced chemosensitivity of the cancer cells. Dicoumarol, a potent inhibitor of the NQO1 enzyme, has been shown to increase sensitivity of CCA cells to chemotherapeutic agents [22]. Furthermore, NQO1 silencing by gene knockdown in conjunction with chemotherapeutic agents has been shown to suppress the replication capacity of CCA cells [23]. In the present study, β-eudesmol suppressed NQO1 enzyme activity in KKU-100 cells with moderate potency compared with dicoumarol, the most potent inhibitor of NQO1 [28]. Direct addition of β-eudesmol to cell lysates significantly inhibited NQO1 activity at all concentrations. At highest concentration (100 μM, 95.56% inhibition), the extent of the inhibitory activity was almost similar to that of dicoumarol (1 μM, 99.21% inhibition). On the other hand, significant suppression of NQO1 protein expression was observed only at the highest concentration (100 μM) compared with that inhibited enzyme activity both in the cells (at the lowest concentration of 30 μM) and cell lysates (at the lowest concentration of 1 μM). Dicoumarol has been shown to exert no or little effect on CCA NQO1 protein expression [42]. It is possible that β-eudesmol-mediated NQO1 suppression was through direct inhibition of the enzyme activity with similar mechanism of that observed with dicoumarol. The suppression of NQO1 activity by dicoumarol is a consequence of its competition with NAD(P)H for binding to NQO1 and prevention of

electron transfer to FAD co-factor, allowing the quinone substrate to bind the enzyme and to be reduced [43]. It is well established that NQO1 functions as a detoxification and antioxidant enzyme that protects cells from oxidative stress. Additionally, it also functions as a p53 wild-type stabilizer by interference with 20s proteasome-mediated degradation of p53 [44]. P53 is a tumor suppressor gene which functions in response to stimulation by DNA damage, oxidative stress, or cell cycle abnormalities [44, 45]. The anticancer and apoptotic activity of P53 involves several mechanisms [46]. In the present study, β-eudesmol was shown to enhance chemosensitivity-induced apoptosis of CCA cells which was linked with suppression of NQO1 activity. So far, the previously reported role of NQO1 suppression on p53 modulation and cell apoptosis remains controversial. Inhibition of NQO1 by natural inhibitor curcumin has been shown to suppress p53 protein levels and p53-induced apoptosis of cancer cells in the NQO1-dependent pathway [26]. On the other hand, dicoumarol or NQO1 knockdown cells was shown to enhance p53 protein levels which was associated with induction of apoptosis in CCA [22, 23] and urogenital cancer cells [20]. The CCA-KKU-100 cell used in the present study was shown to express both the wild-type full-length p53 and the splicing variant of the truncated p53 protein [47]. Interestingly, our results showed that the potentiating effect of NQO1 suppression by β-eudesmol on the cytotoxicity and apoptotic activity of 5-FU and DOX occurred even in such the CCA cells with a high expression ratio of mutant p53/wild-type p53. The exact molecular action on NQO1 activity of β-eudesmol needs further investigation. It is yet to investigate the

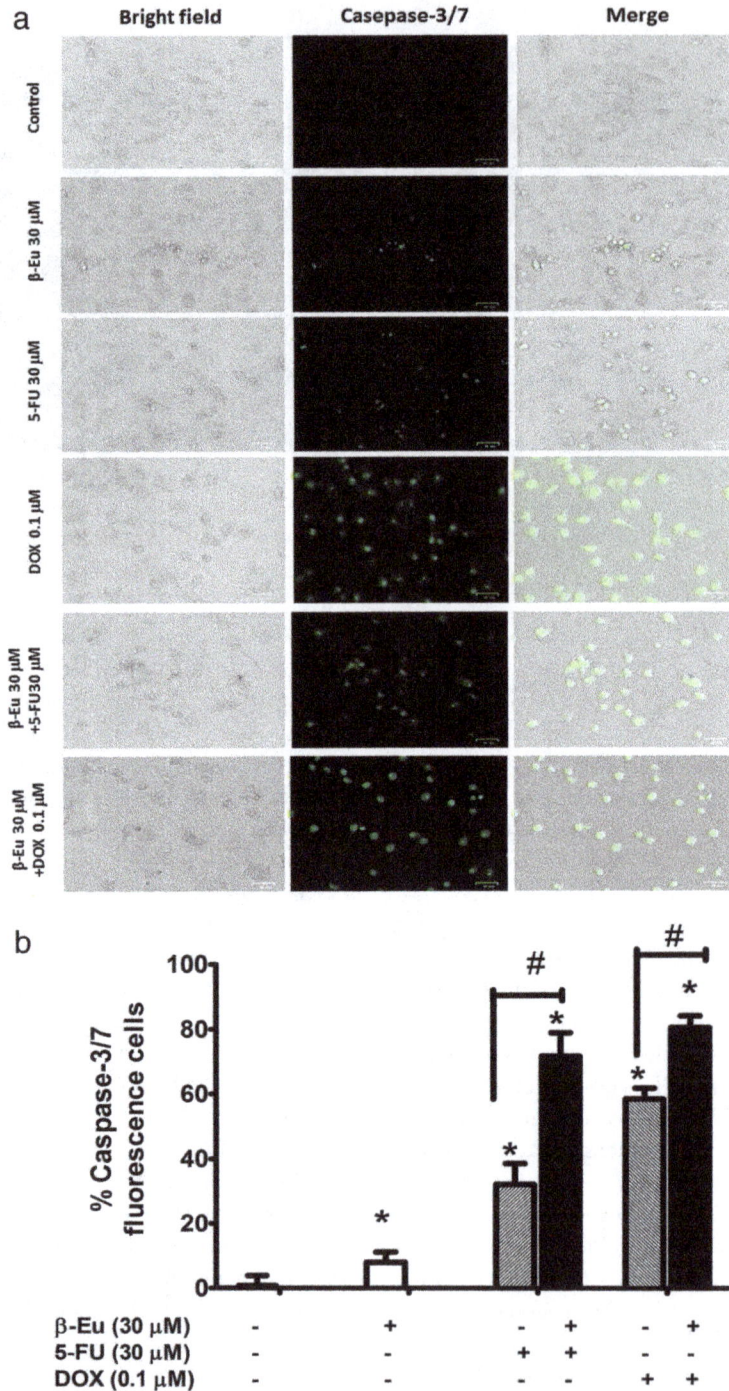

Fig. 6 Caspase-3/7 activation in KKU-100 cells following treatment with β-eudesmol, 5-FU, and DOX, and the combination of β-eudesmol and 5-FU or DOX detected by fluorescence microscopy. **a** KKU-100 cells were treated with 30 μM of β-eudesmol, 30 μM of 5-FU, 0.1 μM of DOX and β-eudesmol (30 μM) combined with 5-FU (30 μM) or DOX (0.1 μM) for 24 h and labeled with CellEvent® Caspase 3/7 Green Detection Reagent and examined under the fluorescence microscope. Left panel, the grey image reveals KKU-100 CCA cells in the field of view. Middle and right panel show apoptotic caspase 3/7 positive cells green fluorescent in the same area of interest. Data are representative of at least 4–5 randomly selected fields' images with similar results. Morphological changes were evaluated under a microscope. There were shrink and blabbing cells treated with β-eudesmol with or without 5-FU or DOX, indicating apoptosis induction. The scale bar corresponds to 40 μm. **b** The graph shows the level of caspase-3/7 activity as the percentage of caspase-3 /7 fluorescent cells expression at 24 h. Data are presented as mean ± SD of three independent experiments, triplicate each. * indicates statistically significant difference with each drug alone (paired t-test, $p < 0.05$). *β-Eu= β-Eudesmol, 5-FU= 5-Fluorouracil, DOX= Doxorubicin*

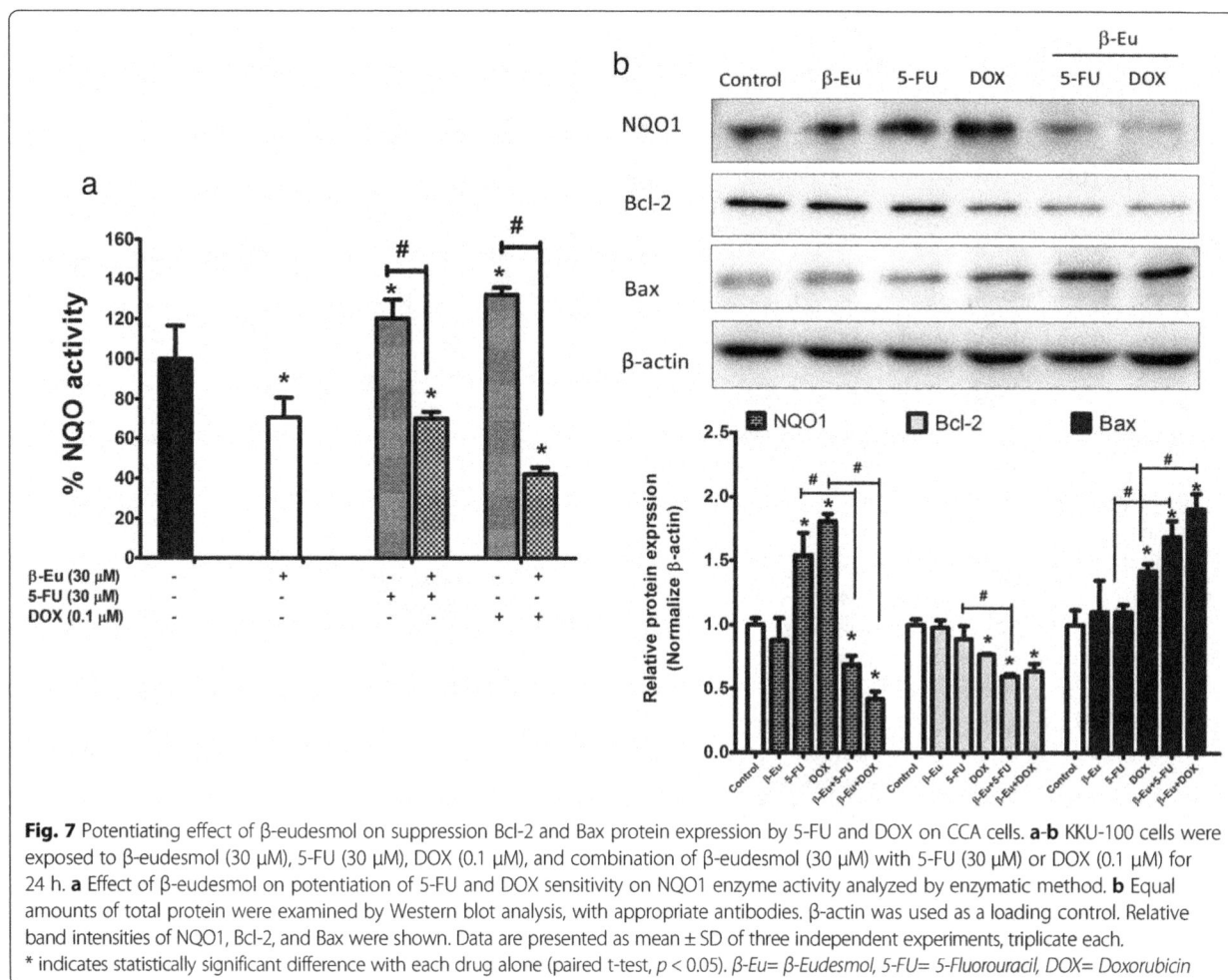

Fig. 7 Potentiating effect of β-eudesmol on suppression Bcl-2 and Bax protein expression by 5-FU and DOX on CCA cells. **a-b** KKU-100 cells were exposed to β-eudesmol (30 μM), 5-FU (30 μM), DOX (0.1 μM), and combination of β-eudesmol (30 μM) with 5-FU (30 μM) or DOX (0.1 μM) for 24 h. **a** Effect of β-eudesmol on potentiation of 5-FU and DOX sensitivity on NQO1 enzyme activity analyzed by enzymatic method. **b** Equal amounts of total protein were examined by Western blot analysis, with appropriate antibodies. β-actin was used as a loading control. Relative band intensities of NQO1, Bcl-2, and Bax were shown. Data are presented as mean ± SD of three independent experiments, triplicate each. * indicates statistically significant difference with each drug alone (paired t-test, $p < 0.05$). β-Eu= β-Eudesmol, 5-FU= 5-Fluorouracil, DOX= Doxorubicin

chemosensitizing effect of NQO1 suppression by β-eudesmol on CCA cells which express other p53 mutation variants.

5-FU and DOX are widely used for chemotherapy of several types of cancer including CCA. However, the effectiveness of both drugs in the treatment of recurrent/ metastatic cancers is limited due to acquired or intrinsic resistance of the cancer cells. β-Eudesmol was shown to suppress NQO1 enzyme activity and protein expression and thereby, potentiating the cytotoxic activity of both drugs in KKU-100 cells. Combination of both conventional drugs with β-eudesmol may be an effective therapeutic strategy for targeting chemoresistant CCA as well as improving therapeutic efficacy and minimizing toxicity of conventional drugs. The enhancement of CCA cell sensitivity has also been reported when conventional chemotherapeutics are used in conjunction with NQO1 knockdown [23].

Metastasis is one of the most important characteristics of cancers indicating poor prognosis and death in cancer patients. The process reflects the ability of cancer cells to break away from the main tumor and enter the bloodstream or lymphatic system. The key steps include degradation of tumor extracellular matrix, cell invasion, and cell migration [48]. Inhibitors of these metastasis-associated processes would, therefore, provide a significant impact on cancer chemoprevention and chemotherapy. Previous studies have shown that NQO1 is one of the enzymes that play an important role in cancer cell migration and invasion of human aortic vascular smooth muscle cells. The NQO1 inhibitor dicoumarol or NQO1 knockdown was shown to suppress matrix metallopeptidase 9 (MMP 9) expression and tumor necrosis factor α (TNF-α)-induced cell migration [49]. In the present study, treatment of KKU-100 cells with β-eudesmol markedly decreased cancer cell migration mediated by 5-FU or DOX. It is of note that this antimigratory effect of β-eudesmol was detected at a concentration that significantly inhibited NQO1 expression (> 40%) with minimal cytotoxic effect to KKU-100 cells. The chemosensitivity enhancing effect of β-eudesmol on the CCA cell could at least in part, be a consequence of its inhibitory effect on CCA cell metastasis.

The process of programmed cell death or apoptosis is generally characterized by a programmed sequence of events leading to the eradication of cells without releasing damaging substances into the surrounding area [50]. Initiation of apoptosis process therefore, benefits cancer cells. The mechanism through which β-eudesmol mediated suppression of NQO1-induced cell death was further explored in the present study. β-Eudesmol was shown to significantly enhance proapoptotic activities of both 5-FU and DOX. During the steps of apoptosis, the cells shrunk despite undamaged membranes. Cells with DNA fragmentation, condensed chromatin, and nuclear pyknosis were detected by DAPI. Combination of β-eudesmol and 5-FU or DOX markedly increased apoptotic bodies. Induction of cell apoptosis by β-eudesmol was also observed in other cancer cells, i.e., human hepatocellular carcinoma [51] and human leukemia cells [52]. Apoptosis process is finely regulated at gene level resulting in the orderly and efficient removal of damaged cells such as those occurring following DNA damage or during development. The balance between the proapoptotic (Bax) and anti-apoptotic (Bcl-2) protein regulators is a critical key point to determine cell apoptosis. The apoptotic activity of various compounds has been evaluated by measuring caspase activity particularly caspase 3/7 activity which is the final step in both the intrinsic or extrinsic pathways of apoptosis [53]. In this study, the combination of β-eudesmol and 5-FU or DOX significantly activated caspase 3/7 activity compared to each drug alone. The β-eudesmol-induced enhancement of chemosensitivity of CCA cells by promoting their apoptosis was shown to be associated with increase of the Bax/Bcl-2 ratio and caspase activation. The Bcl-2 family is a key factor in the regulation of cell homeostasis which is directly associated with cell survival and cell death. The process that promotes pro-apoptotic factor Bax expression or/and decreases anti-apoptotic factor Bcl-2 expression results in the release of cytochrome to the cytosol and subsequently, initiation of caspase 9 and caspase 3 cascades, leading to cell apoptosis [39, 40]. .Our results indicated that β-eudesmol in combination with 5-FU or DOX stimulated the expression of Bax protein while decreasing the expression of Bcl-2.

Conclusions

The cytotoxic activity of β-eudesmol was at least in part, mediated through suppression of NQO1. Induction of cell apoptosis and activation of caspase 3/7, up-regulation of Bax and down-regulation of Bcl-2 proteins could contribute to its cytotoxic and proapoptotic activity. β-Eudesmol may serve as a potential anti-CCA candidate particularly when used in combination with conventional chemotherapeutics. Further investigations in animal models are needed to confirm its potential clinical use.

Abbreviations

5-FU: 5-Fluorouracil; CCA: Cholangiocarcinoma; DMSO: Dimethyl sulfoxide; DOX: Doxorubicin; DTT: Dithiothreitol; FBS: Fetal bovine serum; NQO1: NAD(P)H-quinone oxidoreductase1; PMSF: Phenylmethylsulfonyl fluoride; PVDF: Polyvinylidene difluoride; β-Eu: β-Eudesmol; Tween-20: Polyethylene glycol sorbitan monolaurate

Acknowledgments

We would like to thank Professor Banchob Sripa, Department of Pathology, Faculty of Medicine, Khon Kean University, for providing KKU-100 cell.

Funding

This present study was supported by Chulabhorn International College of Medicine (CICM2015), and Center of Excellence in Pharmacology and Molecular Biology of Malaria and Cholangiocarcinoma, Thammasat University, Thailand (2015).

Authors' contributions

PS and KNB contributed to the conception and design of the entire study. PS carried out most of the experiments, contributed to the data interpretation. SP contributed to the analysis of cell apoptosis and caspase-3/7 activation. KBN provided grant support, funding and the final editing of the manuscript. All contributed to data interpretation, drafting and final editing of the manuscript. All authors read and approved the final manuscript.

Competing interests

The authors declare that they have no competing interests.

References

1. Cardinale V, Semeraro R, Torrice A, Gatto M, Napoli C, Bragazzi MC, et al. Intra-hepatic and extra-hepatic cholangiocarcinoma: new insight into epidemiology and risk factors. World J Gastrointest Oncol. 2010;2(11):407–16.
2. Kamsa-ard S, Wiangnon S, Suwanrungruang K, Promthet S, Khuntikeo N, Kamsa-ard S, et al. Trends in liver cancer incidence between 1985 and 2009, Khon Kaen, Thailand: cholangiocarcinoma. Asian Pac J Cancer Prev. 2011;12(9):2209–13.
3. Sripa B, Pairojkul C. Cholangiocarcinoma: lessons from Thailand. Curr Opin Gastroenterol. 2008;24(3):349–56.
4. Sripa B, Brindley PJ, Mulvenna J, Laha T, Smout MJ, Mairiang E, et al. The tumorigenic liver fluke Opisthorchis viverrini—multiple pathways to cancer. Trends Parasitol. 2012;28(10):395–407.
5. Khan SA, Thomas HC, Davidson BR, Taylor-Robinson SD. Cholangiocarcinoma. Lancet. 2005;366(9493):1303–14.
6. Hezel AF, Zhu AX. Systemic therapy for biliary tract cancers. Oncologist. 2008;13(4):415–23.
7. Fodale V, Pierobon M, Liotta L, Petricoin E. Mechanism of cell adaptation: when and how do cancer cells develop chemoresistance? Cancer J. 2011;17(2):89–95.
8. Holohan C, Van Schaeybroeck S, Longley DB, Johnston PG. Cancer drug resistance: an evolving paradigm. Nat Rev Cancer. 2013;13(10):714–26.
9. Ross D, Kepa JK, Winski SL, Beall HD, Anwar A, Siegel D. NAD(P)H:quinone oxidoreductase 1 (NQO1): chemoprotection, bioactivation, gene regulation and genetic polymorphisms. Chem Biol Interact. 2000;129(1–2):77–97.
10. Siegel D, Ross D. Immunodetection of NAD(P)H:quinone oxidoreductase 1 (NQO1) in human tissues. Free Radic Biol Med. 2000;29(3–4):246–53.

11. Strassburg A, Strassburg CP, Manns MP, Tukey RH. Differential gene expression of NAD(P)H:quinone oxidoreductase and NRH:quinone oxidoreductase in human hepatocellular and biliary tissue. Mol Pharmacol. 2002;61(2):320–5.

12. Dinkova-Kostova AT, Talalay P. NAD(P)H: quinone acceptor oxidoreductase 1 (NQO1), a multifunctional antioxidant enzyme and exceptionally versatile cytoprotection. Arch Biochem Biophys. 2010;501(1):116–23.

13. Joseph P, Long DJ 2nd, Klein-Szanto AJ, Jaiswal AK. Role of NAD(P)H: quinone oxidoreductase 1 (DT diaphorase) in protection against quinone toxicity. Biochem Pharmacol. 2000;60(2):207–14.

14. Cui X, Jin T, Wang X, Jin G, Li Z, Lin L. NAD(P)H:quinone oxidoreductase-1 overexpression predicts poor prognosis in small cell lung cancer. Oncol Rep. 2014;32(6):2589–95.

15. Ji M, Jin A, Sun J, Cui X, Yang Y, Chen L, et al. Clinicopathological implications of NQO1 overexpression in the prognosis of pancreatic adenocarcinoma. Oncol Lett. 2017;13(5):2996–3002.

16. Glorieux C, Sandoval JM, Dejeans N, Ameye G, Poirel HA, Verrax J, et al. Overexpression of NAD(P)H:quinone oxidoreductase 1 (NQO1) and genomic gain of the NQO1 locus modulates breast cancer cell sensitivity to quinones. Life Sci. 2016;145:57–65.

17. Jin Z, Cui X, Zhang Y, Yang Y, Li L, Lin Z, et al. Significance of NAD (P) H: quinone oxidoreductase 1 overexpression in prognostic evaluation of thyroid medullary carcinoma. Zhonghua Bing Li Xue Za Zhi. 2015;44(2):128–9.

18. Lin L, Qin Y, Jin T, Liu S, Zhang S, Shen X, et al. Significance of NQO1 overexpression for prognostic evaluation of gastric adenocarcinoma. Exp Mol Pathol. 2014;96(2):200–5.

19. Buranrat B, Chau-in S, Prawan A, Puapairoj A, Zeekpudsa P, Kukongviriyapan V. NQO1 expression correlates with cholangiocarcinoma prognosis. Asian Pac J Cancer Prev. 2012;13(Suppl):131–6.

20. Matsui Y, Watanabe J, Ding S, Nishizawa K, Kajita Y, Ichioka K, et al. Dicoumarol enhances doxorubicin-induced cytotoxicity in p53 wild-type urothelial cancer cells through p38 activation. BJU Int. 2010;105(4):558–64.

21. Watanabe J, Nishiyama H, Matsui Y, Ito M, Kawanishi H, Kamoto T, et al. Dicoumarol potentiates cisplatin-induced apoptosis mediated by c-Jun N-terminal kinase in p53 wild-type urogenital cancer cell lines. Oncogene. 2006;25(17):2500–8.

22. Buranrat B, Prawan A, Kukongviriyapan U, Kongpetch S, Kukongviriyapan V. Dicoumarol enhances gemcitabine-induced cytotoxicity in high NQO1-expressing cholangiocarcinoma cells. World J Gastroenterol. 2010;16(19):2362–70.

23. Zeekpudsa P, Kukongviriyapan V, Senggunprai L, Sripa B, Prawan A. Suppression of NAD(P)H-quinone oxidoreductase 1 enhanced the susceptibility of cholangiocarcinoma cells to chemotherapeutic agents. J Exp Clin Cancer Res. 2014;33:11.

24. Colucci MA, Reigan P, Siegel D, Chilloux A, Ross D, Moody CJ. Synthesis and evaluation of 3-aryloxymethyl-1,2-dimethylindole-4,7-diones as mechanism-based inhibitors of NAD(P)H:quinone oxidoreductase 1 (NQO1) activity. J Med Chem. 2007;50(23):5780–9.

25. Nolan KA, Zhao H, Faulder PF, Frenkel AD, Timson DJ, Siegel D, et al. Coumarin-based inhibitors of human NAD(P)H:quinone oxidoreductase-1. Identification, structure-activity, off-target effects and in vitro human pancreatic cancer toxicity. J Med Chem. 2007;50(25):6316–25.

26. Tsvetkov P, Asher G, Reiss V, Shaul Y, Sachs L, Lotem J. Inhibition of NAD(P)H:quinone oxidoreductase 1 activity and induction of p53 degradation by the natural phenolic compound curcumin. Proc Natl Acad Sci U S A. 2005;102(15):5535–40.

27. Chen S, Hwang J, Deng PS. Inhibition of NAD(P)H:quinone acceptor oxidoreductase by flavones: a structure-activity study. Arch Biochem Biophys. 1993;302(1):72–7.

28. Chen S, Wu K, Zhang D, Sherman M, Knox R, Yang CS. Molecular characterization of binding of substrates and inhibitors to DT-diaphorase: combined approach involving site-directed mutagenesis, inhibitor-binding analysis, and computer modeling. Mol Pharmacol. 1999;56(2):272–8.

29. Na-Bangchang K, Karbwang J. Traditional herbal medicine for the control of tropical diseases. Trop Med Health. 2014;42(2 Suppl):3–13.

30. Ji L, Ao P, Pan JG, Yang JY, Yang J, Hu SL. GC-MS analysis of essential oils from rhizomes of Atractylodes lancea (Thunb.) DC. and A. Chinensis (DC.) Koidz. Zhongguo Zhong Yao Za Zhi. 2001;26(3):182–5.

31. Duan JA, Wang L, Qian S, Su S, Tang Y. A new cytotoxic prenylated dihydrobenzofuran derivative and other chemical constituents from the rhizomes of Atractylodes lancea DC. Arch Pharm Res. 2008;31(8):965–9.

32. Zhao M, Wang Q, Ouyang Z, Han B, Wang W, Wei Y, et al. Selective fraction of Atractylodes lancea (Thunb.) DC. and its growth inhibitory effect on human gastric cancer cells. Cytotechnology. 2014;66(2):201–8.

33. Mahavorasirikul W, Viyanant V, Chaijaroenkul W, Itharat A, Na-Bangchang K. Cytotoxic activity of Thai medicinal plants against human cholangiocarcinoma, laryngeal and hepatocarcinoma cells in vitro. BMC Complement Altern Med. 2010;10:55.

34. Plengsuriyakarn T, Karbwang J, Na-Bangchang K. Anticancer activity using positron emission tomography-computed tomography and pharmacokinetics of beta-eudesmol in human cholangiocarcinoma xenografted nude mouse model. Clin Exp Pharmacol Physiol. 2015;42(3):293–304.

35. Plengsuriyakarn T, Viyanant V, Eursitthichai V, Picha P, Kupradinun P, Itharat A, et al. Anticancer activities against cholangiocarcinoma, toxicity and pharmacological activities of Thai medicinal plants in animal models. BMC Complement Altern Med. 2012;12:23.

36. Yu F, Harada H, Yamasaki K, Okamoto S, Hirase S, Tanaka Y, et al. Isolation and functional characterization of a beta-eudesmol synthase, a new sesquiterpene synthase from Zingiber zerumbet Smith. FEBS Lett. 2008; 582(5):565–72.

37. Wang CC, Lin SY, Cheng HC, Hou WC. Pro-oxidant and cytotoxic activities of atractylenolide I in human promyeloleukemic HL-60 cells. Food Chem Toxicol. 2006;44(8):1308–15.

38. Salleh NA, Ismail S, Ab Halim MR. Effects of Curcuma xanthorrhiza extracts and their constituents on phase II drug-metabolizing enzymes activity. Pharm Res. 2016;8(4):309–15.

39. Mathema VB, Chaijaroenkul W, Karbwang J, Na-Bangchang K. Growth inhibitory effect of beta-eudesmol on cholangiocarcinoma cells and its potential suppressive effect on heme oxygenase-1 production, STAT1/3 activation, and NF-kappaB downregulation. Clin Exp Pharmacol Physiol. 2017;44(11):1145–54.

40. Prochaska HJ, Santamaria AB. Direct measurement of NAD(P)H:quinone reductase from cells cultured in microtiter wells: a screening assay for anticarcinogenic enzyme inducers. Anal Biochem. 1988;169(2):328–36.

41. Senggunprai L, Kukongviriyapan V, Prawan A, Kukongviriyapan U. Quercetin and EGCG exhibit chemopreventive effects in cholangiocarcinoma cells via suppression of JAK/STAT signaling pathway. Phytother Res. 2014;28(6):841–8.

42. Chen M, Gong L, Qi X, Xing G, Luan Y, Wu Y, et al. Inhibition of renal NQO1 activity by dicoumarol suppresses nitroreduction of aristolochic acid I and attenuates its nephrotoxicity. Toxicol Sci. 2011;122(2):288–96.

43. Asher G, Dym O, Tsvetkov P, Adler J, Shaul Y. The crystal structure of NAD(P)H quinone oxidoreductase 1 in complex with its potent inhibitor dicoumarol. Biochemistry. 2006;45(20):6372–8.

44. Nioi P, Hayes JD. Contribution of NAD(P)H:quinone oxidoreductase 1 to protection against carcinogenesis, and regulation of its gene by the Nrf2 basic-region leucine zipper and the arylhydrocarbon receptor basic helix-loop-helix transcription factors. Mutat Res. 2004;555(1–2):149–71.

45. Asher G, Lotem J, Cohen B, Sachs L, Shaul Y. Regulation of p53 stability and p53-dependent apoptosis by NADH quinone oxidoreductase 1. Proc Natl Acad Sci U S A. 2001;98(3):1188–93.

46. Bouchet BP, Caron de Fromentel C, Puisieux A, Galmarini CM. p53 as a target for anti-cancer drug development. Crit Rev Oncol Hematol. 2006;58(3):190–207.

47. Nutthasirikul N, Limpaiboon T, Leelayuwat C, Patrakitkomjorn S, Jearanaikoon P. Ratio disruption of the 133p53 and TAp53 isoform equilibrium correlates with poor clinical outcome in intrahepatic cholangiocarcinoma. Int J Oncol. 2013;42(4):1181–8.

48. Friedl P, Wolf K. Tumour-cell invasion and migration: diversity and escape mechanisms. Nat Rev Cancer. 2003;3(5):362–74.

49. Lee SO, Chang YC, Whang K, Kim CH, Lee IS. Role of NAD(P)H:quinone oxidoreductase 1 on tumor necrosis factor-alpha-induced migration of human vascular smooth muscle cells. Cardiovasc Res. 2007;76(2):331–9.

50. Su Z, Yang Z, Xu Y, Chen Y, Yu Q. Apoptosis, autophagy, necroptosis, and cancer metastasis. Mol Cancer. 2015;14:48.

51. Bomfim DS, Ferraz RP, Carvalho NC, Soares MB, Pinheiro ML, Costa EV, et al. Eudesmol isomers induce caspase-mediated apoptosis in human hepatocellular carcinoma HepG2 cells. Basic Clin Pharmacol Toxicol. 2013;113(5):300–6.

52. Li Y, Li T, Miao C, Li J, Xiao W, Ma E. beta-Eudesmol induces JNK-dependent apoptosis through the mitochondrial pathway in HL60 cells. Phytother Res. 2013;27(3):338–43.

53. McIlwain DR, Berger T, Mak TW. Caspase functions in cell death and disease. Cold Spring Harb Perspect Biol. 2013;5(4):a008656.

8

Adefovir dipivoxil induced hypophosphatemic osteomalacia in chronic hepatitis B: a comparative study of Chinese and foreign case series

Nan Chen[1†], Jian-bo Zhang[2†], Qiujie Zhang[1†], Yun-peng Zhao[3], Li-yan Li[4], Li-wei Liu[1], Fei Yu[1], Xin Yu[1], Tao Peng[5] and Kuan-xiao Tang[1,6*]

Abstract

Background: Adefovir dipivoxil (ADV)-induced renal tubular dysfunction and hypophosphatemic osteomalacia (HO) have been given great consideration in the past few years. However, no standard guidance is available due to a lack of powerful evidence from appropriate long-term prospective case-control studies and variations in the definition of renal adverse events. The aim of this study is to clarify clinical features of ADV-related HO in Chinese chronic hepatitis B patients with long-term ADV treatment in Chinese and non-Chinese comparative case series.

Methods: Retrieval of case reports was based on Pubmed, CNKI, Wan Fang and VIP databases using the key words adefovir dipivoxil, hypophosphatemia, osteomalacia and Fanconi syndrome. We divided patients into Chinese (C group) and Foreign (F group) groups according to their nationality. Comparisons involving demographics, clinical manifestations, tests, treatment and prognosis were conducted between the two groups.

Results: Of the patients screened, 120 Chinese patients were identified in the C group, and 32 non-Chinese patients were identified in the F group. The average age of the C group was younger than that of the F group (51.89 years ±10.96 years versus 56.47 years ±11.36 years, $t = -2.084$, $P = 0.039$). No significant difference was found in gender (male to female, 3.29:1 versus 3:1, $\chi^2 = 0.039$, $P = 0.844$). Although there was no significant difference in the duration of ADV therapy before ostalgia onset, the C group tended to develop adverse events earlier, by 2–3 years, while the F group developed adverse events at 4–5 years ($Z = -1.517$, $P = 0.129$). Prognosis was good after adjustment of the ADV dose and supplemental administration of phosphate and calcitriol. Time to resolution of tubular dysfunction was commenced at the first month, and Chinese patients were more prone to recover in the first 3 months than non-Chinese patients (91.3% of patients in the C group versus 56.3% in the F group, $Z = -3.013$, $P = 0.003$).

Conclusions: Sufficient attention is required for middle-aged males before and during exposure to long-term ADV therapy, regardless of nationality. The clinical picture, laboratory and radiograph alterations are important clues for those patients and are usually characterized by polyarthralgia, renal tubular dysfunction and mineralization defects. Implementation of an early renal tubular injury index is recommended for patients with higher risk, which would prevent further renal injury.

Keywords: Adefovir dipivoxil, Hypophosphatemia, Osteomalacia, Renal insufficiency, Fanconi syndrome

* Correspondence: tkx610@hotmail.com
†Equal contributors
[1]Department of Geriatrics, Qilu Hospital of Shandong University, Jinan, Shandong, China
[6]Present Address: Department of Geriatrics, Qilu Hospital of Shandong University, No. 107, Wenhua Xi Road, Jinan, Shandong 250012, People's Republic of China
Full list of author information is available at the end of the article

Background

Adefovir dipivoxil (ADV) is a nucleotide analogue of adenosine monophosphate, which is effective in viral suppression for both treatment-naive and lamivudine-resistant chronic HBV-infected patients [1]. Chronic hepatitis B virus (HBV) infection affects more than 350 million people worldwide, with 75% living in the Asia-Pacific region [2]. Moreover, chronic HBV infection continues to be a major health problem because it leads to the development of liver cirrhosis and hepatocellular carcinoma and increases the risk of hepatic disease-related death. Various studies have reported that adefovir dipivoxil (ADV) can cause proximal renal tubular complex dysfunction, hypophosphatemic osteomalacia (HO) and even Fanconi syndrome since it was first used in the long-term treatment of chronic hepatitis B in 2002 [3]. However, several pitfalls remain to be explained. First, a unified definition of ADV-related renal dysfunction has not yet been identified. Some studies used serum creatinine or evaluated glomerular filtration rate (eGFR), which mainly reflects glomerular function as an endpoint [4, 5], while some studies only investigated indexes concerning renal tubular absorption [6, 7]. No evidence from case-control studies including Chinese chronic hepatitis B patients have been reported, and sample sizes of previous studies were relatively small [8, 9]. Furthermore, patients not matching the original clinical settings were included. To further determine the clinical features of ADV-induced HO in Chinese chronic hepatitis B patients, we investigated the demographics, clinical spectrum, laboratory tests, treatment and prognosis of ADV-induced HO through a comparison of Chinese and non-Chinese case series.

Comparative series study

Methods

Search strategy

PubMed, Chinese National Knowledge Infrastructure (CNKI), the Chinese literature database (Wanfang) and the Chinese Science and Technology Journal Database (VIP) [10] from October 2002 to October 2015 were searched for case reports and relevant clinical trials. The key words were adefovir dipivoxil, hypophosphatemia, osteomalacia, Fanconi Syndrome, and renal insufficiency. The language was limited to Chinese and English. Search strategies for PubMed are shown below:

#1: Search "adefovir dipivoxil"[All Fields]; #2: Search "Fanconi Syndrome"[Mesh]; #3: Search "osteomalacia"[Mesh]; #4: Search "hypophosphatemia"[All Fields]; #5: Search "renal insufficiency"[All Fields]; #6: Search (#2 OR #3 OR #4 OR #5) AND #1.

Relevant Chinese characters were used as keywords when searching Chinese databases.

All references from articles obtained through the databases were reviewed manually.

Inclusion criteria included three parts as follows: (1) Case reports or clinical studies reporting specific cases and conference abstracts with no formal published articles. (2) Safety-related events restricted to hypophosphatemia, osteomalacia and Fanconi syndrome. (3) Events listed occurred during the use of ADV in mono-therapy or combination therapy in naïve or rescue treatment for HBV infection.

Exclusion criteria included the following: (1) Published data that were recorded repeatedly or were lacking in details (e.g., without exact values for hypophosphatemia). (2) Clinical articles without specific case reports or including patients co-infected with HIV or hepatitis C. (3) Meta-analyses, systemic reviews and conference speeches with lack of details.

Data selection

Two authors (Nan C and Jian-bo Z) independently screened the titles and abstracts of the collected citations from primary searches. Relevant clinical studies were downloaded for specific case reports, as well as those meeting inclusion criteria. Disagreements between the two authors were resolved by discussion and, if needed, arbitrated by a third author (Kuan-xiao T).

Data extraction

A flow chart of the study selection process and exclusion criteria is shown in Fig. 1. One hundred and thirteen records were identified by the electronic database search. After removing duplicates, 109 articles were screened according to the inclusion/exclusion criteria. The remaining 101 full-text articles were assessed for eligibility. Of these articles, 20 were excluded (see S2 File for a list of reasons for exclusion). The remaining 81 articles were included in the final review. We divided patients into Chinese and Foreign groups according to their nationality (C for the Chinese group and F for the Foreign group). Data such as demographics, history (duration of CHB, hepatitis-related complications and comorbidity) and drug details (antiviral drugs, dose, time of starting and maintaining), clinical manifestation, tests, treatment and prognosis were obtained from published sources. The index of laboratory tests was rated according to the National Cancer Institute Common Toxicity Evaluation Standard (NCICTC) Edition 2.0 [11]. For hypophosphatemia, Grade 1 was defined as 0.60- < 0.80 mmol/L, Grade 2 was defined as 0.30- < 0.60 mmol/L, and Grade 3 was defined as < 0.30 mmol/L. For increased serum creatinine, Grade 1 was defined as ≤132.6 μmol/L (≤1.5 mg/dL), Grade 2 was defined as 132.6 μmol/L- ≤ 176.8 μmol/L (1.5- ≤ 2.0 mg/dL), and Grade 3 was defined as 176.

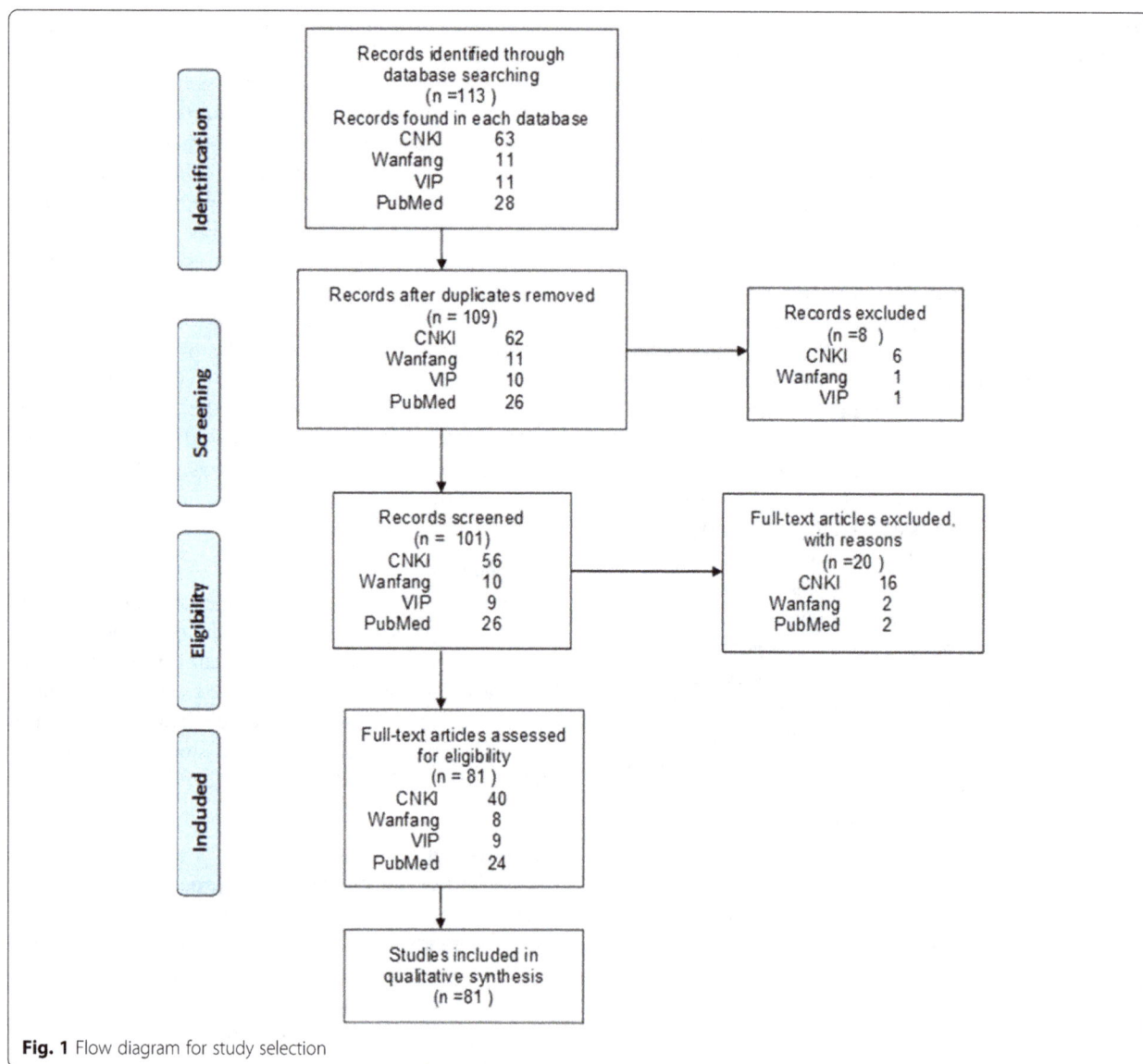

Fig. 1 Flow diagram for study selection

8 μmol/L - ≤ 265.2 μmol/L (2.0- ≤ 3.0 mg/dL). The grade classifications are well accepted [12].

Statistical analysis

Normally distributed data were described as the mean ± standard deviation, while a non-normal distribution was described as the median (inter-quartile range). Two independent sample *t*-tests were used for normally distributed data, while non-parametric tests were used for non-normal data. The count data were analyzed by a *Chi-square* test or *Fisher's exact* test. A *Mann-Whitney U* test of the two independent samples was used in count data with index variables distributed in one-way orderly, while a *Kruskal-Wallis H* test and rank correlation analysis were used for ordinal categories with different properties. A two-tailed P-value < 0.05 was considered to be statistically significant.

Results

Demographics (see Table 1)

There were 152 patients eligible for the study, with 120 patients allocated to the C group and 32 non-Chinese patients allocated to the F group. The C group was significantly younger than the F group (51.89 ± 10.96 years versus 56.47 ± 11.36 years, $t = -2.084$, $P = 0.039$). Of all the patients in both groups, the age distribution illustrated a gender difference, with males being predominant in the middle-aged group (62/116, 53.4%) and females being the majority in the older group (18/36, 50%) ($Z = -3.640$, $P < 0.001$). No similar tendency was detected in between-group comparisons, and there was no significant difference between the groups regarding gender (male to female, 3.29:1 versus 3:1, $\chi^2 = 0.039$, $P = 0.844$) and gender proportion among different age groups (males represented 57.6% versus 37.5% ($Z = -0.831$,

Table 1 Baseline characteristics in the C and F group

Characteristics	Descriptive statistics	C group	F group	Df	P Value
Case number	n	120	32		
Age	Mean ± SD	51.89 ± 10.96	56.47 ± 11.36	150	0.039[a]
	Range	22–79	31–81		
Gender				1	0.844[c]
Male	n (%)	92 (76.7%)	24 (75.0%)		
Female	n (%)	28 (23.3%)	8 (25.0%)		
Period of pain (months)	n	86	17	–	0.098[b]
	Median (Interquartile range)	18 (12–26.5)	13 (5.5–24)		
	Range	1–102	1–72		
ADV total treatment time (months)	n	115	30	–	0.939[b]
	Median (Interquartile range)	60 (36–72)	57 (38–69)		
	Range	5–144	9–132		
ADV treatment time of pain onset (months)	n	87	22	–	0.153[b]
	Median (Interquartile range)	36 (24–48)	47.5 (28–60)		
	Range	2–95	1–90		
BMI (kg/m^2)	n	8	5	11	0.192[a]
	Mean ± SD	21.21 ± 1.85	23.44 ± 3.98		
	Range	19.53–24.70	18.00–28.00		
Initial time of pain relief (months)	n	76	20	–	0.003[b]
	Median (Interquartile range)	1.5 (1–2)	3 (2–6)		
	Range	0.3–6.0	0.5–18.0		
Initial time of serum Phos. Rising (months)	n	53	11	–	0.115[b]
	Median (Interquartile range)	2 (1–3)	3.5 (1.75–6)		
	Range	0.3–12.0	0.5–11.0		

ADV Adefovir Dipivoxil, *BMI* body mass index, *Phos.* phosphate

[a]Two independent sample *t* test

[b]Two independent sample *Mann-Whitney U* test

[c]Fisher's exact test

$P = 0.406$), females represented 46.4% versus 62.5% ($Z = -0.956$, $P = 0.339$)). Asian nationalities accounted for 84.4% in the F group, which were mostly Korean (40.6%) and Japanese (31.3%). The other patients included 2 from France, 2 from Italy and 1 from Spain.

History
ADV history

The average duration of ADV therapy was 60 (36–72) months in C group and 57 (38–69) months in the F group ($Z = -0.076$, $P = 0.939$), while the duration of ADV therapy before ostalgia onset was 36 (24–48) months versus 47.5 (28–60) months ($Z = -1.428$, $P = 0.153$). Two to five years of ADV therapy accounted for most patients in both groups (55.7% versus 63.3%, $Z = -0.346$, $P = 0.729$). Although the differences were not significant, the C group tended to develop ostalgia 1–2 years earlier than the F group ($Z = -1.517$, $P = 0.129$). The ADV dosage was administered at 10 mg daily, except for 3 patients given 20 mg daily and 1 patient given 15 mg daily in the C group.

Other history

The median duration of CHB was 120 (84–195) months in the C group and 132 (46.5–210) months in the F group (only 5 patients recorded). No significant difference was observed in the proportion of liver cirrhosis (95.8% in the C group versus 83.3% in the F group, $P = 0.253$), LAM therapy before exposure to ADV (61.29% versus 76.50%, $\chi^2 = 1.739$, $P = 0.187$) or LAM add-on with ADV (38.71% versus 23.50%, $\chi^2 = 0.849$, $P = 0.357$). In addition, there were 6 different comorbid diseases in the C group, including 11 patients with hypertension, 7 with diabetes, and one each with gout, chronic bronchitis, Turner's syndrome and atopic dermatitis. In the F group, no available details were recorded except that 1 patient had epilepsy and 4 underwent surgery (femoral surgery in 2, kidney transplantation in 1 and subtotal gastrectomy in 1).

Clinical manifestation

Symptoms

All patients presented with persistent ostalgia, occurring originally in the lower limbs (e.g., ankle, knee) and aggravated after load-bearing. Commonly, pain perception progressed gradually from the lower limbs to the thorax, ribs, and upper joints, leading to difficulty in motion, staggering gait and passive position. Moreover, the patients usually complained of fatigue and loss of appetite. Some of them could barely stand up and pursue daily activities. Additionally, it is noted that 14 patients in the C group had non-specific symptoms, such as nocturia and peripheral paresthesia, before the initial onset of ostalgia.

Physical examination

For all patients, body mass index (BMI) was within the normal range (21.21 ± 1.85 kg/m^2 in the C group versus 23.44 ± 3.98 kg/m^2 in the F group, $t = -1.389$, $P = 0.192$). No significant difference was detected in the tenderness distribution of the two groups (see Fig. 2a). Moreover, Fig. 2b shows the detailed data of the abnormal signs recorded in the C group, which showed that a positive orthopedic special test (PST) had the highest incidence, followed by mobility limitation (ML), reduced muscle strength (RMS), and waddling gait.

Examinations

Laboratory examination (Table 2)

Bone mineral metabolism No significant difference was found in the reduction of serum phosphorus between the two groups. A Grade 1 decrease (0.60- < 0.80 mmol/L) was recorded in a total of 32.7% in the C group versus 25.8% in the F group, a Grade 2 (0.30- < 0.60 mmol/L) decrease was recorded in 63.7% versus 67.7%, and a Grade 3 (< 0.30 mmol/L) decrease was recorded in 3.5% versus 6.5% ($Z = -0.880$, $P = 0.379$). In addition, 71.4% versus 81.5% of patients had normal excretion of urine phosphorus ($Z = -0.617$, $P = 0.657$). Moreover, 71.6% versus 63.2% of patients developed hypocalcemia ($Z = -0.720$, $P = 0.472$). Interestingly, 85.7% versus 88.9 and 78.8% versus 83.3% of patients had a normal level of 25-(OH) D3 ($Z = -0.249$, $P = 0.804$) [13–17] and PTH ($Z = -0.289$, $P = 0.772$), respectively. The C group had more information regarding bone biochemical metabolism, and 5.3, 93.8 and 76.9% of patients had increased levels of osteocalcin, Type I tropocollagen amino terminal extension of the peptide (PINP), and special series I type collagen peptide carboxyl end β (β-CTX), respectively, which reflected activation of both osteoblasts and osteoclasts. Though the F group had a higher mean value of alkaline phosphatase (AKP), 81.8% versus 100% of patients had drastically increased AKP. It is not difficult to conclude that patients with ADV-induced HO have hypophosphatemia,

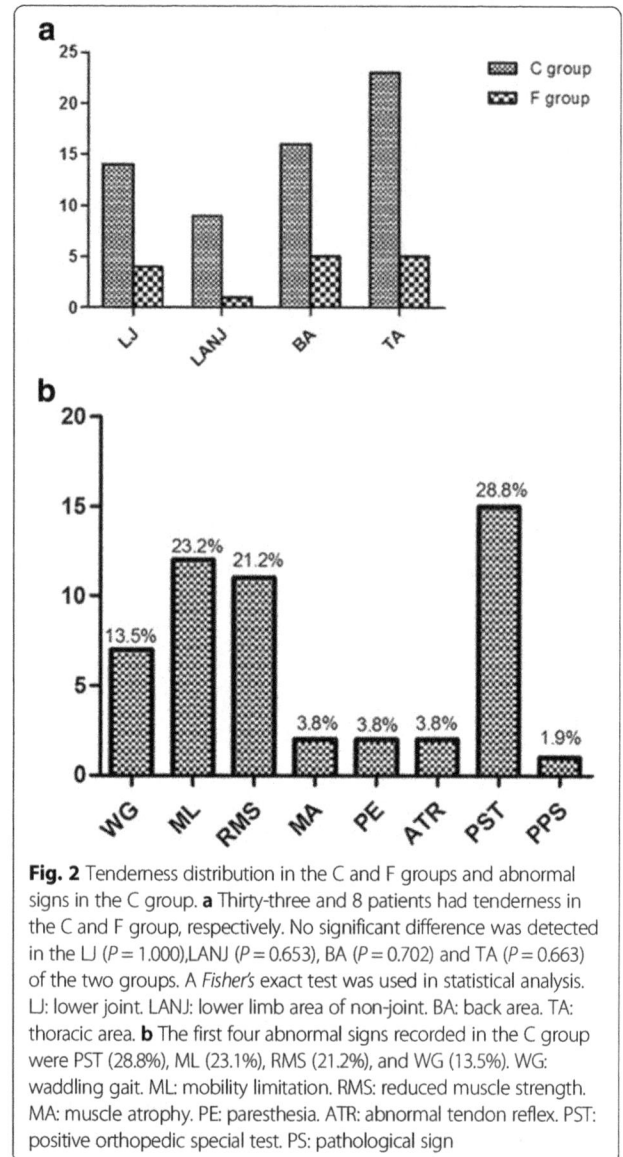

Fig. 2 Tenderness distribution in the C and F groups and abnormal signs in the C group. **a** Thirty-three and 8 patients had tenderness in the C and F group, respectively. No significant difference was detected in the LJ ($P = 1.000$),LANJ ($P = 0.653$), BA ($P = 0.702$) and TA ($P = 0.663$) of the two groups. A *Fisher's* exact test was used in statistical analysis. LJ: lower joint. LANJ: lower limb area of non-joint. BA: back area. TA: thoracic area. **b** The first four abnormal signs recorded in the C group were PST (28.8%), ML (23.1%), RMS (21.2%), and WG (13.5%). WG: waddling gait. ML: mobility limitation. RMS: reduced muscle strength. MA: muscle atrophy. PE: paresthesia. ATR: abnormal tendon reflex. PST: positive orthopedic special test. PS: pathological sign

hypocalcemia, and increased levels of alkaline phosphatase (AKP), which is essentially different from osteoporosis in bone and mineral metabolism, with the latter including over-activated bone reabsorption. Interestingly, most patients had a normal level of 25(OH)VitD3 in both groups.

Biochemical metabolism No significant difference was found in the level blood uric acid, serum creatinine, plasma glucose and serum PH. Hypouricemia was seen in 90.8% of patients in the C group and 100% in the F group ($Z = -1.089$, $P = 0.276$). The C group was more prone to experiencing hypokalemia, with an average serum potassium of 3.48 ± 0.40 mmol/L versus 3.75 ± 0.42 mmol/L ($t = -2.01$, $P = 0.048$). Of note, 88.4% versus 78.9% of patients had increased serum creatinine in Grade 1 ($Z = -1.090$, $P = 0.276$). Interestingly,

Table 2 Biochemical parameters in the C and F group

Biochemical parameters[*]		C group		F group		Df	P value	Ref. range
	n	mean±SD or median (IQ range)	n	mean±SD or median (IQ range)				
Blood								
PH[#]	37	7.36(7.33–7.39)	4	7.32(7.28–7.36)	–	0.109[b]	7.35–7.45
Phos. (mmol/L)	117	0.54 ± 0.15	31	0.49 ± 0.14	146	0.115[a]	0.81–1.45
Ca^{2+} (mmol/L)	81	2.18 ± 0.13	19	2.11 ± 0.28	98	0.305[a]	2.25–2.75
K^+ (mmol/L)	80	3.48 ± 0.40	10	3.75 ± 0.42	88	0.048[a]	3.5–5.5
UA (umol/L)	65	110(90.65–131.85)	13	107(95.20–152.85)	–	0.406[b]	210–420
BG (mmol/L)	33	5.02(4.75–5.36)	4	5.55(4.70–5.93)	–	0.352[b]	3.9–5.6
SCr (umol/L)	69	107.71 ± 28.75	19	115.65 ± 32.20	86	0.302[a]	44.2–88.4
25-(OH)VitD3 (ng/ml) [&]	42	15.45(12.90–21.75)	9	23.50(11.80–29.80)	–	0.236[b]	9–52
PTH (ng/ml)	52	30.56(23.84–48.22)	18	28.37(20.00–46.96)	–	0.657[b]	15–65
AKP (IU/L)	94	240.5(179.8–317.0)	25	698(324.5–1160.0)	–	<0.001[b]	40–150
Urine								
Phos./24 h (mmol/24 h)	35	18.81 ± 10.39	8	21.69 ± 8.98	41	0.473[a]	12.9–42.0
Ca^{2+} /24 h (mmol/24 h)	26	9.23 ± 4.31	9	7.19 ± 4.50	33	0.234[a]	2.5–7.5
Protein/24 h (mmol/24 h)	34	1.00 ± 0.49	10	1.16 ± 0.43	42	0.361[a]	< 0.15
NAG (U/L)	10	35.5 (27.0–55.15)	4	22.8 (13.65–43.35)	–	0.239[b]	2–18
β2-MG (mg/L)	14	13.71 (5.13–81.3)	4	77.1 (50.58–119.32)	–	0.110[b]	< 0.2

[*]Different sample size has been given for different parameters in the C and the F group order
[#]Only 3 patients had urine PH record, they were 6.5, 7.5, 7.5, respectively
[a]Two independent sample t test
[b]Two independent sample Mann-Whitney U test
[&]The range was set according to published reports [13–17]

positive urine glucose was detected in both groups, even in those without diabetes. Both groups had markedly elevated urinary β2-microglobulin (β2-MG). Though no significant differences were noted, the C group had a lower rate of N-acetyl beta D glucose anhydride enzyme (NAG) increase (87.5% versus 100%) and proteinuria over 0.5 g per 24 h (82.4% versus 100%). Furthermore, the C group also had less tendency to develop acidosis despite a median serum PH value (40% versus 83.3%) at the lower limit of the normal range.

A significant inverse correlation between age and serum creatinine was found in the C ($\gamma = -0.820$, $P = 0.005$) and F group ($\gamma = -0.840$, $P = 0.006$). This correlation was not seen in age and serum phosphorus or in serum creatinine and serum phosphorus. For 20 patients with severe proteinuria, no correlation was observed with serum creatinine. Hypophosphatemia, hypouricemia, hypocalcemia, and proximal renal tubular dysfunction were characterized by an increased excretion of urine phosphorus, calcium, β2-MG, NAG, severe proteinuria and renal tubular acidosis, which are commonly present in ADV-related HO. No correlation was found between hypophosphatemia and age or serum creatinine. In contrast to conventional wisdom, serum creatinine did not show a positive trend

with age and was insensitive for the detection of early pathological alterations.

Imaging examination

No significant difference was found in the results of bone mineral density by dual energy X-ray absorptiometry (DEXA), with 65.2% in the C group versus 62.5% in the F group, which had a T score below − 2.5 standard deviation (SD), as well as a distribution of abnormality in the ^{99m}Tc-MDP whole body bone scintigraphy. There were increased multiple foci with radiotracer symmetrically distributed in the area of the lower joints (ankles, knees, sacroiliac joints, and hips), upper joints (shoulders), thorax (ribs), back (spines), and skull. In addition, 4 patients in the C group were diagnosed with neurogenic damage through an electromyogram.

Cytology examination

No comparison was conducted in this situation since there was a significant difference in sample size. Twenty patients in the C group had a renal biopsy, of whom 18 displayed proximal tubular epithelium atrophy and dramatic vacuolization of epithelial cells with a fading of the brush border and 9 had simultaneous glomeruli lesions. The other two patients were diagnosed with IgA nephropathy by electron microscopy. Renal biopsy was reported in only two patients in the F group. One patient had significant renal tubular lesions, while the other had lesions limited to the glomeruli. Three patients had bone biopsies in the F group, and the biopsies mainly showed local osteoid accumulation and a lack of mineralization. One patient had a muscle biopsy in the C and F groups, and no significant abnormality was found in response to myasthenia. Multiple myeloma was excluded for one patient having bone marrow cytology in the C group.

Misdiagnosis and diagnosis
Misdiagnosis
Twenty-seven patients in the C group (Fig. 3) reported misdiagnosis. Osteoporosis (10/27, 18.0%), ankylosing spondylitis (9/27, 16.0%), lumbar disc herniation (6/27, 12.0%), osteoarthritis (4/27, 10.0%) and bone tumors (4/27, 10.0%) were more frequent. For the F group, only 3 patients had misdiagnoses, including osteoporosis, ankylosing spondylitis and Paget's disease.

Diagnosis
All of the patients were diagnosed with hypophosphatemia and developed hypophosphatemic osteomalacia except for 10 patients in the C group who only reported hypophosphatemia. General damage of proximal renal tubular function, namely, Fanconi syndrome, was recorded in 57 patients in the C group versus 16 in the F group.

Treatment and prognosis
Treatment (Table 3)

Antiviral drugs There was a significant difference in the proportion of ADV dosage adjustment; 89% of patients in the C group versus 67.9% in the F group had treatment discontinuation ($\chi^2 = 5.652$, $P = 0.017$), while 4.4% versus 28.6% had reduced ADV dosage or a prolonged dosage interval ($\chi^2 = 13.802$, $P < 0.001$). Furthermore, 56% versus 36.7% of patients replaced ADV with entecavir after ADV discontinuation ($\chi^2 = 3.542$, $P = 0.06$).

Bone mineral metabolism regulation
There was no significant difference in the proportion of phosphate (58.2% versus 71.4%, $\chi^2 = 1.570$, $P = 0.210$) or vitamin D3 (57.1% versus 42.9%, $\chi^2 = 1.758$, $P = 0.185$) supplementation between the two groups. The C group was more prone to supplement with calcium than the F group (51.6% versus 10.7%, $\chi^2 = 14.726$, $P < 0.001$).

Prognosis (Table 4)

Time of symptom remission Significant differences were found in the median time of pain remission (1.5 (1, 2) months in the C group versus 3 (2, 6) months in the F group, $Z = -2.951$, $P = 0.003$), with the C group being more likely to recover in the first 3 months (91.3% of patients in the C group versus 56.3% in the F group, $Z = -3.013$, $P = 0.001$).

Recovery of serology Though no significant difference was observed in the median time of resolution of serum

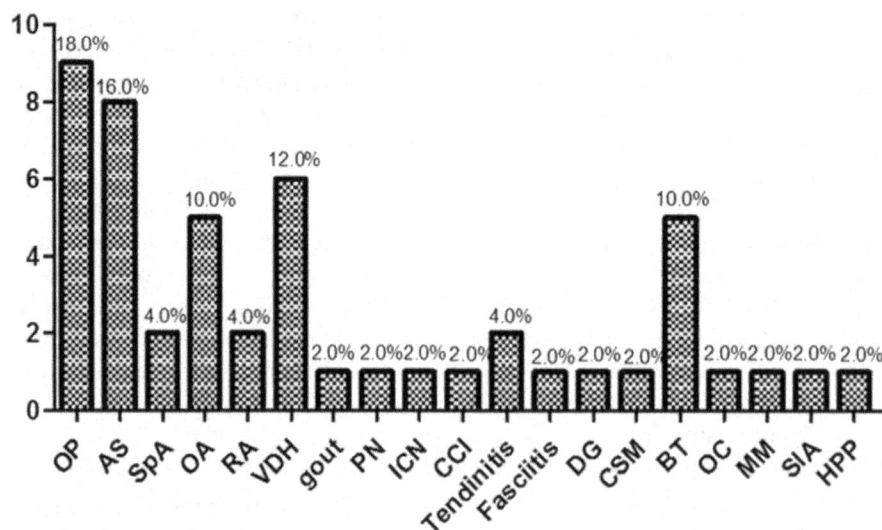

Fig. 3 Misdiagnosis in the C group. Osteoporosis accounted for the most common misdiagnosis (18%), followed by AS (16%), VDH (12%), OA (10%) and BT (10%). OP: osteoporosis. AS: ankylosing spondylitis. SpA: spondyloarthropathy. OA: osteoarthropathy. RA: rheumatoid arthritis. VDH: vertebral disc herniation. PN: peripheral neuropathy. ICN: intercostal neuralgia. CCI: costochondritis. DG: degeneration. CSM: cervical spondylosis myelopathy. BT: bone tumor. OC: osteochondroma. MM: multiple myeloma. SIA: sacroiliac arthritis. HPP: hypopotassium periodic paralysis

Table 3 Treatment in the C and F group*

Treatment	Presence	Absence	Df	P value
cADV[#]			1	0.017[b]
C	81(89.0%)	10(11.0%)		
F	19(67.9%)	9(32.1%)		
rADV			1	0.001[b]
C	4(4.4%)	87(95.6%)		
F	8(28.6%)	20(71.4%)		
ETV			1	0.060[a]
C	51(56.0%)	40(44.0%)		
F	10(35.7%)	18(64.3%)		
Phos.			1	0.210[a]
C	53(58.2%)	38(41.8%)		
F	20(71.4%)	8(28.6%)		
Calcium			1	0.001[a]
C	47(51.6%)	44(48.4%)		
F	3 (10.7%)	25(89.3%)		
Calcitriol			1	0.185[a]
C	52(57.1%)	39(42.9%)		
F	12(42.9%)	16(57.1%)		
BM			1	0.755[b]
C	6(6.6%)	85(93.4%)		
F	3(10.7%)	25(89.3%)		

*Ninety-one and 28 patients had treatment in the C and F group, respectively
cADV ceased Adefovir Dipivoxil, *rADV* reduced Adefovir Dipivoxil, *ETV* entecavir, *Phos.* Phosphate supplement, *Calcium* Calcium supplement, *Calcitriol* Calcitriol supplement, *BM* drugs regulating bone metabolism
[a]*Pearson Chi-square test*
[b]Corrected *Pearson Chi-square test*

Table 4 Time of symptom and serology recovery*

	C group	F group	P-value
Initial time of pain relief (months)			0.001[a]
≤1	37(46.3%)	3(18.8%)	
1<T≤3	36(45.0%)	6(37.5%)	
>3	7(8.8%)	7(43.8%)	
Initial time of serum Phos. Rising (months)			0.099[a]
≤1	19(35.2%)	2(20.0%)	
1<T≤3	25(46.3%)	3(30.0%)	
3<T≤6	6(11.1%)	4(40.0%)	
>6	4(7.4%)	1(10.0%)	

*Eighty and 16 patients recorded the initial time of pain relief in C and F group, respectively, and 54 and 10 patients recorded the initial time of serum Phos. Rising
[a]Two independent sample *Mann-Whitney U* test

phosphorus (2 (1, 3) months in the C group versus 3.5 (1.75, 6) months in the F group, $Z = -1.157$, $P = 0.115$), the C group tended to recover in the first three months (81.5% of patients versus 50%, $Z = -1.649$, $P = 0.099$).

Here, we reported a Chinese woman with generalized bone pain for 8 months without antecedent trauma. The study was approved by the ethics committee of Qilu Hospital of Shandong University, and the study protocol conformed to the ethical guidelines of the 1975 Declaration of Helsinki. The individual in this manuscript had given written informed consent to publish the case details.

The patient was a 43-year-old woman with chronic hepatitis B for more than eight years. ADV was administered from diagnosis until the occurrence of pain initiating from the foot joints eight months ago. No remarkable history of hypertension or renal insufficiency was noted. She experienced progressive bone pain extending from the lower limbs to the lower back and ribs in the next two months. Laboratory tests showed a serum phosphorus level of 0.62 mmol/L, a calcium level of 2.21 mmol/L, and an AKP of 160 U/L. Urine testing revealed proteinuria

and glucosuria. Electrolytes from the urinalysis showed a calcium level of 19.84 mmol/24 h, a potassium level of 74.48 mmol/24 h, and a phosphate level of 35.77 mmol/24 h. Impaired renal tubular reabsorption was noted as a drastic increase of urine micro-albumin (75.8 mg/L) and β2-microglobulin (11.8 mg/L). Bone biochemical metabolism tests showed a decreased level of 25-OH vitamin D with no further abnormalities. DEXA detected a decreased femur neck mineral density (BMD) with a mean Z-score of − 3.0 standard deviations. The whole-body ^{99m}Tc-MDP diphosphonate bone scintigraphy (Fig. 4) showed increased symmetrical uptake in the ankles, knees, hips, sacroiliac joints and multiple ribs and increased diffuse uptake in the limbs, pelvis, spine, sternum and skull. A clinical diagnosis of ADV-induced HO with secondary Fanconi syndrome was suspected. ADV was discontinued and supplementation with oral phosphate, calcium, and vitamin D was started. The patient's symptoms improved after two weeks, and the serum phosphorus increased to 0.63 mmol/L. Systemic pain was adequately relieved one month after discharge. Two months later, all of the symptoms disappeared, and the serum phosphorus returned to normal (no test data available).

Discussion

To the best of our knowledge, this is the first study to investigate the differences among the demographics, clinical manifestation, tests, treatment and prognosis in ADV-related HO between Chinese and non-Chinese CHB patients. Several studies have shown that males older than 50 years are at an increased risk of developing HO [5, 12]. Consistently, middle-aged males were highly vulnerable to HO in our study. Moreover, it seems that being a middle-aged male may be a predictor of HO regardless of nationality. Chinese patients were prone to developing HO earlier, which might due to the difference in sample size. Potential gender-specific association

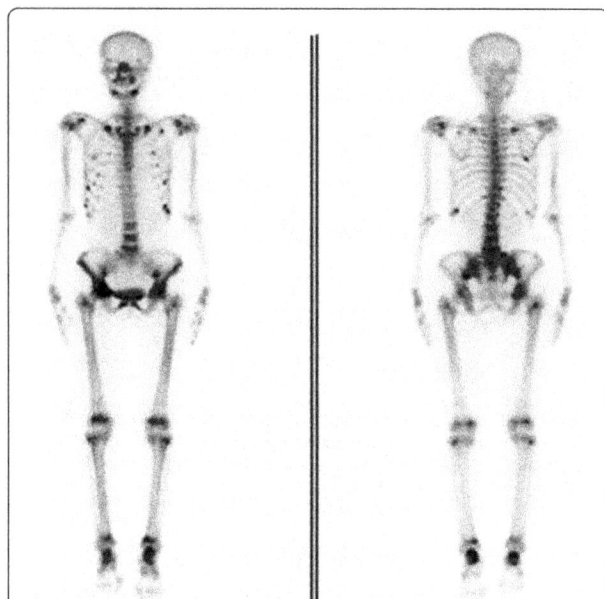

Fig. 4 ^{99m}Tc-MDP diphosphonate bone scintigraphy of the patient discussed above. A technetium bone scan showed multifocal lesions which distributed to the bilateral ankles, knees, hips, pelvis, ribs, and shoulders symmetrically, while the lesions were dispersed in the skull, sternum, spine and limbs

of HO with ADV need to be elucidated in further studies for females. The elderly seemed to be more predisposed to HO. Such considerable age difference in genders regarding the incidence of HO may partly be explained by the variance in bone structure and strength, body fat deposition, sex hormone levels, and the risk of falls between men and women [18]. Intriguingly, the F group is predisposed compared to Asian nationals, probably due to the high incidence of hepatitis B in Asians, race differences and personal genetic susceptibility [19, 20].

Hypophosphatemia mostly occurs one year after ADV therapy in a time- and dosage-dependent manner [12, 21]. As shown in our study, the median course before onset of HO was 3–4 years, with Chinese patients predisposed earlier occurrence, indicating a preexistence of underlying hypophosphatemia. The symptoms of patients varied from mild, such as fatigue, muscle weakness and paresthesia, to severe skeletal pain, disabling myopathy, walking difficulty, and even fractures. However, for some patients, ostalgia never occurred, which might due to differences in duration of CHB, the severity of hypophosphatemia and personal tolerance. Non-specific malnutrition causing muscle atrophy is commonly present in CHB patients with decreased muscle strength, which in turn decreases bone mineral density [22].

Hypophosphatemic osteomalacia (HO) is one of the serious adverse events of ADV, which is mainly related to proximal renal tubular dysfunction. The underlying mechanisms have not been well-explained. ADV is excreted from the kidney in its original form; human organic anion transporter 1 (hOAT1) in the basolateral membrane of the proximal renal tubules [23] and multidrug resistance–associated protein type 2 (MRP2) in the apical membrane [24] control basolateral uptake and luminal excretion, respectively. The polymorphism of genes encoding these two drug transporters may play a role in individual susceptibility [25], leading to generalized dysfunction of proximal renal tubular reabsorption after exposure to ADV. Moreover, ADV has a low-level activity against mitochondrial DNA polymerase-γ when inhibiting HBV-DNA polymerase simultaneously, ultimately leading to mitochondrial dysfunction, impaired oxidative phosphorylation, and tissue injury [26]. Nonetheless, differences in general health and personal tolerance might result in different clinical phenotypes of mitochondrial toxicity [27], leading to differences in the clinical spectrum.

Moreover, it must be outlined that renal abnormalities are frequently observed in patients without any oral antihepatitis B virus treatment. In a cross-section study, Amet et al. [28] found that the prevalence of renal dysfunction in CHB patients was approximately 64.6% and emphasized the necessity for regular monitoring of renal function. Several studies [5, 12, 29, 30] showed middle-aged male patients, especially those with cirrhosis, were more vulnerable, because low-grade renal abnormalities are frequently found in such patients with a history of CHB. Our study showed that over 80% of patients in both groups developed renal tubular dysfunction with elevated β2-MG and NAG. Furthermore, severe proteinuria frequently occurred in the patients, even if serum creatinine was still normal or near normal. The underlying mechanisms are unknown. One study reported that the expression of hepatitis B virus in kidney tissues through an immune-complex mechanism [31] results in direct pathological lesion and chronic immunologic injury. Interestingly, in contrast to common sense, serum creatinine is not positively correlated with age in such patients. However, it should be noted that the extent to which ADV contributed to the observed renal abnormalities was confounded by the concomitant use of nephrotoxic medications, including valproic acid in epilepsy [32], and co-morbid conditions such as diabetes, hypertension and non-alcoholic fatty disease [33].

A small number of patients in both groups were exposed to LAM therapy before ADV or had ADV treatment after LAM intolerance. Whether LAM increases renal toxicity remained undetermined until recently. Recent studies showed that LAM was not a risk factor for renal impairment in either the univariate or multivariate analysis [5]. Additional studies are necessary to elucidate the renal safety of LAM.

Metabolic disturbances of bone are common complications in patients with chronic liver disease, mainly osteoporosis [34]. Our study showed that more than 80% of patients had cirrhosis, over 70% had osteopenia, and over 60% had moderate hypophosphatemia. Though osteoporosis accounted for a large portion of misdiagnoses, a total of 142 (93.4%) patients were diagnosed with osteomalacia. Multiple factors, such as vitamin D deficiency, low levels of osteocalcin, PTH, insulin growth factor-1(IGF-1), hypogonadism, behavioral factors such as low body mass index (BMI), malnutrition [35], and a sedentary lifestyle with physical inactivity [36] are frequently observed in these patients, especially those with cirrhosis. There is no doubt that long-term administration of antiviral therapy in such patients would further increase the risk of bone loss resulting from decreased remodeling of bone in the absence of adequate phosphorus and calcium, leading to softening and distortion of the skeleton. Unexpectedly, over 85% of patients maintained a normal level of 25-(OH) D3 in our study [37], which may be explained by the heterogeneity of the subjects in different reports and by differences in the statistical methods used.

According to our present study, routine renal function tests based on serum creatinine are not sensitive enough to detect early abnormalities of renal structure and function [38]. Previous studies have demonstrated biomarkers such as fractional excretion of filtered phosphate (FEPO4) [39], retinol-binding protein (RBP) and N-acetylglucosamine (NAG) [40] may be used for early renal tubular injury detection during long-term ADV treatment. No complete data can be found in the application of the above indices in our study, which implicates that tests reflecting early kidney injury are still not yet widely implemented in the daily clinical setting. In addition, significant differences found in serum potassium and AKP may due to differences in the sample size and methods used. ADV-related nephrotoxicity manifests as a proximal renal tubular dysfunction and is primarily featured by the onset of gradual decreases in serum phosphorus, usually mild to moderate in severity, and can be accompanied by changes in serum potassium, bicarbonate, uric acid, glycosuria, and proteinuria. Though lacking predictor analysis, we still emphasize the importance of monitoring serum phosphorus, calcium, AKP, urine electrolytes, serum uric acid, urine routine testing, and biomarkers of renal tubular injury (NAG, β2-MG, FEPO4) during long-term ADV therapy. Special care is needed, especially for differential diagnoses, since oeteomalacia and osteoporosis commonly co-exist in such patients, and both are characterized by reduced bone mineral density, diffuse bone pain and susceptibility to fracture. Radiologically, pseudofractures are seen most commonly in stress-bearing bones of

osteomalacia patients in 99mTc-MDP whole body bone scintigraphy. 99mTc-MDP whole body bone scintigraphy would be preferable to diagnose osteomalacia primarily characterized by mineralization defects, despite the ability of DEXA to diagnose osteoporosis.

Treatment of ADV-induced HO is still not well established. Modification of risk factors involving smoking, alcohol and malnutrition is of prime importance. Some studies suggest that changes of the antiviral drug are more favorable than a phosphate regimen for the purpose of bone protection, preferring dosing-interval adjustment [41, 42]. In this respect, our study showed that Chinese patients were more prone to ADV withdrawal, while non-Chinese patients were prone to dosage adjustment. However, comprehensive consideration, including the potential risk for viral breakthrough, aggravation of liver function, therapy cost and tolerance, is essential before adjustment. For most mildly affected patients, dosage interval adjustment or termination is sufficient without further phosphate supplementation, while for severe cases, phosphate supplementation is indispensable. Our study indicated that both groups adopted phosphate supplementation, in combination with vitamin D3 supplementation, whereas Chinese patients more commonly had calcium supplementation. Several patients were treated with drugs that regulate bone metabolism, such as calcitonin. It is important to note that calcitonin is not optimal, since it can reduce renal tubular phosphate reabsorption and inhibit osteoclast activity even though it has obvious analgesic functions [43]. Other drugs affecting proximal renal tubular reabsorption, such as valproic [32], should also be adjusted. Individual differences in bone remodeling period, duration of CHB, and comorbidity (e.g., osteoporosis) may result in different times to remission. Our study showed that the resolution of proximal renal tubular dysfunction started in the first month, and most patients did not resolve completely until three months of treatment, with Chinese patients being prone to resolve earlier. We consider such variable responses to therapy to be a result of race differences and bias in reports. On the whole, ADV-induced abnormalities are reversible after appropriate drug modification, and remission is predictable at the first month of therapy.

In addition, differences in group samples and the absence of multivariable analysis limit the power of our study. A large clinical prospective case-control study is required to further elucidate the risk factors and assist clinical implementation.

There are limitations in this study. First, this is a retrospective study, and it was hard to collect all of the required lab parameters. Second, multivariate analysis is a useful way to show figures more clearly, but considering the loss of effective information, it is impossible to analyze in that way. Third, the smaller population in the F group compared to the Chinese group leads to a deviation error in the conclusions. Further investigation with more detailed information is in process and will be published in the future.

To date, there are no common definition for adequate vitamin D status measured as 25(OH)D serum concentrations, and the range of 25-(OH) D3 varies from article to article. National Institute of Health, Office of Dietary Supplements, considered 25(OH) D levels < 12 ng/ml as 25-(OH) D3 deficiency, and 12-< 20 ng/ml as insufficient and > 20 ng/ml sufficient. However, some researchers and clinicians defined 25-(OH) D3 deficiency as < 20 ng/ml [44]. Besides, explanations of the normal ranges for 25-(OH) D3 in adults and children from ARUP laboratories (one of the major reference laboratories in the USA) are present in http://ltd.aruplab.com/Tests/Pdf/203. In the current study, we collected the information from various case reports and other clinical reports, which is closed to NIH Office of Dietary supplements definition. Moreover, the level of 25-(OH) D3 is a composition of endogenous synthesis of 25-(OH) D3 as well as absorption of exogenous 25-(OH) D3, and variation between different races and even different countries because of diet, geological and other factors might also contribute to the difference for the normal range of 25-(OH) D3.

In conclusion, middle-aged male patients have a higher risk of HO during long-term ADV treatment, especially those with cirrhosis, and Chinese patients are more prone to develop HO earlier than foreign patients. Sufficient attention is needed for older females, regardless of nationality. The clinical picture and laboratory and radiograph alterations are the most important factors in the diagnosis for those suspected of HO and are characterized by polyarthralgia, renal tubular dysfunction, and mineralization defects. Routine tests are not appropriate. Monitoring early indicators reflecting proximal renal tubular function before and during exposure to ADV is paramount, because renal abnormalities are still revisable after prophylactic or therapeutic intervention. Prognosis is good after adjustment of ADV therapy, and phosphate as well as calcium supplementation might be necessary otherwise.

Conclusions

Our results show that attention should be paid to middle-aged males before and during exposure to long-term ADV therapy in both the Chinese patients and selected non-Chinese patients included in our study. Clues such as clinical picture and laboratory and radiograph alterations are necessary for suspected patients, and they are characterized by polyarthralgia, renal tubular dysfunction and mineralization defects. Implementation of an early renal tubular injury index is beneficial for higher-risk patients to avoid further renal injuries.

Abbreviations
ADV: Adefovir dipivoxil; AKP: Alkaline phosphatase; BMI: Body mass index; CHB: Chronic viral hepatitis B; CNKI: Chinese National Knowledge Infrastructure; DEXA: Dual energy X-ray absorptiometry; eGFR: Evaluated glomerular filtration rate; HO: Hypophosphatemic osteomalacia; IGF-1: Insulin growth factor-1; LAM: Lipoarabinomannan; ML: Mobility limitation; MRP2: Multidrug resistance–associated protein type 2; NAG: N-acetyl beta D glucose anhydride enzyme; NAG: N-acetylglucosamine; PST: Positive orthopedic special test; RBP: Retinol-binding protein; RMS: Reduced muscle strength; SD: Standard deviation; VIP: Chinese Science and Technology Journal Database; β-CTX: Collagen peptide carboxyl endβ

Acknowledgments
We would like to thank the patient for letting us share her medical history. We also would like to thank our colleagues, including Mei Cheng, Zhenxia Han, Qian Cai, and Chunli Fu, for the careful diagnosis, treatment and nursing care during the case.

Funding
Special Research Fund of Clinical Medicine of the Chinese Medical Association (13060990484), the Natural Science Foundation of Shandong Province (ZR2015HM074), Key Research and Development Plan of Shandong Province (2016GSF201014), and the Joint Scientific Research Fund of Shandong University (11671315).

Authors' contributions
KXT designed the study. NC and YPZ prepared the first draft of the paper. NC and JBZ were responsible for statistical analysis of the data. QJZ and LYL designed the methodology for searching. NC, QJZ, TP, LWL, FY and XY performed the data collection. All authors revised the paper critically for intellectual content and approved the final version. All authors agree to be accountable for the work and to ensure that any questions relating to the accuracy and integrity of the paper are investigated and properly resolved.

Competing interests
The authors declare that they have no competing interests.

Author details
[1]Department of Geriatrics, Qilu Hospital of Shandong University, Jinan, Shandong, China. [2]Department of Emergency, Qilu Hospital of Shandong University, Jinan, Shandong, China. [3]Department of Orthopedics, Qilu Hospital of Shandong University, Jinan, Shandong, China. [4]Department of Endocrinology and Metabolism, First People's Hospital of Jinan City, Jinan, Shandong, China. [5]Department of Nephrology, Qilu Hospital of Shandong University, Jinan, Shandong, China. [6]Present Address: Department of Geriatrics, Qilu Hospital of Shandong University, No. 107, Wenhua Xi Road, Jinan, Shandong 250012, People's Republic of China.

References
1.   Lim SG, Marcellin P, Tassopoulos N, Hadziyannis S, Chang TT, Tong M, Sievert W, Hu P, Arterburn S, Brosgart CL, et al. Clinical trial: effects of

adefovir dipivoxil therapy in Asian and Caucasian patients with chronic hepatitis B. Aliment Pharmacol Ther. 2007;26(10):1419–28.

2. Lavanchy D. Hepatitis B virus epidemiology, disease burden, treatment, and current and emerging prevention and control measures. J Viral Hepat. 2004; 11(2):97–107.

3. Segovia MC, Chacra W, Gordon SC. Adefovir dipivoxil in chronic hepatitis B: history and current uses. Expert Opin Pharmacother. 2012;13(2):245–54.

4. Ha NB, Ha NB, Garcia RT, Trinh HN, Vu AA, Nguyen HA, Nguyen KK, Levitt BS, Nguyen MH. Renal dysfunction in chronic hepatitis B patients treated with adefovir dipivoxil. Hepatology. 2009;50(3):727–34.

5. Kim YJ, Cho HC, Sinn DH, Gwak GY, Choi MS, Koh KC, Paik SW, Yoo BC, Lee JH. Frequency and risk factors of renal impairment during long-term adefovir dipivoxil treatment in chronic hepatitis B patients. J Gastroenterol Hepatol. 2012;27(2):306–12.

6. Gara N, Zhao X, Collins MT, Chong WH, Kleiner DE, Jake Liang T, Ghany MG, Hoofnagle JH. Renal tubular dysfunction during long-term adefovir or tenofovir therapy in chronic hepatitis B. Aliment Pharmacol Ther. 2012; 35(11):1317–25.

7. Shimizu M, Furusyo N, Ikezaki H, Ogawa E, Hayashi T, Ihara T, Harada Y, Toyoda K, Murata M, Hayashi J. Predictors of kidney tubular dysfunction induced by adefovir treatment for chronic hepatitis B. World J Gastroenterol. 2015;21(7):2116–23.

8. Shimizu Y, Hiraoka A, Yamago H, Shiraishi A, Imai Y, Tatsukawa H, Tanihira T, Miyata H, Ninomiya T, Tokumoto Y, et al. Hypophosphatemia in patients with hepatitis B virus infection undergoing long-term adefovir dipivoxil therapy. Hepatol Res. 2014;44(11):1081–7.

9. Xu LJ, Jiang Y, Liao RX, Zhang HB, Mao JF, Chi Y, Li M, Wang O, Liu XQ, Liu ZY, et al. Low-dose adefovir dipivoxil may induce Fanconi syndrome: clinical characteristics and long-term follow-up for Chinese patients. Antivir Ther. 2015;20(6):603–11.

10. Yang S, Du A, Zhang Y, Shen L. Meta-analysis of personality of child abuse in China. West Indian Med J. 2015; https://doi.org/10.7727/wimj.2015.135.

11. Cancer therapy evaluation program, common toxicity criteria. Version 2.0. CTD, NCI, NIH, DHHS, March 1998, revised March 23, 1998; published date: April 30, 1999; http://clep.cancer.gov/forms/ctcv20_4-30-992.pdf.

12. Tanaka M, Suzuki F, Seko Y, Hara T, Kawamura Y, Sezaki H, Hosaka T, Akuta N, Kobayashi M, Suzuki Y, et al. Renal dysfunction and hypophosphatemia during long-term lamivudine plus adefovir dipivoxil therapy in patients with chronic hepatitis B. J Gastroenterol. 2014;49(3):470–80.

13. Gifre L, Peris P, Monegal A, Martinez de Osaba MJ, Alvarez L, Guanabens N. Osteomalacia revisited : a report on 28 cases. Clin Rheumatol. 2011;30(5):639–45.

14. Wang BF, Wang Y, Wang BY, Sun FR, Zhang D, Chen YS. Osteomalacia and Fanconi's syndrome caused by long-term low-dose adefovir dipivoxil. J Clin Pharm Ther. 2015;40(3):345–8.

15. Law ST, Li KK, Ho YY. Nephrotoxicity, including acquired Fanconi's syndrome, caused by adefovir dipivoxil - is there a safe dose? J Clin Pharm Ther. 2012;37(2):128–31.

16. Kawate H, Taketomi A, Watanabe T, Nomura M, Kato M, Sakamoto R, Ikegami T, Soejima Y, Maehara Y, Takayanagi R. Hypophosphatemic osteomalacia as a long-term complication after liver transplantation. Transplantation. 2011;91(1):e6–8.

17. Wu C, Zhang H, Qian Y, Wang L, Gu X, Dai Z. Hypophosphatemic osteomalacia and renal Fanconi syndrome induced by low-dose adefovir dipivoxil: a case report and literature review suggesting ethnic predisposition. J Clin Pharm Ther. 2013;38(4):321–6.

18. Li M, Xu Y, Xu M, Ma L, Wang T, Liu Y, Dai M, Chen Y, Lu J, Liu J, et al. Association between nonalcoholic fatty liver disease (NAFLD) and osteoporotic fracture in middle-aged and elderly Chinese. J Clin Endocrinol Metab. 2012;97(6):2033–8.

19. Chen YC, Su YC, Li CY, Wu CP, Lee MS. A nationwide cohort study suggests chronic hepatitis B virus infection increases the risk of end-stage renal disease among patients in Taiwan. Kidney Int. 2015;87(5): 1030–8.

20. Chen YC, Su YC, Li CY, Hung SK. 13-year nationwide cohort study of chronic kidney disease risk among treatment-naive patients with chronic hepatitis B in Taiwan. BMC Nephrol. 2015;16:110.

21. Wei Z, He JW, Fu WZ, Zhang ZL. Osteomalacia induced by long-term low-dose adefovir dipivoxil: clinical characteristics and genetic predictors. Bone. 2016;93:97–103.

22. Yadav A, Carey EJ. Osteoporosis in chronic liver disease. Nutr Clin Pract. 2013;28(1):52–64.

23. Ho ES, Lin DC, Mendel DB, Cihlar T. Cytotoxicity of antiviral nucleotides adefovir and cidofovir is induced by the expression of human renal organic anion transporter 1. J Am Soc Nephrol. 2000;11(3):383–93.

24. Schaub TP, Kartenbeck J, Konig J, Spring H, Dorsam J, Staehler G, Storkel S, Thon WF, Keppler D. Expression of the MRP2 gene-encoded conjugate export pump in human kidney proximal tubules and in renal cell carcinoma. J Am Soc Nephrol. 1999;10(6):1159–69.

25. Vigano M, Facchetti F, Dongiovanni P, Valenti L, Soffredini R, Fargion S, Colombo M, Lampertico P. Drug transporter gene polymorphism predicts renal tubular toxicity in patients with chronic hepatitis B on long-term adefovir and lamivudine comnination. Dig Liver Dis. 2010;42:S8.

26. Qi X, Wang J, Chen L, Huang Y, Qin Y, Mao R, Zhang J. Impact of nucleos(t)ide analogue combination therapy on the estimated glomerular filtration rate in patients with chronic hepatitis B. Medicine (Baltimore). 2015; 94(15):e646.

27. Hulgan T, Haas DW, Haines JL, Ritchie MD, Robbins GK, Shafer RW, Clifford DB, Kallianpur AR, Summar M, Canter JA. Mitochondrial haplogroups and peripheral neuropathy during antiretroviral therapy: an adult AIDS clinical trials group study. AIDS. 2005;19(13):1341–9.

28. Amet S, Bronowicki JP, Thabut D, Zoulim F, Bourliere M, Mathurin P, de Ledinghen V, Benhamou Y, Larrey DG, Janus N, et al. Prevalence of renal abnormalities in chronic HBV infection: the HARPE study. Liver Int. 2015; 35(1):148–55.

29. Hartono JL, Aung MO, Dan YY, Gowans M, Lim K, Lee YM, Lee GH, Low HC, Tan PS, Thwin MA, et al. Resolution of adefovir-related nephrotoxicity by adefovir dose-reduction in patients with chronic hepatitis B. Aliment Pharmacol Ther. 2013;37(7):710–9.

30. Tamori A, Enomoto M, Kobayashi S, Iwai S, Morikawa H, Sakaguchi H, Habu D, Shiomi S, Imanishi Y, Kawada N. Add-on combination therapy with adefovir dipivoxil induces renal impairment in patients with lamivudine-refractory hepatitis B virus. J Viral Hepat. 2010;17(2):123–9.

31. Bhimma R, Coovadia HM. Hepatitis B virus-associated nephropathy. Am J Nephrol. 2004;24(2):198–211.

32. Hall AM, Bass P, Unwin RJ. Drug-induced renal Fanconi syndrome. QJM. 2014;107(4):261–9.

33. Guo J, Shao M, Lu F, Jiang J, Xia X. Role of Sirt1 Plays in Nucleus Pulposus Cells and Intervertebral Disc Degeneration. Spine (Phila Pa 1976). 2017; 42(13): E757–66.

34. Lucaci C, Acalovschi M. Hormonal and cytokine implications in the pathophysiology of osteoporosis occurring in chronic liver diseases. Maedica (Buchar). 2012;7(4):358–63.

35. Santos LA, Romeiro FG. Diagnosis and Management of Cirrhosis-Related Osteoporosis. Biomed Res Int. 2016;2016:1423462.

36. Gatta A, Verardo A, Di Pascoli M, Giannini S, Bolognesi M. Hepatic osteodystrophy. Clin Cases Miner Bone Metab. 2014;11(3):185–91.

37. Hao Y, Ma X, Shen Y, Ni J, Luo Y, Xiao Y, Bao Y, Jia W. Associations of serum 25-hydroxyvitamin D3 levels with visceral adipose tissue in Chinese men with normal glucose tolerance. PLoS One. 2014;9(1):e86773.

38. Jia HY, Ding F, Chen JY, Lian JS, Zhang YM, Zeng LY, Xiang DR, Yu L, Hu JH, Yu GD, et al. Early kidney injury during long-term adefovir dipivoxil therapy for chronic hepatitis B. World J Gastroenterol. 2015;21(12):3657–62.

39. Assadi F. Hypophosphatemia: an evidence-based problem-solving approach to clinical cases. Iran J Kidney Dis. 2010;4(3):195–201.

40. Hall AM, Hendry BM, Nitsch D, Connolly JO. Tenofovir-associated kidney toxicity in HIV-infected patients: a review of the evidence. Am J Kidney Dis. 2011;57(5):773–80.

41. Kim du H, Sung DH, Min YK. Hypophosphatemic osteomalacia induced by low-dose adefovir therapy: focus on manifestations in the skeletal system and literature review. J Bone Miner Metab. 2013;31(2):240–6.

42. Shiffman ML, Pol S, Rostaing L, Schiff E, Thabut D, Zeuzem S, Zong J, Frederick D, Rousseau F. Efficacy and pharmacokinetics of adefovir dipivoxil liquid suspension in patients with chronic hepatitis B and renal impairment. J Clin Pharmacol. 2011;51(9):1293–301.

43. Azria M. Possible mechanisms of the analgesic action of calcitonin. Bone. 2002;30(5 Suppl):80S 3S.

44. Holick MF. Vitamin D deficiency. N Engl J Med. 2007;357(3):266–81.

9

Stent thrombosis associated with drug eluting stents on addition of cilostazol to the standard dual antiplatelet therapy following percutaneous coronary intervention

Feng Huang (ID)

Abstract

Background: In this analysis, we aimed to systematically compare stent thrombosis (ST) and its different subtypes following treatment with DAPT (aspirin + clopidogrel) versus TAPT (aspirin + clopidogrel + cilostazol).

Methods: Studies were included if: they were randomized controlled trials (RCTs) comparing TAPT (cilostazol + aspirin + clopidogrel) with DAPT (aspirin + clopidogrel); they reported ST or its subtype including definite, probable, acute, sub-acute and late ST as their clinical outcomes. RevMan software (version 5.3) was used to carry out this analysis whereby odds ratios (OR) and 95% confidence intervals (CI) were generated.

Results: Statistical analysis of the data showed no significant difference in total ST with the addition of cilostazol to the standard DAPT with OR: 0.65, 95% CI: 0.38–1.10; $P = 0.11$, $I^2 = 6\%$. Moreover, when ST was further subdivided and analyzed, still, no significant difference was observed in acute, sub-acute, late, definite and probable ST with OR: 0.48, 95% CI: 0.13–1.74; $P = 0.27$, $I^2 = 0\%$, OR: 0.56, 95% CI: 0.22–1.40; $P = 0.21$, $I^2 = 0\%$, OR: 0.72, 95% CI: 0.23–2.28; $P = 0.58$, $I^2 = 0\%$, OR: 1.18, 95% CI: 0.38–3.69; $P = 0.77$, $I^2 = 3\%$ and OR: 0.75, 95% CI: 0.17–3.55; $P = 0.70$, $I^2 = 0\%$ respectively. No change was observed during a short term (≤ 6 months) and a longer (≥ 1 year) follow-up time period.

Conclusions: This current analysis showed no significant difference in stent thrombosis with the addition of cilostazol to the standard dual antiplatelet therapy during any follow-up time period after PCI.

Keywords: Dual antiplatelet therapy, Triple antiplatelet therapy, Cilostazol, Percutaneous coronary intervention, Stent thrombosis

Correspondence: huangfeng7925@163.com
Institute of Cardiovascular Diseases and Guangxi Key Laboratory Base of Precision Medicine in Cardio-cerebrovascular Diseases Control and Prevention, The First Affiliated Hospital of Guangxi Medical University, Nanning, Guangxi 530021, P. R. China

Background

Nowadays, percutaneous coronary intervention (PCI) is mainly carried out with drug eluting stents (DES). In the year 2017, a clinically interesting meta-analysis of randomized controlled trials showed similar cardiovascular outcomes in patients who were discharged on the same day versus patients who stayed overnight in the hospital following PCI [1]. However, the main shortcoming of DES is the occurrence of stent thrombosis (ST) [2].

In order to minimize ST, the 2014 European Society of Cardiology (ESC) and the European Association of Percutaneous Cardiovascular Interventions (EAPCI) guidelines on myocardial revascularization recommend the use of dual antiplatelet therapy (DAPT) consisting of aspirin and clopidogrel for at least six months in patients with stable coronary artery disease and for at least one year in patients with acute coronary syndrome [3]. However, recent progress in clinical medicine showed the addition of cilostazol (another antiplatelet agent) to DAPT, now called triple antiplatelet therapy (TAPT), to be more effective in comparison to DAPT [4] especially in decreasing repeated revascularization.

Further updated meta-analyses compared the outcomes which were associated with DAPT (aspirin + clopidogrel) and TAPT (cilostazol + aspirin + clopidogrel) [5, 6]. However, ST was never well compared systematically.

In contrast to other previously published meta-analyses, we aimed to systematically compare ST and its different subtypes following treatment with DAPT (aspirin + clopidogrel) versus TAPT (aspirin + clopidogrel + cilostazol) to show any significant difference related to ST.

Methods

Searched databases
The following databases were searched:

1. The Cochrane database;
2. EMBASE (www.sciencedirect.com);
3. MEDLINE;
4. www.ClinicalTrials.gov;
5. Reference lists of relevant publications.

Searched terms
The following terms were searched:

1. Dual antiplatelet therapy versus triple antiplatelet therapy;
2. Cilostazol and percutaneous coronary intervention;
3. Cilostazol and coronary angioplasty;
4. Cilostazol, aspirin and clopidogrel;
5. Triple antiplatelet therapy and percutaneous coronary intervention;
6. DAPT versus TAPT;
7. DAPT versus cilostazol.

Inclusion criteria
Studies were included if:

1. They were randomized controlled trials (RCTs) comparing TAPT (cilostazol + aspirin + clopidogrel) with DAPT (aspirin + clopidogrel);
2. They reported ST (or its subtype including definite, probable, acute, sub-acute and late ST) as their clinical outcomes.

Exclusion criteria
Studies were excluded if:

1. They were meta-analyses, review articles, observational cohorts, case-control studies and letter to editors;
2. TAPT did not consist of cilostazol, but instead, consisted of another antiplatelet or antithrombotic drug such as warfarin;
3. ST was not reported among the clinical outcomes;
4. They were duplicated studies.

Type of patients, outcomes, definitions and follow-ups
Several types of patients with CAD who were treated by PCI were included in this analysis (Table 1):

1. Patients with type 2 diabetes mellitus (T2DM);
2. Patients with obesity;
3. Patients with acute coronary syndrome (ACS);
4. Patients with long coronary lesions (LCL);
5. Patients with coronary bifurcation;
6. Patients with native CAD;
7. Patients with multi-vessel CAD.

ST and its subtypes including (Table 1):

1. Total ST: the total number of any type of ST;
2. Acute ST: less than 1 day;
3. Sub-acute ST: 1 day to 1 month;
4. Late ST: 1 to 12 months or more;
5. Definite ST and;
6. Probable ST were assessed.

Definite and probable ST were defined according to the Academic Research Consortium [7].

The follow-up time periods were as followed:

1. A short term follow up period of 6 months or less.
2. A longer follow up time period of 1 year or more (1–3 years) as shown in Table 1.

Table 1 Types of stent thrombosis which were reported

Studies	Type of stent thrombosis reported	Follow-up period	Type of participants	Type of stent
Ahn2008 [10]	Acute, sub-acute and late ST	6 months	PCI in patients with T2DM	DES
Gao2013 [11]	Definite, probable, acute and late ST	1 year	PCI in patients with obesity	DES
Han2009 [12]	Sub-acute ST	1 month	PCI in patients with ACS	DES
Lee2005 [13]	Acute and sub-acute ST	1 month	PCI in patients with CAD	DES
Lee2010A [14]	Acute, sub-acute, late and very late ST	2 years	PCI in patients with T2DM and LCL	DES
Lee2011 [15]	Acute, sub-acute, late ST	1 year	PCI in patients with LCL	DES
Suh2011 [16]	ST	6 months	PCI in patients with native CAD	DES
Youn2014 [17]	ST, definite and probable ST	3 months and 1 year	PCI in patients with LCL or MVD	DES
Zhu2015 [18]	Sub-acute and late ST	1 year	PCI in patients with ACS	DES
Park2013 [19]	Definite and probable ST	1 month	PCI in patients with CAD	DES

Abbreviations: ST: Stent thrombosis, PCI: Percutaneous coronary intervention, T2DM = type 2 diabetes mellitus, ACS: Acute coronary syndrome, CAD: Coronary artery disease, LCL: Long coronary lesions, MVD: Multi-vessel diseases, DES: Drug eluting stents

Data extraction and quality assessment

The following data were extracted and cross-checked by the reviewer Feng Huang:

1. The type of study (trial or observational cohort);
2. The total number of patients who were treated by DAPT and TAPT respectively;
3. The types of participants;
4. The patients' enrollment time periods;
5. The baseline characteristics of the participants;
6. The follow-up time periods.

Another reviewer (Pravesh Kumar Bundhun) was also involved in the searched process and in data extraction. However, because he did not satisfy all the criteria for authorship, he was only acknowledged at the end of the paper.

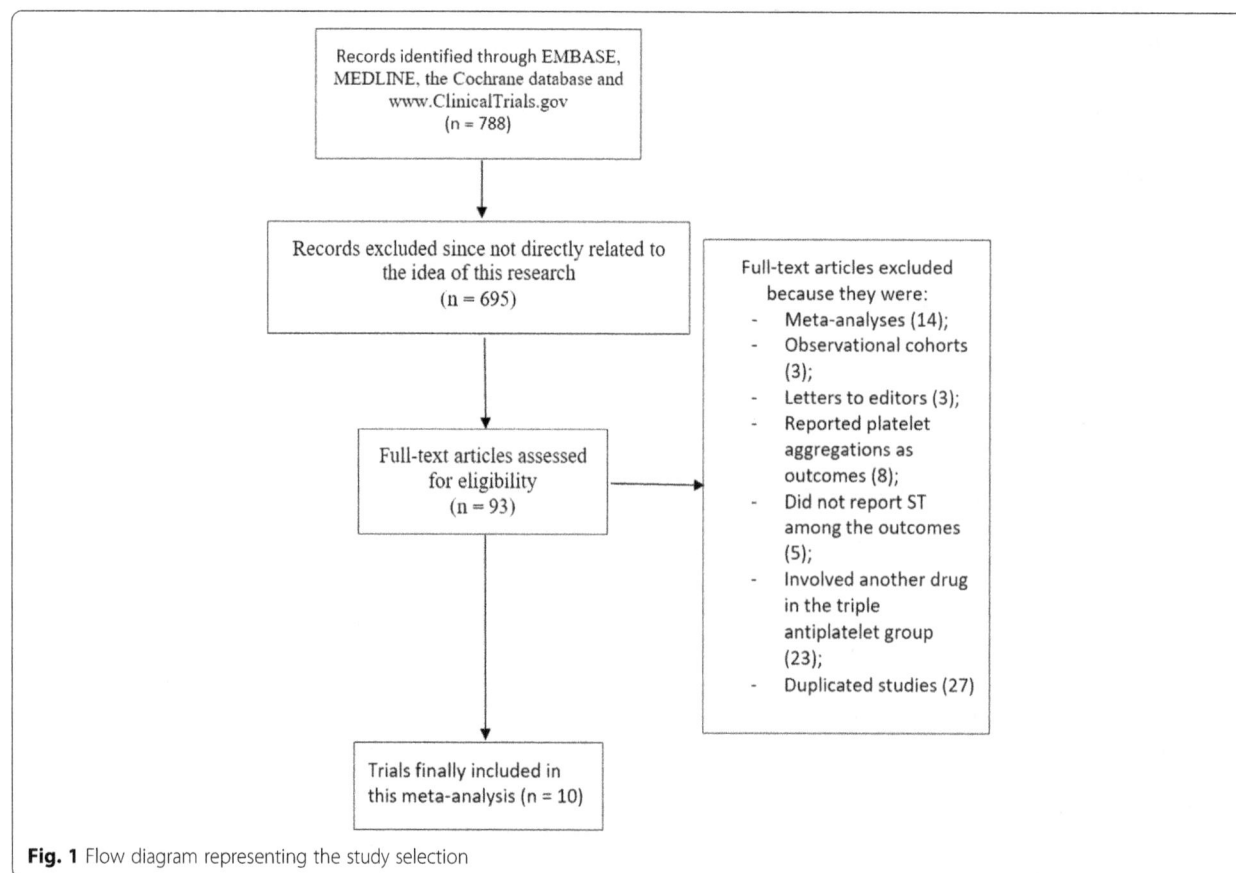

Fig. 1 Flow diagram representing the study selection

Table 2 General features of the studies which were included

Studies	No of patients with DAPT (n)	No of patients with TAPT (n)	Type of study	Year of patients' enrollment	Bias risk grade
Ahn2008 [10]	124	113	RCT	2004–2006	B
Gao2013 [11]	215	213	RCT	–	B
Han2009 [12]	608	604	RCT	–	B
Lee2005 [13]	1597	1415	OS	1998–2003	–
Lee2010A [14]	450	450	RCT	2004–2006	A
Lee2011 [15]	249	250	RCT	2007–2008	A
Suh2011 [16]	458	457	RCT	2006–2009	A
Youn2014 [17]	307	308	RCT	2010–2011	B
Zhu2015 [18]	151	154	RCT	–	B
Park2013 [19]	1876	1879	RCT	2010–2011	B
Total (n)	6035	5843			

Abbreviations: DAPT: Dual anti-platelet therapy, TAPT: Triple antiplatelet therapy, RCT: Randomized controlled trials, OS: Observational studies

The methodological quality was assessed in accordance to the criteria suggested by the Cochrane collaboration (for randomized controlled trials) [8]. Grades were allotted (A to E with a grade A implying a low risk of bias).

Statistical analysis

RevMan analytical software for meta-analysis (version 5.3) was used to carry out this analysis whereby odds ratios (OR) and 95% confidence intervals (CI) were generated.

Heterogeneity was assessed by two simple methods:

1. The Q statistic test whereby a P value less or equal to 0.05 was considered statistically significant;
2. The I^2 statistic test which focused on the value of I^2 (the greater the value, the higher the heterogeneity).

In addition, a fixed effects model ($I^2 < 50\%$) or a random effects model ($I^2 > 50\%$) was used based on the I^2 value which was obtained.

Sensitivity analysis was also carried out by an exclusion method (each trial was excluded one by one and a new analysis was carried out each time and the results were observed for any significant difference).In addition, publication bias was visually estimated through funnel plots.

Since registration for meta-analyses was not compulsory, protocol for this study was not prospectively registered.

Ethics

Ethical approval was not required for such types of research articles.

Results

Searched outcomes

The PRISMA guideline was followed [9]. This search resulted in a total number of 788 articles. Six hundred and ninety-five (695) articles were eliminated since they were not related to this research title. Ninety three (93) full

Table 3 Baseline features of the studies which were included

Studies	Age (years)	Males (%)	HT (%)	Ds (%)	DM (%)	Cs (%)
	DT/TT	DT/TT	DT/TT	DT/TT	DT/TT	DT/TT
Ahn2008 [10]	62.0/61.2	54.7/61.7	54.0/48.9	25.2/19.1	100/100	34.5/39.5
Gao2013 [11]	55.3/57.6	81.9/78.9	54.4/56.3	21.4/24.9	16.2/19.2	42.3/38.5
Han2009 [12]	60.2/59.6	72.9/73.8	56.1/57.9	45.4/45.5	20.1/23.3	–
Lee2005 [13]	59.0/59.0	71.8/71.8	46.1/42.3	27.6/26.8	26.2/23.4	31.9/32.4
Lee2010A [14]	61.0/60.9	60.7/62.2	57.1/57.0	28.5/30.2	62.4/63.3	34.7/31.6
Lee2011 [15]	62.1/60.9	71.5/70.0	64.7/58.4	45.0/42.4	33.7/36.8	30.1/30.4
Suh2011 [16]	64.0/64.8	68.3/68.6	66.6/64.5	–	32.2/35.5	26.8/23.7
Youn2014 [17]	64.2/65.0	64.2/63.0	65.8/68.2	47.6/49.4	30.9/32.5	44.0/48.4
Zhu2015 [18]	60.1/60.2	64.9/66.9	45.7/41.6	57.0/51.3	21.9/17.5	32.5/39.0
Park2013 [19]	63.7/62.8	67.0/69.8	68.6/66.8	62.7/64.2	31.3/31.8	30.8/32.8

Abbreviations: DT: Dual antiplatelet therapy, TT: Triple antiplatelet therapy, HT: Hypertension, ds: Dyslipidemia, DM: Diabetes mellitus, Cs: Current smoker

text articles were assessed for eligibility. Further elimination was carried out due to the following reasons:

1. They were meta-analyses (14);
2. They were observational studies (3);
3. They were letters to editors (3);
4. They reported platelet aggregation as outcomes (8);
5. They did not report ST among the cardiovascular outcomes (5);
6. They involved another drug in the triple antiplatelet group (23);
7. They were duplicated studies (27).

Finally 10 randomized controlled trials [10–19] were confirmed for this analysis as shown in Fig. 1.

General features of the studies which were included

The general features of the studies have been listed in Table 2. Ten randomized controlled trials consisting of a total number of 11, 878 participants (6035 patients were assigned to the DAPT group and 5843 patients were assigned to the TAPT group). The time period for patients' enrollment varied from years 1998 to 2011. A detailed data set for the total number of patients which were extracted from each trial has been shown in Table 2.

As previously stated, the bias risk was assessed in accordance to the criteria suggested by the Cochrane collaboration. A grade 'A' with low risk bias was allotted to three randomized trials, whereas a grade 'B' was allotted to the other remaining 6 trials.

Baseline characteristics of the participants

The baseline features of the participants have been listed in Table 3. The participants had a mean age ranging from 55.3 to 65.0 years. In addition, male patients were predominant in both groups (DAPT and TAPT). Other co-morbidities or risk factors such as hypertension, dyslipidemia, diabetes mellitus and current smoker were also reported in Table 3. According to the data which were presented, no significant difference was observed in the baseline features among those participants who were assigned to the DAPT or TAPT groups.

Main results of this analysis

Results of this analysis have been represented in Table 4.

Statistical analysis of the data showed no significant difference in total ST with the addition of cilostazol to the standard DAPT with OR: 0.65, 95% CI: 0.38–1.10; $P = 0.11$, $I^2 = 6\%$ as shown in Fig. 2.

When ST was further subdivided and analyzed, still, no significant difference was observed in acute, sub-acute, late, definite and probable ST with OR: 0.48, 95% CI: 0.13–1.74; $P = 0.27$, $I^2 = 0\%$, OR: 0.56, 95% CI: 0.22–1.40; $P = 0.21$, $I^2 = 0\%$, OR: 0.72, 95% CI: 0.23–2.28; $P = 0.58$, $I^2 = 0\%$, OR: 1.18, 95% CI: 0.38–3.69; $P = 0.77$,

Table 4 Results of this analysis

Outcomes	OR with 95% CI	P value	I^2 (%)	Statistical model used
ST	0.65 [0.38–1.10]	0.11	6	Fixed effects
Definite ST	1.18 [0.38–3.69]	0.77	3	Fixed effects
Probable ST	0.75 [0.17–3.35]	0.70	0	Fixed effects
Acute ST	0.48 [0.13–1.74]	0.27	0	Fixed effects
Sub-acute ST	0.56 [0.22–1.40]	0.21	0	Fixed effects
Late ST	0.72 [0.23–2.28]	0.58	0	Fixed effects

Abbreviations: OR: Odds ratios, CI: Confidence intervals, ST: Stent thrombosis, RCT: Randomized controlled trials, OS: Observational studies

$I^2 = 3\%$ and OR: 0.75, 95% CI: 0.17–3.35; $P = 0.70$, $I^2 = 0\%$ respectively as shown in Fig. 2.

Another analysis was carried out based on the follow-up time period.

During a short term follow-up time period, total, sub-acute, definite and probable ST were again similarly manifested with OR: 0.55, 95% CI: 0.29–1.07; $P = 0.08$, $I^2 = 0\%$, OR: 0.35, 95% CI: 0.10–1.32; $P = 0.12$, $I^2 = 0\%$, OR: 1.00, 95% CI: 0.27–3.69; $P = 1.00$, $I^2 = 42\%$ and OR: 0.75, 95% CI: 0.17–3.35; $P = 0.70$, $I^2 = 0\%$ respectively as shown in Fig. 3.

During a longer follow-up time period, still no significant difference was observed in total, acute, sub-acute, late, and definite ST with the addition of cilostazol to the standard DAPT, with OR: 1.09, 95% CI: 0.47–2.53; $P = 0.84$, $I^2 = 39\%$, OR: 0.75, 95% CI: 0.17–3.37; $P = 0.71$, $I^2 = 0\%$, OR: 0.99, 95% CI: 0.25–3.97; $P = 0.99$, $I^2 = 0\%$, OR: 0.66, 95% CI: 0.19–2.36; $P = 0.53$, $I^2 = 0\%$, and OR: 3.03, 95% CI: 0.47–19.32; $P = 0.24$, $I^2 = 0\%$ respectively as shown in Fig. 4.

Sensitivity analysis was also carried out. No significant difference in results were obtained when each study was excluded one by one.

Since this analysis consisted of a small volume of studies, publication bias could better be represented by funnel plots. After carefully assessing the funnel plots, no evidence of publication bias was observed across all the trials which assessed the different subtypes of ST in this analysis as shown in Figs. 5 and 6.

Discussion

Even though the ESC/EACTS guidelines recommend DAPT as the treatment of choice following PCI with DES, we aimed to show whether the addition of cilostazol to DAPT might potentially be associated with significantly lower ST.

In this analysis, the addition of cilostazol to the standard DAPT (aspirin and clopidogrel) did not show any significant difference in total ST or any of its subtypes including acute, sub-acute, late, definite and probable ST. No significant difference was

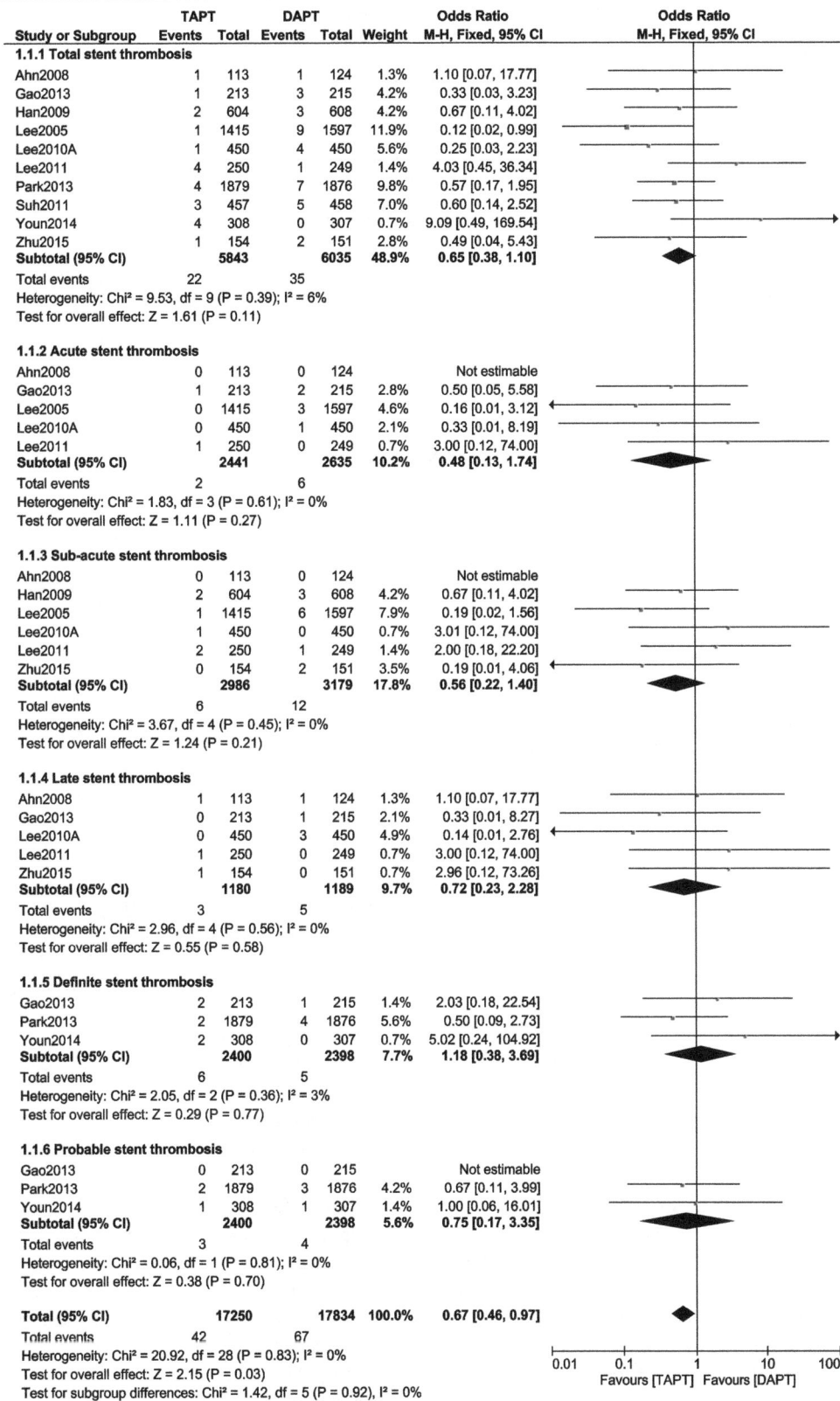

Fig. 2 Stent thrombosis observed with the addition of cilostazol to the standard DAPT

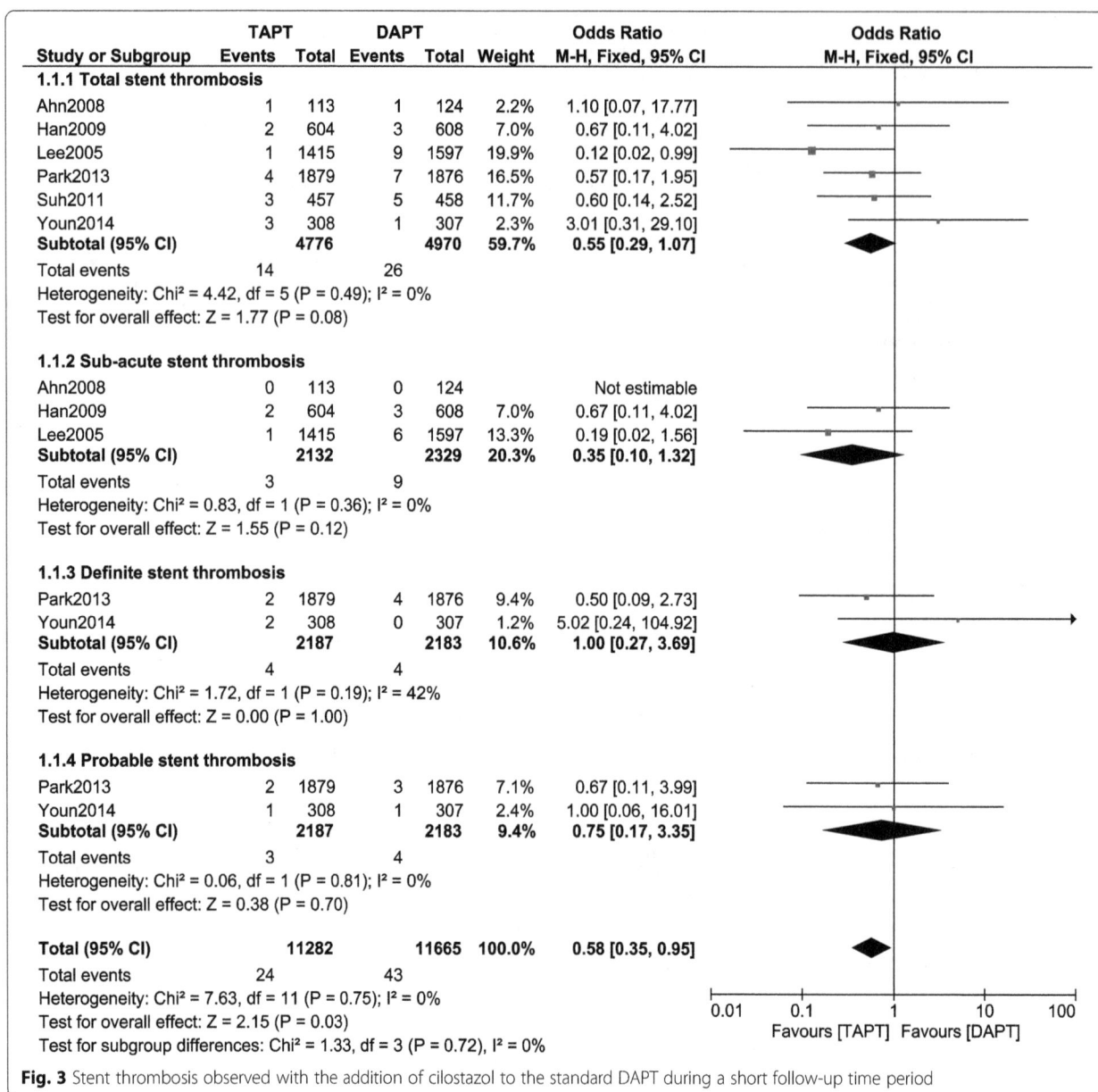

Study or Subgroup	TAPT Events	Total	DAPT Events	Total	Weight	Odds Ratio M-H, Fixed, 95% CI
1.1.1 Total stent thrombosis						
Ahn2008	1	113	1	124	2.2%	1.10 [0.07, 17.77]
Han2009	2	604	3	608	7.0%	0.67 [0.11, 4.02]
Lee2005	1	1415	9	1597	19.9%	0.12 [0.02, 0.99]
Park2013	4	1879	7	1876	16.5%	0.57 [0.17, 1.95]
Suh2011	3	457	5	458	11.7%	0.60 [0.14, 2.52]
Youn2014	3	308	1	307	2.3%	3.01 [0.31, 29.10]
Subtotal (95% CI)		**4776**		**4970**	**59.7%**	**0.55 [0.29, 1.07]**
Total events	14		26			

Heterogeneity: Chi² = 4.42, df = 5 (P = 0.49); I² = 0%
Test for overall effect: Z = 1.77 (P = 0.08)

1.1.2 Sub-acute stent thrombosis						
Ahn2008	0	113	0	124		Not estimable
Han2009	2	604	3	608	7.0%	0.67 [0.11, 4.02]
Lee2005	1	1415	6	1597	13.3%	0.19 [0.02, 1.56]
Subtotal (95% CI)		**2132**		**2329**	**20.3%**	**0.35 [0.10, 1.32]**
Total events	3		9			

Heterogeneity: Chi² = 0.83, df = 1 (P = 0.36); I² = 0%
Test for overall effect: Z = 1.55 (P = 0.12)

1.1.3 Definite stent thrombosis						
Park2013	2	1879	4	1876	9.4%	0.50 [0.09, 2.73]
Youn2014	2	308	0	307	1.2%	5.02 [0.24, 104.92]
Subtotal (95% CI)		**2187**		**2183**	**10.6%**	**1.00 [0.27, 3.69]**
Total events	4		4			

Heterogeneity: Chi² = 1.72, df = 1 (P = 0.19); I² = 42%
Test for overall effect: Z = 0.00 (P = 1.00)

1.1.4 Probable stent thrombosis						
Park2013	2	1879	3	1876	7.1%	0.67 [0.11, 3.99]
Youn2014	1	308	1	307	2.4%	1.00 [0.06, 16.01]
Subtotal (95% CI)		**2187**		**2183**	**9.4%**	**0.75 [0.17, 3.35]**
Total events	3		4			

Heterogeneity: Chi² = 0.06, df = 1 (P = 0.81); I² = 0%
Test for overall effect: Z = 0.38 (P = 0.70)

Total (95% CI)		**11282**		**11665**	**100.0%**	**0.58 [0.35, 0.95]**
Total events	24		43			

Heterogeneity: Chi² = 7.63, df = 11 (P = 0.75); I² = 0%
Test for overall effect: Z = 2.15 (P = 0.03)
Test for subgroup differences: Chi² = 1.33, df = 3 (P = 0.72), I² = 0%

Fig. 3 Stent thrombosis observed with the addition of cilostazol to the standard DAPT during a short follow-up time period

observed even during a short (≤ 6 months) or a longer follow-up time period (≥ 1 year) after PCI.

In 2015, a clinically important meta-analysis which was published in BMC Cardiovascular Disorders compared DAPT with TAPT (cilostazol + aspirin + clopidogrel) in patients with T2DM. In their results, the authors demonstrated a significant reduction in major adverse cardiac events, and revascularization when cilostazol was added to aspirin and clopidogrel [4].

However, even if this current study did not report adverse cardiovascular outcomes, ST which was reported was not significantly different between DAPT and TAPT further supporting this analysis. In addition, this current analysis was far better since

different subtypes of ST were assessed with a higher total number of participants.

A meta-analysis carried out by Zhou et al. showed no significant difference in ST with DAPT and TAPT further supporting this current analysis [20]. Additionally, another meta-analysis of randomized trials with adjusted indirect comparisons still showed no significant difference in ST with the addition of cilostazol to DAPT [21]. Major and minor bleeding events were also not increased [22].

Nevertheless, insights from a recent meta-analysis of randomized trials which aimed to show the efficacy of cilostazol on platelet reactivity and cardiovascular outcomes in patients undergoing PCI showed reduced

Study or Subgroup	TAPT Events	Total	DAPT Events	Total	Weight	Odds Ratio M-H, Fixed, 95% CI	Odds Ratio M-H, Fixed, 95% CI
1.1.1 Total stent thrombosis							
Gao2013	1	213	3	215	11.5%	0.33 [0.03, 3.23]	
Lee2010A	1	450	4	450	15.4%	0.25 [0.03, 2.23]	
Lee2011	4	250	1	249	3.8%	4.03 [0.45, 36.34]	
Youn2014	4	308	0	307	1.9%	9.09 [0.49, 169.54]	
Zhu2015	1	154	2	151	7.7%	0.49 [0.04, 5.43]	
Subtotal (95% CI)		1375		1372	40.3%	1.09 [0.47, 2.53]	
Total events	11		10				
Heterogeneity: Chi² = 6.60, df = 4 (P = 0.16); I² = 39%							
Test for overall effect: Z = 0.21 (P = 0.84)							
1.1.2 Acute stent thrombosis							
Gao2013	1	213	2	215	7.6%	0.50 [0.05, 5.58]	
Lee2010A	0	450	1	450	5.8%	0.33 [0.01, 8.19]	
Lee2011	1	250	0	249	1.9%	3.00 [0.12, 74.00]	
Subtotal (95% CI)		913		914	15.4%	0.75 [0.17, 3.37]	
Total events	2		3				
Heterogeneity: Chi² = 1.07, df = 2 (P = 0.58); I² = 0%							
Test for overall effect: Z = 0.37 (P = 0.71)							
1.1.3 Sub-acute stent thrombosis							
Lee2010A	1	450	0	450	1.9%	3.01 [0.12, 74.00]	
Lee2011	2	250	1	249	3.8%	2.00 [0.18, 22.20]	
Zhu2015	0	154	2	151	9.7%	0.19 [0.01, 4.06]	
Subtotal (95% CI)		854		850	15.5%	0.99 [0.25, 3.97]	
Total events	3		3				
Heterogeneity: Chi² = 1.89, df = 2 (P = 0.39); I² = 0%							
Test for overall effect: Z = 0.01 (P = 0.99)							
1.1.4 Late stent thrombosis							
Gao2013	0	213	1	215	5.8%	0.33 [0.01, 8.27]	
Lee2010A	0	450	3	450	13.5%	0.14 [0.01, 2.76]	
Lee2011	1	250	0	249	1.9%	3.00 [0.12, 74.00]	
Zhu2015	1	154	0	151	1.9%	2.96 [0.12, 73.26]	
Subtotal (95% CI)		1067		1065	23.1%	0.66 [0.19, 2.36]	
Total events	2		4				
Heterogeneity: Chi² = 2.90, df = 3 (P = 0.41); I² = 0%							
Test for overall effect: Z = 0.63 (P = 0.53)							
1.1.5 Definite stent thrombosis							
Gao2013	2	213	1	215	3.8%	2.03 [0.18, 22.54]	
Youn2014	2	308	0	307	1.9%	5.02 [0.24, 104.92]	
Subtotal (95% CI)		521		522	5.7%	3.03 [0.47, 19.32]	
Total events	4		1				
Heterogeneity: Chi² = 0.21, df = 1 (P = 0.64); I² = 0%							
Test for overall effect: Z = 1.17 (P = 0.24)							
Total (95% CI)		4730		4723	100.0%	1.04 [0.60, 1.78]	
Total events	22		21				
Heterogeneity: Chi² = 14.05, df = 16 (P = 0.60); I² = 0%							
Test for overall effect: Z = 0.13 (P = 0.90)							
Test for subgroup differences: Chi² = 1.96, df = 4 (P = 0.74), I² = 0%							

0.01   0.1   1   10   100
Favours [TAPT]   Favours [DAPT]

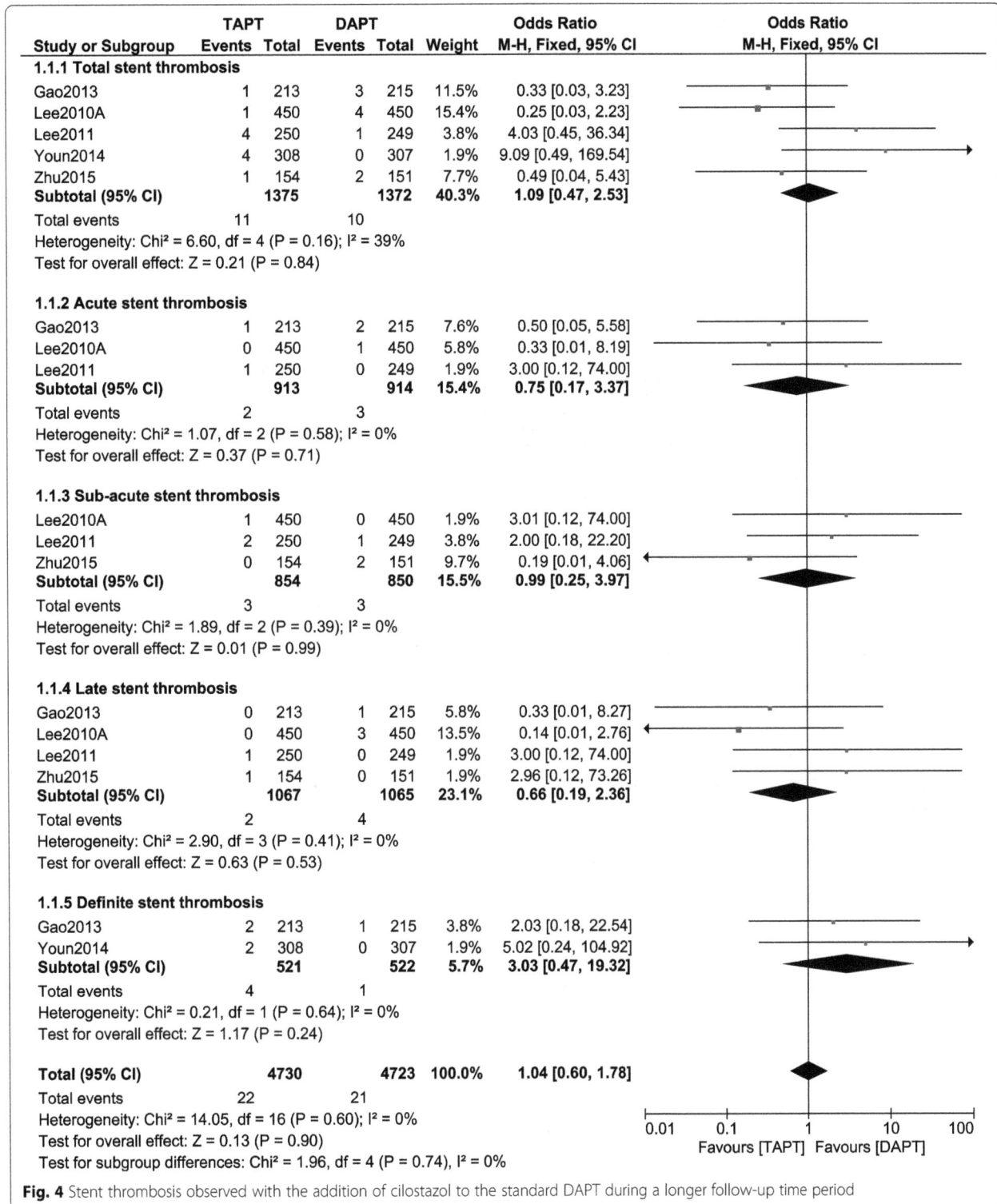

Fig. 4 Stent thrombosis observed with the addition of cilostazol to the standard DAPT during a longer follow-up time period

stent thrombosis with the triple therapy [23]. The result was completely different from our current analysis. However, it should be clearly noted that in their analysis, the authors repeated data from the DECLARE trial (DECLARE-LONG, DECLARE-DM). In addition, in their analysis, bare metal stents were also included, which was not the case in this current analysis whereby only DES were used. Also, they included unpublished studies and their focus was not specifically based on ST. Our focus was centered specifically on ST and was based on published trials.

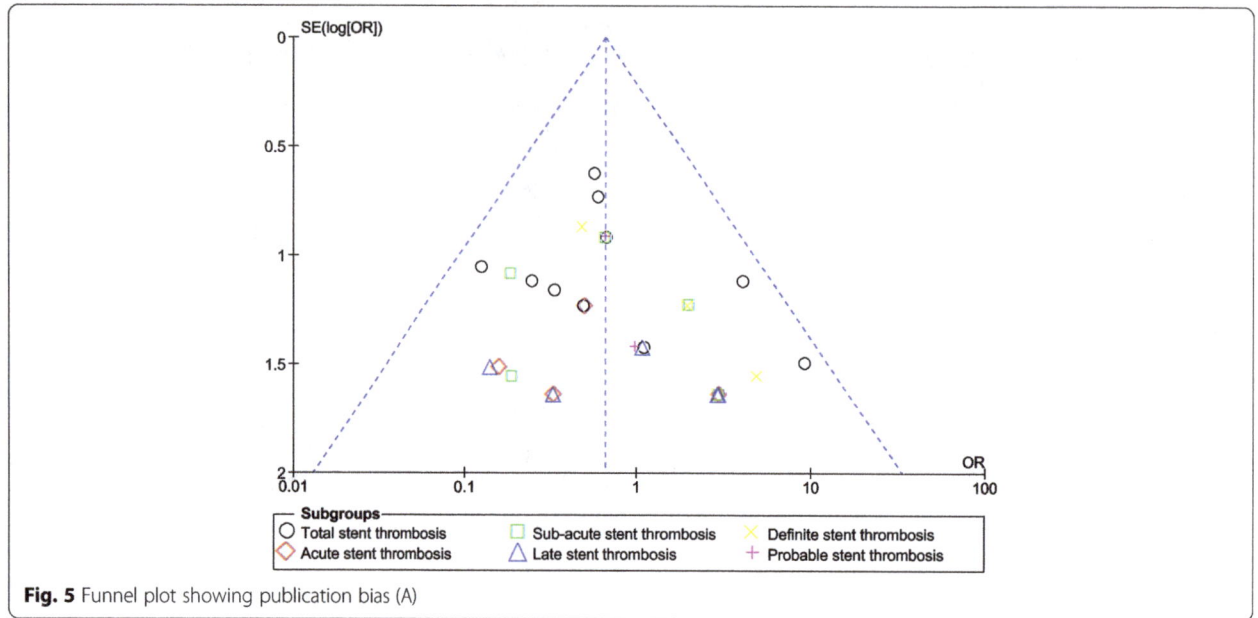

Fig. 5 Funnel plot showing publication bias (A)

Novelty

New features of this analysis included:

1. A high total number of participants;
2. Comparing a detailed outcome of ST (acute, sub-acute, late, definite and probable ST) in one particular paper.
3. The systematical comparison of short term and long-term ST in the general population with CAD undergoing PCI.

Limitations

Limitations were as followed:

1. Even though all the participants were CAD patients with coronary stenting, they were different in terms of subtypes of disease and co-morbidities. A few studies reported patients with diabetes mellitus, obesity, ACS, whereas other studies involved patients with stable CAD, multi-vessel CAD, long coronary lesions, and coronary bifurcation which might affect the results.

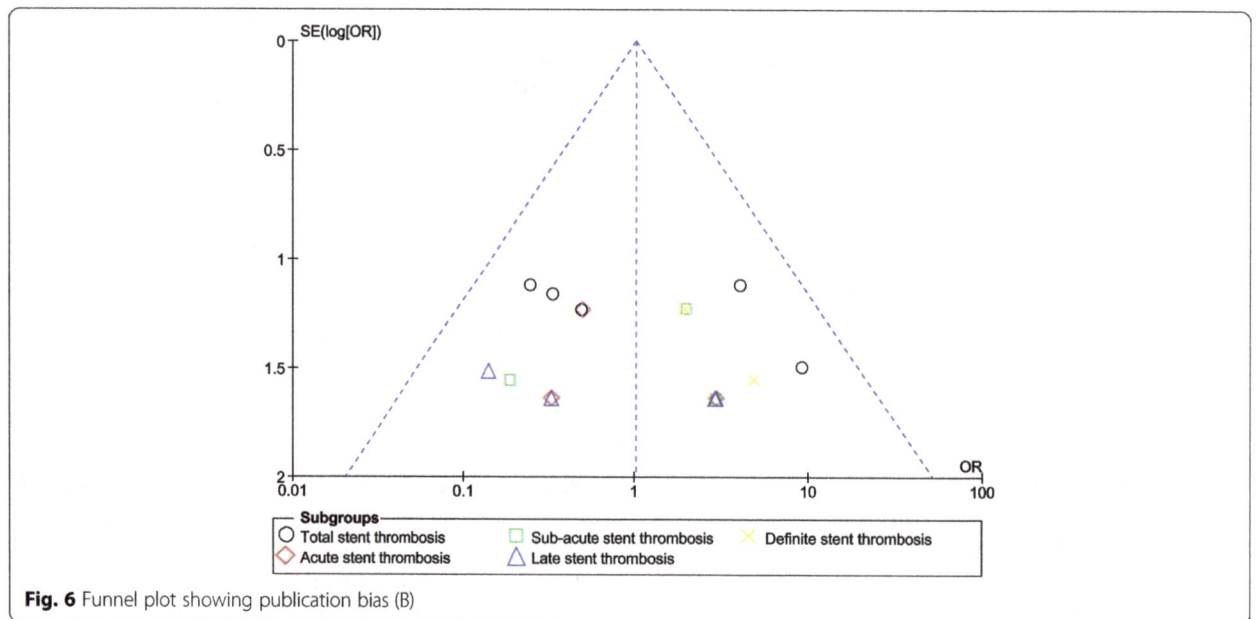

Fig. 6 Funnel plot showing publication bias (B)

2. More data would have significantly improved the results when assessing for definite and probable ST. However, improvement on this aspect was not possible since only few studies reported definite and probable ST among the trials which were included in this analysis.

3. Longer follow-up time periods above 5 years would have further enhanced this analysis. Nevertheless, no studies have evaluated the use of cilostazol in addition to aspirin and clopidogrel for such a longer follow up time period.

4. One observational cohort was also included among the trials.

Conclusions

This current analysis showed no significant difference in stent thrombosis with the addition of cilostazol to the standard dual antiplatelet therapy during any follow-up time period after PCI.

Abbreviations

DAPT: Dual antiplatelet therapy; PCI: Percutaneous coronary intervention; RCT: Randomized controlled trials; ST: Stent thrombosis; TAPT: Triple antiplatelet therapy

Acknowledgements

The author would like to thank Dr. Pravesh Kumar Bundhun (MD), from the Institute of Cardiovascular Diseases, The First Affiliated Hospital of Guangxi Medical University, Nanning, Guangxi, China, for his immense contribution to the search process and data extraction.

Funding

This research was supported by National Natural Science Foundation of China (No. 81560046), Guangxi Natural Science Foundation (No. 2016GXNSFAA380002), Scientific Project of Guangxi Higher Education (No. KY2015ZD028), Science Research and Technology Development Project of Qingxiu District of Nanning (No. 2016058) and Lisheng Health Foundation pilotage fund of Peking (No. LHJJ20158126).

Authors' contributions

FH was responsible for the conception and design, acquisition of data, analysis and interpretation of data, drafting the initial manuscript and revising it critically for important intellectual content. FH wrote and approved the final manuscript.

Competing interests

The author declare that he has no competing interests.

References

1. Bundhun PK, Soogund MZ, Huang WQ. Same day discharge versus overnight stay in the hospital following percutaneous coronary intervention in patients with stable coronary artery disease: a systematic review and meta-analysis of randomized controlled trials. PLoS One. 2017;12(1): e0169807.

2. Bundhun PK, Yanamala CM, Huang WQ. Comparing stent thrombosis associated with Zotarolimus eluting stents versus Everolimus eluting stents at 1 year follow up: a systematic review and meta-analysis of 6 randomized controlled trials. BMC Cardiovasc Disord. 2017;17(1):84.

3. Task Force members, Windecker S, Kolh P, Alfonso F, et al. 2014 ESC/EACTS guidelines on myocardial revascularization: the Task Force on Myocardial Revascularization of the European Society of Cardiology (ESC) and the European Association for Cardio-Thoracic Surgery (EACTS) developed with the special contribution of the European Association of Percutaneous Cardiovascular Interventions (EAPCI). Eur Heart J. 2014;35:2541–619.

4. Bundhun PK, Qin T, Chen MH. Comparing the effectiveness and safety between triple antiplatelet therapy and dual antiplatelet therapy in type 2 diabetes mellitus patients after coronary stents implantation: a systematic review and meta-analysis of randomized controlled trials. BMC Cardiovasc Disord. 2015;15:118.

5. Bangalore S, Singh A, Toklu B, DiNicolantonio JJ, Croce K, Feit F, Bhatt DL. Efficacy of cilostazol on platelet reactivity and cardiovascular outcomes in patients undergoing percutaneous coronary intervention: insights from a meta-analysis of randomised trials. Open Heart. 2014;1(1):e000068.

6. Zhang Y, Tang HQ, Li J, Fu ZX. Efficacy and safety of triple-antiplatelet therapy after percutaneous coronary intervention: a meta-analysis. Chin Med J. 2013;126(9):1750–4.

7. Cutlip DE, Windecker S, Mehran R, et al; Academic Research Consortium. Clinical end points in coronary stent trials: a case for standardized definitions. Circulation 2007;115(17):2344–2351.

8. Higgins JP, Thompson SG, Deeks JJ, et al. Measuring inconsistency in meta-analyses. BMJ. 2003;327:557–60.

9. Liberati A, Altman DG, Tetzlaff J, et al. The PRISMA statement for reporting systematic reviews and meta-analyses of studies that evaluate healthcareinterventions: explanation and elaboration. BMJ. 2009;339:b2700.

10. Ahn Y, Jeong MH, Jeong JW, Kim KH, Ahn TH, Kang WC, Park CG, Kim JH, Chae IH, Nam CW, Hur SH, Bae JH, Kim KY, Oh SK. Randomized comparison of cilostazol vs clopidogrel after drug-eluting stenting in diabeticpatients-clilostazol for diabetic patients in drug-eluting stent (CIDES) trial. Circ J. 2008;72(1):35–9.

11. Gao W, Zhang Q, Ge H, Guo Y, Zhou Z. Efficacy and safety of triple antiplatelet therapy in obese patients undergoing stent implantation. Angiology. 2013;64(7):554–8.

12. Han Y, Li Y, Wang S, Jing Q, Wang Z, Wang D, Shu Q, Tang X. Cilostazol in addition to aspirin and clopidogrel improves long-term outcomes after percutaneouscoronary intervention in patients with acute coronary syndromes: a randomized, controlled study. Am Heart J. 2009;157(4):733–9.

13. Lee SW, Park SW, Hong MK, Kim YH, Lee BK, Song JM, Han KH, Lee CW, Kang DH, Song JK, Kim JJ, Park SJ. Triple versus dual antiplatelet therapy after coronary stenting: impact on stent thrombosis. J Am Coll Cardiol. 2005;46(10):1833–7.

14. Lee SW, Chun KJ, Park SW, Kim HS, Kim YH, Yun SC, Kim WJ, Lee JY, Park DW, Lee CW, Hong MK, Rhee KS, Chae JK, Ko JK, Park JH, Lee JH, Choi SW, Jeong JO, Seong IW, Jon S, Cho YH, Lee NH, Kim JH, Park SJ. Comparison of triple antiplatelet therapy and dual antiplatelet therapy in patients at high risk of restenosis after drug-eluting stent implantation (from the DECLARE-DIABETES and –LONG trials). Am J Cardiol. 2010;105(2):168–73.

15. Lee SW, Park SW, Kim YH, Yun SC, Park DW, Lee CW, Kang SJ, Park SJ, Lee JH, Choi SW, Seong IW, Lee NH, Cho YH, Shin WY, Lee SJ, Lee SW, Hyon MS, Bang DW, Choi YJ, Kim HS, Lee BK, Lee K, Park HK, Park CB, Lee SG, Kim MK, Park KH, Park WJ; DECLARE-LONG II Study Investigators. A randomized, double-blind, multicenter comparison study of triple antiplatelet therapy with dualantiplatelet therapy to reduce restenosis after drug-eluting stent Implantation In long coronarylesions: results from the DECLARE-LONG II (drug-eluting stenting followed by Cilostazol treatment reduces late restenosis in patients with long coronary lesions) trial. J Am Coll Cardiol 2011;57(11):1264–1270.

16. Suh JW, Lee SP, Park KW, Lee HY, Kang HJ, Koo BK, Cho YS, Youn TJ, Chae IH, Choi DJ, Rha SW, Bae JH, Kwon TG, Bae JW, Cho MC, Kim HS. Multicenter randomized trial evaluating the efficacy of cilostazol on ischemic vascularcomplications after drug-eluting stent implantation for coronary heart disease: results of the CILON-T (influence of CILostazol-based triple antiplatelet therapy ON ischemic complication after drug-eluting stenT implantation) trial. J Am Coll Cardiol. 2011;57(3):280–9.

17. Youn YJ, Lee JW, Ahn SG, Lee SH, Choi H, Yu CW, Hong YJ, Kwon HM, Hong MK, Jang Y, Yoon J. Multicenter randomized trial of 3-month cilostazol use in addition to dual antiplatelet therapy afterbiolimus-eluting stent implantation for long or multivessel coronary artery disease. Am Heart J. 2014;167(2):241–248.e1.

18. Zhu HC, Li Y, Guan SY, Li J, Wang XZ, Jing QM, Wang ZL, Han YL. Efficacy and safety of individually tailored antiplatelet therapy in patients with acute coronarysyndrome after coronary stenting: a single center, randomized, feasibility study. J Geriatr Cardiol. 2015;12(1):23–9.

19. Park KW, Kang SH, Park JJ, Yang HM, Kang HJ, Koo BK, Park BE, Cha KS, Rhew JY, Jeon HK, Shin ES, Oh JH, Jeong MH, Kim S, Hwang KK, Yoon JH, Lee SY, Park TH, Moon KW, Kwon HM, Chae IH, Kim HS. Adjunctive cilostazol versus double-dose clopidogrel after drug-eluting stent implantation: the HOST-ASSURE randomized trial (harmonizing optimal strategy for treatment of Coronary Artery Stenosis-Safety & Effectiveness of Drug-Eluting Stents & Anti-platelet Regimen). JACC Cardiovasc Interv. 2013;6(9):932–42.

20. Zhou H, Feng XL, Zhang HY, Xu FF, Zhu J. Triple versus dual antiplatelet therapy for coronary heart disease patients undergoing percutaneous coronary intervention: a meta-analysis. Exp Ther Med. 2013;6(4):1034–40.

21. Chen Y, Zhang Y, Tang Y, Huang X, Xie Y. Long-term clinical efficacy and safety of adding cilostazol to dual antiplatelet therapy for patients undergoing PCI: a meta-analysis of randomized trials with adjusted indirect comparisons. Curr Med Res Opin. 2014;30(1):37–49.

22. Ding XL, Xie C, Jiang B, Gao J, Zhang LL, Zhang H, Zhang JJ, Miao LY. Efficacy and safety of adjunctive cilostazol to dual antiplatelet therapy after stent implantation: an updated meta-analysis of randomized controlled trials. J Cardiovasc Pharmacol Ther. 2013;18(3):222–8.

23. Bangalore S, Singh A, Toklu B, DiNicolantonio JJ, Croce K, Feit F, Bhatt DL. Efficacy of cilostazol on platelet reactivity and cardiovascular outcomes in patients undergoingpercutaneous coronary intervention: insights from a meta-analysis of randomised trials. Open Heart. 2014;1(1):e000068.

10

Prevalence of borrowing and sharing prescription medicines and associated socio-demographic factors: findings from COBERS health centres in northern Uganda

James Henry Obol[1*], Peter Akera[1], Pamela Ochola Atim[1], Sylvia Awor[2], Ronald Wanyama[3], Kenneth Luryama Moi[4], Bongomin Bodo[5], Patrick Olwedo Odong[6], Emmanuel Otto Omony[7], Hussein Oria[8], David Musoke[9] and Felix Kaducu[1]

Abstract

Background: The use of prescription medications without the involvement of medical professionals is a growing public health concern. Therefore this study was conducted to determine the prevalence of borrowing and sharing prescription medicines and associated socio-demographic factors among community members who had sought health care from COBERS health centres.

Methods: We conducted analytical cross – sectional study among former patients who sought treatment during the two months period prior to data collection in nine COBERS health centres. We used cluster proportional-to-size sampling method to get the numbers of research participants to be selected for interview from each COBERS site and logistic regression model was used to assess the associations.

Results: The prevalence of borrowing prescription medication was found to be 35.9% (95% CI 33.5–38.2%) and sharing prescription medication was 32.7% (95% CI 30.4–34.9%). The Socio-demographic factors associated with borrowing prescription medicines were: age group ≤19 years (AOR = 2.64, 95%CI 1.47–4.74, p-value = 0.001); age group 20–29 years (AOR = 2.78, 95%CI 1.71–4.50, p-value≤0.001); age group 30–39 years (AOR = 1.90, 95%CI 1.18–3.06, p-value = 0.009); age group 40–49 (AOR = 1.83, 95%CI 1.15–2.92, p-value = 0.011); being a female (AOR = 2.01, 1.58–2.55, p-value< 0.001); being a Pentecostal by faith (AOR = 1.69, 95%CI 1.02–2.81, p-value = 0.042) and being Employed Salary Earner (AOR = 0.44, 95%CI 0.25–0.78, p-value = 0.005). The socio-demographic factors associated with sharing prescription medicines were: age group ≥19 years (AOR = 4.17, 95%CI 2.24–7.76, p-value< 0.001); age group 20–29 years (AOR = 3.91, 95%CI 2.46–6.29, p-value< 0.001); age group 30–39 years (AOR = 2.94, 95%CI 2.05–4.21, p-value< 0.001); age group 40–49 years (AOR = 2.22, 95%CI 1.29–3.82, p-value = 0.004); being female (AOR = 2.50, 95%CI 1.70–3.47, p-value< 0.001); being Pentecostal by faith (AOR = 2.15, 95%CI 1.15–4.03, p-value = 0.017); and being engaged in business (AOR = 1.80, 95%CI 1.16–2.80, p-value = 0.009).

Conclusion: A high proportion of study participants had borrowed or shared prescription medicines during the two months prior to our study. It is recommended that stakeholders sensitise the community members on the danger of borrowing and sharing prescription medicines to avert the practice.

Keywords: Socio-demographic factors, Borrowing and sharing prescription medicines, COBERS health centres, Gulu University

* Correspondence: obolh@yahoo.com
[1]Department of Public Health, Faculty of Medicine, Gulu University, P.O Box 166, Gulu, Uganda
Full list of author information is available at the end of the article

Introduction

Background

The use of prescription medications without the involvement of medical professionals is a growing public health concern [1, 2]. Borrowing prescription medication is when a patient takes medication which is prescribed for someone else [3, 4] and sharing is a situation of giving one's medications to someone [2]. In our study, borrowing prescription medicine means receiving the medicine with the implied intention of returning the same while sharing prescription medicine is giving part of one's medicine to someone else.

This behaviour is of medical and public health concern because of the many potential adverse consequences [5, 6]. Some of the adverse consequences are resistance to the medicine, wrong dosing or duration of treatment leading to delay in cure of a condition thereby making someone believe that the treatment was ineffective. There is also a likelihood of some adverse events occurring as the result of using the medication [2, 3, 7, 8].

In developed countries, studies have investigated the influence of demographic factors on the rate of medication borrowing. Studies have shown that women share medications more than men but both men and women were likely to borrow medications equally [3, 9]. In Africa, there is little information on the prevalence of prescription medication borrowing and sharing as well as associated socio-demographic factors [3, 9]. Research has shown that the prevalence of prescription medication borrowing increases through adolescence, it peaks in the third decade and then decreases as age increases [4].

Study has shown that the most frequently borrowed prescription medications are opiates and hypnotics [3]. Analgesics had a high lifetime rate at 35% of being borrowed [10]. Results from other researches show that other prescription medications borrowed, were for conditions such as acne, allergy, pain, birth control, asthma amongst others [11, 12].

In developing countries, people are more likely to borrow, share prescription medicine because of the large stock of medicines kept at home for reuse, or given to those who request them [13]. The prevalence and socio-demographic factors that are associated with prescription medication borrowing and sharing in Uganda is scanty. The Uganda Ministry of Health in its 2010 Annual Health Sector Performance Report noted that there had been inherent drug stock out at the health facilities in Uganda [14]. Northern Uganda is just recovering from over two decades of armed conflict, which has led to breakdown of healthcare and social services. The poverty rate is 43.7% while the national average is 19.7% [15]. In the light of the above, we then undertook to explore whether the community members practice the habit of sharing or borrowing prescription medicine; what types of prescription medicines are the most commonly borrowed or shared; and their sources. The information gathered will provide the basis for actions by stakeholders (The Ministry of Health, the Local Government, the Development partners and Gulu University Faculty of Medicine) to combat these habits, which have potentially negative consequences on individual, and community health. Therefore, this study aimed at determining the prevalence of borrowing and sharing prescription medicines as well as associated socio-demographic factors among community members who sought health care from the health centres used for Community Based Education Research and Services (COBERS) by Gulu University. COBERS is an academic program during which 4th year medical students are attached to lower health centres for six (6) weeks every semester. During the COBERS placement, medical students participate in both preventive and curative healthcare services as well as community outreach. Therefore, our findings would help in public health campaign to mitigate the adverse impact of borrowing and sharing prescription medicine in the society. The results would also help to create awareness among all health care professionals in finding out whether the patient has had any medicine prior to coming to the health centre for treatment so that correct dosing can be provided.

Methods

Study design

This was a cross sectional analytical study conducted in March 2014.

Study setting

Gulu University uses 11 health centres for COBERS as part of community attachment by medical students during their fourth year of study. We used nine (9) COBERS sites in this study of which five (5) are health centre levels III and four (4) are health centre level IV. Health centre IIIs and IVs provide both curative and preventive services. The health centres also supervise and support planning and implementation of services by the lower health units that are under their areas of jurisdiction [16].

Study population

The study population were former patients who had sought medical care at the health centres two months prior to data collection. All patients who had received healthcare services from the selected COBERS sites in the last two months before data collection were eligible to participate in the study. We excluded patients referred from other health facilities; those with unknown address; and those who had died.

Sample size estimation and sampling procedure

We used the modified Kish Leslie formula of 1965 [17] to estimate our sample size. Since the proportion of borrowing and sharing prescription medicines were unknown, we used 50% as our proportion of patients borrowing and sharing prescription medicines. The desired level of precision was set at 5% with the standard normal deviate of 1.96 and a design effect of 2.0 to give sample size of 769 in each of the two months. We assumed that 10% of the participants would not consent/assent to be in the study and thus we selected 1692 eligible study participants of which 78 potential participants did not consent/assent were not included in the study.

We purposively selected COBERS health centres because medical students use them during community placement and, using simple random sampling technique without replacement, we selected nine (9) out of eleven (11) health centres as clusters. We used data capturing form to extract information about former patient's addresses from the health management information system (HMIS) of the health centres. We used the list as our sampling frame. We then used cluster proportional to size sampling method to get the number of research participants to be selected for interview from each COBERS site. After we had obtained the numbers of study participants in each cluster, we used simple random sampling technique without replacement to generate research participants for the interview. Using the former patients' bio data, research assistants traced the eligible participants to their homes and interviewed them using a semi-structured questionnaire.

Data collection, quality and data management

We used semi-structure questionnaires with both open-ended questions and closed ended questions (Additional file 1), which research assistants delivered to the respondents, and recorded their responses. The questionnaire was translated into the local language (Acholi) and then back translated into English to ensure that the meaning of the questions were not lost during translation. We recruited six research assistants whom we trained. During the training, we tested the questionnaire in two villages, which were not part of the communities served by the COBERS health centres to minimise errors during data collection. Close monitoring of data collection process was done to ensure that the questionnaires were filled correctly. Data was double entered into Epidata version 3.1, backed up, edited and cleaned by the researcher to ensure data quality.

Data analysis

The data was exported to STATA version 11 (StataCorp, College Station, Texas 77,845 USA) for analysis. Univariate analysis was performed for socio-demographic characteristics and prevalence of borrowing and sharing prescription medicines. Bivariate analysis was done using Chi-squared test to assess for association between the socio-demographic characteristics and prescription medication borrowing/sharing among participants. We used logistic regression model to assess for association between socio-demographic characteristics and borrowing/sharing prescription medicines. We calculated cluster-adjusted odds ratios plus 95% confidence intervals (CI) for the independent variables. We adjusted for clustering of data among communities around each COBERS site. Any socio-demographic characteristic at multivariate analysis with P-value ≤ 0.05 was taken as a significant predictor of borrowing and sharing prescription medicine.

Results

The age of the study participants ranged from 12 to 87 years with median of 31 years with inter-quartile range of 25–42 years. The majority of the participants were in the age range 20 to 29 years; were females; were at primary education level only; were Catholics; were married or cohabiting; and were working as peasant farmers. The factors associated with borrowing prescription medicines at bivariate were:- age groups of participants, sex, religious affiliation and occupation. The factors associated with sharing prescription medicine among participants at bivariate were-age groups, sex, religious affiliation and occupation. Table 1 summarises the socio-demographic factors and chi-square test results for borrowing and sharing prescription medicine.

35.9% (95% CI 33.5–38.2%) of the study participants had borrowed prescription medicines during the study period while 32.7% (95% CI 30.4–34.9%) of the study participants had shared their prescription medicine during the study period. The details are shown in Table 2.

Analgesics (pain killers) and anti-malarial drugs were the most commonly borrowed and shared prescription medicines. The details are shown in Table 3.

The most common sources of borrowed or shared prescription medicine were neighbours and family members. The details are shown in Table 4.

The socio-demographic factors associated with borrowing prescription medicines were: age groups; being female and being a member of the Pentecostal faith. The socio-demographic factors associated with sharing prescription medicines were: age groups; being female; being a member of the Pentecostal faith and being a businessperson. The details are shown in Table 5.

Discussion

The age of our study participants ranged from 12 to 87 years with the median age of 31 years. The results of our study showed that the prevalence of borrowing

Table 1 Socio-demographic factors and Chi-squared test results for borrowing and sharing prescription medicine, $n = 1614$

Variable	Frequency n (%)	Borrowed Prescription Medicine				Shared Prescription medicine			
		Yes (%)	No (%)	X^2	P-value	Yes (%)	No (%)	X^2	P-value
Age groups									
60 and above years	117 (7.2)	27 (23.1)	90 (76.9)	22.17	< 0.001	17 (14.5)	100 (85.5)	44.94	< 0.001
≤ 19 Years	105 (6.5)	43 (41.0)	62 (59.1)			42 (40.0)	63 (60.0)		
20–29 years	532 (33.0)	225 (42.3)	307 (57.7)			216 (40.6)	316 (59.4)		
30–39 years	489 (30.3)	163 (33.3)	326 (66.7)			158 (32.3)	331 (67.7)		
40–49 years	236 (14.6)	78 (33.0)	158 (67.0)			63 (26.7)	173 (73.3)		
50–59 years	135 (8.4)	43 (31.9)	92 (68.2)			31 (23.0)	104 (77.0)		
Sex									
Male	512 (31.7)	124 (24.2)	388 (75.8)	44.28	< 0.001	103 (20.1)	409 (79.9)	53.58	< 0.001
Female	1102 (68.3)	455 (41.3)	647 (58.7)			424 (38.5)	678 (61.5)		
Level of education									
None	377 (23.3)	133 (35.3)	244 (64.7)	9.26	0.056	108 (28.7)	269 (71.4)	7.41	0.119
Primary education	786 (48.7)	305 (38.8)	481 (61.2)			268 (34.1)	518 (65.9)		
Ordinary level education	345 (21.4)	111 (32.2)	234 (67.8)			122 (35.4)	223 (64.6)		
Advanced level education	87 (05.4)	27 (31.0)	60 (69)			26 (29.9)	61 (70.1)		
Tertiary education	19 (01.2)	3 (15.8)	16 (84.2)			3 (15.8)	16 (84.2)		
Religious affiliation									
Catholic	940 (58.2)	325 (34.6)	615 (65.4)	13.09	0.009	290 (30.9)	650 (69.1)	20.71	< 0.001
Protestant	590 (36.6)	221 (37.5)	369 (62.5)			200 (33.9)	390 (66.1)		
Muslim	12 (0.8)	3 (25.0)	9 (75.0)			4 (33.3)	8 (66.7)		
Seventh Day Adventist (SDA)	15 (0.9)	1 (6.7)	14 (93.3)			1 (6.7)	14 (93.3)		
Pentecostal	57 (03.5)	29 (50.9)	28 (49.1)			32 (56.1)	25 (43.9)		
Occupation									
Peasant farmer	1149 (71.2)	426 (37.1)	723 (62.9)	24.27	< 0.001	358 (31.2)	791 (68.8)	42.28	< 0.001
Employed Salary Earning	171 (10.6)	33 (19.3)	138 (80.7)			32 (18.7)	139 (81.3)		
Business	294 (18.2)	120 (40.8)	174 (59.2)			137 (46.6)	157 (53.4)		
Marital status									
Single/Widow/Divorce/Widower	362 (22.4)	122 (33.7)	240 (66.3)	0.96	0.351	108 (29.8)	254 (70.2)	1.68	0.204
Married/Cohabiting	1252 (77.6)	457 (36.5)	795 (63.5)			419 (33.5)	833 (66.5)		

prescription medication was high with 35.9% of the respondents reported to have ever borrowed prescription medicines during the study period. Similarly, the prevalence of sharing prescription medicine was found to be high with 32.7% of the study participants reported to have ever shared prescription medicine during the study

Table 2 Prevalence of borrowing and sharing prescription medicine

Borrowed prescription medicine	Frequency	Percentage	95% CI
No	1035	64.1	
Yes	579	35.9	33.5–38.2%
Shared prescription medicine			
No	1087	67.3	
Yes	527	32.7	30.4–34.9%

period. A systematic review of literature by Beyene et al. shows that the prevalence of prescription medication borrowing ranges from 5%, which is much lower, compared with the result of our study to 51.9%, which is much higher compared with the result of our study [18]. The review further shows that the prevalence of sharing prescription medicine ranges from 6% to 22.9%, which is much lower, compared with result of our study [18]. The prevalence rates of borrowing and sharing prescription medication in this study are 35.9% and 32.7% respectively. This falls in the range of systematic review that reports it from 5 to 51%. However, previous reports from developed countries show the rate of borrowing and sharing to be 25–26% and 22–24% respectively [3, 19, 20]. This could be due to convenience in accessing those medicines or lack of access to medical care [1].

Table 3 Types of prescription medicine borrowed or shared (Multiple responses allowed)

Types of medicine	Borrowed Prescription Medicine		Shared Prescription Medicine	
	Frequency (n)	Percentage (%)	Frequency (n)	Percentage (%)
Analgesics (pain killers)	451	59.8	463	49.8
Anti-malarial drug	231	30.7	262	28.2
Antibiotics	71	9.4	196	21.1
Antiretroviral	1	0.1	2	0.2
Anti-helminthes	0	0.0	1	0.1
Allergies	0	0.0	6	0.6
Total	754	100.0	930	100.0

Our study indicated a much higher prevalence of borrowing and sharing prescription medicine than the findings of most of the above studies. This could be due to inherent drug stocks out at the health facilities as was reported by the Uganda Ministry of Health in its 2010 Annual Health Sector Performance Report [14]. So people would tend to look for medicine from other sources to treat their conditions. In addition, Northern Uganda has been consistently ranked the poorest region in the country in terms of development index because of the over two decades of armed rebellion in the area. This could explain why they borrowed or shared prescription medicine because most people would not afford to pay for health care services in the private health facilities [15].

Medication for relieving pain was the most frequently borrowed and shared prescription medicine and this is consistent with other previous studies [1, 3, 9, 21, 22]. This could be because pain is a symptom that is felt by the patient and it may negatively affect the patient's quality of life from day to day. The second frequently borrowed and shared prescription medicine was anti-malarial medicine. Malaria is ranked number one among the top ten causes of morbidity and mortality for all age groups in Uganda [16]. It usually presents with headache in people who are infected. From the patient's perspective therefore, prompt treatment with anti-malaria

medicine and pain reliever is vital for patients' recovery and relief. This could explain why pain relievers and anti-malarial medicine were the most frequently borrowed and shared prescription medicine. Neighbours, family members and friends were the most common sources of borrowed and shared prescription medicine. This is consistent with other previous research findings from elsewhere [18, 19].

Socio-demographic factors associated with borrowing and sharing prescription medication

In our study, age was found to be significantly associated with borrowing and sharing prescription medicine. The prevalence of borrowing and sharing prescription medicine peaked at the age group 20 to 29 years and then declined with increasing age. This could be due to poverty and the change in life style on becoming independent within the community making people more exposed to diseases such as malaria. Because of high poverty rate, most people are unable to pay for medical expenses in privates' clinic. The government health centres which offer free services always suffer from frequent drug stock outs. Our finding is in contrast with other studies which showed that the prevalence of medication borrowing increases through adolescence, peak during the third decade of life, and then generally declines with increasing age [1, 4].

Table 4 Sources of borrowed and shared out prescription medicine (Multiple responses allowed)

Sources	Borrowed from		Shared with	
	Frequency (n)	Percentage (%)	Frequency (n)	Percentage (%)
Neighbours	435	75.1	338	62.9
Family members	119	20.6	182	33.9
Friends	14	2.4	17	3.2
Village Health Team members	8	1.4	0	0.0
Health workers	1	0.2	0	0.0
Workmates	1	0.2	0	0.0
Fellow HIV-positive patients	1	0.2	0	0.0
Total	579	100.0	537	100.0

Table 5 Multivariate analysis of socio-demographic factors associated with borrowing and sharing prescription medicine

Variable	Frequency n (%)	Borrow Prescription Medicine			Share Prescription medicine		
		AOR	95% CI	P-value	AOR	95% CI	P-value
Age groups							
60 and above years	117 (7.2)	1.00			1.00		
≤ 19 Years	105 (6.5)	2.64	1.47–4.74	0.001	4.17	2.24–7.76	< 0.001
20–29 years	532 (33.0)	2.78	1.71–4.50	< 0.001	3.91	2.46–6.29	< 0.001
30–39 years	489 (30.3)	1.90	1.18–3.06	0.009	2.94	2.05–4.21	< 0.001
40–49 years	236 (14.6)	1.83	1.15–2.92	0.011	2.22	1.29–3.82	0.004
50–59 years	135 (8.4)	1.65	0.94–2.91	0.083	1.87	0.88–3.98	0.103
Sex							
Male	512 (31.7)	1.00			1.00		
Female	1102 (68.3)	2.01	1.58–2.55	< 0.001	2.50	1.70–3.47	< 0.001
Level of education							
None	377 (23.3)	1.00			1.00		
Primary education	786 (48.7)	0.94	0.69–1.27	0.676	0.92	0.73–1.15	0.442
Ordinary level secondary education	345 (21.4)	0.80	0.56–1.45	0.227	1.09	0.71–1.66	0.691
Advanced level high school education	87 (05.4)	0.94	0.51–1.74	0.840	0.98	0.63–1.53	0.946
Tertiary education	19 (01.2)	0.39	0.11–1.36	0.139	0.47	0.19–1.18	0.108
Religious affiliation							
Catholic	940 (58.2)	1.00			1.00		
Protestant	590 (36.6)	1.15	0.93–1.41	0.189	1.11	0.90–1.36	0.340
Muslim	12 (0.8)	0.58	0.16–2.09	0.404	0.89	0.34–2.30	0.807
SDA	15 (0.9)	0.12	0.01–1.09	0.060	0.12	0.01–1.47	0.096
Pentecostal	57 (03.5)	1.69	1.02–2.81	0.042	2.15	1.15–4.03	0.017
Occupation							
Peasant farmer	1149 (71.2)	1.00			1.00		
Employed Salary Earning	171 (10.6)	0.44	0.25–0.78	0.005	0.51	0.23–1.09	0.083
Businessperson	294 (18.2)	1.12	0.84–1.50	0.428	1.80	1.16–2.80	0.009
Marital status							
Single	362 (22.4)	1.00			1.00		
Married/Cohabiting	1252 (77.6)	1.14	0.87–1.47	0.340	1.17	0.87–1.57	0.311

AOR Adjusted Odds Ratio, *Single* Single/Widow/Divorce/Widower, *SDA* Seventh Day Adventist

Furthermore, women are twice as likely to both borrow and share prescription medication compared to men. This agrees with the findings of other previous studies [1, 3, 9, 23]. Research participants who were members of the Pentecostal faith were 1.69 times more likely to borrow prescription medicine than those from other religious faiths (*p*-value = 0.042). They were slightly over two times more likely to share prescription medication than those from other religious faiths (*p*-value = 0.017). This interesting finding requires further investigation. The question arises whether the Pentecostal preaching of sharing or their belief that prohibits the use of Western medicine drives them to borrow and share prescription medicine so as not to people do not see them at health facilities when sick.

The research participants who were gainfully employed and earning salary were 0.44 times less likely to borrow prescription medicine than other participants (*p*-value = 0.005). This could be because employed salary earning persons are able to pay for healthcare services and transport themselves to the nearest health facility in case of emergency. In addition, those people who are employed are literate and tend to be cautious in making decision related to their health. Therefore, they would be less likely to borrow prescription medicine. In addition, job related engagements would make them busy and interact less with other members of the community. Being somewhat detached from the community would make them less likely to borrow prescription medicine in case of need.

Participants who were engaged in business were 1.8 times more likely to share their prescription medicine than other research participants who were either gainfully employed earning salary or peasant farmers (*p*-value = 0.009). This could be because being engaged in business enables one to afford to pay for medical services including prescription medicine and would be willing to help those in need so as to be seen as someone who cares for others in the society.

Our study had some limitations. The study was a cross-sectional survey and so we could not reliably estimate the pattern of prescription medication borrowing and sharing since there could be seasonal variations. Furthermore, because of the cross-sectional nature of the study, we could not draw cause and effect relationship and our results were limited to association only. It should be noted that, although the prevalence of prescription medication borrowing and sharing were high compared to other studies done elsewhere, social desirability bias might have resulted in underreporting resulting in underestimate of the true prevalence of prescription medication borrowing and sharing in the study population especially with regards to antiretroviral (ARV) medicines. Also, we did not probe those who responded that they neither borrowed nor shared prescription medicine if they would consider lending medication or borrowing it themselves should the need arise; or whether they refrain from borrowing and sharing because they were aware of the potential hazards.

Our study has several important inferences among which are that it is a community-based study. It is the first study in Uganda that utilises members of the community who had sought health care from health centres within their locality. The prevalence of prescription medication borrowing and sharing was significantly high in our study. About one in every three-research participants had reportedly borrowed or shared prescription medicine during the study period. This is of particular importance to medical professionals as it provides insight into the prevalence of prescription medication borrowing and sharing among community members who use COBERS health centres for medical care. With these findings, there is need for providers of medical care to always probe for borrowing prescription medicine while taking patient's medication history. This would help in prescribing medications since; in any given day, several of their patients might have borrowed prescription medication and used them irrationally before coming to the facility for treatment. Thus, there is need for medical care providers to always inquire about medication use, and sensitise the patients about the danger of prescription medication borrowing and sharing.

Conclusions

About one third of the participants have borrowed or shared prescription medicine within the study period, which is a high proportion. Factors, which promote borrowing prescription medicine, were-being female, and ages below 50 years while being employed salary earner avert the habit. Factors associated with sharing prescription medicine were- being female, ages below 50 years and person's occupation that is classified as business. Therefore, stakeholders should sensitise community members on the danger of borrowing and sharing prescription medicine so that the practice is averted. We encourage health care providers to always probe for borrowing prescription medicine while taking patient's medication history. This can help in prescribing medications since, in any given day; several of their patients might have borrowed prescription medication and used them before coming to the facility for treatment. There is need for further study to determine the pattern of borrowing and sharing prescription medicine and the reasons for borrowing and sharing prescription medicine.

Abbreviations
AOR: Adjusted Odds Ratio; ARV: Antiretroviral; CI: Confidence Interval; COBERS: Community Based, Education, Research and Services; GU-REC: Gulu University Research Ethics Committee; SDA: Seventh Day Adventist; UNCST: Uganda National Council for Sciences and Technology

Acknowledgements
We acknowledge the financial support provided by MESAU-MEPI, which enables us to conduct this research. We are grateful to our Research Assistants and Health centre staff that helped us in data collection. We are indebted to our research participants who provided us with valuable information. Last but not least is our sincere gratitude to Prof. Mark James Obwolo for helping us copy edit the manuscript.

Funding
The project described was supported by the Medical Education for Equitable Services to All Ugandans - Medical Education Partnership Initiative (MESAU-MEPI) Programmatic Award through Award Number 1R24TW008886 from the Fogarty International Centre.

Authors' contributions
JHO is the PI. He conceived and designed the study, wrote the proposal, reviewed literature, devised data collection tool, carried out field data collection, designed database and carried out data entry, performed statistical analysis of the data, interpreted the results and drafting of manuscript. PA reviewed literature, drafted proposal, edited data collection tool, carried out field data collection and drafting of manuscript. PAO reviewed literature and participated in drafting of manuscript. SA interpreted the results and drafted the manuscript. RW, POO and EOO reviewed literature, interpreted results and drafted the manuscript. KLM edited data collection tool, interpreted results and drafted the manuscript. BB and DM Designed data collection tool, interpreted the results and drafted the manuscript. HO reviewed literature, edited data collection tool, interpreted results and drafted the manuscript. FK interpreted the results and drafted the manuscript. All the authors have read and approved the manuscript for publication in its current form.

Competing interests
The authors declare that they have no competing interests.

Author details

[1]Department of Public Health, Faculty of Medicine, Gulu University, P.O Box 166, Gulu, Uganda. [2]Department of Obstetrics and Gynaecology, Faculty of Medicine, Gulu University, P.O Box 166, Gulu, Uganda. [3]Department of Biochemistry, Faculty of Medicine, Gulu University, P.O Box 166, Gulu, Uganda. [4]Department of Medical Microbiology & Immunology, Faculty of Medicine, Gulu University, P.O Box 166, Gulu, Uganda. [5]Department of Paediatrics and Child Health: Faculty of Medicine, Gulu University, P.O Box 166, Gulu, Uganda. [6]District Health Office, Amuru District Local Government, P.O Box 1074, Gulu, Uganda. [7]District Health Office, Agago District Local Government, P.O Box 1, Agago, Uganda. [8]Department of Pharmacy, School of health Sciences Makerere University, P.O Box 7072, Kampala, Uganda. [9]Department of Pharmacology, Faculty of Medicine, Gulu University, P.O Box 166, Gulu, Uganda.

References

1. Ward L, Patel NM, Hanlon A, Eldakar-Hein S, Sherlinski K, Ward SH. Prescription medication borrowing among adult patients at an urban medical center. J Urban Health. 2011;88:6.

2. Coben JH, Davis SM, Furbee PM, Sikora RD, Tillotson RD, Bossarte RM. Hospitalizations for poisoning by prescription opioids, sedatives, and tranquilizers. Am J Prev Med. 2010;38(5):517–24.

3. Goldsworthy RC, Schwartz NC, Mayhorn CB. Beyond abuse and exposure: framing the impact of prescription-medication sharing. Am J Public Health. 2008;98:1115–21.

4. Daniel KL, Honein MA, Moore CA. Sharing prescription medication among teenage girls: potential danger to unplanned/undiagnosed pregnancies. Pediatrics. 2003;111:1167–70.

5. Forgione DA, Neuenschwander P, Vermeer TE. Diversion of prescription to the black market: what the states are doing to curb the tide. Health Care Finance. 2001;27:65–78.

6. Compton WM, Volkow ND. Abuse of prescription drugs and the risk of addiction. Drug Alcohol Depend. 2006;81:103–7.

7. Ellis J, Mullin J. Prescription medication borrowing and sharing: risk factors and management. Aust Family Physician. 2009;38(10):816–19.

8. Grzybowski S. The black market in prescription drugs. Med Crime Punishment. 2004;364:28–9.

9. Emily PE, Rasmussen SA, Daniel KL, Yazdy MM, Honein MA. Prescription medication borrowing and sharing among women of reproductive age. J Women's Health. 2008;17(7):1073–80.

10. Garnier LM, Arria AM, Caldiera KM, Vincent KB, O'Grady KE, Wish ED. Sharing and selling of prescription medications in a college student sample. J Clin Psychiatry. 2010;71:262–9.

11. Howell L, Kochhar K, Jr SR, Zollinger T, Koehler J, Mandzuk C, Sutton B, Sevilla-Martir J, Allen D. Use of herbal remedies by hispanic patients: do they inform their physician? J Am Board Fam Med. 2006;19(6):566–78.

12. Larson EL, Dilone J, Garcia M, Smolowitz J. Factors which influence latino community members to self-prescribe antibiotics. Nurs Res. 2006;55(2):94–102.

13. Hardon A, Hodgkin C, Fresle D. How to investigate the use of medicines by consumers. Geneva: World Health Organisation; 2004. (WHO/EDM/PAR/2004.2). www.who.int/drugresistance/Manual1_HowtoInvestigate.pdf. Accessed: 11 Mar 2016

14. Ministry of Health Uganda. Annual Health Sector Performance Report for financial year 2009/10. 2010. http://library.health.go.ug/publications/health-workforce-human-resource-management/performance-management/annual-health-secto-3. Accessed 11 Mar 2016.

15. UNDP Uganda annual report. 2014. http://www.ug.undp.org/content/dam/uganda/docs/UNDPUg2014%20-%20POVERTY%20STATUS%20REPORT%20 2014.compressed.pdf. Accessed 11 Mar 2016.

16. Ministry of Health Uganda. Annual Health Sector Performance Report, 2013.

17. Leslie K. Survey sampling. New York: John Wiley and Sons, Inc.; 1965. p. 78–94.

18. Beyene KA, Sheridan J, Aspden T. Prescription medication sharing: a systematic review of the literature. Am J Public Health. 2014;104(4):15–26.

19. Goulding E, Murphy M, Di Blasi Z. Sharing and borrowing prescription medication: a survey of Irish college students. Ir J Med Sci. 2011;180(3):687–90.

20. Gascoyne A, Beyene K, Stewart J, Aspden T, Sheridan J. Sharing prescription medicines: results of a survey of community pharmacy clients in Auckland, New Zealand. Int J Clin Pharm. 2014;36(6):1268–76.

21. Goldsworthy RC, Mayhorn CB. Prescription medication sharing among adolescents: prevalence, risks, and outcomes. J Adolescent Health. 2009;(6):1–4.

22. Ellis Janette, Mullan Judy. Prescription medication borrowing and sharing – risk factors and management Aust Fam Physician 2009;38(10): 816–819.

23. Asa Auta, Banwat B. Samuel and Francis A. Rachael. Prevalence of prescription medication sharing behaviour among students. Int J of Pharm Life Sci 2011; 2(4): 651–654.

11

A randomised, double-blind, placebo-controlled phase 1 study of the safety, tolerability and pharmacodynamics of volixibat in overweight and obese but otherwise healthy adults: implications for treatment of non-alcoholic steatohepatitis

Melissa Palmer[1]* ⓘ, Lee Jennings[1], Debra G. Silberg[2], Caleb Bliss[1] and Patrick Martin[1]

Abstract

Background: Accumulation of toxic free cholesterol in hepatocytes may cause hepatic inflammation and fibrosis. Volixibat inhibits bile acid reuptake via the apical sodium bile acid transporter located on the luminal surface of the ileum. The resulting increase in bile acid synthesis from cholesterol could be beneficial in patients with non-alcoholic steatohepatitis. This adaptive dose-finding study investigated the safety, tolerability, pharmacodynamics, and pharmacokinetics of volixibat.

Methods: Overweight and obese adults were randomised 3:1 to double-blind volixibat or placebo, respectively, for 12 days. Volixibat was initiated at a once-daily dose of 20 mg, 40 mg or 80 mg. Based on the assessment of predefined safety events, volixibat dosing was either escalated or reduced. Other dose regimens (titrations and twice-daily dosing) were also evaluated. Assessments included safety, tolerability, stool hardness, faecal bile acid (FBA) excretion, and serum levels of 7α-hydroxy-4-cholesten-3-one (C4) and lipids.

Results: All 84 randomised participants (volixibat, 63; placebo, 21) completed the study, with no serious adverse events at doses of up to 80 mg per day (maximum assessed dose). The median number of daily bowel evacuations increased from 1 (range 0–4) to 2 (0–8) during volixibat treatment, and stool was looser with volixibat than placebo. Volixibat was minimally absorbed; serum levels were rarely quantifiable at any dose or sampling time point, thereby precluding pharmacokinetic analyses. Mean daily FBA excretion was 930.61 μmol (standard deviation [SD] 468.965) with volixibat and 224.75 μmol (195.403) with placebo; effects were maximal at volixibat doses $\geq$20 mg/day. Mean serum C4 concentrations at day 12 were 98.767 ng/mL (standard deviation, 61.5841) with volixibat and 16.497 ng/mL (12.9150) with placebo. Total and low-density lipoprotein cholesterol levels decreased in the volixibat group, with median changes of $-$0.70 mmol/L (range $-$2.8 to 0.4) and $-$0.6990 mmol/L ($-$3.341 to 0.570), respectively.

(Continued on next page)

* Correspondence: mpalmer@shire.com
[1]Global Development Lead Hepatology, Shire, 300 Shire Way, Lexington, MA 02421, USA
Full list of author information is available at the end of the article

(Continued from previous page)

Conclusions: This study indicates that maximal inhibition of bile acid reabsorption, as assessed by FBA excretion, occurs at volixibat doses of ≥20 mg/day in obese and overweight adults, without appreciable change in gastrointestinal tolerability. These findings guided dose selection for an ongoing phase 2 study in patients with non-alcoholic steatohepatitis.

Keywords: Volixibat, SHP626, LUM002, Non-alcoholic steatohepatitis, Non-alcoholic fatty liver disease, Apical sodium-dependent bile acid transporter (ASBT), Cholesterol, Obesity

Background

Non-alcoholic steatohepatitis (NASH) is a severe, potentially progressive, fatty liver disease characterised histologically by the accumulation of excessive fat in the liver (steatosis) coupled with lobular inflammation and hepatocyte injury, with or without fibrosis [1–3]. A contributing factor to the pathogenesis of NASH is abnormal cholesterol metabolism and the accumulation of free cholesterol in the liver. Free cholesterol is directly toxic to hepatocytes, leading to inflammation and fibrosis [4].

The prevalence of NASH is difficult to establish because definitive diagnosis requires liver biopsy [5, 6]. Estimates of the population prevalence of NASH range from 2% to 5% [7]; observational studies have reported rates of approximately 5% in adults in Finland [8], and 12.2% in middle-aged adults in the US, rising to 22.2% in those with diabetes [5]. The number of people with NASH is growing at an epidemic rate, paralleling the global rise in obesity, with a prevalence of about 33% in people who are obese [6, 9]. Prospective, long-term histological follow-up studies have found that 27–43% of people with NASH develop liver fibrosis and up to 22% develop cirrhosis, depending on the study [10–14]. Progression of NASH can lead to complications such as liver failure, liver cancer, and the need for liver transplantation [15]. In recent registry studies, NASH was the second most common reason for liver transplantation in the USA in 2013 [16], and the most common reason in adults under 50 years of age in 2014 [17]. The incidence of NASH among adults awaiting liver transplantation increased by 170% from 2004 to 2013 [16].

No approved pharmacotherapies with demonstrated long-term efficacy and safety exist for NASH. Treatment guidelines for NASH recommend individualised plans to manage the metabolic comorbidities with lifestyle interventions such as weight loss, dietary changes and physical activity [18, 19]. However, guidance regarding the implementation of lifestyle interventions in the clinical setting is limited [20] and these interventions are rarely successful [19]. Untreated, NASH is associated with significant morbidity and mortality [15]. Accordingly, NASH is a disease with an unmet medical need for therapy.

Volixibat (SHP626; formerly LUM002) is a highly potent, minimally absorbed, competitive inhibitor of the apical sodium-dependent bile acid transporter (ASBT) that is being developed as a potential pharmacological treatment for NASH [21]. We hypothesise that inhibition of bile acid reuptake via ASBT will stimulate de novo synthesis of bile acids from cholesterol (including free cholesterol) in the liver and have positive metabolic, anti-inflammatory, anti-steatotic, and potentially anti-fibrotic effects in patients with NASH. Approximately 95% of bile acids that enter the gut lumen are recycled back to the gallbladder, where they are stored for subsequent release into the duodenum [22]. Inhibition of ASBT on the luminal surface of enterocytes in the terminal ileum increases faecal bile acid (FBA) excretion, with subsequent upregulation of bile acid synthesis in the liver to replenish circulating bile acids. Bile acids promote the micellisation of fats and fat-soluble vitamins to enable intestinal absorption, but also act as signalling molecules in the hepatic lipid and glucose metabolism pathways via receptors including the farnesoid X receptor (FXR) and G protein-coupled bile acid receptor 1 (GPBAR1; also known as TGR5) [23, 24]. Activation of these receptors on enteroendocrine L cells in the intestine stimulates the release of peptide hormones such as glucagon-like peptides 1 and 2 and peptide YY, which have key functions in controlling insulin release from the pancreas, modulating intestinal growth and function and regulating appetite [25–27]. Intestinal bile acid signalling also stimulates the release of fibroblast growth factors (FGFs) such as FGF19 and FGF21 [28], which regulate glucose and lipid metabolism and bile acid synthesis in the liver [29]. In the liver, bile acid signalling via FXR regulates the synthesis of bile acids, cholesterol and fatty acids, as well as controlling serum cholesterol levels [30, 31]. In addition, because bile acids are synthesized in the liver from low-density lipoprotein cholesterol (LDL-C), reduction of cholesterol levels in the liver to decrease, and possibly reverse, hepatocyte damage may be another mechanism of action for volixibat in the treatment of NASH. Indeed, it has been confirmed that serum LDL-C levels can be reduced if the recycling of bile acids via the enterohepatic circulation is inhibited [32].

In animal models, ASBT inhibitors increase bile acid excretion and promote bile acid signalling in the intestine, with resultant modulation of serum and liver bile acid concentrations, serum cholesterol levels, glucose metabolism, and hepatic fatty acid metabolism [33–35].

A previous phase 1 study [36, 37] demonstrated that volixibat, at doses of 0.5–10 mg/day for 28 days, increased FBA excretion compared with placebo, and upregulated the synthesis of new bile acids from cholesterol in the liver and serum, as indicated by dose-dependent increases in levels of serum 7α-hydroxy-4-cholesten-3-one (C4), a marker of synthesis of bile acids from cholesterol. While FBA excretion was greatest with volixibat 10 mg/day, no clear dose–response relationship was discernible at doses of 0.5–5 mg/day [36, 37]. Volixibat also reduced fasting glucose levels, suggesting improvements in glucose homeostasis in the cohort of patients with type 2 diabetes mellitus (T2DM) included in the study. Volixibat treatment commonly resulted in mild to moderate gastrointestinal adverse events (AEs), consistent with its mechanism of action and a drug with minimal systemic absorption [36, 37]. In this, and in a separate phase 1 study assessing the absorption, distribution, metabolism and excretion of [14C]-volixibat following a single 50 mg dose, the drug was minimally absorbed [36–38]. Serum levels of volixibat were below the lower limit of quantification in nearly all samples, so pharmacokinetic parameters for volixibat could not be calculated, even at the maximum administered dose of 50 mg/day [36–38]. The study of radiolabelled volixibat also showed that it is not metabolized and is eliminated from the body almost exclusively via faecal excretion [38].

The adaptive dose-finding phase 1 study described here reports safety, tolerability, and pharmacodynamics data of daily volixibat doses up to 80 mg (range 5-80 mg), once-daily (q.d.) or twice-daily (b.i.d.) dosing, in addition to ascending and descending dose titration regimens, in obese and overweight individuals – a population characteristic of patients with NASH. A pharmacokinetic analysis was also included to assess the systemic exposure of volixibat at doses above those investigated in previous phase 1 studies of volixibat.

Methods

Conduct and ethics

This phase 1 study (ClinicalTrials.gov identifier NCT 02287779) was conducted between 19 January 2015 and 19 June 2015 at a single site in Knoxville, TN, USA. The study was conducted in accordance with International Conference for Harmonisation guidelines for Good Clinical Practice, the principles of the Declaration of Helsinki, and other applicable local ethical and legal requirements. The study protocol was approved by an independent institutional review board and regulatory agency before initiation. Each participant provided written informed consent before commencing any study-specific procedures.

Participants

The study recruited generally healthy men and women aged 18–65 years who were overweight or obese (body mass index 25.0–35.0 kg/m^2 and body weight > 63.5 kg at initial screening). 'Generally healthy' was defined as no evidence of any active or chronic disease following a detailed review of medical and surgical history, a complete physical examination that included monitoring of vital signs and 12-lead electrocardiography (ECG), and clinical laboratory tests (haematology, biochemistry and urinalysis). In addition, all clinical laboratory findings had to be within normal limits or be considered clinically insignificant by the study investigator. Key exclusion criteria were: a history of any haematological, hepatic, respiratory, cardiovascular, renal, neurological or psychiatric disease; gallbladder removal; and current or recurrent disease that could affect the action, absorption or disposition of the study drug, or that could affect the clinical or laboratory assessments. Full inclusion and exclusion criteria are provided in Additional file 1.

Study design

The study comprised the following periods: screening (days − 28 to − 4), check-in (day − 3), diet stabilisation (days − 2 and − 1), treatment (days 1–12), washout (days 13 and 14), final visit (discharge, day 15) and follow-up. All participants followed an identical low-fibre (approximately 10 g/day), medium-fat (approximately 30% energy from lipids) diet that repeated every 48 h (days − 2 to 15). Eligible participants who successfully completed all the required pre-admission assessments and procedures were admitted to the clinical research centre and were randomised before dosing (day 1).

The study was designed to randomise participants 3:1 to receive volixibat ($n = 9$) or matching placebo ($n = 3$) for 12 days in each of up to nine planned multiple-dose cohorts (Fig. 1). Participants were randomly allocated to receive volixibat or placebo using a computer-generated randomisation schedule. Randomisation was stratified within each cohort using a block size of four. Study drugs (volixibat or placebo) were dispensed by an unblinded individual who was not involved in any other study procedure and who had minimal contact with the participants. Volixibat or matching placebo capsules were administered orally with 240 mL water, 30 min before breakfast on days 1–12. For the b.i.d. regimen, the second capsules were administered 10 h after the morning dose and 30 min before the evening meal.

This adaptive dose-finding study was designed with three initial sequential cohorts of participants who received fixed single daily doses of volixibat (cohort 1: 20 mg q.d.; cohort

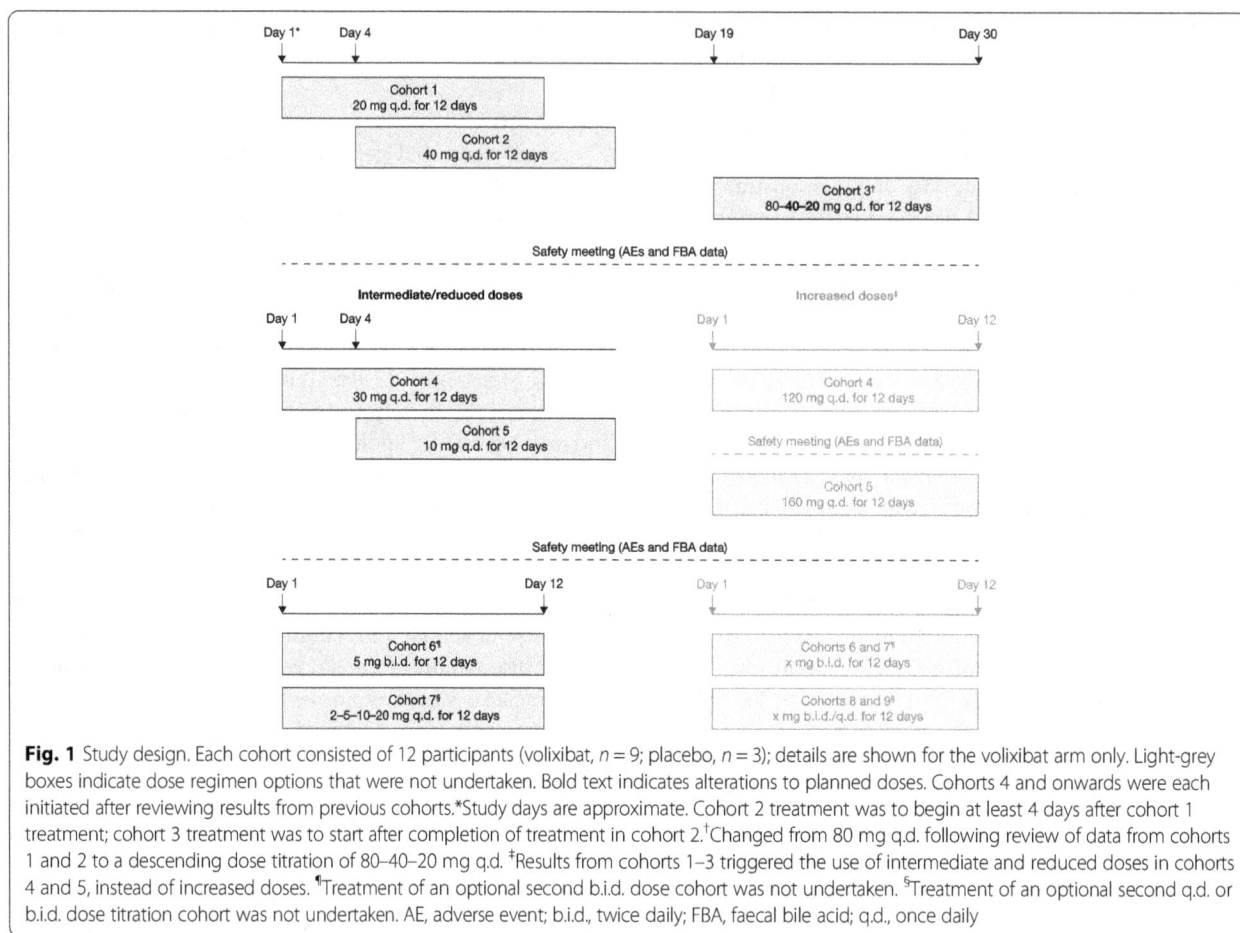

Fig. 1 Study design. Each cohort consisted of 12 participants (volixibat, $n = 9$; placebo, $n = 3$); details are shown for the volixibat arm only. Light-grey boxes indicate dose regimen options that were not undertaken. Bold text indicates alterations to planned doses. Cohorts 4 and onwards were each initiated after reviewing results from previous cohorts.*Study days are approximate. Cohort 2 treatment was to begin at least 4 days after cohort 1 treatment; cohort 3 treatment was to start after completion of treatment in cohort 2.[†]Changed from 80 mg q.d. following review of data from cohorts 1 and 2 to a descending dose titration of 80–40–20 mg q.d. [‡]Results from cohorts 1–3 triggered the use of intermediate and reduced doses in cohorts 4 and 5, instead of increased doses. [¶]Treatment of an optional second b.i.d. dose cohort was not undertaken. [§]Treatment of an optional second q.d. or b.i.d. dose titration cohort was not undertaken. AE, adverse event; b.i.d., twice daily; FBA, faecal bile acid; q.d., once daily

2: 40 mg q.d.; cohort 3: 80 mg q.d.) (Fig. 1). Patients in cohort 2 began treatment 4 days after those in cohort 1; outcomes from cohorts 1 and 2 were evaluated before treatment was started in cohort 3 (19 days after the start of treatment in cohort 1). Modifications to the planned treatment schedule were permitted at the discretion of the investigator and the sponsor's medical monitor, based on assessment of AEs, clinical laboratory data, ECG parameters, vital signs, and FBA excretion. The dose of volixibat was to be escalated in subsequent cohorts, provided that there were no safety or tolerability concerns and that there was a rationale for increasing the dose based on FBA excretion. Dose escalation was halted if any of three predefined safety conditions were met: (1) a serious and severe AE judged by the investigator to be related to treatment; (2) total cholesterol level < 100 mg/dL and LDL-C level ≤ 50 mg/dL on two consecutive days; or (3) clinically important AEs of moderate severity in all participants and severe AEs in at least 25% of participants in a dose cohort. If any of these conditions were met in cohorts 1–3, reduced intermediate doses were to be used for cohorts 4 and 5. Conversely, if none of the conditions were met, the dose of volixibat could be escalated to 120 mg q.d. (cohort 4) and then to 160 mg q.d. (cohort 5), with the possibility of still

higher doses in cohorts 6–9. The study was also designed to assess different dose regimens (titrations or b.i.d. dosing) once the safety, tolerability and FBA excretion profiles had been established for q.d. dosing. If these profiles were similar for an initial b.i.d. dosing regimen compared with the previous q.d. regimens, then a second b.i.d dosing regimen could be examined in an additional cohort, with either an increase or decrease in b.i.d. dose. If appropriate, the study also planned to examine a titration regimen (q.d., b.i.d. or both) and determine the possibility of increasing FBA excretion while improving tolerability.

Participants in each cohort remained in the clinical research centre until discharge on day 15. A follow-up phone call was made 7 ± 2 days after the last dose of study drug to assess AEs, serious AEs and concomitant treatments.

Objectives and outcome measures
The primary objectives of the study were to assess the safety and tolerability of multiple oral doses of volixibat administered q.d. or b.i.d. for 12 days in overweight and obese adults. The secondary objectives were: to evaluate the pharmacodynamics of volixibat using FBA and C4 concentrations and a stool assessment chart; to characterise the

pharmacokinetics of multiple oral doses of volixibat administered q.d. or b.i.d. for 12 days; and to assess the safety and tolerability and characterise the pharmacokinetic profile of volixibat administered in an ascending dose titration regimen. Efficacy was not assessed in the study.

Safety and tolerability assessments

Safety assessments were based on AEs, physical examination, vital signs, clinical laboratory parameters, and ECG parameters. The schedule for all assessments can be found in Additional file 2: Table S1. Treatment-emergent AEs were defined as AEs that started or increased in severity on or after the first dose of study drug and up to the ninth day after treatment cessation. AEs were classified using version 17.1 of the Medical Dictionary for Regulatory Activities. Clinical laboratory assessments included serum biochemistry (at screening and on days − 3, 1, 3, 6, 9, 12, 13, and 15), haematology and urinalysis (at screening and on days − 3, 1, 6, 12, 13, and 15), serum lipid profile (at screening and on days − 3, 1, 9, 13, and 15), blood coagulation (at screening and on days − 3, 6, 13, and 15) and serum fat-soluble vitamin levels (days − 3, 13 and 15) (Additional file 2: Table S1). Blood and urine samples were taken before dosing during the treatment period.

Pharmacokinetic assessments

Blood samples (4 mL) for determination of plasma concentrations of volixibat were obtained at pre-dose and 0.5, 1, 1.5, 2, 3, 4, 6, 8, and 10 h after dosing on day 1; at pre-dose on days 2, 4, 7, and 10; at pre-dose and 0.5, 1, 1.5, 2, 3, 4, 6, 8, and 10 h after dosing on day 12; and on the morning of day 13. Pharmacokinetic parameters were to be determined from plasma concentration–time data for volixibat using non-compartmental analysis, including the maximum observed plasma concentration of volixibat (C_{max}), the time to C_{max} (t_{max}), and the area under the plasma concentration–time curve from time 0 to time t (AUC_{0-t}), where t is the time of the last quantifiable plasma concentration. Plasma concentrations that were below the lower limit of quantification were reported as zero (not quantifiable).

Pharmacodynamic assessments

FBA and serum C4 were measured at Envigo Laboratories, Princeton Research Center, NJ, USA, using standard validated clinical laboratory tests. Blood samples (2 mL) for determination of serum concentrations of C4 were obtained on the morning of day − 1, pre-dose and 5 and 13 h after dosing on day 1, pre-dose on days 6 and 12, and on the morning of day 13.

Stool samples for determination of total FBA excretion were collected at 48-h intervals from 48 h before dosing on day 1 until day 14. Bowel movement frequency was recorded and stool hardness was assessed after each

evacuation using the Bristol Stool Chart (type 1 = hardest stool, type 7 = softest stool) [39].

Data analysis

The planned size of each cohort in this study ($n = 12$) was not based on statistical power calculations. Safety analyses were performed using the safety analysis set, defined as all randomised participants who had received at least one dose of study drug. The pharmacodynamic analysis set was defined as all participants in the safety analysis set with primary pharmacodynamic data that were considered sufficient and interpretable. The pharmacokinetic analysis set included all participants in the safety analysis set with primary pharmacokinetic data that were considered sufficient and interpretable. Statistical analyses were performed using Statistical Analysis System version 9.1.3 or higher (SAS Institute, Inc., Cary, NC, USA). Continuous variables were summarised using the following descriptive statistics: number of participants, mean, median, standard deviation (SD), minimum and maximum. Categorical and count variables were summarised using the number of participants and the percentage of participants in each category.

Results

Treatment cohorts

Each of the seven treatment cohorts in the study consisted of nine participants randomised to receive volixibat (volixibat group) and three randomised to receive placebo (placebo group) for 12 days (Fig. 1). Participants in the volixibat group in cohorts 1 and 2 received 20 mg q.d. and 40 mg q.d., respectively, for 12 days, as planned. Participants in the volixibat group in cohort 3 received the planned dose of 80 mg q.d. on day 1 only. The prespecified safety condition of total cholesterol < 100 mg/dL and LDL-C ≤ 50 mg/dL on two consecutive days was met in one participant in cohort 2, triggering the use of intermediate doses below 40 mg q.d. in subsequent cohorts (this occurrence was not classified as an AE). Furthermore, participants in the volixibat group in cohort 3 received a descending q.d. dose regimen (80 mg on day 1, 40 mg on day 2, 20 mg on days 3–12) instead of the planned 80 mg q.d. Participants in the volixibat group in cohorts 4, 5, and 6 received intermediate doses (30 mg q.d., 10 mg q.d., and 5 mg b.i.d., respectively). A maximal effect based on safety, tolerability and FBA excretion was observed in cohort 2 (20 mg q.d.). Participants in the volixibat group in cohort 7 received an ascending q.d. titration regimen to the dose of maximal effect (2 mg on days 1–3, 5 mg on days 4–6, 10 mg on days 7–9, 20 mg on days 10–12).

Participants and baseline characteristics

In total, 84 adults were randomised to receive volixibat ($n = 63$) or placebo ($n = 21$) and all participants completed the study. All randomised participants received at least one dose of study drug and were included in the safety analysis set. The pharmacodynamic analysis set consisted of 81 participants (placebo, $n = 20$; volixibat, $n = 61$); the remaining three (placebo, $n = 1$; volixibat 5 mg b.i.d., $n = 1$; volixibat 40 mg q.d., $n = 1$) were excluded from the pharmacodynamic analyses because they did not have faecal evacuations when pharmacodynamic outcomes were to be assessed. The pharmacokinetic analysis set was null because sufficient and interpretable primary pharmacokinetic data were not available for any participant.

Demographic and baseline characteristics were generally similar across the treatment groups (Table 1). At study entry, participants had a mean (± SD) age of 40.1 ± 10.93 years and a mean body mass index of 29.44 ± 2.210 kg/m^2 and a mean weight of 90.51 ± 9.976 kg, and 78/84 (92.9%) were men.

Pharmacokinetic analyses
Sufficient and interpretable primary pharmacokinetic data were not available because serum levels of volixibat were rarely above the lower limit of quantification (0.0500 ng/mL) at any of the sampling time points.

Pharmacodynamic analyses
FBA excretion
During treatment (days 1–12), the mean daily total FBA excretion was approximately fourfold greater in participants receiving volixibat than in those receiving placebo in all cohorts combined (Fig. 2a). The mean (± SD) FBA excretion after the first dose of study drug was 930.61 ± 468.965 µmol in the volixibat group, compared with 224.75 ± 195.403 µmol in the placebo group. Mean increases in FBA excretion from baseline (days – 1 and – 2) to days 11–12 in the volixibat group exceeded 600 µmol

in all cohorts, while a small mean (± SD) increase from baseline (51.55 ± 180.371 µmol) was observed in the placebo group (Fig. 2b). Within the q.d. dosing cohorts, the greatest increases in FBA excretion from baseline to days 11–12 occurred at volixibat doses of 20 mg or higher. With b.i.d. dosing at 5 mg, FBA excretion was comparable to the maximal effect obtained at 20 mg q.d. or higher, and about one-third greater than that obtained at 10 mg q.d.

Serum C4 concentrations
On day 12, 13 h after morning dosing, mean (± SD) serum C4 concentrations were approximately sixfold higher in participants receiving volixibat (98.767 ± 61.5841 ng/mL) than in those receiving placebo (16.497 ± 12.9150 ng/mL) (Fig. 3a). In the volixibat treatment group, the highest mean (± SD) serum C4 concentration on day 12 (13 h post dose) occurred in the 2–5–10–20 mg q.d. cohort (152.989 ± 81.6364 ng/mL). Mean serum C4 concentrations in the volixibat group increased by at least 46.9 ng/mL from baseline to day 12 (13 h post dose) in all cohorts, compared with a mean (± SD) decrease of 0.967 (± 22.3963) ng/mL in the placebo group (Fig. 3b).

Bowel movements and stool hardness
Before treatment (day – 1), the daily frequency of bowel movements and stool hardness were similar in the volixibat and placebo groups (Fig. 4). The frequency of bowel movements in all participants receiving volixibat increased from a median of 1 per day (range 0–4) at baseline (day – 1) to a median of 2 (range, 0–8) on day 12 (the last day of treatment). The increase in bowel movement frequency was not dose dependent. No meaningful changes in bowel movement frequency were observed in the placebo group during the treatment period.

Table 1 Demographic and baseline characteristics

| Parameter | Placebo (n = 21) | Volixibat | | | | | | | |
		5 mg b.i.d. (n = 9)	10 mg = q.d. (n = 9)	20 mg q.d. (n = 9)	2–5–10–20 mg q.d. (n = 9)	30 mg q.d. (n = 9)	40 mg q.d. (n = 9)	80–40–20 mg q.d. (n = 9)	Total (n = 63)
Age, years	41.5 (9.47)	37.1 (15.40)	46.2 (7.61)	33.3 (9.82)	46.2 (7.82)	44.6 (10.70)	36.6 (8.92)	33.2 (11.34)	39.6 (11.41)
Men, n (%)	18 (85.7)	9 (100)	7 (77.8)	9 (100)	9 (100)	8 (88.9)	9 (100)	9 (100)	60 (95.2)
BMI, kg/m^2	29.65 (1.426)	27.81 (1.614)	29.53 (2.087)	29.49 (2.587)	29.67 (3.399)	30.96 (1.368)	28.91 (1.898)	29.27 (2.971)	29.38 (2.422)
Race, n (%)									
White	8 (38.1)	4 (44.4)	4 (44.4)	4 (44.4)	7 (77.8)	3 (33.3)	9 (100)	4 (44.4)	35 (55.6)
Black or African American	12 (57.1)	5 (55.6)	5 (55.6)	5 (55.6)	2 (22.2)	6 (66.7)	0	5 (55.6)	28 (44.4)
American Indian or Alaska native	1 (4.8)	0	0	0	0	0	0	0	0

Values are mean (standard deviation) unless otherwise stated. Data are from the safety analysis set
b.i.d., twice daily; BMI, body mass index; q.d., once daily

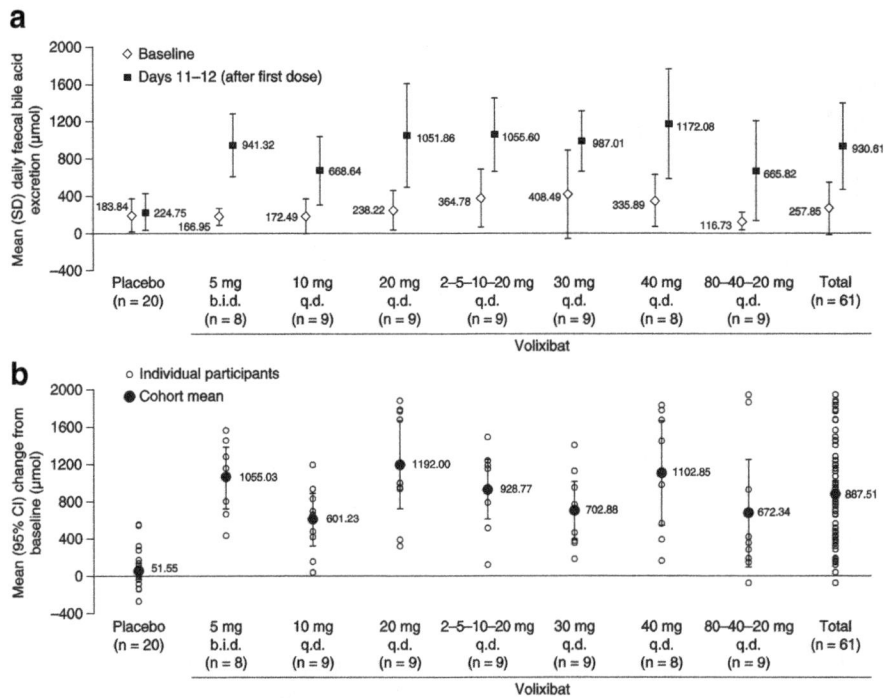

Fig. 2 Mean daily faecal bile acid excretion (**a**) at baseline and days 11–12, and (**b**) change from baseline to days 11–12. Baseline was days − 2 and − 1 for this data set. Data are from the pharmacodynamic analysis set. b.i.d., twice daily; CI, confidence interval; q.d., once daily; SD, standard deviation

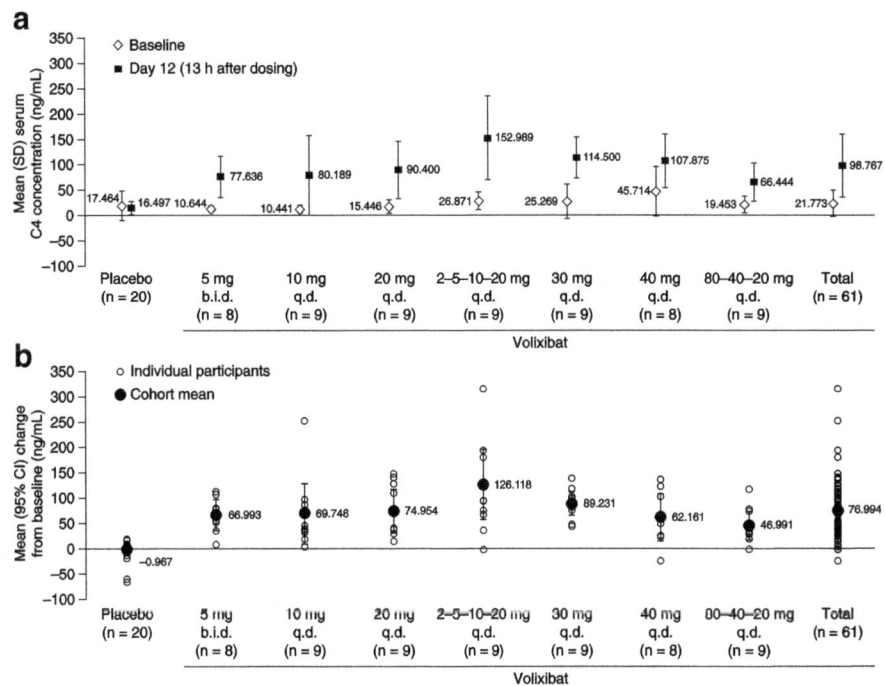

Fig. 3 Absolute serum 7α-hydroxy-4-cholesten-3-one (C4) concentration at (**a**) baseline and 13 h after dosing on day 12, and (**b**) change from baseline to 13 h after dosing on day 12. Baseline was the last observation before the first dose of study drug. Data are from the pharmacodynamic analysis set. b.i.d., twice daily; CI, confidence interval; q.d., once daily; SD, standard deviation

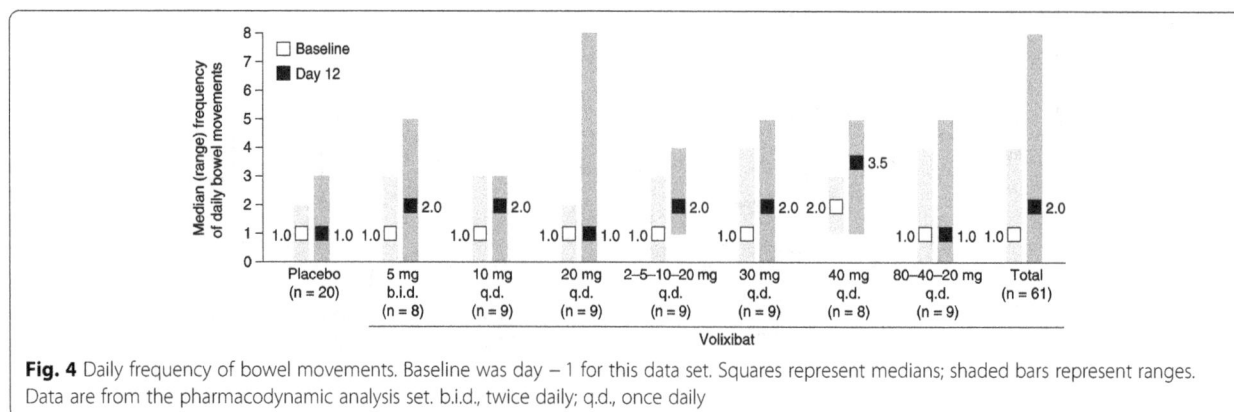

Fig. 4 Daily frequency of bowel movements. Baseline was day − 1 for this data set. Squares represent medians; shaded bars represent ranges. Data are from the pharmacodynamic analysis set. b.i.d., twice daily; q.d., once daily

The proportion of participants with stool samples rated as type 6 or 7 on the Bristol Stool Chart was numerically higher in the volixibat groups than in the placebo group during treatment (Additional file 3: Figure S1). In the volixibat group, this ranged from 41/61 participants (67.2%) on day 1 to 56/61 (91.8%) on day 11. In the placebo group, this ranged from 1/20 participants (5.0%) to 4/20 (20.0%) on days 5–10. During washout, bowel movement frequencies and stool hardness returned to pretreatment values in both the placebo and volixibat groups.

Clinical laboratory parameters
Blood lipids
The median reduction in serum total cholesterol levels from baseline to the final on-treatment assessment in the volixibat group (− 0.70 mmol/L; range − 2.8 to 0.4) was numerically greater than in the placebo group (− 0.20 mmol/L; − 1.0 to 1.7) (Table 2). Median baseline total cholesterol levels were 5.10 mmol/L (range 3.0 to 7.9) in the volixibat group and 5.50 mmol/L (3.7 to 7.5) in the placebo group. Median LDL-C levels decreased in the volixibat group during treatment (− 0.6990 mmol/L; range − 3.341 to 0.570), compared with a small increase in the placebo group (0.0260 mmol/L; − 1.088 to 1.838). Median baseline LDL-C levels were 3.0560 (range 1.321 to 5.594) in the volixibat group and 3.3930 (1.554 to 5.672) in the placebo group. No clinically meaningful changes in levels of triglycerides, high-density lipoprotein cholesterol or very low-density lipoprotein cholesterol were observed.

Blood glucose
No clinically meaningful changes in serum glucose levels were found during the study. At day 13, the median change in glucose concentration was − 0.20 mmol/L (range − 0.9 to 0.7) in the volixibat group and 0.00 mmol/L (− 1.5 to 0.7) in the placebo group, from median baseline concentrations of 5.20 mmol/L (3.9 to 5.9) and 5.30 mmol/L (4.2 to 7.3), respectively.

Fat-soluble vitamins
Clinically meaningful changes in the serum levels of vitamins A, D, E and K (as measured by prothrombin international normalised ratio [PT/INR]) were not seen during the study. Median changes in vitamin A levels at day 13 in the volixibat and placebo groups were 6.0 µg/dL (range − 19 to 31) and 4.0 µg/dL (− 22 to 18), respectively, from median baseline levels of 52.0 µg/dL (29 to 86) and 51.0 µg/dL (31 to 80), respectively. Median changes in vitamin D levels at day 13 in the volixibat and placebo groups were − 0.90 ng/mL (range − 7.4 to 8.8) and 0.50 ng/mL (− 7.3 to 6.2), respectively, from median baseline levels of 19.40 ng/mL (4.5 to 39.4) and 20.30 ng/mL (9.1 to 34.7), respectively. Median changes in vitamin E levels at day 13 in the volixibat and placebo groups were 1.00 mg/L (range − 9.6 to 8.9) and 0.90 mg/L (− 3.4 to 5.0), respectively, from median baseline levels of 9.80 mg/L (5.4 to 19.9) and 9.80 mg/L (5.7 to 16.3), respectively. Vitamin K as measured by PT/INR was unchanged at day 13 in the volixibat and placebo groups (median change of 0.00 in both groups [overall range − 0.3 to 0.8]), from a median baseline value of 1.00 (0.9 to 1.2) in both groups.

Alanine aminotransferase
The only clinically meaningful changes in serum biochemistry, haematology or urinalysis parameters were in serum levels of alanine aminotransferase (ALT). In the volixibat group, the median ALT level at the final on-treatment assessment had increased by 4.0 U/L (range − 44 to 78) from baseline, while a decrease was observed in the placebo group (− 2.0 U/L; − 19 to 25). During treatment, four participants had ALT levels that exceeded twice the upper limit of normal (normal range 0–55 U/L): ALT elevations started on day 3 in one participant, on day 6 in another participant, and after treatment discontinuation (on day 13) in the other two. One participant had concurrent ALT and γ glutamyl-transferase (GGT) elevations that met potentially clinically important (PCI) criteria during the

Table 2 Changes in blood lipid parameters from baseline to final on-treatment assessment

Parameter, mmol/L	Placebo (n = 21)	Volixibat							Total (n = 63)
		5 mg b.i.d. (n = 9)	10 mg q.d. (n = 9)	20 mg q.d. (n = 9)	2–5–10–20 mg q.d. (n = 9)	30 mg q.d. (n = 9)	40 mg q.d. (n = 9)	80–40–20 mg q.d. (n = 9)	
Total cholesterol	−0.20 (−1.0, 1.7)	−0.90 (−2.0, 0.3)	−0.40 (−2.8, 0.4)	−0.70 (−2.0, −0.1)	−0.10 (−0.8, 0.2)	−0.60 (−1.4, 0.3)	−1.30 (−1.8, −0.1)	−1.00 (−1.5, −0.6)	−0.70 (−2.8, 0.4)
LDL cholesterol	0.0260 (−1.088, 1.838)	−0.9190 (−1.502, −0.233)	−0.2975 (−2.719, 0.570)	−0.7520 (−1.761, −0.130)	−0.4925 (−0.699, 0.156)	−0.6990 (−1.451, 0.103)	−1.2690 (−3.341, −0.337)	−0.8030 (−1.476, −0.518)	−0.6990 (−3.341, 0.570)
HDL cholesterol	−0.030 (−0.49, 0.73)	−0.050 (−0.38, 0.23)	−0.080 (−0.85, 0.18)	0.000 (−0.26, 0.18)	0.120 (−0.03, 0.33)	0.130 (0.00, 0.23)	0.030 (−0.21, 0.33)	−0.050 (−0.16, 0.16)	0.000 (−0.85, 0.33)
Triglycerides	0.000 (−2.49, 1.00)	0.190 (−0.11, 3.05)	0.210 (−0.50, 2.08)	−0.130 (−0.68, 1.45)	−0.120 (−0.31, 1.20)	0.060 (−0.10, 0.32)	−0.010 (−0.76, 1.24)	−0.200 (−0.45, 0.05)	−0.010 (−0.76, 3.05)
VLDL cholesterol	0.0 (−1, 1)	0.0 (0, 1)	0.0 (−1, 1)	0.0 (0, 1)	0.0 (−1, 0)	0.0 (0, 1)	0.0 (−1, 2)	0.0 (−1, 0)	0.0 (−1, 2)

Values are median (range). Baseline was the last observation before the first dose of study drug. Data are from the safety analysis set

b.i.d, twice daily; HDL, high-density lipoprotein; LDL, low-density lipoprotein; q.d., once daily; VLDL, very low-density lipoprotein

treatment period, and one had concurrent ALT, aspartate aminotransferase and GGT elevations that met PCI criteria after treatment discontinuation (AST, days 14–15; GGT, days 13–18). None of these four participants with ALT elevations had elevations in bilirubin or prothrombin international normalised ratio. Furthermore, no clear dose–response relationship was evident, and ALT elevations had returned to normal or were returning to normal at the last evaluation.

AEs

Overall, AEs were reported for the majority of participants (placebo, 14/21 [66.7%]; volixibat, 63/63 [100%]). No serious AEs or deaths were reported, and no participant discontinued treatment because of an AE. With the exception of one severe case of upper abdominal pain in a participant receiving volixibat 20 mg q.d., all AEs were mild or moderate in severity. The most commonly reported class of AEs was gastrointestinal, and the single most common AE was diarrhoea, reported for all 63 participants who received volixibat and for 11/21 participants (52.4%) who received placebo (Table 3). Diarrhoea AEs included events described as loose stools (136/182 events in the volixibat group and all 27 events in the placebo group) and events described as diarrhoea (46/182 events in the volixibat group). The majority of participants who received volixibat (39/63) experienced diarrhoea AEs from the first day of treatment. Almost all the AEs that were considered by the investigator to be related to the study drug were gastrointestinal (volixibat, 210/219 events; placebo, 28/34 events). There was no apparent relationship between the incidence of gastrointestinal AEs and volixibat dose. No changes in clinical laboratory parameters, including serum lipid profile, were reported as AEs except for one mild AE of increased hepatic enzyme (ALT) in one participant.

Table 3 Summary of treatment-emergent AEs

AEs, no. of events, n (%)	Placebo (n = 21)	Volixibat							
		5 mg b.i.d. (n = 9)	10 mg q.d. (n = 9)	20 mg q.d. (n = 9)	2–5–10–20 mg q.d. (n = 9)	30 mg q.d. (n = 9)	40 mg q.d. (n = 9)	80–40–20 mg q.d. (n = 9)	Total (n = 63)
Any AE	36, 14 (66.7)	44, 9 (100)	35, 9 (100)	46, 9 (100)	30, 9 (100)	21, 9 (100)	33, 9 (100)	22, 9 (100)	231, 63 (100)
AEs related to study drug	34, 12 (57.1)	39, 9 (100)	32, 9 (100)	45, 9 (100)	30, 9 (100)	18, 9 (100)	33, 9 (100)	22, 9 (100)	219, 63 (100)
AEs occurring in > 1 participant overall									
Gastrointestinal disorders									
Diarrhoea[a]	27, 11 (52.4)	33, 9 (100)	27, 9 (100)	32, 9 (100)	26, 9 (100)	16, 9 (100)	26, 9 (100)	22, 9 (100)	182, 63 (100)
Anorectal discomfort	0	1, 1 (11.1)	0	0	0	2, 2 (22.2)	1, 1 (11.1)	0	4, 4 (6.3)
Nausea	0	1, 1 (11.1)	1, 1 (11.1)	2, 1 (11.1)	1, 1 (11.1)	0	0	0	5, 4 (6.3)
Abdominal pain	1, 1 (4.8)	0	1, 1 (11.1)	2, 2 (22.2)	0	0	0	0	3, 3 (4.8)
Abdominal pain, upper	0	0	0	3, 3 (33.3)	0	0	0	0	3, 3 (4.8)
Gastrointestinal sounds, abnormal	0	0	1, 1 (11.1)	0	1, 1 (11.1)	0	1, 1 (11.1)	0	3, 3 (4.8)
Vomiting	0	1, 1 (11.1)	0	2, 1 (11.1)	1, 1 (11.1)	0	0	0	4, 3 (4.8)
Defaecation urgency	0	0	0	2, 2 (22.2)	0	0	0	0	2, 2 (3.2)
Nervous system disorders									
Headache	2, 2 (9.5)	1, 1 (11.1)	0	1, 1 (11.1)	1, 1 (11.1)	0	3, 2 (22.2)	0	6, 5 (7.9)
General disorders and administrative site conditions									
Application site irritation	1, 1 (4.8)	0	1, 1 (11.1)	1, 1 (11.1)	0	0	0	0	2, 2 (3.2)
Pyrexia	0	2, 2 (22.2)	0	0	0	0	0	0	2, 2 (3.2)

Values are the number of events, followed by the number and percentage of participants experiencing the event [m, n (%)]. Data are from the safety analysis set
[a]Includes events described as 'loose stools' or 'diarrhoea'
AE, adverse event; b.i.d., twice daily; q.d., once daily

Vital signs

The only clinically meaningful changes in vital signs or ECG parameters related to participants' weight. A reduction in median weight was observed at day 15 in both treatment groups. In the volixibat group, reductions in median weight were observed in all cohorts except for the 2–5–10–20 mg q.d. cohort. Compared with a change of − 1.20 kg (range, − 7.20 to 1.9) in the placebo group, reductions were numerically greater in the cohorts receiving volixibat 20 mg q.d. (− 3.60 kg [range − 6.6 to − 0.4]), 80–40–20 mg q.d. (− 3.5 kg [− 6.9 to − 0.6]), 40 mg q.d. (− 2.90 kg [− 5.7 to − 0.7]), and 30 mg q.d. (− 2.30 kg [− 4.9 to 0.3]). At day 15, the proportion of participants with a PCI reduction in weight (≥5% from baseline) was 11/63 (17.5%) in the volixibat group and 1/21 (4.8%) in the placebo group, with the highest proportion occurring in the 20 mg q.d. cohort (4/9; 44.4%) and the lowest in the 2–5–10–20 mg q.d. cohort (0/8; 0%). No clear relationship between dose and degree of weight reduction was evident.

Discussion

This double-blind, randomised, placebo-controlled, multiple-dose, phase 1 study characterised the safety, tolerability, and pharmacodynamics of oral volixibat in overweight and obese adults. In agreement with a previous phase 1 study of volixibat [36, 37], inhibition of ASBT was generally found to be well tolerated and resulted in increased FBA excretion and bile acid synthesis (indicated by increased serum C4 levels). Furthermore, reductions in total cholesterol and LDL-C levels were numerically greater in the volixibat group than in the placebo group but there was no evidence of an effect on glucose levels. In a previous phase 1 study of volixibat in adults with T2DM [36, 37], fasting glucose levels were nominally significantly lower with volixibat than with placebo, with a trend towards improved insulin sensitivity, but there was no evidence for an effect on cholesterol levels [36, 37]. Taken together, the decreased cholesterol levels in normoglycaemic patients with obesity in the present study and the decreased fasting glucose levels in normolipidaemic patients with T2DM in the previous phase 1 study suggest that volixibat may have both anti-dyslipidaemic and anti-dysglycaemic effects in patients with NASH, who typically have obesity, T2DM, or both [40].

Consistent with previous studies of volixibat at doses up to 50 mg [36–38], in the present study volixibat at doses up to 80 mg was minimally absorbed. Due to the lack of sufficient and interpretable primary pharmacokinetic data, pharmacokinetic parameters could not be calculated for volixibat. The minimal absorption of volixibat is most likely due its benzothiepine-based structure including a negatively charged sulfonate moiety [41], which is thought to prevent an interaction with the intestinal cell membrane. The low bioavailability of volixibat is expected considering its mechanism of action as a local inhibitor in the intestinal lumen. Importantly, high systemic exposure of volixibat is neither necessary nor desirable in the treatment of diseases such as NASH, because the local inhibition of bile acid reabsorption in the small intestine results in a series of systemic downstream reactions involved in cholesterol and glucose metabolic processes. Furthermore, the low bioavailability of volixibat reduces the potential for interactions with other pharmacotherapies that are likely to be administered for associated comorbidities in patients with NASH.

The most commonly reported AEs were gastrointestinal, mainly diarrhoea or loose stools. Elevation of the concentration of bile acids in the colon increases mucus secretion, stimulates colonic contractions and reduces colonic transit time [42]. Only one participant receiving volixibat had a severe AE of abdominal pain (at a dose of 20 mg q.d.). The observed AE outcomes were consistent with those seen in a previous phase 1 study, in which diarrhoea was the most frequently reported AE in participants receiving volixibat 10 mg q.d. for 28 days [36, 37]. Neither ascending nor descending volixibat titration (2–5–10–20 mg q.d. or 80–40–20 mg q.d.) provided any clinically significant improvement in tolerability.

Daily oral volixibat for 12 days inhibited bile acid reabsorption, as indicated by increases in FBA excretion and the median frequency of bowel movements relative to baseline and placebo. An associated upregulation of bile acid synthesis from cholesterol was demonstrated by increases in serum C4 concentration relative to baseline and placebo. Furthermore, median reductions in total blood cholesterol and LDL-C levels were numerically greater in patients receiving volixibat than in those receiving placebo. In a previous phase 1 study that investigated daily volixibat doses of 0.5, 1, 5 and 10 mg for 28 days, the greatest increases in FBA excretion and serum C4 concentration were found in the volixibat 10 mg q.d. cohort [36, 37]. In the present study, there was evidence of a dose-dependent effect of volixibat on FBA excretion in the q.d. dose cohorts. The highest mean increases in FBA excretion after the first dose of volixibat occurred in the 20 mg q.d. and 40 mg q.d. cohorts, and FBA excretion in the 10 mg q.d. cohort was approximately two-thirds of the maximal effect. The present study also investigated whether b.i.d. dosing was more effective than q.d. dosing. In patients receiving volixibat 5 mg b.i.d., FBA excretion was similar to the maximum levels seen with q.d. dosing, although in practice the occurrence of diarrhoea after the second dose is likely to limit the feasibility of a b.i.d. dosing regimen.

Due to the lack of primary pharmacokinetic data, a traditional exposure-response analysis using PK/PD modelling was not possible. However, the study provides an alternative approach to the characterization of a dose-response relationship of volixibat, with response based on a marker for potential clinical efficacy (FBA excretion) and on tolerability. The results show that a volixibat dose of 20 mg q.d. resulted in near-maximal increases in FBA excretion, with no apparent relationship between volixibat dose and the incidence of gastrointestinal AEs.

A median increase in ALT level (4.0 U/L higher than baseline) was observed in the volixibat group but not in the placebo group. These mild, asymptomatic ALT elevations, which were not dose dependent, may be an expected and transient effect of ASBT inhibitors, resulting from increased hepatic cholesterol turnover, rather than an adverse effect of the drug [43, 44]. Phase 2 studies of volixibat will investigate this possibility further.

Fat-soluble vitamin deficiency was not reported in this 12-day study. Because bile acids play a crucial role in the absorption of fat-soluble vitamins, further evaluation of vitamin A, D, E and K levels is warranted in ongoing trials of longer duration.

Conclusion

This phase 1 study of volixibat in overweight and obese adults involved a short treatment period and a small sample size, factors that may limit interpretation of the results. Nevertheless, the promising safety and tolerability profile of volixibat, combined with the observed effects on bile acids and lipid metabolism, warrant further clinical development of this ASBT inhibitor. Based on the results of this trial and other phase 1 studies of volixibat [36, 37], as well as preclinical studies of ASBT inhibition [45], a 48-week, double-blind, placebo-controlled, phase 2 study in adults with NASH (ClinicalTrials.gov Identifier: NCT02787304) has been started. The study aims to assess the effects of volixibat 5, 10 and 20 mg q.d. compared with placebo on liver histology, serum liver-related biochemistry, serum lipids and metabolic indicators (blood glucose, insulin, glycated haemoglobin), in addition to safety and tolerability.

Abbreviations

AE: adverse event; ALT: alanine aminotransferase; ASBT: apical sodium-dependent bile acid transporter; AUC_{0-t}: area under the plasma concentration–time curve from time 0 to time t; b.i.d.: twice-daily; CI: confidence interval; C_{max}: maximum observed plasma concentration; ECG: electrocardiography; FGF: fibroblast growth factor; FXR: farnesoid X receptor; GGT: γ glutamyl-transferase; GPBAR1: G protein-coupled bile acid receptor 1; HDL-C: high-density lipoprotein cholesterol; LDL-C: low-density lipoprotein cholesterol; NASH: non-alcoholic steatohepatitis; PCI: potentially clinically important; PT/INR: prothrombin international normalised ratio; q.d.: once daily; SD: standard deviation; T2DM: type 2 diabetes mellitus; t_{max}: time to maximum observed plasma concentration; VLDL-C: very low-density lipoprotein cholesterol

Acknowledgements

We thank the volunteers and investigators who participated in the study, including the principal investigator, William Smith MD (New Orleans Center for Clinical Research, University of Tennessee Medical Center, Knoxville, TN, USA).

Funding

This study was funded by Shire Development LLC. Under the direction of the authors and funded by Shire International GmbH, Dr. E Gandhi of Oxford PharmaGenesis, Oxford, UK provided writing assistance for this publication. Editorial assistance in formatting, proofreading, copy editing and fact checking was also provided by Oxford PharmaGenesis with funding from Shire International GmbH.

Authors' contributions

MP contributed to drafting of the manuscript, data collection and analysis. LJ was involved in study design and conduct of research. DGS contributed to study design, conduct of research, data collection or analysis and drafting of manuscript. CB contributed to data collection or analysis and drafting of the manuscript. PM was involved in study design, conduct of research, data collection or analysis, and drafting of the manuscript. All authors approved the final version of the article including the authorship list.

Competing interests

All authors are employees of Shire and may own stock or stock options. This study was funded by Shire Development LLC. Volixibat is a Shire investigational medical product. Shire develops and markets treatments for gastrointestinal and metabolic diseases, including NASH.

Author details

[1]Global Development Lead Hepatology, Shire, 300 Shire Way, Lexington, MA 02421, USA. [2]Shire International GmbH, Zahlerweg 10, 6301 Zug, Switzerland.

References

1. Chalasani N, Younossi Z, Lavine JE, Diehl AM, Brunt EM, Cusi K, Charlton M, Sanyal AJ. The diagnosis and management of non-alcoholic fatty liver disease: practice guideline by the American Association for the Study of Liver Diseases, American College of Gastroenterology, and the American Gastroenterological Association. Hepatology. 2012;55(6):2005–23.
2. Masuoka HC, Chalasani N. Nonalcoholic fatty liver disease: an emerging threat to obese and diabetic individuals. Ann N Y Acad Sci. 2013;1281:106–22.
3. Rinella ME. Nonalcoholic fatty liver disease: a systematic review. JAMA. 2015; 313(22):2263–73.
4. Musso G, Gambino R, Cassader M. Cholesterol metabolism and the pathogenesis of non-alcoholic steatohepatitis. Prog Lipid Res. 2013;52(1):175–91.
5. Williams CD, Stengel J, Asike MI, Torres DM, Shaw J, Contreras M, Landt CL, Harrison SA. Prevalence of nonalcoholic fatty liver disease and nonalcoholic steatohepatitis among a largely middle-aged population utilizing ultrasound and liver biopsy: a prospective study. Gastroenterology. 2011;140(1):124–31.
6. Zezos P, Renner EL. Liver transplantation and non-alcoholic fatty liver disease. World J Gastroenterol. 2014;20(42):15532–8.
7. Bhala N, Jouness RI, Bugianesi E. Epidemiology and natural history of patients with NAFLD. Curr Pharm Des. 2013;19(29):5169–76.
8. Hyysalo J, Mannisto VT, Zhou Y, Arola J, Karja V, Leivonen M, Juuti A, Jaser N, Lallukka S, Kakela P, et al. A population-based study on the prevalence of NASH using scores validated against liver histology. J Hepatol. 2014;60(4):839–46.
9. Vernon G, Baranova A, Younossi ZM. Systematic review: the epidemiology and natural history of non-alcoholic fatty liver disease and non-alcoholic steatohepatitis in adults. Aliment Pharmacol Ther. 2011;34(3):274–85.
10. Ekstedt M, Franzen LE, Mathiesen UL, Thorelius L, Holmqvist M, Bodemar G, Kechagias S. Long-term follow-up of patients with NAFLD and elevated liver enzymes. Hepatology. 2006;44(4):865–73.
11. Wong VW, Wong GL, Choi PC, Chan AW, Li MK, Chan HY, Chim AM, Yu J, Sung JJ, Chan HL. Disease progression of non-alcoholic fatty liver disease: a prospective study with paired liver biopsies at 3 years. Gut. 2010;59(7):969–74.
12. Fassio E, Alvarez E, Dominguez N, Landeira G, Longo C. Natural history of nonalcoholic steatohepatitis: a longitudinal study of repeat liver biopsies. Hepatology. 2004;40(4):820–6.
13. Adams LA, Sanderson S, Lindor KD, Angulo P. The histological course of nonalcoholic fatty liver disease: a longitudinal study of 103 patients with sequential liver biopsies. J Hepatol. 2005;42(1):132–8.

14. McPherson S, Hardy T, Henderson E, Burt AD, Day CP, Anstee QM. Evidence of NAFLD progression from steatosis to fibrosing-steatohepatitis using paired biopsies: implications for prognosis and clinical management. J Hepatol. 2015;62(5):1148–55.

15. Angulo P. Nonalcoholic fatty liver disease. N Engl J Med. 2002;346(16):1221–31.

16. Wong RJ, Aguilar M, Cheung R, Perumpail RB, Harrison SA, Younossi ZM, Ahmed A. Nonalcoholic steatohepatitis is the second leading etiology of liver disease among adults awaiting liver transplantation in the United States. Gastroenterology. 2015;148(3):547–55.

17. Banini BA. Nonalcoholic steatohepatitis (NASH) has surpassed hepatitis C as the leading etiology for listing for liver transplant: implications for NASH in children and young adults. In: American College of Gastroenterology Annual Scientific Meeting (Congress Abstract 46). 2016. https://www.eventscribe.com/2016/ACG/QRcode.asp?Pres=199366 Accessed 17 Nov 2017.

18. European Association for the Study of the Liver. European Association for the Study of diabetes, European Association for the Study of obesity: EASL-EASD-EASO clinical practice guidelines for the management of non-alcoholic fatty liver disease. J Hepatol. 2016;64(6):1388–402.

19. Kassirer JP, Angell M. Losing weight – an ill-fated new Year's resolution. N Engl J Med. 1998;338(1):52–4.

20. Hallsworth K, Avery L, Trenell MI. Targeting lifestyle behavior change in adults with NAFLD during a 20-min consultation: summary of the dietary and exercise literature. Curr Gastroenterol Rep. 2016;18(3):11.

21. Keller B, Dorenbaum A, Wynne D, Gedulin B, Setchell K, Olek E, Levin N, Kennedy C. Effect of apical sodium-dependent bile acid transporter (ASBT) inhibition on serum and fecal bile acids in healthy volunteers (congress abstract 55). Falk Symposium. 2014;194

22. Shneider BL. Intestinal bile acid transport: biology, physiology, and pathophysiology. J Pediatr Gastroenterol Nutr. 2001;32(4):407–17.

23. Halilbasic E, Claudel T, Trauner M. Bile acid transporters and regulatory nuclear receptors in the liver and beyond. J Hepatol. 2013;58(1):155–68.

24. Hylemon PB, Zhou H, Pandak WM, Ren S, Gil G, Dent P. Bile acids as regulatory molecules. J Lipid Res. 2009;50(8):1509–20.

25. Drucker DJ, Nauck MA. The incretin system: glucagon-like peptide-1 receptor agonists and dipeptidyl peptidase-4 inhibitors in type 2 diabetes. Lancet. 2006;368(9548):1696–705.

26. Dunning BE, Foley JE, Ahren B. Alpha cell function in health and disease: influence of glucagon-like peptide-1. Diabetologia. 2005;48(9):1700–13.

27. Gutzwiller JP, Goke B, Drewe J, Hildebrand P, Ketterer S, Handschin D, Winterhalder R, Conen D, Beglinger C. Glucagon-like peptide-1: a potent regulator of food intake in humans. Gut. 1999;44(1):81–6.

28. Cyphert HA, Ge X, Kohan AB, Salati LM, Zhang Y, Hillgartner FB. Activation of the farnesoid X receptor induces hepatic expression and secretion of fibroblast growth factor 21. J Biol Chem. 2012;287(30):25123–38.

29. Pournaras DJ, Glicksman C, Vincent RP, Kuganolipava S, Alaghband-Zadeh J, Mahon D, Bekker JH, Ghatei MA, Bloom SR, Walters JR, et al. The role of bile after roux-en-Y gastric bypass in promoting weight loss and improving glycaemic control. Endocrinology. 2012;153(8):3613–9.

30. Lambert G, Amar MJ, Guo G, Brewer HB Jr, Gonzalez FJ, Sinal CJ. The farnesoid X-receptor is an essential regulator of cholesterol homeostasis. J Biol Chem. 2003;278(4):2563–70.

31. Modica S, Gadaleta RM, Moschetta A. Deciphering the nuclear bile acid receptor FXR paradigm. Nucl Recept Signal. 2010;8:e005.

32. Halilbasic E, Baghdasaryan A, Trauner M. Nuclear receptors as drug targets in cholestatic liver diseases. Clin Liver Dis. 2013;17(2):161–89.

33. Chen L, Yao X, Young A, McNulty J, Anderson D, Liu Y, Nystrom C, Croom D, Ross S, Collins J, et al. Inhibition of apical sodium-dependent bile acid transporter as a novel treatment for diabetes. Am J Physiol Endocrinol Metab. 2012;302(1):E68–76.

34. Gedulin B. Apical sodium-dependent bile transport inhibitors (ASBTi) exhibit potent antidiabetic activity in ZDF rats. 49th EASD Annual Meeting.

35. West KL, Zern TL, Butteiger DN, Keller BT, Fernandez ML. SC-435, an ileal apical sodium co-dependent bile acid transporter (ASBT) inhibitor lowers plasma cholesterol and reduces atherosclerosis in Guinea pigs. Atherosclerosis. 2003;171(2):201–10.

36. Tiessen RG, Kennedy C, Keller B, Levin N, Acevedo L, Gedulin C, van Vliet A, Dorenbaum A, Palmer M. Randomized controlled trial: safety, tolerability, pharmacokinetics and pharmacodynamics of apical sodium-dependent bile acid transporter inhibition with volixibat in healthy adults and patients with type 2 diabetes mellitus. BMC Gasteroenterology. 2017; [ms submitted]

37. Tiessen RG, Kennedy C, Keller BT, Levin N, Acevedo L, Wynne D, Gedulin B, van Vliet A, Olek E, Dorenbaum A: LUM002 positive metabolic profile shown after administration of 10mg for 28 days in type 2 diabetes mellitus patients leading to potential treatment for patients with nonalcoholic steatohepatitis (NASH). Hepatology 2014; 60(S1):629A.

38. Siebers N, Palmer M, Silberg DG, Jennings L, Bliss C, Martin PT. Absorption, Distribution, Metabolism, and excretion of [14C]-Volixibat in healthy men: phase 1 open-label study. Eur J Drug Metab Pharmacokinet. 2017; https://doi.org/10.1007/s13318-017-0429-7. [Epub ahead of print]

39. Lewis SJ, Heaton KW. Stool form scale as a useful guide to intestinal transit time. Scand J Gastroenterol. 1997;32(9):920–4.

40. Chiang DJ, Pritchard MT, Nagy LE. Obesity, diabetes mellitus, and liver fibrosis. Am J Physiol Gastrointest Liver Physiol. 2011;300(5):G697–702.

41. Tremont SJ, Lee LF, Huang HC, Keller BT, Banerjee SC, Both SR, Carpenter AJ, Wang CC, Garland DJ, Huang W, et al. Discovery of potent, nonsystemic apical sodium-codependent bile acid transporter inhibitors (part 1). J Med Chem. 2005;48(18):5837–52.

42. Wilcox C, Turner J, Green J. Systematic review: the management of chronic diarrhoea due to bile acid malabsorption. Aliment Pharmacol Ther. 2014; 39(9):923–39.

43. Chalasani N. Statins and hepatotoxicity: focus on patients with fatty liver. Hepatology. 2005;41(4):690–5.

44. Herzog E, Pragst I, Waelchli M, Gille A, Schenk S, Mueller-Cohrs J, Diditchenko S, Zanoni P, Cuchel M, Seubert A, et al. Reconstituted high-density lipoprotein can elevate plasma alanine aminotransferase by transient depletion of hepatic cholesterol: role of the phospholipid component. J Appl Toxicol. 2016; 36(8):1038–47.

45. Rao A, Kosters A, Mells JE, Zhang W, Setchell KD, Amanso AM, Wynn GM, Xu T, Keller BT, Yin H, et al. Inhibition of ileal bile acid uptake protects against nonalcoholic fatty liver disease in high-fat diet-fed mice. Sci Transl Med. 2016;8(357):357ra122.

12

Characterization of differential patient profiles and therapeutic responses of pharmacy customers for four ambroxol formulations

Peter Kardos[1], Kai-Michael Beeh[2], Ulrike Sent[3], Tobias Mueck[3], Heidemarie Gräter[3] and Martin C. Michel[4*] (ID)

Abstract

Background: Ambroxol relieves cough symptoms based on its secretagogue, anti-inflammatory, anti-oxidant, anti-bacterial, anti-viral, immunomodulatory and local anesthetic effects. The present study was designed to explore differential patient profiles and efficacy against acute respiratory symptoms of four formulations registered as over-the-counter medicines.

Methods: Nine hundred sixty-five pharmacy customers purchasing one of four branded ambroxol formulations (extended release capsules, adult syrup, pediatric syrup and soft pastilles) filled a questionnaire including a patient-adapted version of the Bronchitis Severity Scale, several questions on degree of impairment by acute cough, time to onset of symptom relief and duration of treatment. Data on pediatric syrup users were entered by their parents. Based on the exploratory character of the study, no hypothesis-testing statistical analysis was applied.

Results: Users of the pediatric syrup and the pastilles reported somewhat less severe baseline symptoms. The patient-adapted Bronchitis Severity Scale proved feasible as a self-administered tool. Among BSS items, ambroxol formulations improved chest pain while coughing to the largest and sputum to smallest degree (− 75% vs. -40%). Reported efficacy was comparable among formulations with minor differences in favor of the pediatric syrup. Time to onset of symptom relief was less than 60 min in more than 90% of patients and occurred prior to known systemic t_{max}. Time to onset was the parameter with the greatest differences between formulations, being reported fastest with pastilles and pediatric syrup and, as expected, slowest with extended release capsules. All ambroxol formulations were well tolerated.

Conclusions: We conclude that over-the-counter formulations of ambroxol exhibit comparable user profiles and efficacy. Differences in speed of onset of symptom relief may involve not only those in systemic pharmacokinetics but also local anesthetic effects of immediate release formulations. Differences between pediatric and adult syrup may in part reflect reporting bias.

Keywords: Ambroxol, Acute cough, Pharmacy setting, Non-interventional study

* Correspondence: marmiche@uni-mainz.de
[4]Department of Pharmacology, Johannes Gutenberg University, Obere Zahlbacher Str. 67, 55131 Mainz, Germany
Full list of author information is available at the end of the article

Background

The secretolytic agent ambroxol, a metabolite of bromhexine, enhances mucus clearance, facilitates expectoration and eases productive cough based on secretagogue activity, stimulation of pulmonary surfactant production and stimulation of mucociliary transport [1, 2]. It also has anti-inflammatory and anti-oxidant [3, 4] and anti-bacterial and anti-viral properties [2, 5]. Recently, ambroxol was shown to also exhibit immunomodulatory effects in a murine asthma model, where it normalized airway hyperresponsiveness and reduced eosinophils and Th2-related cytokines in bronchoalveolar lavage [6]. Finally, ambroxol affects lysosomal function, which may be beneficial in lysosomal storage diseases [7] or Parkinson's disease [8], but the relevance of this finding remains to be tested clinically. While all of the above effects are assumed to occur by a systemic action, ambroxol also has local anesthetic effects, which are mediated by blockade of Na^+ channels in the cell membrane [9, 10] and probably responsible for its effects in the treatment of sore throat.

Ambroxol is registered for secretolytic treatment of acute and chronic bronchopulmonary diseases associated with a disturbance of mucus formation and transport in adults and children. While many of the clinical studies demonstrating the efficacy and tolerability of ambroxol have been generated prior to the introduction of Good Clinical Practice, a recent review has identified 92 clinical studies of acceptable quality [4]. Randomized, placebo-controlled short-term (up to 2 weeks of treatment) studies showed efficacy against endpoints such as ease of expectoration, phlegm loosening, sputum volume and sputum viscosity [11–13]. Moreover, more recent studies have demonstrated the efficacy of ambroxol lozenges in the treatment of sore throat [14].

Since originally obtaining marketing authorization in Germany in 1978, ambroxol became available in many countries and in multiple formulations. Some of them have meanwhile become available as over-the-counter medications. These include branded formulations of extended release (ER) capsules, pastilles, and syrups for adult and pediatric use. The pediatric and adult syrup formulations are identical in composition except for aromas. This multitude of formulations in part reflects medical science, i.e. that syrups inherently are more effective against cough than tablets – irrespective of their active pharmacological ingredients [15]; it also reflects customer preferences and commercial considerations.

Methods

The present study was designed to explore the different profiles of patients obtaining various ambroxol-containing formulations (Mucosolvan®; ER capsules, soft pastilles, adult syrup or pediatric syrup) as over-the-counter medications and their respective efficacy and tolerability against acute respiratory symptoms within the given indication. In line with the exploratory character of the survey, there was no a-priori hypothesis which formulation may be more effective for which type of patient. Additional goals were to explore a patient-adapted version of the Bronchitis Severity Scale (BSS) [16, 17] for use in a pharmacy setting, efficacy relative to duration of treatment, and treatment satisfaction. Finally, we aimed to obtain additional information on the tolerability of the four formulations of ambroxol based on real world evidence.

In this observational study, a total of 126 participating pharmacies were asked to invite customers aged 18 years or older having purchased one of the four products containing branded formulations of ambroxol (ER capsules, soft pastilles, adult syrup or pediatric syrup) to participate in an anonymous survey. Participants purchased the respective product on their own or according to the pharmacist' recommendation. In case of a parent purchasing the pediatric syrup for a child, the parent was asked to participate on behalf of the child. The study protocol had instructed pharmacies only to invited customers to participate in the survey after a purchase decision had been made. Each pharmacy could recruit up to three customers per formulation. Recruitment was between 7.10.2016 and 4.5.2017. Participants received a € 5 coupon for future purchases from an online retailer as compensation for time spent filling the survey.

Precondition for participation was the purchase of one of the four ambroxol-containing products intended for current treatment of own common respiratory symptoms within the given indication or, for pediatric syrup, those of a child; the person purchasing the product had to have an age ≥ 18 years and be willing and able to independently, plausible and timely complete the questionnaire. The participants could return the survey in a sealed envelope either to the pharmacy or send it postage-free to a contract research organization. The package leaflet and/or the consulting pharmacist provided instructions on appropriate use.

The survey captured demographics and baseline symptoms of the participants prior to start of treatment. Captured demographic variables included gender, age and smoking status (smoking status of parent for pediatric syrup users). Symptom severity was assessed by a patient-adapted version of the BSS, a validated score which rates five key symptoms (cough, sputum, rattles (replacing rales on auscultation), chest pain while coughing and dyspnea) on a scale from 0 to 4 [16, 17]. Additional questions asked for the lead symptom (choice of dry cough, cough with moderate sputum (< 1 teaspoon/day), cough with much sputum (≥ 1 teaspoon/day) and cough bouts), daytime cough frequency (0–2, 3–4 and > 4 times/h), nightly awakening due to cough (0, 1, 2, 3 or ≥ 4 times/night), and degree of impairment for four conditions (falling asleep, exhaustion, ability to concentrate, performing daily tasks; each rated on a Likert scale from 0 to 3 as applies fully, applies mostly, applies partly or does not apply).

The survey also captured when treatment was started relative to onset of symptoms (upon first signs of cough, on day 1–2, on day 3–5 or on day 6), how long it was used (1, 2, 3, 4 or 5 days) and how quickly improvement of symptoms was noticed (0–15, > 15–30, > 30–60 and > 60 min or very fast, fast, moderately fast, slow). It also asked for BSS, frequency of cough, frequency of waking up due to cough in the night, and degree of impairment for five conditions (see above). Final questions were related patient assessment of global treatment success, tolerability and satisfaction with treatment.

Information on adverse events (AE) was collected based on a very broad operational definition as pre-specified in the study protocol. This included reporting of any AE via a healthcare professional on the AE form provided to the participating pharmacies; worsening of any item in the disease symptom or disease-associated impairment score (except for cough with expectoration, which is part of the mechanism of action of ambroxol); global efficacy or global tolerability rated as "poor"; deviation from package leaflet with regard to age range (< 12 years for ER capsules, < 6 years for pastilles).

Data analysis was performed using SAS (version 9.2, SAS Institute Inc., Cary, NC, USA). If one or two of the five BSS items had not been provided, the total BSS was extrapolated from the available items; other missing data were not replaced. In line with the exploratory character of the analyses and recent recommendations [18], no hypothesis-testing statistical analyses were performed. Data on categorical variables are reported as % of participants exhibiting a given parameter. Data on quantitative parameters are reported as means ± SD. Data collection and analysis was performed by Winicker Norimed GmbH (Nuremberg, Germany), a contract research organization, based on a statistical analysis plan developed by the authors. Ethical committee approval was neither required nor recommended for this type of research in Germany at the time it was performed.

Results

Baseline data

A total of 965 customers participated in the survey, equally distributed across the four formulations (Table 1). Twenty-four users were excluded from all analyses due to strong suspicion of incorrect answers; therefore, all analyses are based on a total of 941 subjects. Key demographic data are shown in Table 1. Users of the four ambroxol preparations differed somewhat in baseline symptom severity as determined by the adapted BSS (Table 2). Thus, users of the ER capsules and the adult syrup had a similar total BSS (10.0 and 10.1), whereas users of the pediatric syrup and pastilles were similar to each other but had a lower total BSS (8.7 and 8.8). While all four groups reported similar cough and sputum, the users of the ER capsules and adult syrup had more chest pain while coughing and more dyspnea. In the total cohort, total BSS increased with age (0–5 years: 8.2 ± 3.6, 6–11 years: 8.1 ± 3.1, 12–17 years: 9.3 ± 3.7, ≥18 years: 10.2 ± 3.8), which was largely driven by an age-dependent worsening of expectorations and chest pain while coughing. In the group of all ambroxol users, the most frequent lead symptom was cough with moderate sputum reported by 40.5%, cough with much sputum by 30.1%, cough bouts by 16.4% and dry cough by 13.0%. Daytime coughing frequency and number of nightly awakenings due to cough were comparable across ambroxol formulations; if anything, ER capsule users reported a somewhat greater frequency of both (Figs 1 and 2). Participants reported the strongest impairment in the ability to fall asleep due to cough (Fig. 3) and for exhaustion (Fig. 4), followed by ability to concentrate (Fig. 5) and least impairment for ability to execute daily tasks (Fig. 6). Users of the four ambroxol preparations reported comparable degrees of impairment; if anything, use of the pediatric syrup was associated with the largest impairment of ability to concentrate and to fall asleep.

Treatment outcomes

Across all ambroxol formulations, treatment started upon first signs of cough in 9.1% of patients, on day 1–2 in 51.1%, on day 3–5 in 33.6% and on day 6 or later in 6.2%, indicating its primary use for the treatment of acute cough in line with the intention of the study. Start of treatment was comparable among preparations, but

Table 1 Demographic data of participating subjects. Note that smoking status for the pediatric formulation refers to that of parent (most heavily smoking one if different between parents). Data are means ± SD or percentages of given group

	ER capsules	Adult syrup	Pediatric syrup	Pastilles	Total
n	231	233	244	233	941
Gender, % male	38.0	31.8	40.9	38.2	37.2
Age, years	41.2 ± 15.4	39.3 ± 17.5	12.8 ± 12.8	35.7 ± 15.1	32.0 ± 19.1
Smoking status, % regular/occasional/non-smoker	22.4/17.5/60.1	21.6/18.9/59.5	4.5/8.0/87.5	17.2/12.7/70.1	18.1/15.2/66.7

Table 2 Baseline data, end of treatment data and intra-individual change of items and total score of the Bronchitis Severity Scale (BSS). Possible maximum for individual items is 4, for total score 20. Data are mean ± SD. Numbers of responders for a given item differed somewhat between items but ranged between 92 and 99% in all cases

	ER capsules	Adult syrup	Pediatric syrup	Pastilles	Total
Baseline data					
Cough	2.9 ± 0.7	2.9 ± 0.8	2.9 ± 0.7	2.7 ± 0.7	2.8 ± 0.7
Sputum	2.2 ± 1.0	2.1 ± 1.0	1.9 ± 1.0	2.0 ± 1.0	2.0 ± 1.0
Rattles	1.8 ± 1.1	1.9 ± 1.1	1.6 ± 1.1	1.4 ± 1.1	1.7 ± 1.1
Chest pain while coughing	1.8 ± 1.1	1.8 ± 1.1	1.4 ± 1.1	1.6 ± 1.1	1.6 ± 1.1
Dyspnea	1.5 ± 1.1	1.5 ± 1.2	1.0 ± 1.0	1.1 ± 1.1	1.3 ± 1.1
Total score	10.0 ± 3.8	10.1 ± 3.9	8.7 ± 3.5	8.8 ± 3.8	9.4 ± 3.8
Post-treatment data					
Cough	1.4 ± 0.7	1.3 ± 0.7	1.2 ± 0.6	1.2 ± 0.7	1.3 ± 0.7
Sputum	1.4 ± 1.0	1.3 ± 1.0	1.1 ± 0.9	1.1 ± 1.0	1.2 ± 1.0
Rattles	0.6 ± 0.8	0.6 ± 0.8	0.4 ± 0.7	0.5 ± 0.7	0.5 ± 0.7
Chest pain while coughing	0.6 ± 0.8	0.6 ± 0.8	0.3 ± 0.6	0.5 ± 0.7	0.5 ± 0.7
Dyspnea	0.5 ± 0.7	0.5 ± 0.7	0.3 ± 0.6	0.4 ± 0.6	0.4 ± 0.7
Total score	4.5 ± 3.0	4.1 ± 3.1	3.3 ± 2.5	3.7 ± 2.9	3.9 ± 2.9
Intra-individual change					
Cough	−1.5 ± 0.9	−1.6 ± 0.9	−1.7 ± 0.8	−1.5 ± 0.8	−1.6 ± 0.9
Sputum	−0.8 ± 1.4	−0.9 ± 1.4	−0.8 ± 1.3	−0.8 ± 1.3	−0.8 ± 1.3
Rattles	−1.2 ± 1.0	−1.3 ± 1.0	−1.2 ± 1.0	−0.9 ± 0.9	−1.2 ± 1.0
Chest pain while coughing	−1.2 ± 1.1	−1.3 ± 1.0	−1.0 ± 1.0	−1.1 ± 0.9	−1.2 ± 1.0
Dyspnea	−1.0 ± 1.0	−1.0 ± 0.9	−0.7 ± 0.9	−0.8 ± 0.9	−0.9 ± 0.9
Total score	−5.5 ± 3.8	−6.0 ± 3.8	−5.4 ± 3.3	−5.2 ± 3.3	−5.5 ± 3.6

tended to be earlier with pediatric syrup and pastilles than with adult syrup or ER capsules (day 1–2: 59.0 and 50.6% vs. 46.8 and 47.6%, day 3–4: 31.1 and 21.2% vs. 36.9 and 37.2%). Mean duration of treatment was 4.3 ± 0.9 days, with little difference between formulations, also supporting the idea that these over-the-counter formulations of ambroxol are largely used for treatment of acute cough.

Time to start of symptom relief among all participants was within 1–15 min in 12.2% of patients, within 15–30 min in 38.4%, 30–60 min in 37.2% and > 60 min in 12.1%. While most users of the pediatric syrup (43.4%) and of the pastilles (45.2%) reported a time to onset of 15–30 min, most users of the adult syrup (42.1%) and the ER capsules (47.8%) reported start of symptom relief within 30–60 min. Correspondingly, a subjective start of symptom relief was reported as very fast, fast, moderately fast and slow in 11.1, 47.6, 34.4 and 6.9%, respectively. In comparison of the preparations, a very fast start of improvement was reported most frequently with the pediatric syrup (11.6%) and the pastilles (19.6%) and less frequently with adult syrup (7.8%) and the ER capsules (5.3%); correspondingly, a moderately fast start was reported most frequently with the adult syrup (35.3%) and the ER

capsules (43.0%) and less frequently with the pediatric syrup (31.8%) and the pastilles (27.8%).

Across all formulations, treatment with ambroxol reduced the BSS by 5.5 points (mean end-of-treatment score), i.e. by 59% (Table 2). The strongest improvements were reported for chest pain while coughing (− 1.2; 75%), followed by rattles (− 1.2; 71%), dyspnea (− 0.9; 69%) and cough (− 1.6; 57%), whereas sputum was reduced least (− 0.8; 40%). Compared to ER capsules and pastilles (59%), the improvement was slightly larger with pediatric syrup (62%) and slightly smaller with adult syrup (55%). A similar pattern was observed for each item of the BSS. A post-hoc analysis compared the number of responders as defined by an at least 20, 30% or 40% reduction of the BSS between ambroxol formulations. Responder rate for the 20% reduction was 88.6, 89.5, 92.1 and 91.6% for ER capsules, adulty syrup, pediatric syrup and pastilles, respectively. Corresponding numbers for a 30% reduction were 80.3, 82.0, 87.1 and 84.5%, and for a 40% reduction 70.7, 73.7, 80.9 and 73.0%.

The frequency of daytime coughing was markedly reduced by all ambroxol formulations (Fig. 1). Among all participants, 82.1% reported 0–2 coughs/h, 15.0% 3–4 coughs/h and 2.9% > 4 coughs/h after treatment.

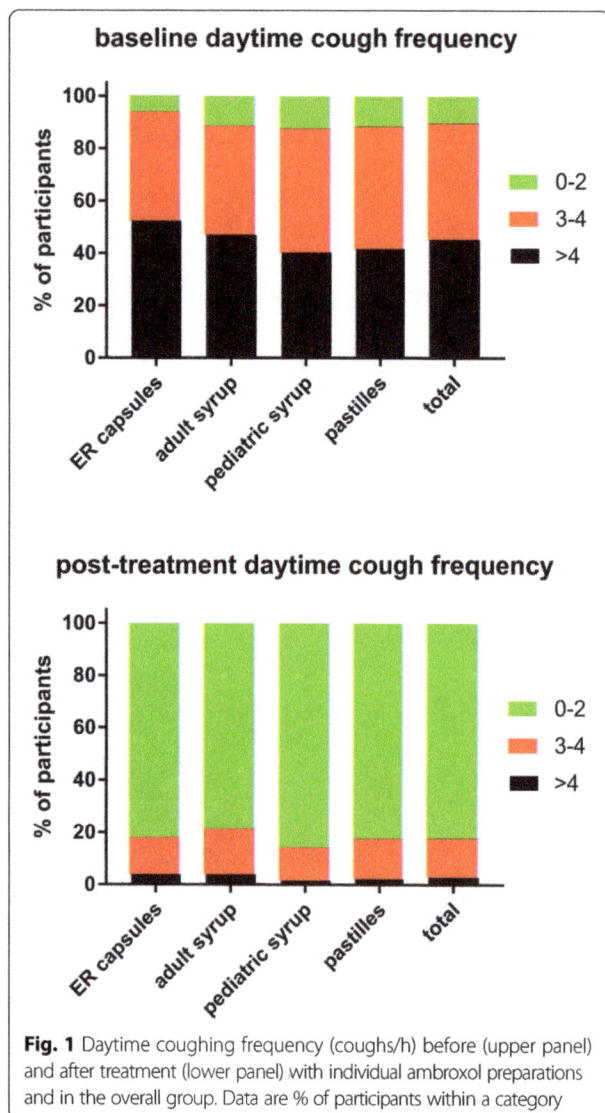

Fig. 1 Daytime coughing frequency (coughs/h) before (upper panel) and after treatment (lower panel) with individual ambroxol preparations and in the overall group. Data are % of participants within a category

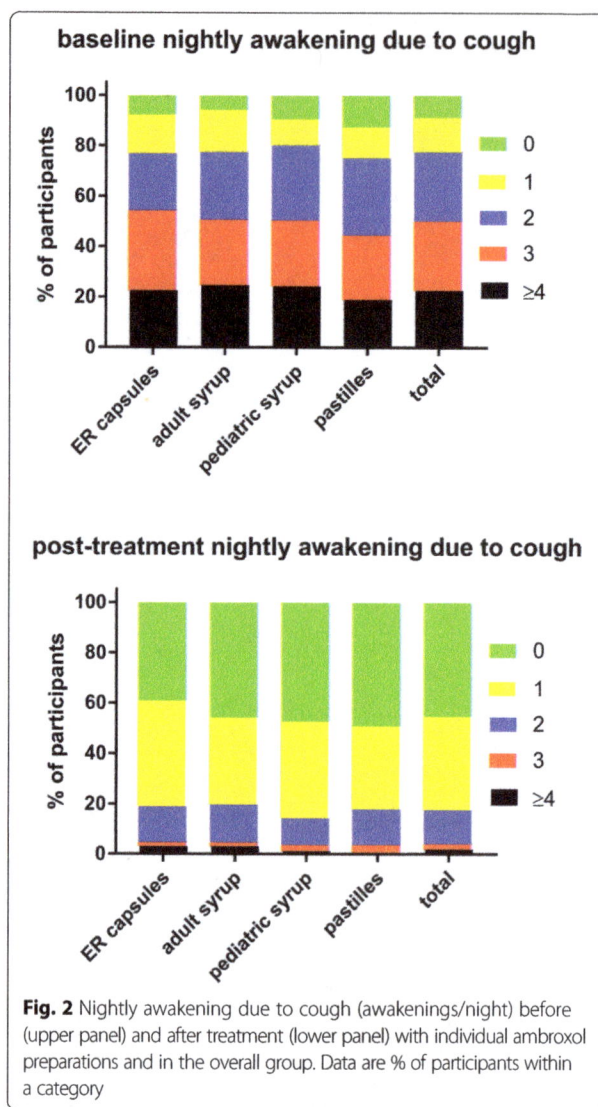

Fig. 2 Nightly awakening due to cough (awakenings/night) before (upper panel) and after treatment (lower panel) with individual ambroxol preparations and in the overall group. Data are % of participants within a category

Notably, 21.2% of subjects with > 4 coughs/h at baseline went to 3–4 and 74.3% to 0–2 coughs/h; similarly, 87.5% of those with 3–4 coughs/h at baseline went to 0–2. The number of nightly awakenings due to cough was also markedly reduced by all ambroxol formulations (Fig. 2). Notably, 31.6% of patients with ≥4 awakenings/night at baseline went to 2, 33.0% to 1 and 23.1% to 0 awakenings/night; similarly, 15.8% of those with 3 awakenings/night went to 2, 56.4% to 1 and 23.9% to 0 awakenings/night. This shift pattern for both daytime coughing frequency and nightly awakening was comparable for all ambroxol preparations (Figs 1 and 2).

Treatment with all four ambroxol preparations markedly improved bronchitis-associated impairments, i.e. ability to fall asleep due to cough (Fig. 3) and exhaustion (Fig. 4), followed by ability to concentrate (Fig. 5) and least impairment for ability to execute daily tasks (Fig. 6). Thus, 51.4% of those reporting to have a fully impaired ability to

fall asleep due to cough at baseline across all ambroxol formulations had no impairment at all after treatment (Fig. 3). Similarly, 45.1% reporting being fully impaired by exhaustion had no impairment after treatment (Fig. 4), 55.1% reporting being fully impaired in their ability to concentrate had no impairment after treatment (Fig. 5) and 60% reporting fully impaired in their ability to perform daily tasks had no impairment after treatment (Fig. 6).

Participants rated global efficacy of ambroxol across formulations as very good, good, moderate or poor in 36.1, 57.5, 6.0 and 0.4% of cases, respectively (Fig. 7). While these estimates were comparable across formulations, ratings were slightly more favorable for the pediatric syrup and the pastilles (Fig. 7). Interestingly, the percentage of patients rating efficacy as very good increased with duration of treatment; thus, it was 31.0% in 2-day users, 34.0% in 3-day users, 34.4% in 4-day

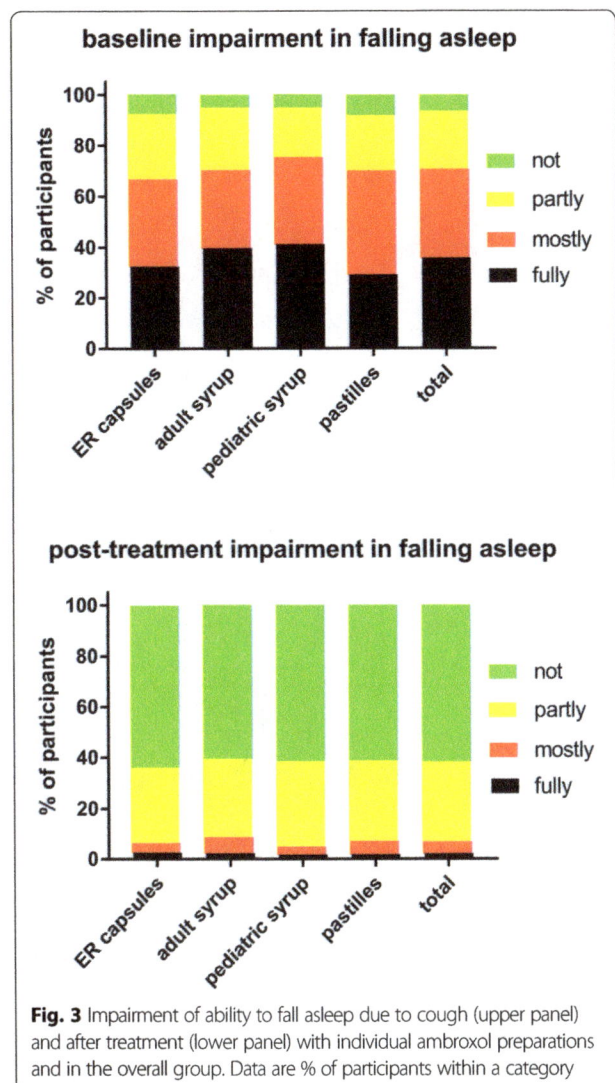

Fig. 3 Impairment of ability to fall asleep due to cough (upper panel) and after treatment (lower panel) with individual ambroxol preparations and in the overall group. Data are % of participants within a category

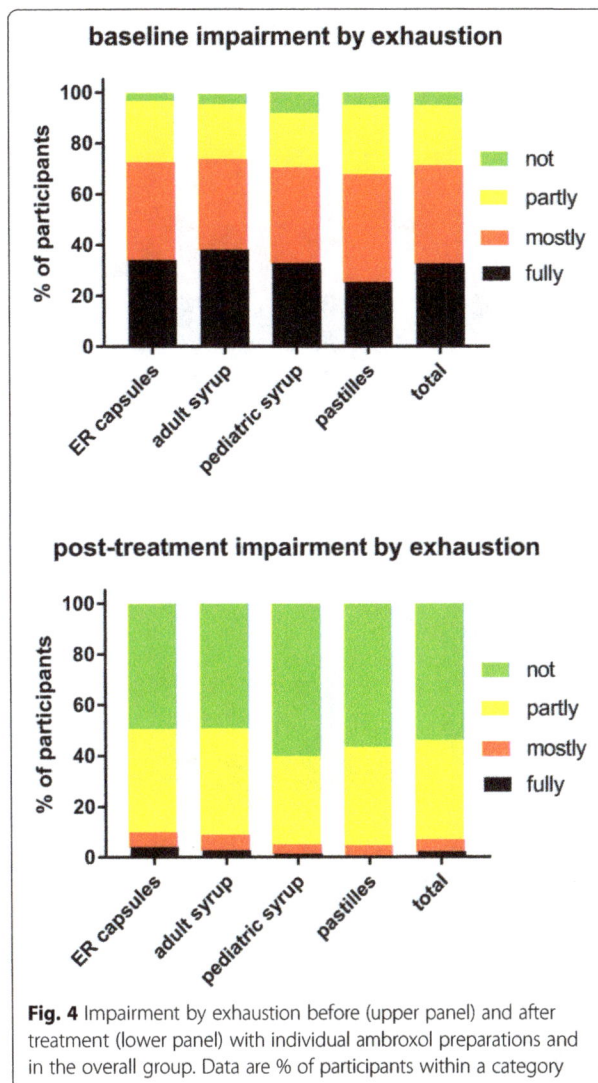

Fig. 4 Impairment by exhaustion before (upper panel) and after treatment (lower panel) with individual ambroxol preparations and in the overall group. Data are % of participants within a category

users and 38.0% in 5-day users. This trend was similarly observed with all formulations. Patients rated global tolerability of ambroxol as very good, good, moderate or poor in 56.4, 41.2, 2.1 and 0.3% of cases, respectively (Fig. 7). While these estimates were comparable across preparations, ratings were slightly more favorable for the pastilles and the pediatric syrup (Fig. 7).

Based on the very broad operational definition of AE (see Methods), AEs were registered in 99 patients (10.3%); none of them had a fatal outcome or was considered serious. This included two cases of diarrhea (0.2%), three with poor global tolerability (0.3%) and four with poor global efficacy (0.4%); the other 90 cases were based on worsening of items in the symptom and impairment scores.

Discussion

Ambroxol has multiple mechanisms of action; while most of them including secretolytic, anti-inflammatory and anti-oxidant activity are assumed to occur by systemic exposure [4], Na$^+$ channel blockade in the treatment of sore throat is assumed to occur by a local effect [9, 10]. However, symptom reduction by syrup and pastilles may partly also involve local effects, for instance in the pharynx as part of the cough inhibition. Against this background, we have surveyed pharmacy customers obtaining different formulations of ambroxol as over-the-counter medication to explore specific profiles of patient groups selecting these formulations as well as their corresponding efficacy and tolerability in a real-world setting.

Critique of methods and feasibility

Our data are based on a survey of pharmacy customers purchasing one of four branded ambroxol containing products. The resulting data are not expected to have the same quality as those collected by a physician or other healthcare professional. Moreover, the use of

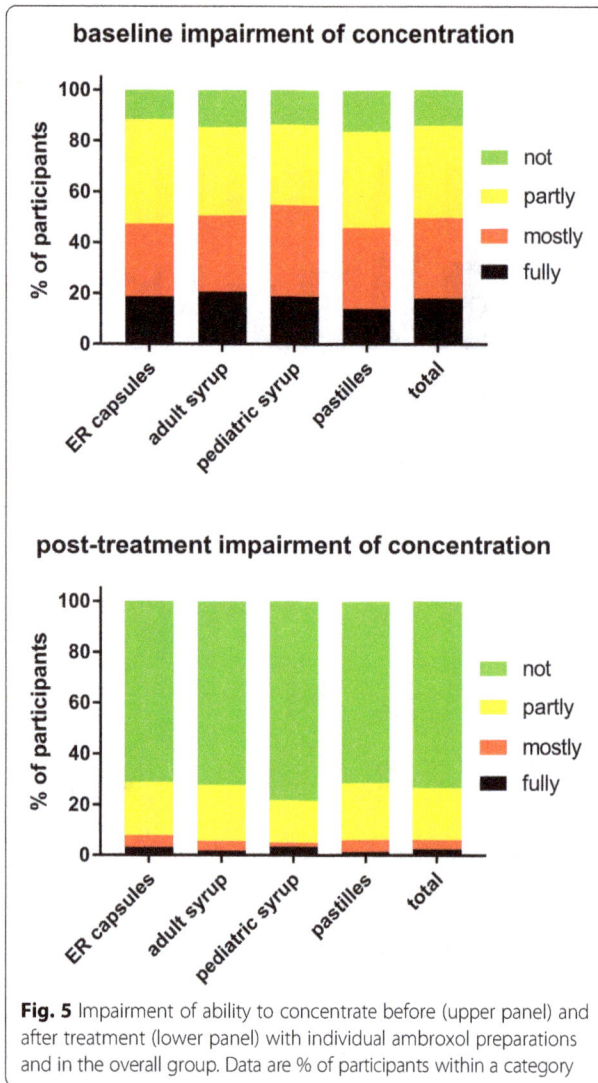

Fig. 5 Impairment of ability to concentrate before (upper panel) and after treatment (lower panel) with individual ambroxol preparations and in the overall group. Data are % of participants within a category

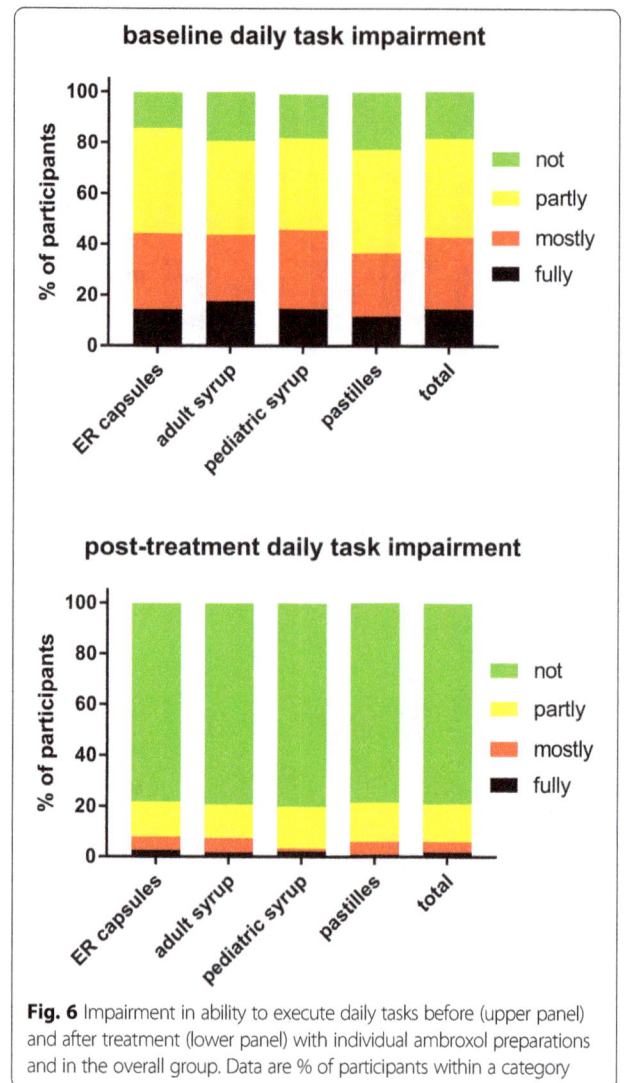

Fig. 6 Impairment in ability to execute daily tasks before (upper panel) and after treatment (lower panel) with individual ambroxol preparations and in the overall group. Data are % of participants within a category

anonymous reponses implies that source data verification was not possible. However, we deem this setting suitable to obtain real-world evidence for over-the-counter medications. Moreover, our previous work using other airway-related over-the-counter medications has demonstrated the external validity of this approach for generating real-world evidence for non-prescription medicines [19, 20].

Our study design did not include a control group, e.g. placebo, for three reasons: Firstly, the efficacy and tolerability of ambroxol has been demonstrated in numerous controlled trials [4]. Therefore, there was no need to re-establish this using a placebo group. Second, such a control group would have interfered with the non-interventional character of our study. Third, the primary intention of our survey was the comparison between ambroxol formulations. Therefore, our data should not be interpreted as proof of efficacy or tolerability but rather as complementary to previously reported controlled studies.

It flows from the non-interventional character of our study that we do not have specific data on ingested doses. While we can assume that ambroxol administration was in line with dosing recommendations of the package insert, this limits comparison of formulations based on exposure data. As the primary aim of the study was explorative, no a priori hypotheses existed; accordingly, no hypothesis-testing statistical tests were applied based on recent recommendations [18].

We have used a patient-adapted version of the BSS to obtain key data (Table 2). The BSS has been validated as a tool for controlled trials [16, 17]. One of the items in the BSS is "rales on auscultation", which obviously needs to be assessed by a healthcare professional. As this would counter the intention to generate real-world evidence, we have replaced this item by the subjective patient-assessed symptom of "rattles". Our data show that pharmacy customers can use this adapted version of the BSS as a self-administered tool.

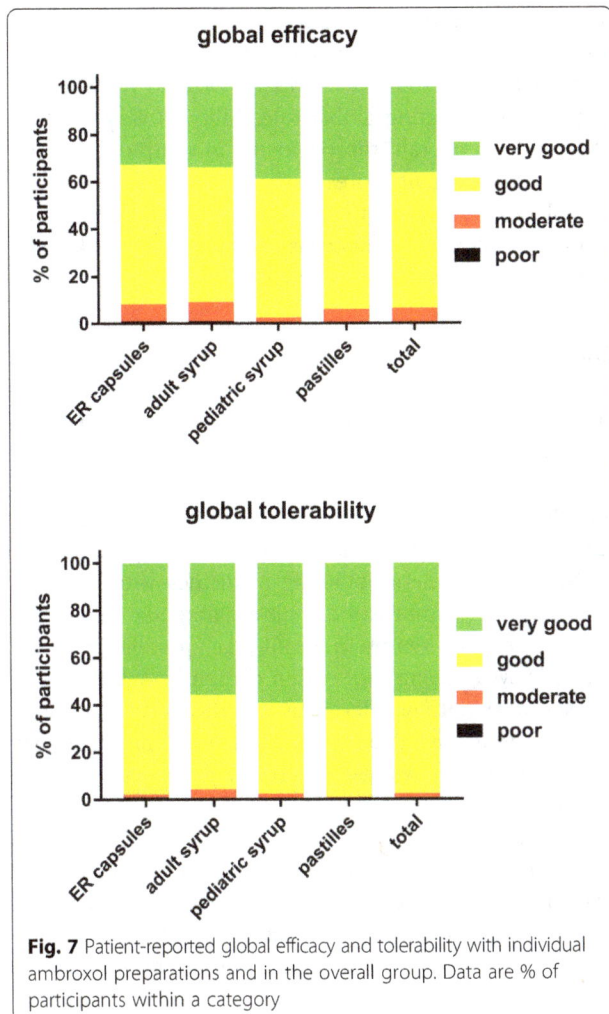

Fig. 7 Patient-reported global efficacy and tolerability with individual ambroxol preparations and in the overall group. Data are % of participants within a category

Based on the efficacy and safety of ambroxol in controlled studies in both adults and children [4, 11–13], our study included a pediatric syrup which yielded somewhat different results than the adult syrup, particularly for time to onset of symptom relief. Several factors may have contributed to such reported differences. Firstly, the vast majority of the users were children and adolescents, but some users have been adults as indicated by the age of 12.8 ± 12.8 years of users of the pediatric syrup (Table 1). This does not represent inappropriate use because the pharmacologically active content is identical to the adult syrup and the package insert of the pediatric syrup also includes dosing recommendations for adults. Nonetheless, it limits interpretation of these data. Second, users of the pediatric syrup tended to have less severe baseline symptoms than those of the adult syrup. Third, the pathophysiology of cough may differ between children and adults. Forth, and perhaps most importantly, data on children were not reported by the patient but by their parents. Previous studies have shown that parental reporting of children's

cough may be biased, for instance smoking parents under-reported night-time cough in their children [21]. However, parent reporting of effects of cough on the quality of life in children has been validated as reliably according to other studies [22]. Therefore, interpretation of data obtained with the pediatric syrup needs to consider potential bias from inclusion of some adult users, differences in baseline severity as well as reporting bias.

Baseline data

Among pooled users of all four ambroxol formulations, cough with moderate and with much sputum production were the most frequently mentioned lead symptoms, accounting for more than 70% of all patients, whereas only 13% reported dry cough as their lead symptom. Accordingly, patients rated the severity of cough higher than that of any other item of the BSS (Table 2). This is not surprising because 45% of participants reported to experience an average of four or more coughs per hour during daytime (Fig. 1). Similarly, 36 and 35% reported "full" or "mostly" impairment of falling asleep (Fig. 3). Awakening four or more times during the night due to coughing was reported in less than 25% of subjects (Fig. 2). While this indicates that coughing impairs falling asleep more frequently than staying asleep, it should be noted that patients experience nighttime cough as a much greater burden than daytime cough [23]. In contrast, users of ambroxol reported full impairment of their ability to concentrate or to execute daily tasks in only 18 and 15% of cases, respectively.

Among formulations for intended use in adults, there was a consistent trend that users of soft pastilles had the least severe symptoms at baseline, be it for the adapted BSS or any of the symptoms shown in Figs 1, 2, 3, 4, 5 and 6. This may reflect that pastilles generally are considered a rather mild form of treatment, perhaps even seen as acting purely locally, whereas capsules and adult syrup are perceived to act systemically. Such perception may have caused a selection bias among those with less severe symptoms.

Treatment data

The present data as reported by pharmacy customers are in line with those from controlled clinical studies [4, 11–13], confirming the efficacy and tolerability of ambroxol in a real-world setting. Moreover, they demonstrate that the patient-adapted version of the BSS is suitable as a self-assessment tool. However, in the absence of reports on effects of ambroxol on BSS in controlled trials, this does not substitute for a formal validation of this version.

The primary aim of the present study had been a comparison of four ambroxol formulations. Focusing on the BSS as efficacy parameter and considering differences in baseline severity among user groups, efficacy was comparable between the formulations. If anything, the pediatric syrup was reported to be slightly more effective and the adult syrup slightly less effective. A similar pattern was also observed for the questions on impairment by the respiratory symptoms. Several factors may have contributed to minor differences in reported efficacy. These include local effects of syrups and pastilles related to local anesthetic action [9, 10], antitussive effects of syrups irrespective of active pharmacological ingredients [15, 24] as well as selection and reporting biases; factors specific for users of the pediatric syrup have been discussed above.

About 90% of participants reported the onset of effect to require no more than 60 min, showing a fast onset of all formulations. This is earlier than the systemic pharmacokinetic t_{max} of the ambroxol formulations, which is 1–2.5 h for all immediate release formulations [25] and 6.5 h for ER capsules [26]. This difference may in part be explained by local effects of the syrups and pastilles, but also points to a possible placebo component in reported time to onset of symptom relief.

Time to onset of symptom relief is the parameter differing most notably between formulations. Thus, compared to the adult syrup, users of pediatric syrup and pastilles reported a somewhat faster and those of the ER capsules a somewhat slower onset of symptom relief. A slower onset of action of the ER capsules is compatible with their later systemic pharmacokinetic t_{max} (6.5 vs. 1–2.5; [26]). A faster onset of action after ingestion of first dose with pastilles may be explained by a longer local contact time in the pharynx, allowing for a greater contribution of local anesthetic effects [9, 10]. Factors possibly involved in specific differential findings in users of the pediatric syrup have been discussed above.

Across all formulations, reported efficacy of treatment increased to some degree with duration of use, i.e. efficacy was rated as very good by 31.0% of subjects using ambroxol for 1 day only, with a step-wise increase to 38.0% in 5-day users. Based on a terminal elimination half-life of 7–11 h [25–27], pharmacokinetic steady-state is not expected to occur earlier than late on the second day of treatment, making earlier full efficacy unlikely. On the other hand, subjects stopping treatment after the first day (other than for adverse events, a situation not reported in this study) are likely to represent a biased sample of patients with very good symptom improvement. As symptoms of acute bronchitis may spontaneously resolve within few days, it is difficult to assess the relative roles of bias vs. reaching pharmacokinetic steady state in the absence of a placebo control group.

Tolerability assessment in a non-controlled study is difficult due to lack of a control group. This particularly applies if any worsening of symptoms or condition-associated impairments is counted as AE, as was done in our study. Such worsening accounted for most of the reported AEs. This is reflected by 97.3% of all participants rating global tolerability as very good or good and the overall improvements in symptom and associated impairment scores at the group level. Therefore, the tolerability data from the present study are not providing new signals or concerns relative to the established tolerability and safety of ambroxol.

Conclusions

The present non-interventional, exploratory study based on effects reported by pharmacy customers confirms the efficacy and tolerability of ambroxol in controlled clinical studies [4, 11–13] in a real-world setting. It establishes that the patient-adapted version of the BSS is suitable for self-assessment, but its validity in this setting remains to be tested. Customers obtaining medicines with different formulations of ambroxol exhibit a differential qualitative and quantitative symptom profile, i.e. pastilles and the pediatric syrup being more often chosen by subjects with less severe symptoms. Nevertheless, efficacy and tolerability of the four formulations tested here was rather similar and, if anything, somewhat greater with pastilles and pediatric syrup, perhaps reflecting the lesser severity of baseline symptoms. We consider it likely that bias of patient perception is involved in these minor differences. The largest difference between formulations was reported time to onset of symptom relief; this may also at least partly reflect patient perceptions as it can only partly be explained by different pharmacokinetic profiles. In a more general view, our data support the concept that symptom relief in over-the-counter self-medication settings are likely to reflect a combination of pharmacodynamic effects and patient perception.

Abbreviations

AE: Adverse event; BSS: Bronchitis severity scale; ER: Extended release

Funding

The underlying study had been funded by Boehringer Ingelheim, part of the analysis has been funded by Sanofi-Aventis. The sponsoring companies as organizations had no role in design of the study, collection, analysis and interpretation of the data, or in the writing of the manuscript. However, three of the authors (US, TM and HG) are employees of the sponsor and worked on this project as part of their employment.

Authors' contributions

PK and KMB led the medical interpretation of the data. US, TM and HG designed the study. MCM led the pharmacological interpretation of the data and drafted the manuscript. All authors contributed to the statistical analysis plan, have commented on the manuscript draft in various stages and approved the final manuscript.

Competing interests

In the last 5 years, PK served on advisory boards for AstraZeneca, Chiesi, GlaxoSmithKline, Menarini, Novartis, Takeda and Teva; received lecture fees from AstraZeneca, Boehringer Ingelheim, Cipla, Menarini, Novartis and Teva; participated in sponsored clinical trials from AstraZeneca, Boehringer Ingelheim and Novartis and has been reimbursed for attending scientific symposia from AstraZeneca, Boehringer Ingelheim, Menarini and Novartis.

KMB declares that no personal payments were received from any pharmaceutical entity in the past 5 years. KMB is a full-time employee of insaf Respiratory Research Institute. His institution has received compensation for services on advisory boards or consulting for Ablynx, Almirall, AstraZeneca, Berlin Chemie, Boehringer, Chiesi, Cytos, Mundipharma, Novartis, Pohl Boskamp, Zentiva. His institution has received compensation for speaker activities in scientific meetings supported by Almirall, AstraZeneca, Berlin Chemie, Boehringer, Cytos, ERT, GSK, Novartis, Pfizer, Pohl Boskamp, Takeda. The institution has further received compensation for design and performance of clinical trials from Almirall, Altana/Nycomed, AstraZeneca, Boehringer, Cytos, GSK, Infinity, Medapharma, MSD, Mundipharma, Novartis, Parexel, Pearl Therapeutics, Pfizer, Revotar, Teva, Sterna, and Zentiva.

US, TM and HG are employees of Sanofi Aventis.

MCM is a past employee of Boehringer Ingelheim and currently a consultant to Sanofi-Aventis.

Author details

¹Group Practice, Center for Allergy, Respiratory and Sleep Medicine, Red Cross Maingau Hospital, Frankfurt am Main, Germany. ²insaf Respiratory Resarch Institute, Wiesbaden, Germany. ³Medical Affairs Consumer Healthcare, Sanofi-Aventis Deutschland GmbH, Frankfurt-Hoechst, Germany. ⁴Department of Pharmacology, Johannes Gutenberg University, Obere Zahlbacher Str. 67, 55131 Mainz, Germany.

References

1. Disse BG, Ziegler HW. Pharmacodynamic mechanism and therapeutic activity of Ambroxol in animal experiments. Respiration. 1987;51(Suppl 1):15–22.

2. Paleari D, Rossi GA, Nicolini G, Olivieri D. Ambroxol: a multifaceted molecule with additional therapeutic potentials in respiratory disorders of childhood. Expert Opin Drug Discov. 2011;6:1203–14. https://doi.org/10.1517/17460441.2011.629646.

3. Beeh KM, Beier J, Esperester A, Paul LD. Antiinflammatory properties of Ambroxol. Eur J Med Res. 2008;13:557–62.

4. Malerba M, Ragnoli B. Ambroxol in the 21st century: pharmacological and clinical update. Expert Opin Drug Metab Toxicol. 2008;4:1119–29. https://doi.org/10.1517/17425255.4.8.1119.

5. Yamaya M, Nishimura H, Lk N, Ota C, Kubo H, Nagatomi R. Ambroxol inhibits rhinovirus infection in primary cultures of human tracheal epithelial cells. Arch Pharm Res. 2014;37:520–9. https://doi.org/10.1007/S12272-013-0210-7.

6. Takeda K, Miyahara N, Matsubara S, Taube C, Kitamura K, Hirano A, Tanimoto M, Gelfand EW. Immunomodulatory effects of Ambroxol on airway Hyperresponsiveness and inflammation. Immune Netw. 2016;16:165–75. https://doi.org/10.4110/In.2016.16.3.165.

7. Fois G, Hobi N, Felder E, Ziegler A, Miklavc P, Walther P, Radermacher P, Haller T, Dietl P. A new role for an old drug: Ambroxol triggers lysosomal exocytosis via Ph-dependent Ca^{2+} release from acidic Ca^{2+} stores. Cell Calcium. 2015;58:628–37. https://doi.org/10.1016/J.Ceca.2015.10.002

8. Mcneill A, Magalhaes J, Shen C, Chau KY, Hughes D, Mehta A, Foltynie T, Cooper JM, Abramov AY, Gegg M, et al. Ambroxol improves lysosomal biochemistry in Glucocerebrosidase mutation-linked Parkinson disease cells. Brain. 2014;137:1481–95. https://doi.org/10.1093/Brain/Awu020.

9. Gaida W, Klinder K, Arndt K, Weiser T. Ambroxol, a Nav1.8-Preferring Na+ Channel Blocker, Effectively Suppresses Pain Symptoms In Animal Models Of Chronic, Neuropathic And Inflammatory Pain. Neuropharmacol. 2005;49:1220–7. https://doi.org/10.1016/J.Neuropharm.2005.08.004

10. Leffler A, Reckzeh J, Nau C. Block of sensory neuronal Na$^+$ channels by the Secreolytic Ambroxol is associated with an interaction with local anesthetic binding sites. Eur J Pharmacol. 2010;630:19–28. https://doi.org/10.1016/J.Ejphar.2009.12.027

11. Olivieri D, Zavattini G, Tomasini G, Daniotti S, Bonsignore G, Ferrara G, Carnimeo N, Chianese R, Catena E, Marcatili S, et al. Ambroxol for the prevention of chronic bronchitis exacerbations: long-term multicenter trial. Respiration. 1987;51(Suppl 1):42–51.

12. Cegla UH. Long-term therapy over 2 years with Ambroxol (Mucosolvan) retard capsules in patients with chronic bronchitis. Prax Klin Pneumol. 1988;42:715–21.

13. Matthys H, De Mey C, Carls C, Rys A, Geib A, Wittig T. Efficacy and tolerability of Myrtol standardized in acute bronchitis. A multi-Centre, randomised, double-blind, placebo-controlled parallel group trial vs. cefuroxime and Ambroxol. Arzneimittelforschung. 2000;50:700–11.

14. De Mey C, Peil H, Kölsch S, Bubeck J, Vix J-M. Efficacy and safety of Ambroxol lozenges in the treatment of acute uncomplicated sore throat. Arzneimittelforschung. 2008;58:557–68. https://doi.org/10.1055/S-0031-1296557.

15. Eccles R. Mechanisms of the placebo effect of sweet cough syrups. Respir Physiol Neurobiol. 2006;152:340–8. https://doi.org/10.1016/J.Resp.2005.10.004

16. Kardos P, Lehrl S, Kamin W, Matthys H. Assessment of the effect of pharmacotherapy in common cold/acute bronchitis – the bronchitis severity scale (Bss). Pneumologie. 2014;68:542–6. https://doi.org/10.1055/S-0034-1377332.

17. Lehrl S, Matthys H, Kamin W, Kardos P. The Bss - a valid clinical instrument to measure the severity of acute bronchitis. J Lung Pulmon Resp Res. 2014;1:00016. https://doi.org/10.15406/Jlprr.2014.01.00016.

18. Motulsky HJ. Common misconceptions about data analysis and statistics. Naunyn Schmiedeberg's Arch Pharmacol. 2014;387:1017–23. https://doi.org/10.1007/S00210-014-1037-6.

19. Kardos P, Schütt T, Mück T, Schumacher H, Michel MC. Pathophysiological Factors In The Relationship Between Chronological Age And Calculated Lung Age As Detected In A Screening Setting In Community-Dwelling Subjects. Front Med. 2016;3:2. https://doi.org/10.3389/Fmed.2016.00002.

20. Klimek L, Schumacher H, Schütt T, Gräter H, Mück T, Michel MC. Factors Associated With Efficacy Of An Ibuprofen/Pseudoephedrine Combination Drug In Pharmacy Customers With Common Cold Symptoms. Int J Clin Pract. 2017;71:E12907. https://doi.org/10.1111/Ijcp.12907.

21. Dales RE, White J, Bhumgara C, Mcmullen E. Parental reporting of Children's Coughin is biased. Eur J Epidemiol. 1997;13:541–5.

22. Anderson-James S, Newcombe PA, Marchant JM, O'grady KA, Acworth JP, Stone DG, Turner CT, Chang AB. An acute cough-specific quality-of-life questionnaire for children: development and validation. J Allergy Clin Immunol. 2015;135:1179–85.E1174. https://doi.org/10.1016/J.Jaci.2014.08.036.

23. Hsu J, Stone R, Logan-Sinclair R, Worsdell M, Busst C, Chung K. Coughing frequency in patients with persistent cough: assessment using a 24 hour ambulatory recorder. Eur Respir J. 1994;7:1246–53.

24. Eccles R. The powerful placebo in cough studies? Pulm Pharmacol Ther. 2002;15:303–8. https://doi.org/10.1006/Pupt.2002.0364

25. Jiang B, Chen J-L, Lou H-G, Yu L-Y, Shen H-H, Ruan ZR. Pharmacokinetic and bioequivalence study of three oral formulations of Ambroxol 30 mg: a randomized, three-period crossover comparison in healthy volunteers. Int J Clin Pharmacol Ther. 2014;52:920–6.

26. Fan G, Hu J, Lin M, An D. Multiple dose pharmacokinetics and relative bioavailability in the human body of orally administered Ambroxol hydrochloride Systained-release capsules. Chin Pharmacol Bull. 2000;16:469–71.

27. Rojpibulstit M, Kasiwong S, Juthong S, Phadoongsombat N, Faroongsarng D. Ambroxol lozenge bioavailability. Clin Drug Investig. 2003;23:273–80. https://doi.org/10.2165/00044011-200323040-00007.

13

Efficacy and safety of adding rivaroxaban to the anti-platelet regimen in patients with coronary artery disease

Jun Yuan (iD)

Abstract

Background: Rivaroxaban, a direct factor Xa inhibitor, has seldom been used in patients with coronary artery disease. In this analysis, we aimed to systematically compare the efficacy and safety of rivaroxaban in addition to the anti-platelet regimen in patients with coronary artery disease.

Methods: Online databases (MEDLINE, EMBASE, Cochrane database, www.ClinicalTrials.gov and Google scholar were searched for randomized controlled trials which were exclusively based on patients with coronary artery disease; and which compared efficacy (cardiovascular outcomes) and safety (bleeding outcomes) outcomes with the addition of rivaroxaban to the other anti-platelet agents. Analysis was carried out by the RevMan 5.3 software whereby odds ratios (OR) and 95% confidence intervals (CI) were generated following data input.

Results: Four trials with a total number of 40,148 patients were included (23,231 participants were treated with rivaroxaban whereas 16,919 participants were treated with placebo) in this analysis. Patients' enrollment period varied from years 2006 to 2016. The current results showed addition of rivaroxaban to significantly lower composite endpoints (OR: 0.81, 95% CI: 0.74–0.88; $P = 0.00001$). In addition, all-cause death, cardiac death, myocardial infarction, and stent thrombosis were also significantly reduced (OR: 0.82, 95% CI: 0.72–0.92; $P = 0.0009$), (OR: 0.80, 95% CI: 0.69–0.92; $P = 0.002$), (OR: 0.87, 95% CI: 0.77–0.98; $P = 0.03$) and (OR: 0.73, 95% CI: 0.55–0.97; $P = 0.03$) respectively. However, stroke was not significantly different.

However, TIMI defined minor and major bleeding were significantly higher with rivaroxaban (OR: 2.27, 95% CI: 1.47–3.49; $P = 0.0002$) and (OR: 3.44, 95% CI: 1.13–10.52; $P = 0.03$) respectively. In addition, intracranial hemorrhage and bleeding which was defined according to the International Society on Thrombosis and Hemostasis criteria were also significantly higher with rivaroxaban (OR: 1.63, 95% CI: 1.04–2.56; $P = 0.03$) and (OR: 1.80, 95% CI: 1.45–2.22; $P = 0.00001$) respectively. Nevertheless, fatal bleeding was not significantly different.

Conclusions: Addition of rivaroxaban to the anti-platelet regimen was effective in patients with coronary artery disease, but the safety outcomes were doubtful. Further future trials will be able to completely solve this issue.

Keywords: Rivaroxaban, Coronary artery disease, Dual anti-platelet therapy, Stent thrombosis, Minor bleeding, Major bleeding

Correspondence: nnyuanjun@163.com
Department of Cardiology, The People's Hospital of Guangxi Zhuang
Autonomous Region, Nanning 530021, Guangxi, China

Background

Rivaroxaban, a direct factor Xa inhibitor, has seldom been used in patients with stable coronary artery disease. Even if recently published studies have already compared rivaroxaban with dabigatran in patients with atrial fibrillation [1], the use of rivaroxaban in patients with coronary artery disease or following percutaneous coronary intervention (PCI) is still under study.

The PIONEER-AF-PCI Trial which consists of 2100 participants, is an exploratory, open-labelled, randomized, multi-center clinical study which is being carried out to assess the safety of rivaroxaban and vitamin K antagonist treatment strategy in patients with non-valvular atrial fibrillation who will require PCI [2]. Also, the RT-AF trial which is also an open-labelled study enrolling patients with non-valvular atrial fibrillation who will require coronary stenting, and who will require either triple therapy (warfarin, clopidogrel and aspirin) or dual therapy (rivaroxaban and ticagrelor) following intervention, is still under investigation [3] whereas the COMMANDER HF Trial, which is an International prospective, randomized, doubled-blind, placebo-controlled study comparing rivaroxaban with placebo in patients with heart failure and coronary artery disease, has not been published yet [4].

Plaque rupture and thrombosis are major concerns in patients with atherosclerosis. Dual antiplatelet therapy (DAPT) with aspirin and clopidogrel is considered the standard antiplatelet regimen especially after coronary intervention with drug eluting stents [5]. However, a more potent regimen was urgently needed due to limitations of these usual anti-platelet agents.

Recently, Bundhun et al. showed the addition of cilostazol to the standard DAPT in patients with acute coronary syndrome to be effective [6]. However, the unwanted safety outcomes which persisted with the use of cilostazol resulted in drug discontinuation indicating that other more effective agents would be required.

In this analysis, we aimed to systematically compare the efficacy and safety of rivaroxaban in addition to the anti-platelet regimen in patients with coronary artery disease.

Methods

Searched databases

The following databases were searched for randomized controlled trials:

1. MEDLINE/PubMed;
2. EMBASE (www.sciencedirect.com);
3. Cochrane database;
4. www.ClinicalTrials.gov;
5. Google scholar.

Searched terms

The online databases were carefully searched for English language publications (from November to December 2017). Publications included the titles with their associated abstract or full-text articles.

Keywords which were used in the search process included:

1. Rivaroxaban and coronary artery disease;
2. Rivaroxaban and percutaneous coronary intervention;
3. Rivaroxaban and dual anti-platelet therapy;
4. Rivaroxaban and aspirin and clopidogrel;
5. Xarelto and percutaneous coronary intervention;
6. Rivaroxaban and drug eluting stents.

Inclusion and exclusion criteria

Studies were included based on the following criteria:

1. They were exclusively randomized controlled trials;
2. They were exclusively based on patients with coronary artery disease;
3. They compared outcomes which were observed with the addition of rivaroxaban to other anti-platelets;
4. They reported adverse cardiovascular (efficacy) and bleeding (safety) outcomes as their endpoints.

Studies were excluded if:

1. They were non-randomized controlled trials (observational cohorts, meta-analysis and systematic reviews, case studies);
2. They involved patients who were treated for other conditions (peripheral artery disease, non-valvular atrial fibrillation);
3. They did not report adverse cardiovascular or bleeding outcomes;
4. They were duplicated studies.

Outcomes, definition and follow-ups

The outcomes (Table 1) which were assessed were as followed:

1. Composite endpoint: consisting of a combination of cardiac death, myocardial infarction, stroke and or stent thrombosis;
2. All-cause mortality;
3. Myocardial infarction (MI);
4. Cardiac death;
5. Stent thrombosis;
6. Stroke;
7. Thrombolysis in myocardial infarction (TIMI) defined minor and major bleedings [7];

Table 1 Outcomes which were assessed

Trials	Outcomes reported	Follow-up periods	Drugs which were used	Dosage of rivaroxaban
ATLAS-ACS 2 TIMI 51 [11]	Cardiac death + stroke + MI (composite endpoint), cardiac death, MI, stroke, all-cause death, ST, TIMI minor and major bleeding, Intracranial hemorrhage, fatal bleeding	13 to 31 months	Rivaroxaban + DAPT versus DAPT (aspirin + clopidogrel)	2.5 mg or 5 mg twice daily
GEMINI-ACS-1 [12]	Cardiac death + stroke + MI + ST (composite endpoint), cardiac death, MI, stroke, all-cause death, ST (definite + probable), TIMI minor and major bleeding, fatal bleeding, intracranial hemorrhage, ISTH major bleeding	1 year	Ribaroxaban + clopidogrel/ ticagrelor versus aspirin + clopidogrel/ticagrelor	2.5 mg twice daily
COMPASS [13]	Cardiac death + stroke + MI (composite endpoint), all-cause death, cardiac death, stroke, MI, fatal bleeding, intracranial hemorrhage, major bleeding according to ISTH criteria	23 months	Rivaroxaban + aspirin versus aspirin alone	2.5 mg or 5 mg twice daily
ATLAS-ACS-TIMI 46 [14]	TIMI minor and major bleeding, death + MI + stroke (composite endpoint)	6 months	Rivaroxaban + DAPT or aspirin versus DAPT (aspirin + clopidogrel)	5 to 20 mg once daily or the same total dose given twice daily

MI myocardial infarction, *ST* stent thrombosis, *TIMI* thrombolysis in myocardial infarction, *ISTH* International Society on Thrombosis and Hemostasis, *DAPT* dual anti-platelet therapy

8. Fatal bleeding: defined as severe life-threatening bleeding;
9. Intracranial hemorrhage;
10. Bleeding which was defined by the International Society on Thrombosis and Hemostasis (ISTH) [8].

The follow-up periods ranged from 6 months to 31 months as shown in Table 1.

Data extraction and review

The following data were extracted by the author Jun Yuan:

1. Type of study;
2. Time period of patients' enrollment;
3. Total number of patients in the experimental and control groups respectively;
4. The methodological quality of the trials;
5. The baseline features of the participants;
6. The adverse cardiovascular and bleeding outcomes;
7. The total number of events which were reported in each subgroup.

Data were also searched, extracted, screened and checked by Dr. Guang Ma Xu whom we have acknowledged at the end of the manuscript.

The review protocol was not prospectively registered.

The methodological quality of each trial was assessed based on the criteria which has been suggested/recommended by the Cochrane Collaboration [9] whereby scores were given depending on the risk of bias which was reported, and the highest which was 12 points indicated lowest risk of bias.

The PRISMA Guideline was followed [10].

Statistical analysis

This analysis was carried out by the most common software which has been used for decades to carry out meta-analyses: The RevMan 5.3 software. Following data input through the software, odds ratios (OR) with 95% confidence intervals (CI) were generated.

Heterogeneity was assessed by:

1. The Q statistic test whereby a P value less or equal to 0.05 was considered as statistically significant.
2. The I^2 statistical test whereby heterogeneity was increased with increasing I^2.

Two statistical effect models were applied based on the value of I^2:

If I^2 was less than 50%, a fixed effects model was used. However, if I^2 was > 50%, a random effects model was used.

Sensitivity analysis was carried out by an exclusion method whereby each trial was excluded one by one and a new analysis was generated each time to observe any significant change in the results.

In addition, publication bias was assessed through the funnel plot which was generated by the software.

Results

Searched outcomes

Search which was carried out from online (electronic) databases resulted in a total number of 298 publications. A pre-assessment was carried out whereby 259 articles were excluded since they were not related to the scope of this research. Thirty-nine (39) full-text articles were assessed for eligibility. Further elimination was carried out based on the following criteria:

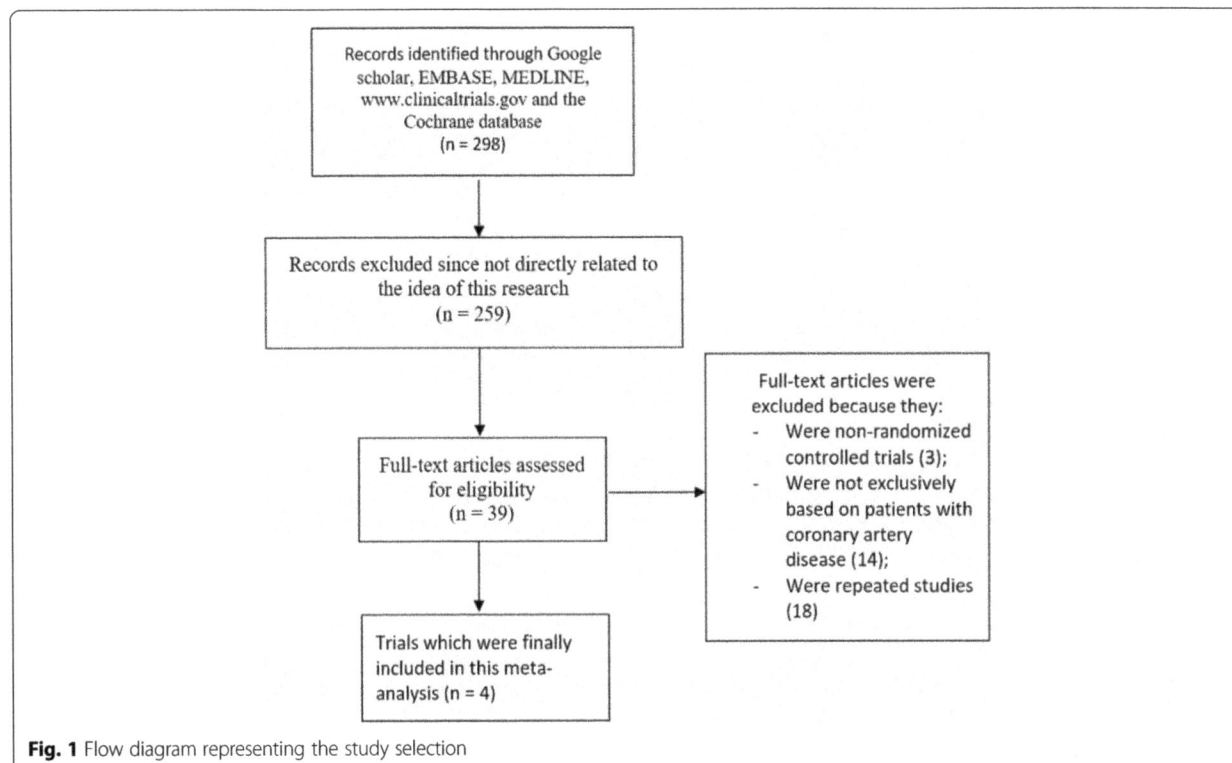

Fig. 1 Flow diagram representing the study selection

1. They were non-randomized controlled trials (3);
2. They were not exclusively based on patients with coronary artery disease (14);
3. They were repeated studies (18).

Finally, only 4 trials [11–14] were selected for this meta-analysis (Fig. 1).

General features of the trials

The general features of the trials have been listed in Table 2. A total number of 40, 148 patients were included in this analysis (23,231 participants were treated with rivaroxaban whereas 16,919 participants were treated with placebo). Patients' enrollment period varied from the year 2006 to the year 2016 as shown in Table 2.

After a careful assessment of the risk of bias, all the four trials were allotted a score of 10 out of 12, representing a low risk of bias.

Baseline features of the participants

The baseline features of the participants have been listed in Table 3. The average age varied from 57.2 to 68.2 years. Majority of the participants were male patients. The percentage of patients with high blood pressure, dyslipidemia, diabetes mellitus and a smoking history has been represented in Table 3. According to the data given, no significant difference was observed in patients

who were assigned to the experimental or the control groups.

Main results of this analysis

The main results of this analysis were shown in Table 4.

Results of this analysis showed that addition of rivaroxaban to the anti-platelet regimen significantly lowered composite endpoints (OR: 0.81, 95% CI: 0.74–0.88; $P = 0.00001$, $I^2 = 19\%$). In addition, all-cause death, cardiac death, MI, and stent thrombosis were also significantly reduced (OR: 0.82, 95% CI: 0.72–0.92; $P = 0.0009$, $I^2 = 0\%$), (OR: 0.80, 95% CI: 0.69–0.92; $P = 0.002$, $I^2 = 0\%$), (OR: 0.87, 95% CI: 0.77–0.98; $P = 0.03$, $I^2 = 10\%$) and (OR: 0.73, 95% CI: 0.55–0.97; $P = 0.03$, $I^2 = 28\%$) respectively as shown in Fig. 2.

Table 2 General features of the trials which were included

Trials	No of patients treated by rivaroxaban (n)	No of patients in the placebo group (n)	Time period of patients' enrollment	Bias risk score
ATLAS-ACS 2 TIMI 51	10,229	5113	2008–2011	10
GEMINI-ACS-1	1519	1518	2015–2016	10
COMPASS	9152	9126	2013–2016	10
ATLAS-ACS-TIMI 46	2331	1160	2006–2008	10
Total no of patients (n)	23,231	16,917		

Table 3 Baseline features of the participants

Trials	Age (years) R/placebo	Males (%) R/placebo	HT (%) R/placebo	Ds (%) R/placebo	DM (%) R/placebo	Cs (%) R/placebo
ATLAS-ACS 2 TIMI 51	61.9/61.5	74.6/75.0	67.4/67.5	48.7/48.2	32.1/31.8	–
GEMINI-ACS-1	62.0/63.0	75.0/75.0	71.0/75.0	56.0/56.0	29.0/30.0	32.0/34.0
COMPASS	68.3/68.2	67.5/68.2	75.5/75.4	–	37.7/38.1	3.80/3.70
ATLAS-ACS-TIMI 46	57.2/57.8	77.6/76.3	57.4/56.9	44.4/43.6	19.4/19.1	61.9/62.6

R rivaroxaban group, *HT* hypertension, *Ds* dyslipidemia, *DM* diabetes mellitus, *Cs* current smoker

However, stroke was not significantly different (OR: 0.77, 95% CI: 0.43–1.38; $P = 0.38$) as shown in Fig. 3.

Bleeding outcomes (safety outcomes) were also assessed. The current results showed TIMI defined minor and major bleeding to be significantly higher with rivaroxaban (OR: 2.27, 95% CI: 1.47–3.49; $P = 0.0002$, $I^2 = 0\%$) and (OR: 3.44, 95% CI: 1.13–10.52; $P = 0.03$, $I^2 = 74\%$) respectively as shown in Figs. 4 and 5.

Intracranial hemorrhage and bleeding which was defined according to the ISTH criteria were also significantly higher with rivaroxaban (OR: 1.63, 95% CI: 1.04–2.56; $P = 0.03$, $I^2 = 44\%$) and (OR: 1.80, 95% CI: 1.45–2.22; $P = 0.00001$, $I^2 = 0\%$) respectively. However, fatal bleeding was similarly manifested (OR: 1.19, 95% CI: 0.74–1.91; $P = 0.48$, $I^2 = 0\%$) as shown in Fig. 4.

Sensitivity analysis and publication bias

Consistent results were obtained through sensitivity analyses. In addition, based on a visual assessment of the funnel plot, which was a better way to illustrate publication bias in an analysis including a small volume of studies, there was low to moderate evidence of publication bias across all the studies that compared the outcomes assessing efficacy and safety with the addition of rivaroxaban to the anti-platelet

Table 4 Results of this analysis

Outcomes which were assessed	OR with 95% CI	P value	I² (%)
Composite endpoint	0.81 [0.74–0.88]	0.00001	19
All-cause mortality	0.82 [0.72–0.92]	0.0009	0
Cardiac death	0.80 [0.69–0.92]	0.002	0
Myocardial infarction	0.87 [0.77–0.98]	0.03	10
Stent thrombosis	0.73 [0.55–0.97]	0.03	28
Stroke	0.77 [0.43–1.38]	0.38	81
TIMI defined minor bleeding	2.27 [1.47–3.49]	0.0002	0
TIMI defined major bleeding	3.44 [1.13–10.52]	0.03	74
Intracranial bleeding	1.63 [1.04–2.56]	0.03	44
Fatal bleeding	1.19 [0.74–1.91]	0.48	0
ISTH bleeding	1.80 [1.45–2.22]	0.00001	0

TIMI thrombolysis in myocardial infarction, *ISTH* International Society on Thrombosis and Hemostasis, *OR* odds ratios, *CI* confidence intervals

regimen in patients with coronary artery disease as shown in Fig. 6.

Discussion

Antiplatelet and anti-thrombotic therapies are vital in patients with coronary artery disease especially after PCI. DAPT (aspirin and clopidogrel) has been used for decades in patients who were implanted with bare metal stents and drug eluting stents [15]. However, more potent drugs or adjuvants were still required to overcome the limitations observed with the commonly used anti-platelet agents.

Recently, Bundhun et al. showed addition of cilostazol to the standard DAPT to be associated with significantly lower adverse outcomes including revascularization [6]. However, cilostazol was associated with unwanted safety outcomes. This was the main reason for drug discontinuation among several of the participants who were randomized to take part in the study. For example, cilostazol was observed to be associated with more headache, diarrhea, skin rashes and tachycardia/palpitations [16] when compared to the other anti-platelet agents. In addition, cilostazol is apparently contraindicated in congestive heart failure [16]. Even if significance was not reached, cilostazol use in the triple anti-platelet regimen was associated with a higher risk of major and minor bleeding when compared to DAPT without cilostazol [17].

In this analysis, rivaroxaban was added to DAPT or to aspirin alone in patients with coronary artery disease, and the efficacy and safety outcomes were assessed in comparison to placebo. Current results showed significantly lower death, myocardial infarction, and stent thrombosis associated with the addition of rivaroxaban to the anti-platelet regimen. However, when the safety outcomes were assessed, TIMI defined minor and major bleedings, intracranial bleeding as well as bleeding which was defined according to the ISTH criteria were significantly increased. In other words, the addition of rivaroxaban to the antiplatelet drug regimen was effective, but the safety outcomes appeared critical.

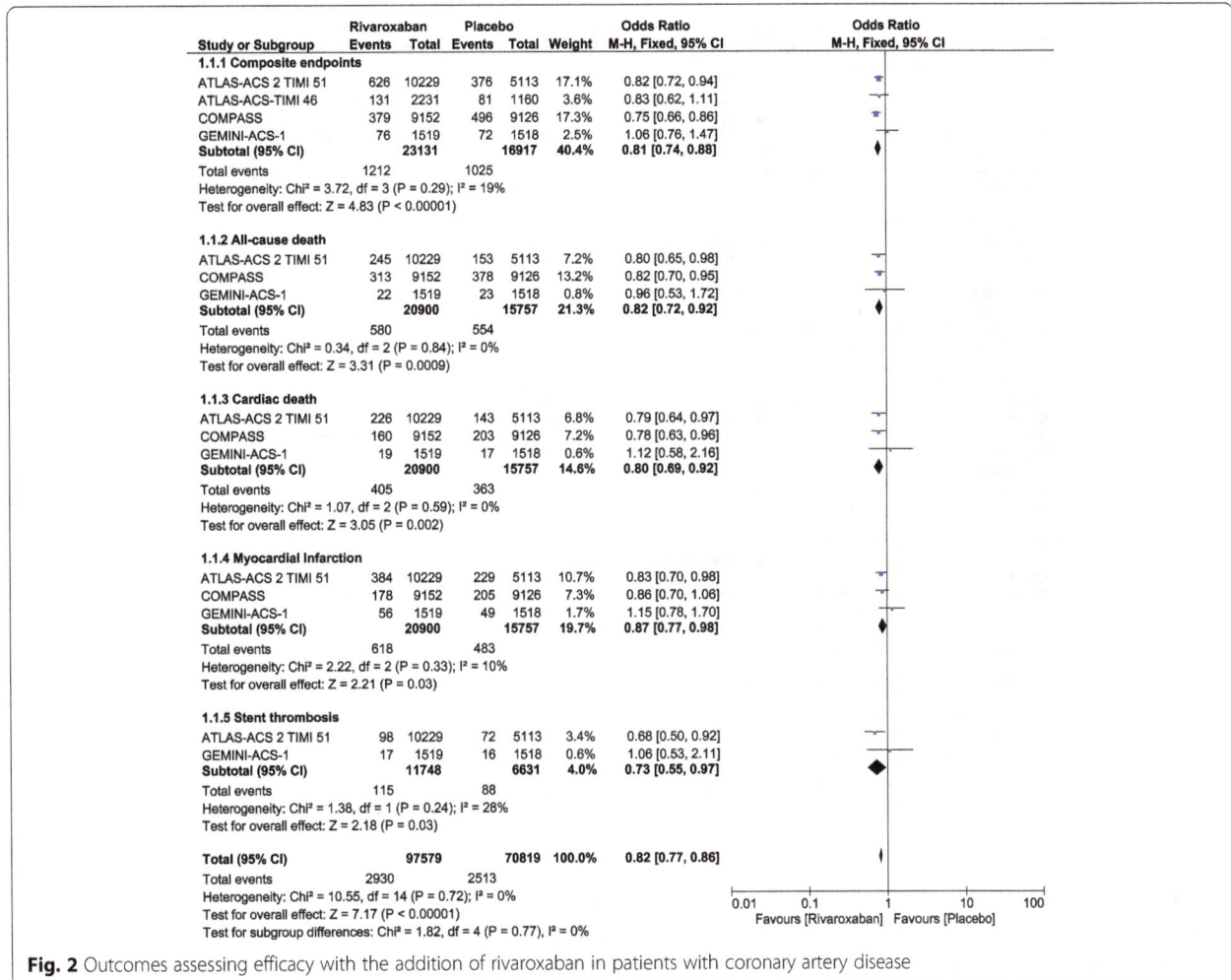

Fig. 2 Outcomes assessing efficacy with the addition of rivaroxaban in patients with coronary artery disease

In the X-PLORER Trial, whereby 111 participants were enrolled (October 2011 to March 2013), rivaroxaban was used during the invasive procedure in patients with stable coronary artery disease [18]. The authors found rivaroxaban to effectively suppress the activation of coagulation following stenting. TIMI defined minor and major bleedings as well as bleeding defined by the Academic Research Consortium (ARC) were not elevated during a follow up period of 30 days. Nevertheless, the X-PLORER Trial was different from our current analysis in terms of shorter follow-up period, and this direct factor Xa inhibitor was used only during the procedure.

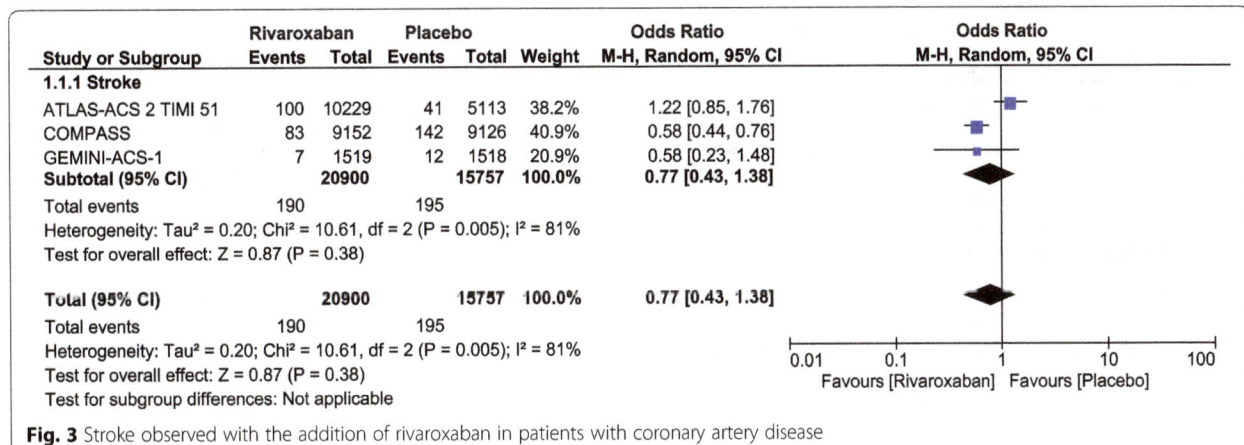

Fig. 3 Stroke observed with the addition of rivaroxaban in patients with coronary artery disease

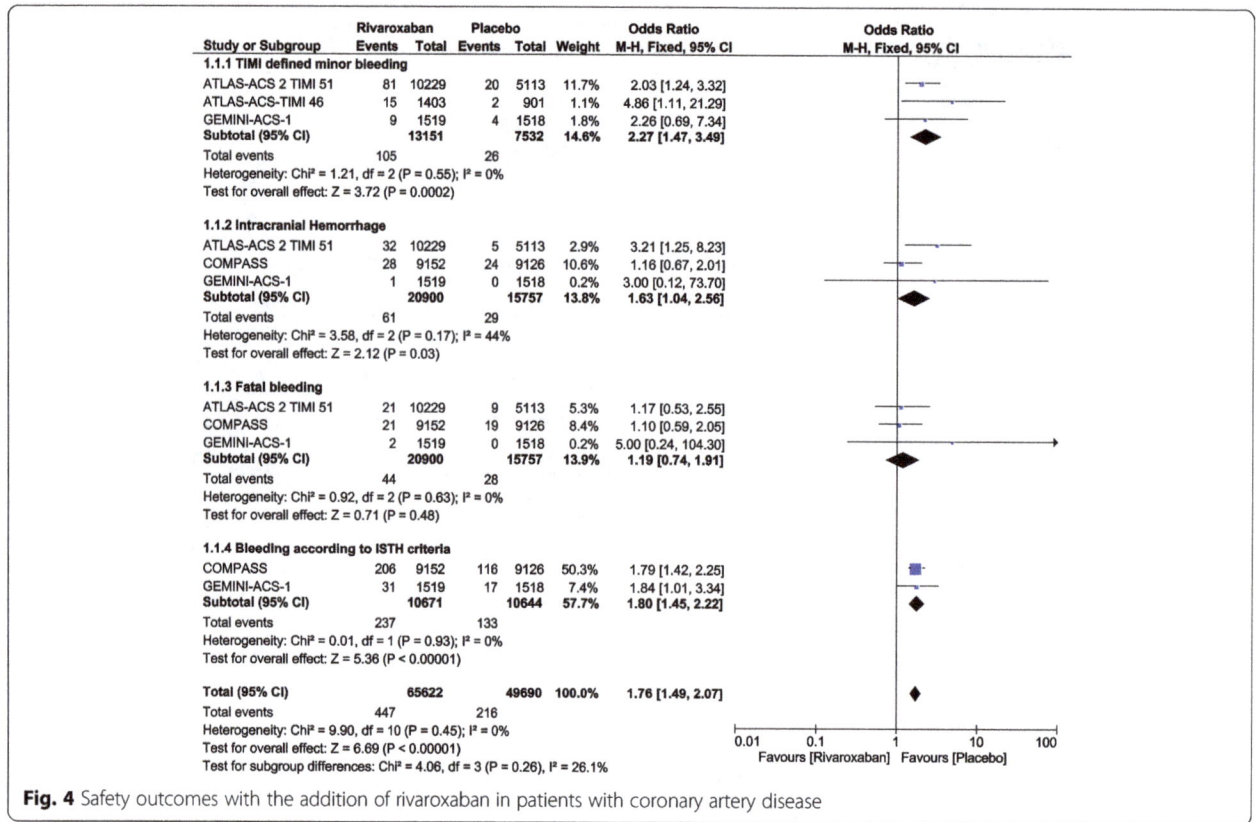

Fig. 4 Safety outcomes with the addition of rivaroxaban in patients with coronary artery disease

Similar to this analysis, the ATLAS-ACS 2 TIMI 51 Trial showed a reduction in mortality and stent thrombosis with the addition of rivaroxaban along with DAPT following PCI in patients with acute coronary syndrome [19].

In contrast, the GEMINI-ACS-1 trial which consisted of 3037 participants showed rivaroxaban to exhibit similar significant bleeding to that of aspirin and clopidogrel [12]. However, it should be noted that the study had a shorter follow-up duration time period of 291 days and the total number of participants was also less in comparison to other studies. In addition, the participants only received 2.5 mg rivaroxaban twice daily in comparison to other studies whereby the dosage was doubled.

Another review even suggested substituting aspirin for rivaroxaban (2.5 mg twice daily) due to a similar bleeding risk [20]. However, since it was a phase II study, the authors specified that a larger phase III trial will be able to confirm their findings.

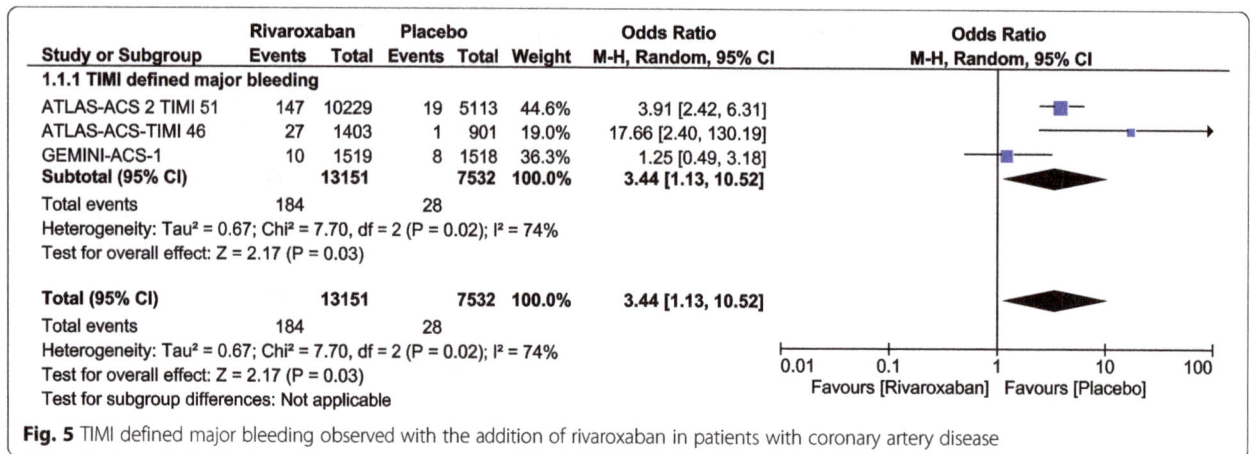

Fig. 5 TIMI defined major bleeding observed with the addition of rivaroxaban in patients with coronary artery disease

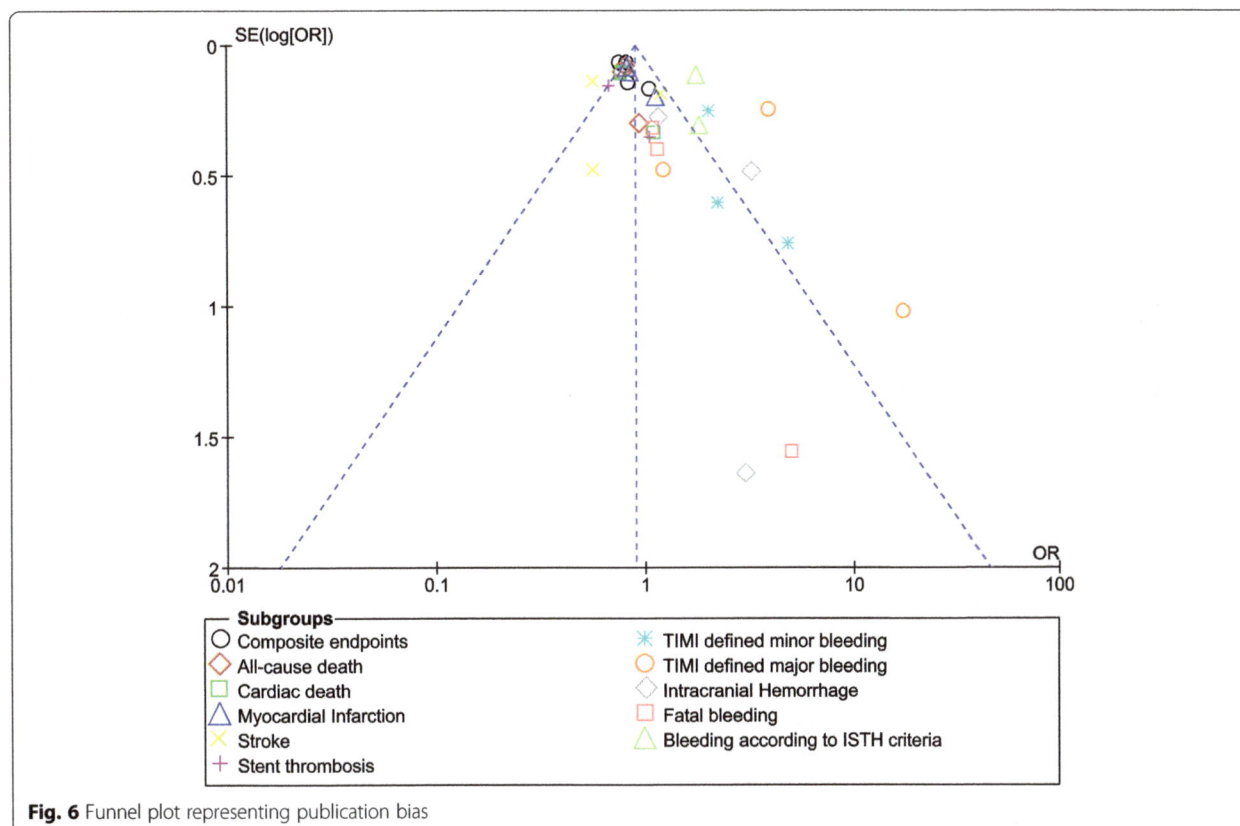

Fig. 6 Funnel plot representing publication bias

Novelty

This research article is new in the following ways:

1. It is the first study to systematically analyze the addition of rivaroxaban to the anti-platelet regimen in patients with coronary artery disease;
2. This idea is new in clinical medicine, and is still being studied;
3. Only data which were obtained from randomized trials (good data) have been included;
4. A very low level of heterogeneity was observed among almost all the subgroups that assessed the efficacy and safety endpoints.

Limitations

Limitations were as followed:

1. This analysis consisted of a limited number of trials and participants;
2. The placebo involved different drug regimens in different trials. Two trials involved DAPT in the placebo group. However, one trial involved only aspirin, and another one consisted only of clopidogrel or ticagrelor. This might have had an effect on the results;
3. Different trials had different follow-up periods which might have influenced the results;

4. Other bleeding outcomes such as bleeding defined by the academic research consortium, and GUSTO bleeding, could not be assessed because they were reported in only one study.
5. Dosage of rivaroxaban might have also influenced the results.

Conclusions

Addition of rivaroxaban to the anti-platelet regimen was effective in patients with coronary artery disease, but the safety outcomes were doubtful. Further future trials will be able to completely solve this issue.

Abbreviations
DAPT: Dual anti-platelet therapy; PCI: Percutaneous coronary intervention; RCT: Randomized controlled trials; TIMI: Thrombolysis in myocardial infarction

Acknowledgements
The author would like to thank Dr. Guang Ma Xu (MD), from the Department of Cardiology, The People's Hospital of Guangxi Zhuang Autonomous Region, Nanning, Guangxi, China, for his immense contribution to the search process and data extraction.

Authors' contributions
JY was responsible for the conception and design, acquisition of data, analysis and interpretation of data, drafting the initial manuscript and

revising it critically for important intellectual content. JY wrote and approved the final manuscript.

Competing interests

The author declares that he has no competing interests.

References

1. Bundhun PK, Soogund MZ, Teeluck AR, Pursun M, Bhurtu A, Huang WQ. Bleeding outcomes associated with rivaroxaban and dabigatran in patients treated for atrial fibrillation: a systematic review and meta-analysis. BMC Cardiovasc Disord. 2017;17(1):15.
2. Gibson CM, Mehran R, Bode C, Halperin J, Verheugt F, Wildgoose P, van Eickels M, Lip GY, Cohen M, Husted S, Peterson E, Fox K. An open-label, randomized, controlled, multicenter study exploring two treatment strategies of rivaroxaban and a dose-adjusted oral vitamin K antagonist treatment strategy in subjects with atrial fibrillation who undergo percutaneous coronary intervention (PIONEER AF-PCI). Am Heart J. 2015; 169(4):472–8.e5.
3. Gao F, Shen H, Wang ZJ, Yang SW, Liu XL, Zhou YJ. Rationale and design of the RT-AF study: combination of rivaroxaban and ticagrelor in patients with atrial fibrillation and coronary artery disease undergoing percutaneous coronary intervention. Contemp Clin Trials. 2015;43:129–32.
4. Zannad F, Greenberg B, Cleland JG, Gheorghiade M, van Veldhuisen DJ, Mehra MR, Anker SD, Byra WM, Fu M, Mills RM. rationale and design of a randomized, double-blind, event-driven, multicentre study comparingthe efficacy and safety of oral rivaroxaban with placebo for reducing the risk of death, myocardialinfarction or stroke in subjects with heart failure and significant coronary artery disease followingan exacerbation of heart failure: the COMMANDER HF trial. Eur J Heart Fail. 2015;17(7):735–42.
5. Task Force members, Windecker S, Kolh P, Alfonso F, et al. 2014 ESC/EACTS guidelines on myocardial revascularization: the Task Force on Myocardial Revascularization of the European Society of Cardiology (ESC) and the European Association for Cardio-Thoracic Surgery (EACTS) developed with the special contribution of the European Association of Percutaneous Cardiovascular Interventions (EAPCI). Eur Heart J. 2014;35:2541–619.
6. Bundhun PK, Qin T, Chen MH. Comparing the effectiveness and safety between triple antiplatelet therapy and dual antiplatelet therapy in type 2 diabetes mellitus patients after coronary stents implantation: a systematic review and meta-analysis of randomized controlled trials. BMC Cardiovasc Disord. 2015;15:118.
7. The Thrombolysis in Myocardial Infarction (TIMI) trial. Phase I findings. TIMI study group. N Engl J Med. 1985;312(14):932–6.
8. Schulman S, Angerås U, Bergqvist D, Eriksson B, Lassen MR, Fisher W. Subcommittee on Control of Anticoagulation of the Scientific and Standardization Committee of the International Society on Thrombosis and Haemostasis. Definition of major bleeding in clinical investigations of antihemostatic medicinal products in surgical patients. J Thromb Haemost. 2010;8(1):202–4.
9. Higgins JP, Thompson SG, Deeks JJ, et al. Measuring inconsistency in meta-analyses. BMJ. 2003;327:557–60.
10. Liberati A, Altman DG, Tetzlaff J, et al. The PRISMA statement for reporting systematic reviews and meta-analyses of studies that evaluate healthcareinterventions: explanation and elaboration. BMJ. 2009;339:b2700.
11. Mega JL, Braunwald E, Wiviott SD, Bassand JP, Bhatt DL, Bode C, Burton P, Cohen M, Cook-Bruns N, Fox KA, Goto S, Murphy SA, Plotnikov AN, Schneider D, Sun X, Verheugt FW, Gibson CM. ATLAS ACS 2–TIMI 51 Investigators. Rivaroxaban in patients with a recent acute coronary syndrome. N Engl J Med. 2012;366(1):9–19.
12. Ohman EM, Roe MT, Steg PG, SK J, et al. Clinically significant bleeding with low-dose rivaroxaban versus aspirin, in addition to P2Y12inhibition, in acute coronary syndromes (GEMINI-ACS-1): a double-blind, multicentre, randomized trial. Lancet. 2017;389(10081):1799–808.
13. Eikelboom JW, Connolly SJ, Bosch J, et al. Rivaroxaban with or without aspirin in stable cardiovascular disease. N Engl J Med. 2017;377(14):1319–30.
14. Mega JL, Braunwald E, Mohanavelu S, Burton P, Poulter R, Misselwitz F, Hricak V, Barnathan ES, Bordes P, Witkowski A, Markov V, Oppenheimer L, Gibson CM. ATLAS ACS-TIMI 46 study group. Rivaroxaban versus placebo in patients with acute coronary syndromes (ATLAS ACS-TIMI 46): a randomised, double-blind, phase II trial. Lancet. 2009;374(9683):29–38.
15. Bundhun PK, Yanamala CM, Huang F. Should a prolonged duration of dual anti-platelet therapy be recommended to patients with diabetes mellitus following percutaneous coronary intervention? A systematic review and meta-analysis of 15 studies. BMC Cardiovasc Disord. 2016;16(1):161.
16. Liu Y, Shakur Y, Yoshitake M, Kambayashi JJ. Cilostazol (pletal): a dual inhibitor of cyclic nucleotide phosphodiesterase type 3 and adenosine uptake. Cardiovasc Drug Rev. 2001;19(4):369–86.
17. Bangalore S, Singh A, Toklu B, DiNicolantonio JJ, Croce K, Feit F, Bhatt DL. Efficacy of cilostazol on platelet reactivity and cardiovascular outcomes in patients undergoingpercutaneous coronary intervention: insights from a meta-analysis of randomised trials. Open Heart. 2014;1(1):e000068.
18. Vranckx P, Leebeek FW, Tijssen JG, Koolen J, Stammen F, Herman JP, de Winter RJ, van T Hof AW, Backx B, Lindeboom W, Kim SY, Kirsch B, van Eickels M, Misselwitz F, Verheugt FW. Peri-procedural use of rivaroxaban in elective percutaneous coronary intervention to treat stablecoronary artery disease. The X-PLORER trial. Thromb Haemost. 2015;114(2):258–67.
19. CM G, Chakrabarti AK, Mega J, Bode C, Bassand JP, Verheugt FW, Bhatt DL, Goto S, Cohen M, Mohanavelu S, Burton P, Stone G, Braunwald E, ATLAS-ACS 2 TIMI 51 Investigators. Reduction of stent thrombosis in patients with acute coronary syndromes treated with rivaroxaban in ATLAS-ACS 2 TIMI 51. J Am Coll Cardiol. 2013;62(4):286–90.
20. Huynh K. Acute coronary syndromes: similar bleeding risks with low-dose rivaroxaban versus aspirin. Nat Rev Cardiol. 2017;14(5):252–3.

14

Effect of CYP3 A4, CYP3 A5 and ABCB1 gene polymorphisms on the clinical efficacy of tacrolimus in the treatment of nephrotic syndrome

Min Li[1†], Min Xu[1†], Wei Liu[2*] and Xin Gao[1*]

Abstract

Background: The efficacy of tacrolimus (TAC) is variable in the treatment of nephrotic syndrome (NS), which might be related to genetic variation among patients. Therefore, we aim to investigate the effects of CYP3 A4, CYP3 A5 and ABCB1 gene polymorphisms on the clinical efficacy of TAC in the treatment of NS patients.

Methods 100 NS patients were treated with TAC and prednisone and followed up for 3 months. Genotype differences (CYP3 A4*1G, CYP3 A5*3, ABCB1 1236C > T and ABCB1 2677G > T/A) were detected by Sanger sequencing. The clinical efficacy was evaluated by the 24 h urinary protein quantitation, albumin, renal function and the degree of edema. Multivariable logistic regression was used to analyze the effect of gene polymorphisms on the clinical efficacy of TAC.

Results: There were 35 patients (35%) with complete remission, 43 patients (43%) with partial remission, 22 patients (22%) without remission, and no patients with recurrence. For CYP3A4, there were 56, 42, and 2 patients with *1/*1, *1/*1G and *1G/*1G genotype, respectively. For CYP3A5, there were 8, 36 and 56 cases with *1/*1, *1/*3 and *3/*3 genotype, respectively. For ABCB1 C1236T, there were 10, 44, and 46 cases with 1236CC, 1236CT and 1236TT genotype, respectively. For ABCB1 G2677 T/A, there were 13, 57, and 30 patients with 2677GG genotype, 2677GT/GA genotype and 2677TT/AA/TA genotype, respectively. The mutant allele frequencies of CYP3A4*1G, CYP3A5*3, ABCB1 C1236T and ABCB1 G2677 T/A were 23%, 74%, 68% and 58.5%, respectively. Results reveal that the gene polymorphisms of CYP3A4 and CYP3A5 and CCB do not affect the clinical efficacy of TAC. For ABCB1 C1236T, TT genotype can increase the effectiveness 12.085 times compared with CC and CT genotype ($P = 0.018$, OR = 12.085, 95%CI 1.535–95.148). For ABCB1 G2677 T/A, the clinical efficacy of patients with mutant genotype is 8.683 times than that of wild-type and heterozygous patients ($P = 0.042$, OR = 8.683, 95%CI 1.080–69.819). Overweight patients can improve the clinical efficacy by 15.838 times ($P = 0.020$, OR = 15.838, 95%CI 1.550–161.788).

Conclusions: ABCB1 C1236T, ABCB1 G2677 T/A genotype and BMI are probably the factors influencing the clinical efficacy of TAC in treating patients with NS.

Keywords: CYP3 A4*1G, CYP3 A5*3, ABCB1C1236T, ABCB1 G2677 T/A, TAC, Clinical efficacy

* Correspondence: 285687995@qq.com; lm89551@163.com
†Equal contributors
²Department of Medicine, The 88th Hospital of PLA, Taian, People's Republic of China
¹Department of Nephrology, The 88th Hospital of PLA, Taian, People's Republic of China

Background

Nephrotic syndrome (NS) is a common condition in renal medicine which has high morbidity in middle aged and elderly people. The response to treatment varies greatly in NS patients, and some of them may develop into renal failure. Tacrolimus (TAC), an inhibitor of calcium phosphatase, also named FK506, is used in the treatment of NS in recent years [1, 2]. The pharmacokinetics of TAC is variable among individuals. The safety range between effective dose and toxic dose is narrow, and it is easy to be affected by gene polymorphisms and other combined drugs. Therefore, it is very important to monitor the blood concentration of TAC in clinical treatment. Drug genomics studies showed that TAC was mainly metabolized by drug metabolism enzyme CYP3A4/5, and then transported by the P glycoprotein (P-gp) [3, 4]. Therefore, CYP3A4, CYP3A5 and P-gp gene polymorphisms are responsible for individual differences in clinical efficacy of TAC [5, 6]. Specifically, the National Health and Family Planning Commission of People's Republic of China gives a formula for TAC dose in Chinese population [4].

The CYP3 A4*1G (rs2242480) is the major site of the single nucleotide polymorphisms (SNPs) and closely related to the metabolism of TAC. The mutation occurs at the 10th intron (G > A; the wild type: CYP3 A4*1/*1; the heterozygous type: CYP3 A4*1/*1G; the mutant type: CYP3 A4*1G/*1G) [5, 7, 8]. The CYP3 A5 also has multipled SNPs and most attention has been paid to the site of CYP3 A5*3 (rs776746). The mutation occurs at the 3rd intron (A > G; the wild type: CYP3 A5 *1/*1; the heterozygous type: CYP3 A5*1/*3; the mutant type: CYP3 A5*3/*3) [9, 10]. ABCB1 gene, which encodes P-gp, is also known as multidrug resistance gene. The two most common SNPs in the protein coding region are rs1128503 (1236C > T; the wild type: ABCB1 1236 CC; the heterozygous type: ABCB1 1236 CT; the mutant type: ABCB1 1236 TT)) and rs2032582 (2677G > T/A; the wild type: ABCB1 2677GG; the heterozygous type: ABCB1 2677GT/GA; the mutant type: ABCB1 2677TT/AA/TA) [11, 12]. The existing literature investigating these gene polymorphisms have been mainly derived from cohorts of renal transplant patients. There is a widespread view that CYP3A5 nonexpressers (CYP3 A5*3/*3 carriers) require lower mean TAC doses and exhibit higher concentration/dose ratios in renal transplant patients [3, 13]. However, the effect of the CYP3A4*1G, ABCB1 1236C > T and 2677G > T/A genetic polymorphisms on TAC pharmacokinetics in renal transplant recipients is controversial [12, 14]. As for NS patient, little is known about these gene polymorphisms in the clinical efficacy of TAC.

Therefore, in order to guide the rational use of clinical medicine, we further investigate the effect of CYP3 A4, CYP3 A5 and ABCB1 gene polymorphisms on the clinical efficacy of patients with NS in Chinese population in this study.

Methods

Object of study

A total of 100 NS patients with a mean age of 37.28 ± 17.0 years between January and November 2016 were included in this study. They all live in or around Tai'an. NS aetiology was determined by renal biopsy. Glomerular filtration rate (GFR) was greater than 80 mL/min/1.73m^2 in all patients. 18.5–25 kg/m^2 is considered to be the normal range for BMI in adults, and 6–19 kg/m^2 in children. Urine routine, 24 h urinary protein, blood routine, liver function, renal function, blood lipid and blood sugar were also detected.

Ethical consideration

We received approval from the Medical Ethics Committee of the 88th Hospital of PLA (Chinese People's Liberation Army) for undertaking this study. The study was designed to be secure and fair to patients while minimizing risk of harm to participants. The included participants provided written informed voluntary consent and participants under the age of 18 years had written consent obtained from their parents. Participants had the right to withdraw from the study at any time.

Therapeutic regimen

All the patients were treated with TAC and prednisone. TAC was given at the dose of 0.05 mg kg^{-1} day^{-1} for both adults and children, divided twice from oral application at intervals of 12 h [3, 15–17]. Prednisone was used 0.5 mg/kg daily initially. After 8 weeks of treatment, the amount of prednisone was reduced by 5 mg every two weeks to 20 mg. Then, the dose of 20 mg/d was maintained for 2 months and the rest of the prednisone gradually reduced to complete withdrawal [3].

Evaluation of safety

Evaluation of safety is to observe the safety of the TAC in the study. Referring to the relevant literatures, the main side effects of TAC were closely observed in the present study, including abnormality of glucose tolerance, infection, renal toxicity, gastrointestinal adverse reactions, elevated blood pressure and liver toxicity, etc. Once the uncontrollable adverse reactions are found, we should stop TAC immediately.

Clinical evaluation criteria

The patients were followed up for 3 months. The clinical efficacy was evaluated by the 24 h urinary protein quantitation, albumin (ALB), renal function and the degree of edema. Evaluation criteria are divided into complete remission (CR), partial remission (PR), no remission (NR) and recrudescence [6, 9]. (1) CR: Urine protein < 0.3 g/d, ALB > 35 g/L, edema disappeared and stable renal function. (2) PR: Urine protein 0.3 ~ 3.5 g/d or decreased > 50%, ALB > 30 g/L, edema disappeared and stable renal function. (3) NR: Urine protein > 3.5 g/d and ALB < 30 g/L with edema or deterioration of renal function. (4) Recrudescence: When reaching CR or PR, proteinuria > 3.5 g/d and ALB < 30 g/L, accompanied by edema or deterioration of renal function appear again. CR + PR are considered to be effective and NR + recurrence are treated as ineffective (Table 1).

Gene determination and sequencing
Blood was collected in heparin anticoagulation tube, and then DNA was extracted (Invitrogen, Carlsbad, CA, USA). Sanger sequencing was used to detect the genotypes of CYP3 A4*1G, CYP3 A5*3, ABCB1 C1236T and ABCB1 G2677 T/A. PCR amplification conditions were as follows: pre-denaturation at 94 °C for 2 min, denaturation at 94 °C for 30 s, anneal at 60 °C for 30 s, and extension at 72 °C for 20 s for a total of 38 cycles. At last, extension was performed at 72 °C for 2 min [7]. The primer F, primer R and the purified DNA were delivered to Shenzhen Hua Da Technology Company for sequencing.

Sequencing map analysis
After all the samples were sequenced, the National Center for Biotechnology Information was used to search the sequencing map of CYP3A4*1G (Additional file 1: Fig. S1), CYP3A5*3 (Additional file 2: Fig. S2), ABCB1 C1236T (Additional file 3: Fig. S3) and G2677 T/A (Additional file 4: Fig. S4). CYP3 A4 genes were sequenced by forward sequencing method. The genes of CYP3 A5, ABCB1 C1236T and ABCB1 G2677 T/A were sequenced by reverse sequencing method.

Statistical analysis
SPSS 18 software was used for statistical analysis. Concordance of genotype distribution with Hardy-Weinberg equilibrium was assessed using the χ^2 test. Logistic regression analysis was used to compare the effects of CYP3 A4, CYP3 A5, ABCB1 C1236T, ABCB1 G2677 T/A, CCB and BMI on the clinical efficacy of TAC in the treatment of NS patients. We used the enter method, that was, the full model method, and all variables were entered into the equation to screen meaningful variables. Clinical efficacy was used as dependent variable and the following indicators were used as covariates (Table 1).

Results
Characteristics of patients
The characteristics of patients were given in Table 2. There were 10 cases of children. Among them, one children was 6 years old and the rest were between 15 and 18 years old. The average age were 15.90 ± 3.54 years, and the average weight were 49.4 ± 11.7 kg. NS could be divided into a variety of different pathological types. The population of this study included membranous nephropathy (MN) (36 cases, 36%), mesangial proliferative glomerulonephritis (MsPGN) (11 cases, 11%), minimal change nephropathy (MCN) (15 cases, 15%), focal segmental glomerulosclerosis (FSGS) (5 cases, 5%), systemic lupus erythematosus (SLE) (16 cases, 16%) and Henoch - Schonlein purpura nephritis (HSPN) (7 cases, 7%).

Clinical efficacy of TAC
There were 35 patients (35%) with CR, 43 patients (43%) with PR, 22 patients (22%) with NR, and no patients with recurrence. The overall rate of effective treatment was 78% (78/100) (Table 3).

The outcomes of patient with different pathological causes were as follows. For MN, there were 9 patients with CR, 17 patients with PR, and 10 cases with NR. In MsPGN, the number of patients with CR, PR, and NR was 6, 4 and 1, respectively. There were 15 people in the MCN group, including 10 cases of CR, 4 cases of PR, and 1 case with NR. All of 5 patients with FSGS were not relieved. As for SLE, the number of people was 5,16,5 in CR, PR, and NR groups, respectively. There were 5 patients with CR and 2 cases with PR among 7 patients with HSPN.

Table 1 Assignment of logistic regression analysis

Factors	Assignment description
CYP3 A4	CYP3 A4*1/*1 = 0, CYP3 A4*1/*1G + CYP3 A4*1G/*1G = 1
CYP3 A5	CYP3 A5*1/*1+ CYP3 A5*1/*3 = 0,CYP3 A5*3/*3 = 1
ABCB1 C1236T	CC + CT = 0,TT = 1
ABCB1 G2677 T/A	GG + GT + GA = 0,TT + TA + AA = 1
CCB	Not applied CCB = 0, applied CCB = 1
BMI	the normal range = 0, the abnormal range that is overweight =1

Table 2 Characteristics of patients

Variable	Value
Age, range (mean ± SD)	6–63 (37.28 ± 17.0)
Children/adults	10/ 90
Females, n (%)	25 (53.2)
Weight (kg), range (mean ± SD)	33.5–103 (63.5 ± 11.3)
BMI (kg/m²), range (mean ± SD)	19.0–33.6 (23.9 ± 2.8)
GFR (mL/min/1.73m²), range (mean ± SD)	83.4–177.0 (115 ± 34.9)
Using CCB (cases)(%)	12 (12%)

BMI: body mass index; GFR: glomerular filtration rate

Table 3 Remission rate of different diseases

Disease types	CR (cases)	PR (cases)	NR (cases)	Total	Effective rate (%)
MN	9	17	10	36	72.2
MsPGN	6	4	1	11	90.9
MCN	10	4	1	15	93.3
FSGS	0	0	5	5	0
SLE	5	16	5	26	80.7
HSPN	5	2	0	7	100
Total	35	43	22	100	78% (78/100)

MN: membranous nephropathy; MsPGN: mesangial proliferative glomerulonephritis; MCN: minimal change nephropathy; FSGS: focal segmental glomerulosclerosis; SLE: systemic lupus erythematosus; HSPN: Henoch - Schonlein purpura nephritis;

Genetic equilibrium test

For CYP3A4, there were 56 patients with *1/*1 genotype, 42 patients with *1/*1G genotype, and only 2 cases with *1G/*1G. For CYP3A5, there were 8 patients with *1/*1 genotype, 36 patients with *1/*3 genotype, and 56 cases with *3/*3. For ABCB1 C1236T, there were 10 patients with 1236CC genotype, 44 patients with 1236CT genotype, and 46 cases with 1236TT. For ABCB1 G2677 T/A, there were 13 patients with 2677 GG genotype, 57 patients with 2677 GT/GA genotype, and 30 cases with 2677 TT/AA/TA. In 100 patients, the frequencies of CYP3 A4*1G, CYP3 A5*3, ABCB1 C1236T and ABCB1 G2677 T/A mutant allele were 23%, 74%, 68% and 58.5%, respectively (Table 4). Through Hardy-Weinberg inspection and analysis, the results showed that the frequency of each gene reached genetic equilibrium ($P > 0.05$). The study data could be representative of the whole group.

The effect of CYP3 A4, CYP3 A5, ABCB1, CCB and BMI on the clinical efficacy of TAC

Multivariate logistic regression analysis (Table 5) showed that the factors that influence the effect of clinical treatment included ABCB1 1236 mutant type TT ($P = 0.018$, OR = 12. 085, 95%CI 1.535–95.148), ABCB1 G2677 T/A gene mutation type TT or TA or AA ($P = 0.042$, OR = 8.683, 95%CI 1.080–69.819) and BMI ($P = 0.020$, OR = 15.838 95%CI 1.550–161.788) at the 0.05 level. For ABCB1 C1236T, TT genotype can increase the effectiveness of clinical treatment 12.085 times compared with CC and CT genotype. As for ABCB1 G2677 T/A, the clinical efficacy of patients with mutant genotype is 8.683 times than that of wild-type and heterozygous patient. Overweight patients can increase the clinical efficacy by 15.838 times than that of whose BMI was in normal range. However, CYP3A4, CYP3A5 and CCB do not directly affect the clinical efficacy of TAC ($P = 0.125$, $P = 0. 397$, $P = 0.357$, respectively).

Adverse reactions

In the group of 100 patients receiving TAC treatment, adverse drug reactions occurred at 8 cases in different degrees, namely, 2 cases of patients with central nervous system response (hand tremor), 4 patients with elevated blood sugar and 2 patients with dyspnea. The incidence of side effects was about 8%.

Discussion

We found evidence that ABCB1 C1236T, ABCB1 G2677 T/A and BMI are factors which may influence the clinical therapeutic effects of TAC on NS patients. We have not found that CYP3 A4, CYP3 A5 and whether the use of the CCB class antihypertensive drugs have impacts on the clinical treatment of patients with NS. These results indicate that detecting the above mentioned genes, especially ABCB1 C1236T and G2677 T/A, is important for the clinical implications of TAC, and that weight should also be taken into account. As a result, we should test genotypes in NS patients routinely prior to treatment to tailor treatment.

TAC, a kind of immunosuppressive drugs, can combine FK506 binding protein 12 (FKBP-12) and play a role in immune suppression [18, 19]. Pharmacokinetic characteristics of TAC were different among individuals, which could be influenced by the genetic factors such as single nucleotide polymorphisms (SNP), haplotype and DNA methylation [20]. In the CYP3A subfamily, CYP3 A4 and CYP3 A5 enzymes are responsible for TAC metabolism. P-gp encoded by the ABCB1 gene is responsible for transferring the drug from the cell to the outside [7, 12, 21]. Previous studies have focused on the effects of gene polymorphisms of CYP3 A4 and CYP3 A5 and ABCB1 genes on TAC metabolism in other setting and we have not found the relevant literature on NS. Therefore, more investigations should be performed to evaluate the effect of these related gene polymorphisms on the clinical efficacy of TAC in the treatment of NS patients.

Table 4 CYP3 A4, CYP3 A5 and ABCB1 genetic equilibrium test of genetic polymorphisms

SNP	Number of examples (theoretical)	Genotype frequency	Allele frequency	χ^2	P
CYP3 A4					
*1/*1	56 (59.29)	0.56	*1 = 0.77	3.45	0.06
*1/*1G	42 (35.42)	0.42			
*1G/*1G	2 (5.29)	0.02	*1G = 0.23		
CYP3 A5					
*1/*1	8 (6.76)	0.08	*1 = 0.26	0.42	0.52
*1/*3	36 (38.48)	0.36			
*3/*3	56 (54.76)	0.56	*3 = 0.74		
ABCB1 C1236T					
CC	10 (10.24)	0.10	C = 0.32	0.012	0.91
CT	44 (43.52)	0.44			
TT	46 (46.24)	0.46	T = 0.68		
ABCB1 G2677 T/A					
GG	13 (17.22)	0.13	G = 0.415	3.03	0.08
GT/A	57 (48.56)	0.57			
AA/TT/TA	30 (34.22)	0.30	T/A = 0.585		

ABCB1 gene is also known as multidrug resistance gene [8]. Some studies show that ABCB1 polymorphisms have nothing to do with the clinical efficacy of TAC [3, 9]. However, some studies have shown that ABCB1 1236 C > T can increase the blood concentration of TAC in the cell [7, 22]. Moreover, part of studies have come to the conclusion that the effect of TAC in patients with 2677G > T/A mutation genotype is better [4]. According to multi-factor logistic regression analysis in this study, we found that rs1128503 (1236C > T), rs2032582 (2677G > T/A) mutation carriers of these two loci were positively correlated with clinical efficacy of TAC in NS patients (Table 5).

We next try to interpret the mechanisms that ABCB1 C1236T and G2677 T/A genes affect the efficacy of TAC. ABCB1 1236C > T causes the codon to change from GGC to GGT. All of the genes encode glycine, which does not change the amino acid sequence of P-gp and belongs to synonymous mutation [21]. As we found that the mutated genotype of ABCB1 C1236T can increase the effectiveness compared with wild-type and

heterozygous genotype, synonymous mutation might have a certain role in regulating the metabolism of TAC. ABCB1 2677G > T/A can result in 839 amino acid residue from alanine to threonine or serine, making it from lipotropy to hydrophily and then affecting the transport function of P-gp and protein expression [21]. As a result, the clinical efficacy of patients with mutant genotype of ABCB1 G2677 T/A was much more better than that of wild-type and heterozygous patients, which was observed in our present study.

A number of studies have shown that non-genetic factors such as body weight, drug interactions and the disease status of patients can also lead to individual differences in drug response [10, 12]. In this study, the dosage of TAC was calculated according to body weight. Patients with the same height and different weight were given different TAC dosage. The BMI of the patients in this study was in the normal range or above the normal range. We found that BMI is a factor affecting the clinical efficacy of patients with NS. Overweight patients can improve the clinical efficacy by 15.838 times than that of whose BMI is in normal range.

A meta-analysis suggested that the CYP3 A4*1G genetic polymorphism played an important role in renal transplant recipients and CYP3 A4*1/*1 carriers exhibited higher C_0/Dose ratios than CYP3 A4*1G [14]. But some literatures indicated that the effect of CYP3 A4 genetic variability is not so well established [21]. Kurzawski et al. [10] finds that the CYP3A5 gene is an important factor in determining the dose requirement for TAC and individuals with CYP3A5*1 allele have

Table 5 The results of logistic regression analysis

Factors	β	SE	χ2	p	OR	95%CI
CYP3 A4	1.208	0.424	2.531	0.125	3.347	0.819–13.670
CYP3 A5	1.057	1.218	0.717	0.397	2.877	0.249–33.217
ABCB1 1236	2.492	1.053	5.603	0.018	12.085	1.535–95.148
ABCB1 2677	2.161	1.064	4.130	0.042	8.683	1.080–69.819
CCB	−1.349	1.464	0.849	0.357	0.260	0.015–4.572
BMI	2.762	1.186	5.428	0.020	15.838	1.550–161.788

higher TAC metabolism and lower blood TAC concentration. However, we found no significant correlation between CYP3 A4, CYP3 A5 genotype and clinical efficacy of TAC. The possible reasons are as follows. First, there may be other factors affecting the metabolism of CYP3A4 and CYP3A5 enzymes in patients with NS. Second, it is possible that the sample size is smaller, which leads to some deviation from the actual situation.

TAC plays a major role in clinical treatment by demethylation or hydroxylation of CYP450 enzyme. Thus, CYP450 enzyme inhibitors and inducers can also affect the TAC concentration and then have a certain impact on clinical efficacy. In our study, some patients took CCB antihypertensive drugs, which are a kind of CYP450 enzyme inhibitors, and did not take other CYP450 enzyme inhibitors and inducers, such as antibiotics, antifungal agents, antiviral drugs, psychiatric drugs and rifomycins [6]. In logistic regression, the application of CCB were used as covariates and clinical efficacy was used as dependent variable in this study. For the CCB, we concluded that the effect of it was not obvious in clinical treatment.

Previous studies showed that the mutation frequency of CYP3 A4 gene in Chinese population is about 30.8% [20]. In our present study, the mutation frequency was about 23%. The mutation frequency of CYP3 A5*3 is about 70% - 90% in Chinese population [11]. In the study, we found the CYP3A5 to be an unusual gene because the frequency of the variant allele (G) was higher (74%) than the wildtype (A) frequency (26%). 1236C > T ranges in allele frequency from 30 to 93% depending upon the ethnic population, and 2677G > T/A allele frequency varies as much as 2–65% among world population [22]. The frequencies of mutation in this study were 68% (1236C > T) and 58.5% (2677G > T/A), respectively.

We studied the effect of CYP3 A4, CYP3 A5, ABCB1 gene polymorphisms on the clinical efficacy of TAC in the treatment of NS and came up with the conclusion that ABCB1 C1236T and ABCB1 G2677 T/A could influence the clinical efficacy of TAC in the treatment of NS patients. However, there are also some limitations about the study. The inadequacy of this study is that the sample size is small, only 100 patients, and they are basically in the same region. There may be a linkage between the genes, which has a complicated effect on the pharmacokinetics of TAC, and the effects of various factors should be considered comprehensively. In the future, we need to expand the size of samples, confirm further study, and extend the time of follow-up.

Conclusions

In summary, the results of this study reveal that the gene mutations of CYP3A4 and CYP3A5 and CCB may not directly affect the clinical efficacy of TAC. However,

ABCB1 C1236T, ABCB1 G2677 T/A genotype and BMI are probably the factors influencing the clinical efficacy of TAC in treating patients with NS. Therefore, our study provides evidence that there may be a potential role for gene detection in tailoring therapy for patients with NS in order to improve response to treatment.

Additional files

Additional file 1: CYP3 A4*1G gene sequencing map (forward sequencing). A: CYP3 A4 *1/*1 (wild type); B: CYP3 A4 *1/*1G (heterozygous type); C: CYP3 A4 *1G/*1G (mutant type). (TIFF 916 kb)

Additional file 2: CYP3 A5*1 gene sequencing map (forward sequencing). A: CYP3 A5 *1/*1 (wild type); B: CYP3 A5 *1/*3 (heterozygous type); C: CYP3 A5 *3/*3 (mutant type). (TIFF 1142 kb)

Additional file 3: ABCB1 C1236T gene sequencing map (reverse sequencing). A: ABCB1 1236 GG (wild type); B: ABCB1 1236 AG (heterozygous type); C: ABCB1 1236 AA (mutant type). (TIFF 833 kb)

Additional file 4: ABCB1 G2677T/A gene sequencing map (reverse sequencing). A: ABCB1 2677CC (wild type); B: ABCB1 2677CT (heterozygous type); C: ABCB1 2677CA (heterozygous type); D: ABCB1 2677TT (mutant type); E: ABCB1 2677AT (mutant type); F: ABCB1 2677AA (mutant type). (TIFF 1876 kb)

Abbreviations
GFR: Glomerular filtration rate; NS: Nephrotic syndrome; P-gp: P-glycoprotein; SNP: Single Nucleotide Polymorphisms; TAC: Tacrolimus

Acknowledgements
XJY and QJY were responsible for DNA extraction, PCR and analysis of sequencing map. FL and CZ helped to collect samples. We thank them for their contributions. We also thank them for their contribution to the article. We also appreciate the participation of patients with NS.

Funding
This study was funded by natural science foundation of Shandong province, China (Grant No.ZR2015HQ028) and a project of medical and health technology development program in Shandong province, China (Grant No. 2016WS0724). These funds are used for the design of the study and collection, analysis, and interpretation of data and in writing the manuscript.

Authors' contributions
XG and WL conceived of the study and participated in the design. ML was responsible for collecting samples and statistical analysis. MX helped to perform the statistic analysis, draft the manuscript and modify the article. All authors read and approved the final manuscript.

Competing interests
The authors declare that they have no financial or non-financial competing interests.

References

1. Lavjay Butani, Rajendra Ramsamooj. Experience with tacrolimus in children with steroid-resistant nephrotic syndrome[J]. Pediatr Nephrol 2009 Aug; 24(8): 1517–1523.

2. Ayako Wakamatsu, Yoshiyasu Fukusumi, Eriko Hasegawa, Masayuki Tomita, Toru Watanabe, Ichiei Narita, Hiroshi Kawachi. Role of calcineurin (CN) in kidney glomerular podocyte: CN inhibitor ameliorated proteinuria by inhibiting the redistribution of CN at the slit diaphragm [J]. Physiol Rep 2016 Mar; 4(6): e12679.

3. Chen Kai. Effects of CYP3A4/5 and MDR1 gene polymorphisms on tacrolimus and liver and kidney function in early stage after liver transplantation [D]. Luzhou Medical College, 2013.

4. Guidelines for the detection of drug metabolizing enzymes and drug target genes (Trial) overview. J Practical organ transplantation. 2015;05:257–67.

5. Wei Wei Xie. Study on the correlation between ABCB1 gene polymorphism and depression and antidepressant efficacy [D]. In: Central South University; 2013.

6. Cusinato DA, Lacchini R, Romao EA, Moyses-Neto M, Coelho EB. Relationship of CYP3A5 genotype and ABCB1 diplotype to tacrolimus disposition in Brazilian kidney transplant patients. Br J Clin Pharmacol. 2014;78:364–72.

7. Luo X, Zhu LJ, Cai NF, Zheng LY, Cheng ZN. Prediction of tacrolimus metabolism and dosage requirements based on CYP3A4 phenotype and CYP3A5(*)3 genotype in Chinese renal transplant recipients. Acta Pharmacol Sin. 2016;37:555–60.

8. Zhang JJ, Liu SB, Xue L, Ding XL, Zhang H, Miao LY. The genetic polymorphisms of POR*28 and CYP3A5*3 significantly influence the pharmacokinetics of tacrolimus in Chinese renal transplant recipients. Int J Clin Pharmacol Ther. 2015;53:728–36.

9. Li Y. Study on the distribution of ABCB1 gene polymorphism in patients with epilepsy and its correlation with the efficacy of antiepileptic drugs [D]: Fudan University; 2010.

10. Kurzawski M, Dabrowska J, Dziewanowski K, Domanski L, Peruzynska M, Drozdzik M. CYP3A5 and CYP3A4, but not ABCB1 polymorphisms affect tacrolimus dose-adjusted trough concentrations in kidney transplant recipients. Pharmacogenomics. 2014;15:179–88.

11. Nikisch G, Eap CB, Baumann P. Citalopram enantiomers in plasma and cerebrospinal fluid of ABCB1 genotyped depressive patients and clinical response: a pilot study. Pharmacol Res. 2008;58:344–7.

12. Brambila-Tapia AJ. MDR1 (ABCB1) polymorphisms: functional effects and clinical implications. Revista de investigacion clinica; organo del Hospital de Enfermedades de la Nutricion. 2013;65:445–54.

13. Yan L, Li Y, Tang JT, An YF, Wang LL, Shi YY. Influence of CYP3A4, CYP3A5 andMDR-1 polymorphisms on tacrolimus pharmacokinetics and earlyrenal dysfunction in liver transplant recipients[J]. Gene. 2013;512(2):226–31.

14. Shi WL, Tang HL, Zhai SD. Effects of the CYP3A4*1B genetic polymorphism on the pharmacokinetics of tacrolimus in adult renal transplant recipients: a meta-analysis. PLoS One. 2015;10:e0127995.

15. Liu S, Li X, Li H, Liang Q, Chen J, Chen J. Comparison of tripterygium wilfordii multiglycosides and tacrolimus in the treatment of idiopathic membranous nephropathy: a prospective cohort study[J]. BMC Nephrol. 2015;16:200.

16. Butani L, Ramsamooj R. Experience with tacrolimus in children with steroid-resistant nephrotic syndrome[J]. Pediatr Nephrol. 2009;24:1517–23.

17. Qin H-Z, Liu L, Liang S-S, Shi J-S, Zheng C-X, Hou Q, Lu Y-H, Le W-B. Evaluating tacrolimus treatment in idiopathic membranous nephropathy in a cohort of 408 patients[J]. BMC Nephrol. 2017;18:2.

18. Li Y, Yan L, Shi Y, Bai Y, Tang J, Wang L. CYP3A5 and ABCB1 genotype influence tacrolimus and sirolimus pharmacokinetics in renal transplant recipients. SpringerPlus. 2015;4:637.

19. de Jonge H, de Loor H, Verbeke K, Vanrenterghem Y, Kuypers DR. In vivo CYP3A4 activity, CYP3A5 genotype, and hematocrit predict tacrolimus dose requirements and clearance in renal transplant patients. Clin Pharmacol Ther. 2012;92:366–75.

20. Rong G, Jing L, Deng-Qing L, Hong-Shan Z, Shai-Hong Z, Xin-Min N. Influence of CYP3A5 and MDR1(ABCB1) polymorphisms on the pharmacokinetics of tacrolimus in Chinese renal transplant recipients[J]. Transplant Proc. 2010;42: 3455–8.

21. Anglicheau D, Verstuyft C, Laurent-Puig P, Becquemont L, Schlageter M. H, Cassinat, B, Beaune P, Legendre C, Thervet E. Association of the multidrug resistance-1 genesingle-nucleotide polymorphisms with the tacrolimus dose requirements in renal transplant recipients[J]. JAm SocNephrol, 2003; 14 (7): 1889.

22. Ben Fredj N, Chaabane A, Chadly Z, Hammouda M, Aloui S, Boughattas NA, Skhiri H, Aouam K. Tacrolimus therapeutic drug monitoring in Tunisian renal transplant recipients: effect of post transplantation period[J]. Trans- pIImmunol. 2013;28:198–202.

15

Determinants of anti-retroviral regimen changes among HIV/AIDS patients of east and west Wollega zone health institutions

Amsalu Bokore[1]*（iD), Belay Korme[1] and Getu Bayisa[2]

Abstract

Background: Human Immunodeficiency Virus (HIV) is one of the main causes of morbidity and mortality; because of this it continues to be a major global public health concern. It has believed to kill more than 34 million lives so far. Sub Saharan Africa constitutes about 70% of people living with HIV among the 37 million on the globe. This region, accounted for more than two third of the global new HIV infections and about 15 million (40%) were receiving antiretroviral therapy (ART) at the end of 2014 throught the world. ART has fundamentally changed the treatment of HIV and transformed this infection from a disease of high mortality to chronic and medically managed disease. The issues of drug induced toxicities & complexity of current highly active antiretroviral therapy (HAART) regimens has remained of great concern. The aim of this study was to determine factors leading to antiretroviral regimen changes among HIV/AIDS Patients in the study area.

Methods: A facility based retrospective cross-sectional study was conducted from April 28, 2017 to May 30, 2017 in the ART clinics of east and west Wollega zone health institutions using a pre-tested data collecting form and chart review. The sample included the 243 patients whose medication had been switched.

Results: Majority 145 (59.67%) of the patients had been on ART for > 10 years duration. More than half 126(51.9%) of the patients had received tuberculosis (TB) treatment and almost three out of five patients (57.2%) had received isoniazid & cotrimoxazole prophylaxis. The most common reason for regimen change was peripheral neuropathy 146(60.1%) and the most common medication for this reason was stavudine, lamivudine and neverapine based 108(44.44%).

Conclusions: The number of patients who changed ARV drug in our resource constrained setting present a challenge to the restricted treatment choices that we currently own. Less toxic and better-tolerated HIV treatment options should be available and used more frequently.

Keywords: HIV/AIDS, HAART, ARV drug, Regimen change, Wollega

* Correspondence: bokore.amsalu@yahoo.com
[1]Nekemte referral hospital, Nekemte, Ethiopia
Full list of author information is available at the end of the article

Background

Human immunodeficiency virus (HIV) annihilates and compromises the function of immune cells. Immunity of infected individuals gradually depletes and susceptibility to a wide range of infections and diseases would be boosted. Acquired immunodeficiency syndrome (AIDS) is the most advanced stage of HIV infection, which can take from 2 to 15 years to develop depending on the individual and it can be explained by the progression of opportunistic infections, or other intense clinical manifestations and certain cancers [1, 2].

HIV is one of the main causes of morbidity and mortality; because of this it continues to be a major global public health concern. It has believed to kill more than 34 million lives so far. Sub Saharan Africa constitutes about 70% of people living with HIV among the thirty seven million on the globe. This region, accounted for more than two third of the global new HIV infections in 2014 with only 12% of the global population. Globally people receiving ART were about fifteen million (40%) among those living with HIV of which about fourteen million were in low- and middle –income countries and nearly one million were children [2].

Ethiopia is among the countries most affected by HIV/AIDS with prevalence of 1.9% for women and 1.0% for men in 2011 [3] and it is also in a low generalized HIV epidemic with significant heterogeneity among regions and population groups [4]. The existence of HIV infection in Ethiopia was recognized in the early 1980s with the first two AIDS cases reported in 1986. The predominant strain is HIV-1 subtype C, predominantly spread through unprotected heterosexual intercourse [5]. Since 2000 the epidemic has declined [6] and recent figures show that HIV infection has significantly decreased over the years in the country [4].

Highly active antiretroviral therapy (HAART) has fundamentally changed the treatment of HIV and changed this infection from a disease of high mortality to chronic and medically managed disease which is a radical change in controlling the hardship of HIV/AIDS. However drug resistance and side effects were the great concern in these advancements [7]. Revolution in the care of patients with HIV/AIDS occurred due to the innovation of potent HAART in around 2000. The qualities of life of people living with HIV/AIDS (PLWHA) have improved and these treatments have dramatically reduced rates of mortality and morbidity among these patients. This result was also confirmed by World health organization (WHO) progress report. ARV drugs produce these effects by restoration of number and quality of cluster of difference (CD4) cells and suppressing viral replication [8].

The goal of ART is to attain maximal and durable suppression of the viral replication. Viral suppression enables recovery of the immune response and thereby reduces risk of opportunistic infections (OIs) and death [1].

The decision to initiate ART for adults and adolescents depend on: WHO stage 3 and 4 disease irrespective of CD4 cell count, CD4 count ≤500cells/mm^3 irrespective of WHO clinical stage and active tuberculosis (TB) co-infection with HIV irrespective of CD4 cell count according to standard treatment guideline of Ethiopia [6].

Triple combination therapy has been in use for more than two decades globally. Currently, the preferred first regimen triple therapy in Ethiopia consists of, two Nucleoside Reverse Transcriptase Inhibitors (NRTIs) and one Protease Inhibitor (PI) or a Non-Nucleoside Reverse Transcriptase Inhibitor (NNRTI) or a triple therapy of three NRTIs. Based on the guideline, common ART regimens in the country are; Tenofovir (TDF)/ Emtricitabine (FTC)/ Efavirenz (EFV) or Nevirapine (NVP); alternatives are TDF/ Lamivudine (3TC) /EFV or NVP, Zidovudine (ZDV)/3TC/EFV or NVP. Other options are Abacavir (ABC)/3TC/NVP, ABC/3TC/EFV and ABC/3TC/ZDV. The second line regimen consists of ZDV ±3TC + Lopinavir/ritonavir (LPV/r) (or Atazanavir/ritonavir (ATV/r)), ZDV + ABC + LPV/r (or ATV/r), TDF/3TC ± ZDV + LPV/r (or ATV/r), ABC/ Didanosine (ddI) /LPV/r (or ATV/r), EFV or NVP / LPV/r (or ATV/r) [1, 9].

Changes of multiple medications in HAART regimens were commonly required simultaneously. These changes may be due to co morbidity with other chronic diseases, a desire for pregnancy, poor adherence, stock out of drugs, treatment failure, long term toxicity or acute toxicity. The approaches to change ART regimens depend largely on amount of previous ART experience, available treatment options and reason for change. For example effective treatment can be accomplished by substituting another agent for the drug which has unpleasant effect in the regimen when it develops to certain drugs in the regimen [7, 10].

The issues of drug toxicities and complexity of current HAART regimens has remained of great concern despite ARTs being of much help to the health of HIV/AIDS patients. Suboptimal therapy, discontinuation, and treatment failure can be resulted from treatment toxicities and adherence problems [11]. The consequence of these may complicate the management and lead to toxicity, loss to follow-up, compromise the effectiveness of HAART regimens, drug interactions and drug resistance [12].

Knowledge of the determinants of ART change may help to minimize the risk factors. These benefits in decreasing the rate of regimen change, treatment failure, drug resistance, and improve the quality of life of the patient. Antiretroviral treatment change should be done when necessary to spare the future treatment options. The approach to patients who need to switch will differ depending on several issues, including ART experience and available options. Regimen substitution requires adjustment in learning the new medication about the treatment dosing, time of intake and deal with many individual based inconveniences, which might be challenging and reason for non-adherence [10, 13].

Data on modification of HAART and factors associated with ARV drug regimen change are limited among HIV/AIDS patients in Ethiopia. Most of the surveys used were on small sample of patients who were on ART for less than three years. As a result it is important to understand common reasons of ARV drug switch in patients on long period exposure to ART.

Therefore, this study attempts to investigate the major determinants of HAART regimen change among HIV/AIDS patients in east and west Wollega zone health institutions by using cross-sectional study.

Objective
General objective

✓ To assess determinants of antiretroviral regimen change among HIV/AIDS patients in east and west Wollega zone health institutions, Oromia region, west Ethiopia.

Specific objectives

✓ To assess determinants of antiretroviral regimen change among HIV/AIDS positive patients.
✓ To identify the pattern of initial ART regimens and the subsequent changes.
✓ To assess the relationship between patient characteristics and reasons for initial ART change.

Methods
Study area, design, and period
The study was conducted in the ART clinics of east and west Wollega zone health institutions, Oromia region, west Ethiopia; Nekemte town which is the capital of east Wollega is located 328 km where as Gimbi town which is the capital of west Wollega is 438 Km western to Addis Ababa [14].

The area is well known by its coffee production. The economy of the people is based on subsistence farming and livestock rearing. The climatic condition of the area is 'woinadega' (semi-desert) and it is found at 2080 m above sea level.

A facility based retrospective cross-sectional study was conducted by reviewing patient information sheets and physician diagnostic cards to assess reasons for HAART regimen change. The study was conducted from April 28, 2017 to May 30, 2017.

Source and study population
All HIV/AIDS positive patients who were greater than 18 years and on HAART in east and west Wollega zone health institutions ART Clinic from April 28, 2007 to April 28, 2017 were the source population. All HIV/AIDS positive patients greater than 18 years who had undergone HAART regimen change in east and west Wollega zone health institutions ART Clinic in between April 28, 2007 to April 28, 2017 were the study population.

Inclusion and exclusion criteria
Inclusion criteria:

✓ Patients on follow up in the ART clinic who had undergone HAART regimen change until the study period.
✓ Patients on follow up in the ART clinic who were on second line regimen when the study was undergone.
✓ HIV/AIDS patients who were greater than18 years.
✓ Patients receiving HAART regimen for at least 6 months at the beginning of the study period

Exclusion criteria:

✓ Patient information cards with incomplete information (Patient information card which had no one or more of information like information on demographics, WHO clinical stage, CD4 count, initiation regimen and changed regimen, duration of initial therapy, and causes for regimen change).
✓ Patients with less than 6 months on HAART regimen.
✓ Patients who didn't switch HAART regimen.
✓ Under eighteen year old HIV/AIDS patients.
✓ Deceased patients
✓ Transfer out patients

Sample population
A total of 243 patients who had undergone HAART regimen change in the ART clinics of east and west Wollega zone health institutions from April 28, 2007 to April 28, 2017 were included in the study while patients below 18 years were excluded from the study. Patient information cards that showed a change in the initial treatment regimen were assessed and analyzed, to identify the common reasons that resulted in a change from the initial treatment regimen.

Study variables
Independent variables

✓ Socio-demographic characteristics: age at initiation, sex, marital status, educational status.

✓ Disease related variables: baseline WHO stage, base line CD4, and baseline weight.

✓ ART related variables: types of initial regimen

Dependent variables

✓ Reasons for change

Data procedure and management

Data collection procedure

Data abstraction form was developed based on the objectives of the study. It contained socio-demographic, clinical information and ART information such as, CD4 count, WHO stage, initial regimen, date on which treatment was started, date of ARV drug switch, duration of initial ARV therapy before first switch, regimen switched to, and causes for regimen change. The types of toxicity and treatment failure reasons were included. If there was ARV drug switch for the second and third time it was recorded in a similar manner. For data collection four 10th grade completed students were recruited. One pharmacist and one druggist from each health institutions were also recruited as supervisors.

Data collectors recruitment and training

Data collectors were recruited and trained methods of data collection prior to the start of actual data collection.

Data quality assurance/control

Training was provided for supervisors and data collectors and they were standardized. Data abstraction form was pre-tested on randomly selected patient information cards to identify any drawbacks in Shambu hospital which is found in Horro Gudru Wollega zone before the actual survey and improvements were made. The principal investigator supervised the data collection. Every questionnaire was checked for completeness and logical consistency.

Data processing and analysis

The data were coded and entered in to a computer using statistical Package for the Social Sciences (SPSS) software for windows version 20 and the analysis was performed after the data were cleaned, edited and processed. Distribution of Patients such as percentages and their number by socio demographic characteristics and other relevant variables in the study were described using descriptive analysis.

Ethical considerations

An official letter was written by department of pharmacy, college of public health and medical sciences, Wollega University to zonal and woreda health offices of east and west Wollega zone Administration to get permission. After permission to conduct the study was obtained, data has been collected in one of refilling rooms at ART Clinic by safe keeping of records.

Only numerical identifications were used as a reference, confidentiality and anonymity of subject was maintained by not recording and identifying details, such as name or any other personal details. No disclosure of any name of the patients, the healthcare provider or drug product was made in relation to the finding.

Operational definitions

ABC based regimen: regimen containing abacavir as one of the NRTI backbones and may have different NNRI or PI bases.

Antiretroviral drug switch/change: it is the change of one or two ARV drugs from the initial drug regimens.

AZT based regimen: regimen containing zidovudine as one of the NRTI backbones and may have different NNRI or PI bases.

Table 1 Socio-demographic characteristics of HIV/AIDS patients who changed their HAART regimen in east and west Wollega zone health institutions, April 28, 2007 to April 28, 2017

Demographic Characteristics	N (%)
Age in years	
20–34	19(7.8)
35–49	174(71.6)
≥ 50	50(20.6)
Sex	
Female	127(52.3)
Male	116(47.7)
Marital status	
Single	18(7.4)
Married	154(63.4)
Divorced	12(4.9)
Widowed	59(24.3)
Educational status	
No formal education	74(30.5)
Primary school education	92(37.9)
Secondary school education	52(21.4)
Higher institute education	25(10.3)
Family size	
Less than five	96(39.5)
5–10	86(35.4)
> 10	61(25.1)
Place of Residence	
Urban	209(86)
Rural	34(14)

Table 2 Clinical characteristics of HIV/AIDS patients who changed their HAART regimen in east and west Wollega zone health institutions, April 28, 2007 to April 28, 2017

		On initiation of ART	Before ART switch	On data collection
WHO clinical stage	stage I	17	60	237
	stage II	40	55	6
	stage III	180	126	0
	stage IV	6	2	0
	Total	243	243	243
CD4 count (cells/ml)	< 200	180	42	27
	200–350	60	54	26
	> 350	03	147	190
	Total	243	243	243
Weight (kg)	< 45	51	24	24
	45–60	164	155	137
	> 60	28	64	82
	Total	243	243	243

Co morbidity: is defined as the occurrence of one or more additional disorders which are on drug therapy with HIV/AIDS simultaneously (TB, diabetes, hypertension).

d4T based regimen: regimen containing Stavudine as one of the NRTI backbones and may have different NNRI or PI bases.

TDF based regimen: regimen containing Tenofovir as one of the NRTI backbones and may have different NNRI or PI bases.

Toxicity: is defined as the occurrence of adverse events such as diarrhea, nausea, vomiting, anemia, rash, fatigue, peripheral neuropathy, lipodystrophy, metabolic disturbances, CNS abnormalities or any other unwanted effect related to HAART.

Transfer out: Patients who changed their follow up to other health institution.

Results

Socio-demographic characteristics of patients whose ART regimen changed

The mean age of patients was 43.68(SD ± 8.2) years. Majority of the patients 174(71.6%) were in the age range of 35–49 years and more than half 127(52.3%) of the patients were females. About 154(63.4%) of the patients were married. In this study only 77(31.7%) of the patients received greater than secondary school education. Regarding the family size 96(39.5%) of the patients had < 5 family size whereas 61(25.1%) had > 10 family size. Regarding place of residence 209(86%) were urban dwellers where as 34(14%) were rural dwellers as shown in (Table 1).

Clinical characteristics of patients whose ART regimen was changed

During initiation of ART 180(74.1%) of the patients were on WHO clinical stage III; whereas WHO stage after the ART switch was stage I for 237(97.53%) of patients. Similarly more than two third 180(74.1%) of patients had baseline CD4 count less than 200 cells/µL on initiation but most 190(78.19%) of patients had > 350 cells/µL after ART switch. In addition, the weight of the majority 164(67.5%) of patients during initiation of ART was between 45 and 60 kg (Table 2). Majority 145 (59.67%) of the patients had been on ART for > 10 years duration (Fig. 1). About 126(51.85%) of the patients had received TB treatment whereas 117(48.15%) of the patients did not receive TB treatment. Regarding OI

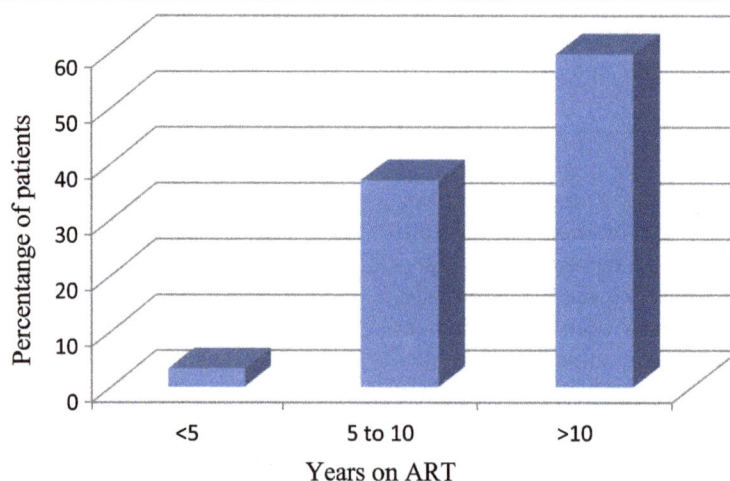

Fig. 1 Years of stay on ART of HIV/AIDS patients who changed their HAART regimen in east and west Wollega zone health institutions, April 28, 2007 to April 28, 2017

Table 3 OI prophylaxis taken by study population in east and west Wollega zone health institutions, April 28, 2007 to April 28, 2017

Type of OI prophylaxis	Frequency	Percent
Cotrimoxazole & Isoniazid	139	57.2
Cotrimoxazole	95	39.1
Neither	9	3.7
Total	243	100.0

prophylaxis 139(57.2%) of the patients received Cotrimoxazole and Isonazid prophylaxis (Table 3).

Patterns of initial ART regimen and regimen switched to/changed regimen

Majority of the patients 159(65.4%) started their initial ART on D4t-3TC-NVP regimens, followed by D4t-3TC-EFV 55 (22.6%). Only 12% of patients started initial ART regimen on AZT based regimen (Table 4).

The HAART regimen of majority of the patients 168(69.14%) was changed to TDF based regimen. Whereas about 69(28.4%) of the patients initial HAART regimen was changed to AZT based regimen and only 6(2.5%) patients initial HAART regimen was changed to ABC based regimen (Table 5).

Reasons for ART change

The main reason for antiretroviral regimen change was Peripheral neuropathy 146(60.1%) followed by hepatotoxicity, d4t faith out, CNS toxicity, Anemia, Rash etc. (Table 4). The most common reason for regimen change was peripheral neuropathy 146(60.1%) and the most common medication for this reason was stavudine, lamivudine and neverapine based 108(44.44%) (Table 6 and 7).

Discussion

The present retrospective cross sectional study of HIV/AIDS patients who changed their HAART regimen in east and west Wollega zone health institutions described the pattern of ART regimen and the common reasons for ARV drug switch. Such studies would be helpful in understanding the complexity of ART use of patients in

Table 4 HAART regimen at initiation among HIV/AIDS patients who changed their HAART regimen in east and west Wollega zone health institutions, April 28, 2007 to April 28, 2017

Initial HAART regimen	Frequency	Percent
D4t-3TC-NVP	159	65.4
D4t-3TC-EFV	55	22.6
AZT-3TC-NVP	14	5.8
AZT-3TC-EFV	15	6.2
Total	243	100.0

Table 5 Patterns of ART switch of HIV/AIDS patients who changed their HAART regimen in east and west Wollega zone health institutions, April 28, 2007 to April 28, 2017

ART drugs after switching	Frequency	Percent
AZT + 3TC + NVP	47	19.3
AZT + 3TC + EFV	16	6.6
TDF + 3TC + EFV	56	23.05
TDF + 3TC + NVP	98	40.33
ABC+ ddi + LPV/R	6	2.5
AZT + 3TC + ATV/R	6	2.5
TDF + 3TC + LPV/R	10	4.1
TDF + 3TC + ATV/R	4	1.6
Total	243	100.0

health institutions which might have different co morbidities.

Majority of the study population 145 (59.67%) had been on ART for > 10 years. This finding indicated longer duration as compared to other studies as all patients stayed on ART for less than 3 years in Bedelle [15] and in Addis Ababa about 98% of patients stayed on ART for less than one and half years and in Dessie only 6% patients stayed on ART for more than 2 years [10, 16].

The main reason for initial ARV drug switch in the present study was toxicity which was known as peripheral neuropathy and it accounted for more than 60% of HAART regimen change. This finding was in agreement with the study conducted in some parts of Ethiopia [10]. The other reasons for HAART regimen change were hepatotoxicity 22(9.1%), anemia 16(6.6%) and rash15 (5.3%). The combined sum of hepatotoxicity, anemia and peripheral neuropathy was more than 80%, which was much higher than the studies done in United Kingdom (35%) [17] and India (27%) [18]. However, it was almost similar to the studies conducted in other parts of Ethiopia as it was 75.8% in Mekelle [19] and 66% in Dessie [16]. But there was a significant heterogeneity on the type of toxicities in these studies.

Table 6 Common reasons for modification of regimens of study population in east and west Wollega zone health institutions, April 28, 2007 to April 28, 2017

Reason for regimen change	Frequency	Percent
Peripheral neuropathy	146	60.1
Hepatotoxicity	22	9.1
d4t phase out	18	7.4
CNS toxicities	16	6.6
Anemia	16	6.6
Rash	15	5.3
Others	10	4.9

Table 7 Common reasons for modification by first treatment regimens among study population in east and west Wollega zone health institutions, April 28, 2007 to April 28, 2017

Patterns of ART Regimen	Reasons for ART regimen change										Total
	Anemia	Rash	Peripheral neuropathy	Hepatotoxicity	Diarrhea	CNS toxicities	stigma disclosure	d4t phase out	jaundice	Burning/ numbness	
d4t-3TC-NVP	5	8	108	16	0	4	0	16	0	2	159
d4t-3TC-EFV	0	3	30	6	0	10	2	2	0	2	55
AZT-3TC-NVP	4	0	2	0	4	2	0	0	2	0	14
AZT-3TC-EFV	7	2	6	0	0	0	0	0	0	0	15
Total	16	13	146	22	4	16	2	18	2	4	243

Change of the entire regimen from first-line to second-line is required in case of treatment failure. In order to increase likelihood of treatment success and minimize the risk of cross-resistance the new second-line regimen should involve drugs that keep activity against the patient's virus strain and should preferably include at least three new drugs, one or more from a new class [12]. The preferred strategy for second-line ART for adults is using a boosted PI and two NRTI combinations when NNRTI-containing regimens were used in first-line ART [8]. Patients from low-income countries were less likely to change two or more drugs and to change to a protease-inhibitor-containing regimen when compared with patients from high-income countries [20].

The study also found that there was high prevalence of TB as almost three out of five patients (57%) had received isoniazid & cotrimoxazole prophylaxis and more than half (52%) of the patients had been treated for TB [16, 19]. NVP has high interaction with Rifampicin which is strong liver enzyme (CYP 3A4) inducer where by therapeutic level of NVP is decreased up to 40% which necessitates switch to EFV. Additive hepatotoxicity effects also exists when NVP and Rifampicin were used together according to findings of some studies which is another requirement to switch from NVP to EFV as the latter has lesser adverse drug reaction with Rifampicin [21].

Conclusions

The number of patients who changed ARV drug in our resource constrained setting present a challenge to the restricted treatment choices that we currently own. The main reasons for ART switch were toxicity among which Peripheral neuropathy and hepatotocity were the leading toxicity for ART switch. Less toxic and better-tolerated HIV treatment options should be available and used more frequently in east and west Wollega zone health institutions. Patient should be evaluated regularly after a treatment change to assess for potential concerns with the new regimen, medication tolerance and to assess the effectiveness. Information is needed on patterns of resistance across the population to recommend future therapy options. Therefore national and health institution based surveillance of antiretroviral drug resistance should be conducted. It helps to know the resistance pattern and select the locally effective treatments. National level study on reasons for regimen change should be done to help drug suppliers and policy makers to improve and solve the problem. The reasons of ARV drug switch observed in this cross sectional study should be investigated further in longitudinal multicenter studies of ART utilization.

Abbreviations

3TC: Lamivudine; ABC: Abacavir; ART: Antiretro Viral Therapy; ARV: Antiretroviral; ATV/R: Atazanavir/Ritonavir; AZT: Zidovudine; CD4: Cluster of Difference; CNS: Central Nervous System; CYP: Cytochrome p-450; d4T: Stavudine; ddl: Didanosine; EFV: Efavirenz; FTC: Emitricibine; HAART: Highly Active Antiretroviral Therapy; LPV/R: Lopinavir/Ritonavir; NNRTI: Nucleoside Reverse Transcriptase inhibitor; NRTI: Nucleoside Reverse Transcriptase inhibitor; NVP: Nevirapine; OI: Opportunistic Infection; PI: Protease Inhibitors; PLWHA: People Living With HIV/AIDS; SD: Standard deviation; TB : Tuberculosis; TDF: Tenofovir; VL: Viral Load; WHO: World Health Organization

Acknowledgments

The authors would like to express their sincere gratitude to Wollega University for their support for the accomplishment of this study. The authors are also thankful for officials of east and west Wollega zone health offices for delivering necessary information for this study. We would also like to thank supervisors and data collectors for taking their precious time to collect the data. We are also thankful for staff members of ART clinics from which the data was collected.

Funding

No funding was obtained for this study.

Authors' contributions

The authors' responsibilities were as follows: AB designed and supervised the study, and ensured quality of the data and made a substantial contribution to the local implementation of the study assisted in the analysis and interpretation of the data. BK participated in the design of the study, performed the data collection and the statistical analysis. GB also designed and supervised the study, and made a substantial contribution to the local implementation of the study. We want to ensure that all authors have performed all important points specified on criteria and guidelines for authorship and all authors read and approved the final manuscript.

Authors' information

AB is graduated from Jimma University with bachelor of pharmacy, from Unity University with bachelor of arts degree in economics and from Wollega University with masters of public health and has published many original research articles in an international journals, is currently working at Nekemte referral hospital chronic care pharmacy, P.O. Box 25, Nekemte, Ethiopia. BK is graduated from Wollega University with bachelor of pharmacy, is currently working at Nekemte referral hospital chronic care pharmacy, P.O. Box 25, Nekemte, Ethiopia. GB has also published many original research articles in an international journals, is currently a lecturer at Wollega University College of health and medical sciences, department of pharmacy, P.O. Box 395, Nekemte, Ethiopia.

Competing interests

The authors declare that they have no competing interests.

Author details

[1]Nekemte referral hospital, Nekemte, Ethiopia. [2]Wollega University, Nekemte, Ethiopia.

References

1. Food, Medicine and Health Care Administration and Control Authority (FMHACA); Standard Treatment Guidelines for general hospitals; 3rd edition; Addis Ababa. Ethiopia 2014.
2. World Health organization (WHO); Fact Sheet; 2015.
3. Central Statistical Agency Ethiopia and ICF International. Ethiopia demographic and health survey. Addis Ababa, Ethiopia and Calverton, Maryland: Central Statistical Agency and ICF International; 2012.
4. World Health Organization (WHO). HIV/AIDS Progress in 2014; Update Ethiopia, WHO country office for Ethiopia UNECA compound; Addis Ababa, Ethiopia; March 2015.
5. Federal democratic republic of Ethiopia. Country progress reports on HIV/ AIDS; Addis Ababa, Ethiopia; 2012.
6. Federal Ministry of Health (MOH). Health Sector Development Program IV: (2010/11–2014/15), Final draft. Addis Ababa, Ethiopia: MOH. p. 2010.
7. Wilkin T, Marshall G, Gulick M. Switching antiretroviral therapy why, when and how. J Acquir Immune Defic Syndr. 2010;12:782–9.
8. World Health organization (WHO). Global update on HIV treatment: results, impact and opportunities, brief summary. Kuala Lumpur, Malaysia: WHO; 2013a.
9. Federal Ministry of Health (MOH). Guideline for implantation of the antiretroviral therapy program in Ethiopia. Addis Ababa, Ethiopia: MOH; 2007.
10. Jima T, Angamo M, Wabe N. Causes for antiretroviral regimen change among HIV/AIDS patients in Addis Ababa. Ethiopia Tanzania Journal of Health Research. 2013;15(1):1–9.
11. Park B, Choe G, Kim H, et al. Early modification of initial HAART regimen associated with poor clinical outcome in HIV patients. AIDS Res Hum Retrovir. 2010;23(8):794–800.
12. Hendrickson S, Jacobson P, Nelson W, et al. Host genetic influences on highly active antiretroviral therapy efficacy and AIDS free survival. J Acquire Immune Deficient Syndrome. 2008;48(3):263–71.
13. Demessie R, Mekonnen A, Amogne W, et al. Knowledge and adherence to antiretroviral therapy among adult people living with HIV / AIDS at TikurAnbessa specialized hospital, Ethiopia. International Journal of Basic & Clinical Pharmacology. 2014;3(2):320–30.
14. Nekemte town health Office (NTHO) Census 2009.
15. Mekonnen Y, Molla G. Reason for regimen change among HIV patients on initial highly active antiretroviral therapy in Bedele. Journal of Biotechnology and Bio safety. 2014;2(4):116–22.
16. Mulugeta A, Chane T. Causes of antiretroviral drug changes among patients on antiretroviral therapy. Int J Pharm Sci Res. 2012;3(1):120–5.
17. Messou E, Anglaret X, Duvignac J, et al. Antiretroviral treatment changes in adults from Côte d'Ivoire: the roles of tuberculosis and pregnancy. AIDS (London, England). 2010;24(1):93–9.
18. Sandeep B, Vansant C, Raghunandan M, et al. Factors influencing the substitution of antiretroviral therapy in human immunodeficiency virus/ acquired immunodeficiency syndrome patients on first line highly active antiretroviral therapy. Asian Journal of Pharmaceutical and Clinical Research. 2014;7(5):117–20.
19. Bayou T, Woldu M, Gebre Meskel G, et al. Factors determinant for change of initial antiretroviral treatment regimen among patients on ART follow-up clinic of Mekelle hospital, Mekelle, Ethiopia. International Journal of Basic & Clinical Pharmacology. 2014;3(1):44.
20. Zhou J, Kumarasamy N, Boyd M, et al. Deferred modification of antiretroviral regimen following documented treatment failure in Asia: Results from the TREAT Asia HIV Observational Database (TAHOD). HIV Medicine. 2010;11(1): 31–9.
21. Hawkins C, Achenbach C, Fryda W, et al. Antiretroviral durability and tolerability in HIV-infected adults living in urban Kenya. J Acquir Immune Defic Syndr. 2009;45(3):304–10.

16

Rituximab impedes natural killer cell function in Chronic Fatigue Syndrome/Myalgic Encephalomyelitis patients: A pilot in vitro investigation

Natalie Eaton[1,2]* (iD), Hélène Cabanas[1,2], Cassandra Balinas[1,2], Anne Klein[1,2], Donald Staines[1,2] and Sonya Marshall-Gradisnik[1,2]

Abstract

Background: A recent in vitro pilot investigation reported Rituximab significantly reduced natural killer (NK) cell cytotoxicity in healthy donors. Chronic fatigue syndrome/Myalgic encephalomyelitis (CFS/ME) is a debilitating disorder of unknown etiology. A consistent finding is a significant reduction in NK cell cytotoxicity. Rituximab has been reported having questionable potential therapeutic benefits for the treatment of CFS/ME, however, the potential effects of Rituximab on NK cell cytotoxicity in CFS/ME patients are yet to be determined.

Methods: A total of eight CFS/ME patients (48.63 ± 15.69 years) and nine non-fatigued controls (NFC) (37.56 ± 11.06 years) were included using the Fukuda case definition. Apoptotic function, lytic proteins and degranulation markers were measured on isolated NK cells using flow cytometry following overnight incubation with Rituximab at 10 μg/ml and 100 μg/ml.

Results: There was a significant reduction in NK cell lysis between CFS/ME patients and NFC following incubation with Rituximab at 100 μg/ml at 12.5:1 and 6.25:1 effecter-target (E:T) ratios ($p < 0.05$). However, there was no significant difference for NFC following incubation with Rituximab at 10 μg/ml and 100 μg/ml.
There was no significant difference between CFS/ME patients and NFC for granzyme A and granzyme B prior to incubation with Rituximab and following overnight incubation with Rituximab at 10 μg/ml. There was a significant decrease in granzyme B in CFS/ME patients compared to NFC with 100 μg/ml of Rituximab prior to K562 cells stimulation ($p < 0.05$). There was a significant increase in CD107a ($p < 0.05$) and CD107b expression ($p < 0.01$) in NFC after stimulation with K562 cells prior to incubation with Rituximab. There was a significant increase in CD107b expression between CFS/ME patients and NFC prior to incubation with Rituximab and without stimulation of K562 cells ($p < 0.01$). Importantly, there was a significant increase in CD107b following overnight incubation with 100 μg/ml of Rituximab in NFC prior to K562 cells stimulation ($p < 0.01$).

Conclusion: This study reports significant decreases in NK cell lysis and a significant increase in NK cell degranulation following Rituximab incubation in vitro in CFS/ME patients, suggesting Rituximab may be toxic for NK cells. Caution should be observed in clinical trials until further investigations in a safe and controlled in vitro setting are completed.

Keywords: Chronic fatigue syndrome, Myalgic encephalomyelitis, Rituximab, Natural killer cells, Lytic proteins, Degranulation, Cytotoxicity

* Correspondence: n.eaton@griffith.edu.au
[1]School of Medical Science, Griffith University, QLD, Gold Coast, Australia
[2]The National Centre for Neuroimmunology and Emerging Diseases, Menzies Health Institute Queensland, Griffith University, QLD, Gold Coast, Australia

Background

CFS/ME is a debilitating disorder hallmarked by unexplained debilitating fatigue accompanied by immune, neurological, musculoskeletal, cardiovascular and gastrointestinal symptoms [1]. The diagnosis of CFS/ME is complex and relies on case definition for diagnostic criteria [1–3]. The underlying etiology of CFS/ME remains unknown; however, a significant reduction of NK cell cytotoxicity is a key and consistently reported feature of CFS/ME [4–14].

CFS/ME is believed to affect approximately 200,000 Australians [15] having a global prevalence of 0.2–6.4% [16]. CFS/ME is reported more commonly in women than in men, with 75% of patients being female [17] and predominantly affecting 30- to 40-year-olds in developed countries [16]. However, due to inconsistencies in CFS/ME case definitions the true prevalence is difficult to determine.

NK cells are effector lymphocytes of the innate immune system that eliminate pathogens and malignant cells, activate immune cells and provide cytokine producing functions [18]. NK cells have tightly regulated cytotoxic activity against stress and antibody-coated cells [18–22]. The majority of human peripheral NK cells are $CD56^{dim}$ NK cell subset bearing the low-affinity Fc-γ-receptor CD16 [23]. CD16 binds to the Fc portion of immunoglobulin (Ig) G and mediates antibody-dependent cellular cytotoxicity (ADCC) [23–26]. NK cell cytotoxicity (NKCC) involves numerous steps including adhesion to the target cell, activations of surface receptors, polarization of secretory granules and release of lytic proteins, including granzyme A and granzyme B, to induce apoptosis of the target cell [7, 21, 27].

NK cell activation is tightly regulated by activating receptors that recognise pathogen-derived, stress-induced and tumour specific ligands [20]. CD16 plays a prominent role as an activating receptor for NK cells [28]. NK cell activation initiates calcium (Ca^{2+})-dependent signal transduction through receptor cytoplasmic tails that contain immunoreceptor tyrosine-based activation motifs (ITAM) [11, 22, 29–31]. Ligation of ITAM-bearing receptor complexes results in the recruitment and activation of mitogen-activated protein kinase (MAPK) phosphorylation cascade [29]. The phosphorylation of kinases induces the polarization of NK cell granules via the microtubule-organizing centre (MTOC) [32, 33]. Granule polarization ensures granule contents are released facing the target cell. NK cell cytotoxic granules are responsible for the storage and secretion of lytic proteins including perforin, a membrane-disrupting protein, and granzymes, a family of proteases [11, 27]. The secretion of perforin is suggested to create pores within the target cell membrane to facilitate endocytosis mechanisms, in which granzymes can enter the target cell to trigger apoptosis by cleaving pro-apoptotic caspases and influence nuclear damage [5, 7, 27, 34, 35].

Importantly, reduced NK cell function is the most consistently reported finding in both severe and moderate CFS/ME patients [4–14]. Impaired NKCC in CFS/ME patients is evident through delayed degranulation [7, 36, 37] and decreased lytic proteins, predominantly granzyme B [5, 11, 36, 38, 39]. The increase in NK cell degranulation in CFS/ME patients may suggest an inability to induce sufficient cytotoxic lysis or continued activation due to insufficient lytic proteins. Therefore, using flow cytometry to investigate expression of degranulation markers, CD107a and CD107b, and intracellular lytic proteins, granzyme A and granzyme B, is critical when investigating the cytotoxic activity of NK cells [40].

Rituximab (RTX), is a chimeric antibody that targets CD20 present on healthy and malignant B lymphocytes. RTX can trigger target cell death through three effector functions: 1) programmed cell death, 2) induction of complement-mediated cytotoxicity, and 3) ADCC mediated by Fc receptor-bearing immune cells such as NK cells [41]. RTX works to opsonize the CD20 surface marker on B lymphocytes, this stimulates the recruitment of NK cells and ligation with CD16. The activation of CD16 to the Fc portion of RTX activates Ca^{2+}-dependent elimination of B lymphocytes through ADCC.

Limited investigations have examined the potential role of therapeutic interventions in CFS/ME patients. We and others have reported elevated $CD20^+$ B lymphocytes in CFS/ME patients [9, 42–44]. Moreover other investigators have employed anti-CD20 therapy as a possible therapeutic approach for the treatment of CFS/ME [45–47], where CFS/ME patients received two infusions at 500 mg/m^2 of RTX two weeks apart. Clinical improvement was self-reported in sixty-four and 67 % of participants in these two separate studies [45, 47]; however this improvement was only maintained in 26.6% of patients twelve months post administration.

Importantly, a recent study conducted by Merkt et al. reported that in vitro treatment of NK cells with RTX at a concentration of 10 µg/ml resulted in significant inhibition of NK cell cytotoxic activity from healthy control donors [41]. This investigation also reported a significant reduction of lytic proteins, predominantly granzyme B, and phenotypical and functional changes to CD16 [41] in NK cells following RTX incubation from non-fatigued controls donors.

The effect of RTX on NK cells in malignancies and rheumatic diseases is documented [41, 48–50]. However, the possible role of RTX modulating NK cell cytotoxicity in CFS/ME patients is unknown as Lunde et al. only investigated NK cell subset numbers in CFS/ME patients receiving 500 mg/m^2 of RTX [51]. Therefore, this investigation aimed to examine NK cell cytotoxic activity, lytic proteins and degranulation following incubation of RTX at varying concentrations with NK cells from CFS/ME patients in a controlled and safe laboratory setting in vitro.

Methods

Study Participants

Participants were sourced from the National Centre for Neuroimmunology and Emerging Diseases (NCNED) research database for CFS/ME. Participants were aged between 18 and 65 years, and recruited from South East Queensland and Northern on New South Wales where ME/CFS patients were defined by the 1994 Center for Disease Control and Prevention criteria for CFS/ME. NFC were healthy volunteers that reported no incidence of CFS/ME or fatigue and were in good health without evidence of illness or co-morbidities. Participants were screening according to routine pathology tests and completed a comprehensive questionnaire corresponding with the International Consensus Criteria (ICC) [1]. Participants were excluded from this study if history of smoking, alcohol abuse, autoimmune diseases, cardiac disease, diabetes or co-morbidities were reported.

Six of the eight CFS/ME patients documented minor interventions aimed to control symptoms including cognitive impairment, sleep disturbances, periodic gastro-intestinal symptoms and pain. No participants reported chronic immunosuppressant therapy, immunomodulators or any current medications that may potentially affect the immunological findings reported in the results of this pilot investigation.

Peripheral Blood Mononuclear Cells Isolation and Natural Killer Cells Isolation

Participants donated 85 ml of whole blood which was collected in ethylendiaminetetraacetic acid (EDTA) tubes between 8:00 am and 11:00 am. Routine full blood analysis was analyzed from 5 ml of blood within 4 h of collection for red blood cell counts, lymphocytes and granulocytes using an automated cell counter (ACT differential analyser; Beckman Coulter, Brea, CA, USA) (Table 1). Participants were screened and excluded if blood parameters were outside the normal range.

Peripheral blood mononuclear cells (PBMCs) were isolated from 80 ml of whole blood by centrifugation over a density gradient medium (Ficoll-Paque Premium; GE Healthcare, Uppsala, Sweden). PBMCs were stained with trypan blue (Invitrogen, Carlsbad, CA) to determine cell count and cell viability, and adjusted to a final concentration of 5×10^7 cells/ml.

NK cells were isolated from PBMCs using an EasySep Negative Human NK Cell Isolation Kit (Stem Cell Technologies, Vancouver, BC, Canada). NK cells purity was measured after staining with CD56 (0.25 µg/5 µl) and CD3 (0.25 µg/20 µl) antibodies for 20 min at room temperature and analyzed using a LSR-Fortessa X20 flow

Table 1 Blood parameters and patient demographic measured in CFS/ME patients and NFC groups

	NFC (n = 9)	CFS/ME (n = 8)	P value
Age (years)	37.56 ± 11.06	48.63 ± 15.69	0.503
Gender			
Male n(%)	3(33.3)	1 (12.5)	
Female n(%)	6 (66.7)	7 (87.5)	
Pathology			
White Cell Count ($\times 10^9$/L)	5.94 ± 1.61	5.45 ± 1.09	0.664
Neutrophils ($\times 10^9$/L)	3.54 ± 1.49	3.36 ± 0.82	0.847
Lymphocytes ($\times 10^9$/L)	1.87 ± 0.38	1.70 ± 0.49	0.248
Monocytes ($\times 10^9$/L)	0.32 ± 0.11	0.32 ± 0.06	0.962
Eosinophils ($\times 10^9$/L)	0.18 ± 0.09	0.18 ± 0.12	0.885
Platelet ($\times 10^9$/L)	240.78 ± 47.65	258.88 ± 37.13	0.413
Haemoglobin (g/L)	132.67 ± 8.51	135.38 ± 7.82	0.384
Haematocrit	0.37 ± 0.10	0.42 ± 0.03	0.191
Red Cell Count ($\times 10^{12}$/L)	4.53 ± 0.34	4.49 ± 0.34	0.923
MCV fl	89.67 ± 2.74	92.88 ± 5.11	0.222

Results from white and red blood cell parameters measured in CFS/ME and control groups. Comparisons of blood parameters between the CFS/ME and NFC revealed no significant differences. No significant differences were observed in patient age distribution. Data presented as mean ± standard deviation. *Abbreviations: NFC, non-fatigued controls; CFS/ME, chronic fatigue syndrome; ME, Myalgic encephalomyelitis*

cytometer (Becton Dickinson [BD] Biosciences, San Diego, CA, USA). NK cells purity was 99.85% ± 0.24% and 99.46% ± 0.91% for CFS/ME and NFC, respectfully (Fig. 1).

Rituximab Treatment

NK cells were treated with concentrations of 10 µg/ml as previously reported [41] and 100 µg/ml of RTX

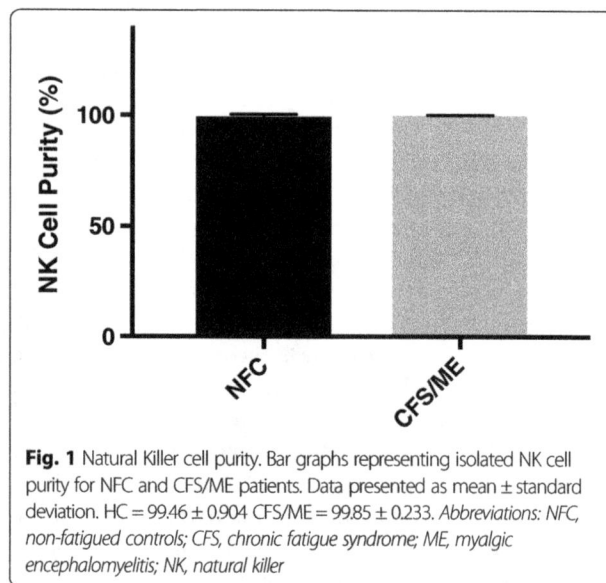

Fig. 1 Natural Killer cell purity. Bar graphs representing isolated NK cell purity for NFC and CFS/ME patients. Data presented as mean ± standard deviation. HC = 99.46 ± 0.904 CFS/ME = 99.85 ± 0.233. *Abbreviations: NFC, non-fatigued controls; CFS, chronic fatigue syndrome; ME, myalgic encephalomyelitis; NK, natural killer*

(Rituxan, Genentech, CA, USA) and incubated for 24 h at 37 °C with 5% CO_2 in RPMI-1640 (Invitrogen Life Technologies, Carlsbad, CA, USA) supplemented with 10% fetal bovine serum (FBS) (Invitrogen Life Technologies, Carlsbad, CA, USA).

Natural Killer Cell Cytotoxicity Assay

NK cytotoxic activity was conducted as previously described [52]. NK cells were labelled with Paul Karl Horan (PKH-26) (3.5 μl/test) (2×10^{-6} M) for 5 min (Sigma-Aldrich, St. Louis. MO, USA) and incubated with K562 cells for 4 h at 37 °C with 5% CO_2 in RPMI-1640 supplemented with 10% FBS. The concentration of NK cells and K562 cells were adjusted to 5×10^5 cells/ml and 1×10^6 cells/ml, respectively. During incubation, cells were combined at E:T ratios of 12.5:1 and 6.25:1 in addition to controlling samples. Control and RTX treated cells were stained using Annexin V (2.5 μl/test) (BD Bioscience, San Jose, CA, USA) and 7-amino-actinomycin (7-AAD) (2.5 μl/test) (BD Bioscience, San Jose, CA, USA) to determine apoptosis using flow cytometry analysis recording 10,000 events (Additional file 1). E:T ratio of 12.5: 1, 6.25 and control were used to assess cytotoxic activity [38, 40, 53]. NK cytotoxic activity was calculated as percent specific death of the K562 cells for the two E:T ratios as previously described [40, 52]. The percentage of target cell lysis was calculated from:

$$Cytotoxicity\,(\%) = \frac{(early\,stage\,apoptosis + late\,stage\,apoptosis + dead\,K562\,cells)}{All\,K562\,Cells} \times 100$$

Natural Killer Cell Lytic Proteins Assay

Intracellular staining was used to measure granzyme A and granzyme B as previously described [7]. NK cells and K562 cells were plated and placed in the incubator at 37 °C for 4 h with 5% CO_2 at E:T 25:1 in RPMI-1640 supplemented with 10% FBS. NK cells were incubated with Monensin (0.67 μl/ml) and Brefeldin A (1 μl/ml) (BD Bioscience, San Jose, CA, USA) to interfere with degranulation and intracellular cytokine transport from the endoplasmic reticulum. NK cells were stained with monoclonal antibodies for granzyme A FITC (0.5 μg/20 μl) and granzyme B BV450 (0.125 μg/5 μl) (BD Bioscience, San Jose, CA, USA) for 30 min at 4 °C. Both control and treated NK cells were measured using flow cytometric analysis recording 10,000 events (Additional file 1).

Natural Killer Cell Degranulation Assay

NK cell surface expression of CD107a and CD107b was measured as a marker for NK cell degranulation and determined as previously described [54]. NK cell concentration was adjusted to 1×10^5 cells/ml and incubated in the presence of CD107a APC (0.06 μg/5 μl) and CD107b FITC (1 μg/20 μl) (BD Bioscience, San Jose, CA, USA)

and stimulated by K562 cells (1×10^4 cells/ml) for 4 h at 37 °C with 5% CO_2 at E:T 25:1 in RPMI-1640 supplemented with 10% FBS. NK cells required the addition of monensin (0.67 μl/ml) to prevent degranulation and Brefeldin A (1 μl/ml) to block exocytosis of cytokines. Both control and treated cells were measured using flow cytometric analysis recording 10,000 events.

Statistical Analysis

Pilot data from this investigation were analyzed using SPSS version 24 (IBM Corp, Version 24, Armonk, NY, USA) and GraphPad Prism, version 7 (GraphPad Software Inc., Version 7, La Jolla, CA, USA). All data sets were tested for normality using the Shapiro–Wilk test. The independent Mann–Whitney U test was used to identify any significant differences in the NK cell parameters between the CFS/ME and NFC groups. Significance was set at $p < 0.05$ and the data are presented as mean ± standard deviation unless otherwise stated.

Results

Participant characteristics, blood parameters and NK cell purity

There were eight CFS patients (48.63 ± 15.69 years), of which seven were females, who met the 1994 Fukuda definition (mean age [years] ± Standard deviation [SD]). There were nine NFC (37.56 ± 11.06 years), of which six were females. There were no significant differences between groups for age (Table 1). All participants in both groups were of European descent and were residents of Australia at the time of blood collection. Comparison of group ages and blood parameters between CFS/ME patients and NFC found no significant differences (Table 1). Isolated NK cell purity was determined using flow cytometry, where NK cell purity for CFS/ME patients was 99.85 ± 0.233 and NFC was 99.46 ± 0.904 (Fig. 1).

Rituximab leads to significant difference in cytotoxic activity of NK cells

Cytotoxic activity was determined using flow cytometry to assess NK cell lysis of the tumour target K562 cell line for both NFC ($n = 9$) and CFS/ME patients ($n = 8$). There was a significant reduction in NK lysis in CFS/ME patients compared to NFC following incubation with RTX at 100 μg/ml (Fig. 2a) ($p < 0.05$) and NK lysis in CFS/ME patients compared to NFC following RTX at 10 μg/ml (Fig. 2b) ($p < 0.05$). There was no significant difference in NK cell lysis for NFC following overnight incubation with RTX at 10 μg/ml and 100 μg/ml (Fig. 2a).

Rituximab leads to significant decrease in NK cell lytic protein granzyme B

Of the nine NFC, four of these were selected for lytic protein analysis due to concentration of NK cells

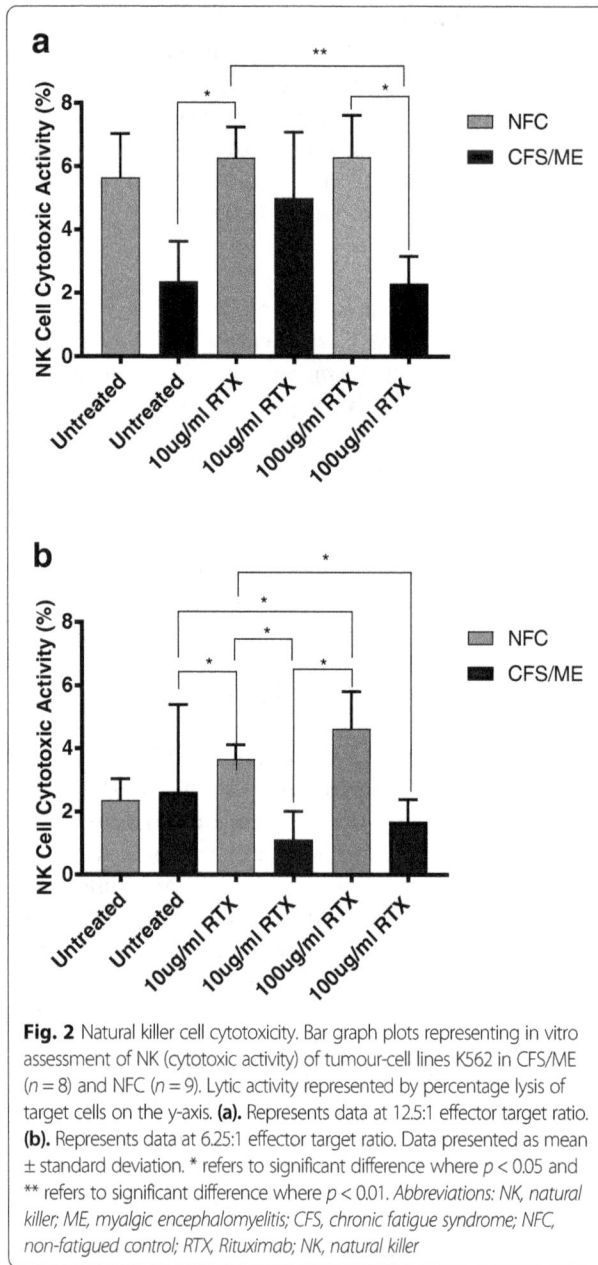

Fig. 2 Natural killer cell cytotoxicity. Bar graph plots representing in vitro assessment of NK (cytotoxic activity) of tumour-cell lines K562 in CFS/ME ($n = 8$) and NFC ($n = 9$). Lytic activity represented by percentage lysis of target cells on the y-axis. **(a).** Represents data at 12.5:1 effector target ratio. **(b).** Represents data at 6.25:1 effector target ratio. Data presented as mean ± standard deviation. * refers to significant difference where $p < 0.05$ and ** refers to significant difference where $p < 0.01$. *Abbreviations: NK, natural killer; ME, myalgic encephalomyelitis; CFS, chronic fatigue syndrome; NFC, non-fatigued control; RTX, Rituximab; NK, natural killer*

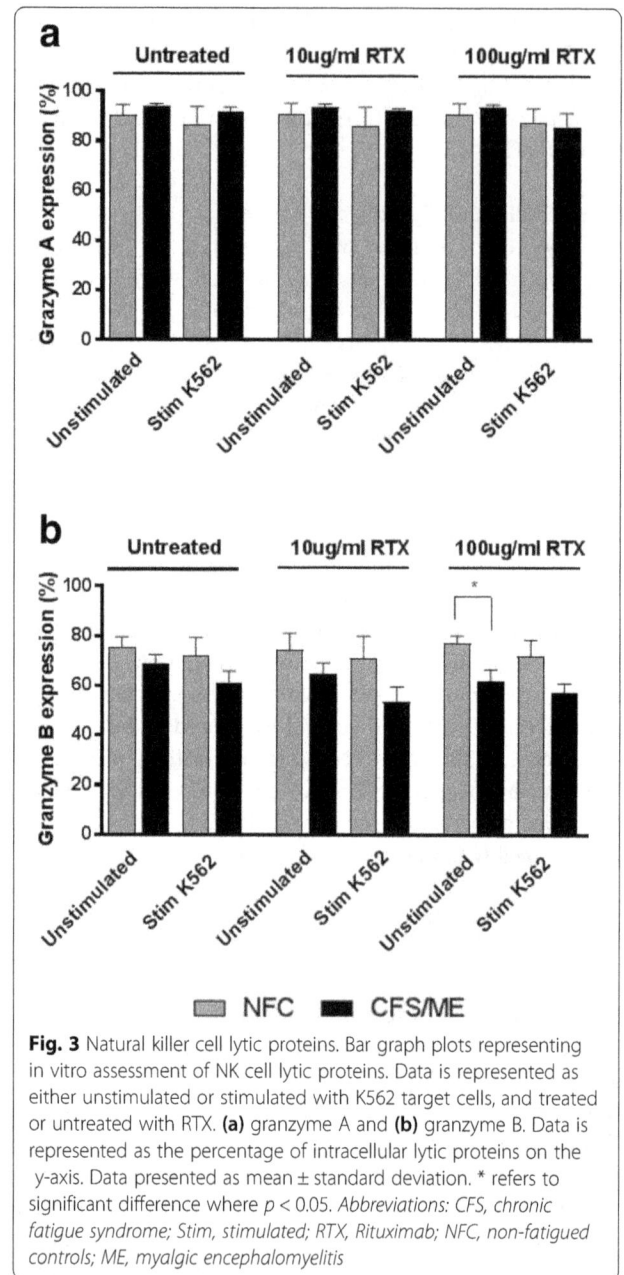

Fig. 3 Natural killer cell lytic proteins. Bar graph plots representing in vitro assessment of NK cell lytic proteins. Data is represented as either unstimulated or stimulated with K562 target cells, and treated or untreated with RTX. **(a)** granzyme A and **(b)** granzyme B. Data is represented as the percentage of intracellular lytic proteins on the y-axis. Data presented as mean ± standard deviation. * refers to significant difference where $p < 0.05$. *Abbreviations: CFS, chronic fatigue syndrome; Stim, stimulated; RTX, Rituximab; NFC, non-fatigued controls; ME, myalgic encephalomyelitis*

following isolation. There was no significant difference between groups for lytic proteins for NFC ($n = 4$) and CFS/ME patients (n = 8) at baseline prior to overnight incubation with RTX for granzyme A (Fig. 3a) and granzyme B (Fig. 3b). No significant difference was shown for lytic proteins following overnight incubation with RTX at 10 μg/ml as well as for granzyme A following overnight incubation with 100 μg/ml of RTX (Fig. 3a). Importantly, there was a significant decrease in granzyme B between NFC and CFS/ME patients incubated with 100 μg/ml of RTX prior to stimulation using K562 cells, while there was no significant change following K562 cell stimulation (Fig. 3b).

Rituximab leads to a significant increase in Natural Killer cell degranulation

Of the nine NFC, six participants were used for degranulation due to the concentration of NK cells following isolation. There was no significant difference between groups for degranulation for NFC ($n = 6$) and CFS/ME patients ($n = 7$) at baseline prior to overnight incubation with RTX for CD107a (Fig. 4a). There was a significant difference in CD107a expression in NFC when stimulated with K562 cell line prior to overnight incubation with RTX ($p < 0.05$). There was an increase in degranulation observed in NFC prior to K562 cell stimulation following overnight incubation with RTX approaching statistical significance.

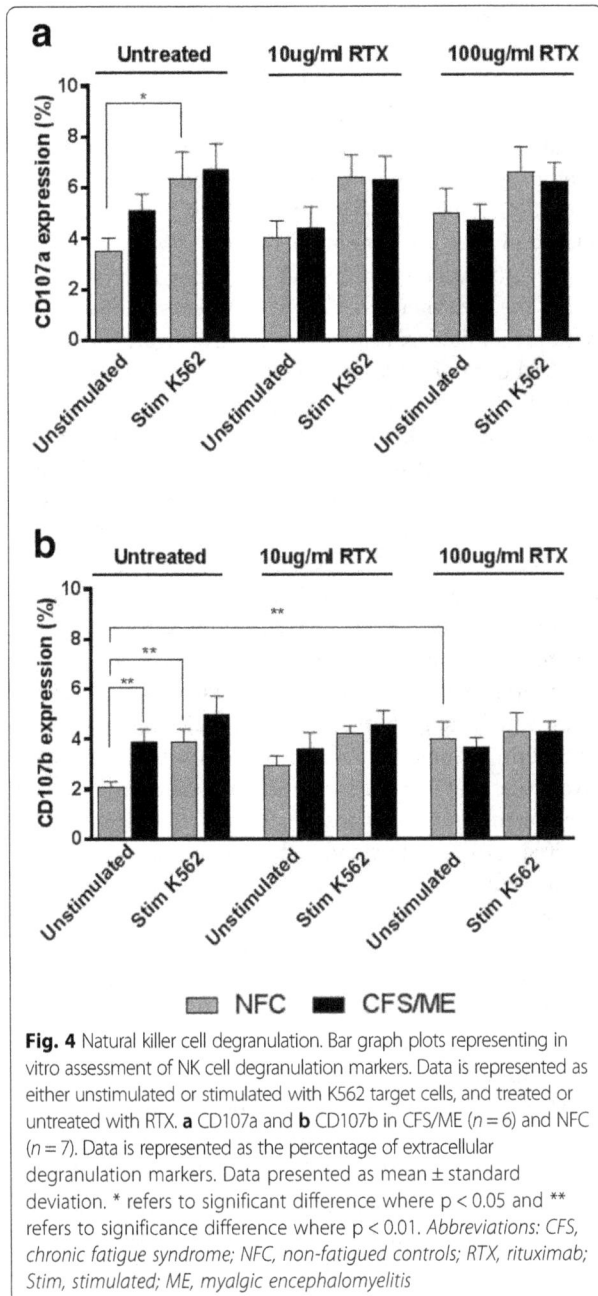

Fig. 4 Natural killer cell degranulation. Bar graph plots representing in vitro assessment of NK cell degranulation markers. Data is represented as either unstimulated or stimulated with K562 target cells, and treated or untreated with RTX. **a** CD107a and **b** CD107b in CFS/ME (*n* = 6) and NFC (*n* = 7). Data is represented as the percentage of extracellular degranulation markers. Data presented as mean ± standard deviation. * refers to significant difference where p < 0.05 and ** refers to significance difference where p < 0.01. *Abbreviations: CFS, chronic fatigue syndrome; NFC, non-fatigued controls; RTX, rituximab; Stim, stimulated; ME, myalgic encephalomyelitis*

Similarly, there was a significant difference observed within and between groups for CD107b expression prior to incubation with RTX (Fig. 4b). Importantly, there was an increase in CD107b expression between NFC after stimulation with K562 cells. There was a significant increase in CD107b expression in CFS/ME patients in comparison to NFC at baseline prior to incubation with RTX and without stimulation of K562 cells ($p < 0.01$). Importantly, there was a significance increase in CD107b following overnight incubation with 100 µg/ml of RTX observed in NFC prior to K562 cell stimulation ($p < 0.01$).

Discussion

This is the first study to investigate NK cell cytotoxic activity following in vitro incubation with RTX at 10 µg/ml and 100 µg/ml in CFS/ME patients and NFC. The present study examined cytotoxic and apoptotic mechanisms through lysis of target K562 cells, intracellular staining of lytic proteins including granzyme A and granzyme B, and extracellular straining of degranulation markers, CD107a and CD107b.

We report novel findings as there were significant reductions in NK cell lysis in CFS/ME patients compared with NFC following incubation with RTX at 100 µg/ml at 12.5:1 E:T ($p < 0.05$). Significance was also observed between groups at 6.25:1 E:T for 10 µg/ml of RTX. A decrease was observed in CFS/ME patients compared with NFC at 100 µg/ml of RTX, however this was not significant possibly due to the small sample size. Previous in vitro investigations using RTX at different concentrations ranging from 10 µg/ml to 200 µg/ml have reported reduced cytotoxic activity of NK cells isolated from healthy donors, chronic lymphocytic leukaemia (CLL) patients and non-Hodgkin lymphoma patients [41, 48, 50]. The significant decrease in cytotoxic activity observed in this study suggests that in vitro RTX at 100 µg/ml impedes NK cell function. Studies completed by us and other researchers have reported significantly reduced NKCC in CFS/ME patients [4–14]. Therefore, RTX may have adverse outcomes for CFS/ME patients as reduced NK cell function impairs the ability to clear virus-infected and malignant cells.

This current investigation did not report significant difference in NFC for NK cell lysis of target K562 cells. In contrast, Merkt et al. reported significant decrease in NK cell cytotoxic activity of healthy donors ($n = 3$) [41]. Additionally, Capuano et al. reported defective NK cell cytotoxic response in healthy donors and CLL patients [50]. However, these studies are not without limitations with the low sample numbers and limited screening definition of healthy control. Without clear indication of criteria for healthy control inclusion in these studies, it can be assumed that these participants may be susceptible to reduced NK cell function. The NFC participating in our current investigation are included using a detailed questionnaire derived from the Fukuda, Canadian Consensus Criteria and ICC [1–3]. Additionally, investigations by Merkt et al. and Capuano et al. used the chromium (Cr)-51 release assay. The ^{51}Cr-release assay is used to measure cytotoxic activity, however, comparisons with flow cytometric analysis have shown cytometric methods to be more sensitive with higher lysis generated [52, 55].

Lytic proteins are apoptotic-inducing proteins released from cytotoxic granules in NK cells. Intracellular staining was used to investigate granzyme A and granzyme B using flow cytometric analysis. We report a significant decrease in granzyme B in CFS/ME patients compared with NFC following incubation with 100 µg/ml of RTX prior to stimulation using K562 target cells ($p < 0.05$). Previous work performed by our group and other researchers have reported a significant reduction in granzyme B in NK cells isolated from CFS/ME patients when stimulated with K562 target cells [5, 36, 38, 39]. Granzyme B is responsible for apoptosis activation by cleaving substrates at aspartic acid leading to caspase-3 activation [56]. Importantly, the decrease in granzyme B following incubation with RTX at 100 µg/ml prior to NK cell stimulating using K562 cells demonstrates that RTX can influence cytolytic activity of NK cells.

Previous research has reported that lytic proteins negatively correlate with degranulation, suggesting a decrease in lytic proteins is associated with an increase in degranulation markers [40]. Degranulation is a critical process by which cytotoxic granules polarize towards the immune synapse to release lytic proteins towards the target cell [27]. Extracellular staining was used to investigate degranulation markers CD107a and CD107b using flow cytometric analysis. We report a significant difference in CD107a expression in NFC when stimulated with K562 cells prior to overnight incubation with RTX ($p < 0.05$) and conversely a significant increase in CD107b expression was found in NFC after stimulation with K562 target cells ($p < 0.01$). Importantly, we reported for the first time a significant increase in CD107b expression in CFS/ME patients in comparison to NFC prior to incubation with RTX and without stimulation of K562 cells ($p < 0.05$). Previous research has reported significant increase in CD107a in NK cells isolated from CFS/ME patients compared with NFC following stimulation with K562 cells [36, 37, 53]. Huth et al. suggested that the increase in degranulation markers in CFS/ME patients suggests continued activation due to inability to induce sufficient cytotoxic lysis of target cells [53].

Finally, we also report novel findings where a significant increase in CD107b expression following overnight incubation with 100 µg/ml of RTX was observed in NFC prior to K562 cell stimulation ($p < 0.01$). Therefore, this suggests that RTX may stimulate Ca^{2+} influx required for NK cell degranulation. Additionally, as there were no significant changes in CD107a following overnight incubation with RTX at 10 µg/ml and 100 µg/ml, our results are not consistent with previous research completed by Merkt et al. who reported an increase in degranulation in healthy donors ($n = 6$) treated with 10 µg/ml of RTX [41]. However, limited information was provided regarding the methodology of degranulation assays in that study. Additional in vitro studies using RTX have shown that continued NK cell activation causes CD16 down regulation, therefore impairing NK cell cytotoxic activity [41, 48, 49]. As there were no

significant changes for CFS/ME patients when incubated overnight with RTX at 10 µg/ml for CD107a and CD107b, and CD107a with RTX at 10 µg/ml, this suggests that RTX does not improve NK cell degranulation. Further research is needed to determine whether RTX changes intracellular signalling of MAPK and ERK1/2 phosphorylation which is reported to be delayed in CFS/ME patients [53].

Our results demonstrate that RTX may have no benefit for the treatment of CFS/ME patients. Additionally, there are limited pharmacokinetic investigations for the standard dose of RTX for the treatment of CFS/ME. The standard dose of RTX is 375 mg/m^2 two weeks apart for non-Hodgkin Lymphoma patients [57, 58]. Herlt et al. suggests that patients treated for autoimmune diseases require a lower dose of RTX as a single infusion with 100 mg/m^2 effectively induces B lymphocyte depletion [58]. For the phase II clinical trial on CFS/ME patients by Fluge et al. RTX infusions were administered to patients at 500 mg/m^2 two weeks apart. Additional maintenance infusions were given after 3, 6, 10 and 15 months with two patients receiving as high as 11 doses, which suggests that CFS/ME patients receive only short term therapeutic effects from RTX treatment [47]. Given the literature in CFS/ME and autoimmunity is inconsistent and inconclusive, further investigations are required to understand the immunological and pharmaceutical mechanisms of RTX in non-malignant diseases.

The novel, preliminary findings of our study provide a rationale for further investigations into a larger cohort to investigate the possible therapeutic role of RTX on NK cell function, notably NK cytotoxicity. The results from this study highlight the importance of in vitro investigations during clinical trials. Furthermore, the reduction in NK cell lysis between NFC and CFS/ME patients with 100 µg/ml of RTX may indicate that RTX impedes NKCC. Further investigation is required for NK cell phenotypes and for CD16 polymorphisms due to their role in efficacy of RTX therapy as high-affinity polymorphisms correlate with better clinical responses to RTX [49].

This current investigation highlights the possible role of RTX in vitro and may not necessarily recreate in vivo conditions. Two ex vivo investigations reported that RTX significantly increased NK cell degranulation [59] and reduced CD16-dependent NKCC [60] in lymphoma patients. Cox et al. suggested that downregulation CD16 impairs RTX recognition that facilitates NKCC. Moreover, the decision to incubate isolated NK cells for 24 h with RTX is supported by previous investigators [41]. The current findings from this investigation are supported by previous research where prolonged treatment in vivo and in vitro with RTX leads to functional impairment of NK cells [41, 50, 59, 60]. Therefore, high doses of RTX may impair NK cell functionality.

Conclusion

This investigation, using isolated NK cells and flow cytometry, is novel as it is the first to investigate the effects of RTX on the NK cells of CFS/ME patients. The results of this study demonstrate significant differences between NFC and CFS/ME patients following overnight incubation with 100 μg/ml of RTX. Our results suggest that RTX may have toxicological effects on NK cells isolated from CFS/ME patients. Further in vitro investigations aimed at examining the effect of RTX on isolated NK cell cytotoxic function in CFS/ME patients are warranted.

Abbreviations

7-AAD: 7-amino-actinomycin; BD: Becton Dickinson; Ca²⁺: Calcium; CFS: Chronic fatigue syndrome; E:T: Effecter-target; EDTA: ethylendiaminetetraacetic acid; FBS: Fetal bovine serum; ICC: International Consensus Criteria; Ig: Immunoglobulin; ITAM: Immunoreceptor tyrosine-based activation motif; MAPK: Mitogen-activated protein kinase; ME: Myalgic Encephalomyelitis.; MTOC: Microtubule-organising centre.; NCNED: National Centre for Neuroimmunology and Emerging Diseases.; NFC: Non-fatigued controls.; NK: Natural killer.; NKCC: Natural killer cell cytotoxicity.; PBMC: Peripheral blood mononuclear cells.; PKH: Paul Karl Horan.; RTX: Rituximab.

Acknowledgements

Not applicable.

Funding

This research was supported by funding from the Stafford Fox Medical Research Foundation, Mr Douglas Stutt, Blake Beckett Foundation, Alison Hunter Memorial Foundation. Patient Donors and Change for ME Charity.

Authors' contributions

The authors in this article were involved in the design, drafting and development of this manuscript. NE analyzed and interpreted the patient data regarding NK cell lysis, NK cell degranulation and NK cell lytic proteins. HC performed experiment for NK cell degranulation. CB performed experiment for NK cell lytic proteins. NE performed experiment for NK cell lysis. AK analyzed and interpreted patient questionnaire responses and determined eligibility for study inclusion in addition to patient blood collection. SMG and DS designed all experiments. All authors read and approved the final manuscript.

Competing interest

The authors declare that they have no competing interest.

References

1. Carruthers BM, et al. Myalgic encephalomyelitis: international consensus criteria. J Intern Med. 2011;270(4):327–38.
2. Fukuda K, et al. The chronic fatigue syndrome: a comprehensive approach to its definition and study. Ann Intern Med. 1994;121(12):953–9.
3. Carruthers BM, et al. Myalgic encephalomyelitis/chronic fatigue syndrome: clinical working case definition, diagnostic and treatment protocols. Journal of chronic fatigue syndrome. 2003;11(1):7–115.
4. Siegel SD, et al. Impaired natural immunity, cognitive dysfunction, and physical symptoms in patients with chronic fatigue syndrome: preliminary evidence for a subgroup? J Psychosom Res. 2006;60(6):559–66.
5. Maher KJ, Klimas NG, Fletcher MA. Chronic fatigue syndrome is associated with diminished intracellular perforin. Clinical & Experimental Immunology. 2005;142(3):505–11.
6. Brenu EW, et al. Longitudinal investigation of natural killer cells and cytokines in chronic fatigue syndrome/myalgic encephalomyelitis. J Transl Med. 2012;10(1):88.
7. Huth T, et al. Pilot study of natural killer cells in chronic fatigue syndrome/myalgic encephalomyelitis and multiple sclerosis. Scand J Immunol. 2016; 83(1):44–51.
8. Nijs J, Frémont M. Intracellular immune dysfunction in myalgic encephalomyelitis/chronic fatigue syndrome: state of the art and therapeutic implications. Expert Opin Ther Targets. 2008;12(3):281–9.
9. Natelson BH, Haghighi MH, Ponzio NM. Evidence for the presence of immune dysfunction in chronic fatigue syndrome. Clin Diagn Lab Immunol. 2002;9(4):747–52.
10. Curriu M, et al. Screening NK-, B-and T-cell phenotype and function in patients suffering from Chronic Fatigue Syndrome. J Transl Med. 2013;11(1):68.
11. Brenu E, et al. Natural killer cells in patients with severe chronic fatigue syndrome. Autoimmunity Highlights. 2013;4(3):69–80.
12. Fletcher MA, et al. Biomarkers in chronic fatigue syndrome: evaluation of natural killer cell function and dipeptidyl peptidase IV/CD26. PLoS One. 2010;5(5):e10817.
13. Brenu EW, et al. Immune and hemorheological changes in chronic fatigue syndrome. J Transl Med. 2010;8(1):1.
14. Ojo-Amaize EA, Conley EJ, Peter JB. Decreased natural killer cell activity is associated with severity of chronic fatigue immune dysfunction syndrome. Clin Infect Dis. 1994;18(Supplement 1):S157–9.
15. Johnston S, et al. The prevalence of chronic fatigue syndrome/ myalgic encephalomyelitis: a meta-analysis. Clin Epidemiol. 2013;5:105–10.
16. Rimbaut S, et al. Chronic fatigue syndrome–an update. Acta Clin Belg. 2016; 71(5):273–80.
17. Prins JB, Van der Meer JW, Bleijenberg G. Chronic fatigue syndrome. Lancet. 2006;367(9507):346–55.
18. Vivier E, et al. Functions of natural killer cells. Nat Immunol. 2008;9(5):503–10.
19. Trapani JA, et al. Proapoptotic functions of cytotoxic lymphocyte granule constituents in vitro and in vivo. Curr Opin Immunol. 2000;12(3):323–9.
20. Stanietsky N, Mandelboim O. Paired NK cell receptors controlling NK cytotoxicity. FEBS Lett. 2010;584(24):4895–900.
21. Lanier LL. Up on the tightrope: natural killer cell activation and inhibition. Nat Immunol. 2008;9(5):495–502.
22. Stewart CA, et al. Recognition of peptide–MHC class I complexes by activating killer immunoglobulin-like receptors. Proc Natl Acad Sci U S A. 2005;102(37):13224–9.
23. Moretta L. Dissecting CD56dim human NK cells. Blood. 2010;116(19):3689–91.
24. Lanier LL, Ruitenberg J, Phillips J. Functional and biochemical analysis of CD16 antigen on natural killer cells and granulocytes. J Immunol. 1988; 141(10):3478–85.
25. Cooper MA, Fehniger TA, Caligiuri MA. The biology of human natural killer-cell subsets. Trends Immunol. 2001;22(11):633–40.
26. Stabile H, et al. Multifunctional human CD56low CD16low natural killer cells are the prominent subset in bone marrow of both healthy pediatric donors and leukemic patients. Haematologica. 2015;100(4):489–98.
27. Smyth MJ, et al. Activation of NK cell cytotoxicity. Mol Immunol. 2005; 42(4):501–10.
28. Bryceson YT, et al. Synergy among receptors on resting NK cells for the activation of natural cytotoxicity and cytokine secretion. Blood. 2006; 107(1):159–66.
29. Lanier LL. Natural killer cell receptor signaling. Curr Opin Immunol. 2003; 15(3):308–14.
30. Smith HR, et al. Recognition of a virus-encoded ligand by a natural killer cell activation receptor. Proc Natl Acad Sci. 2002;99(13):8826–31.
31. Pegram HJ, et al. Activating and inhibitory receptors of natural killer cells. Immunol Cell Biol. 2011;89(2):216–24.
32. Bryceson YT, et al. Molecular mechanisms of natural killer cell activation. Journal of innate immunity. 2011;3(3):216–26.
33. Reefman E, et al. Cytokine secretion is distinct from secretion of cytotoxic granules in NK cells. J Immunol. 2010;184(9):4852–62.
34. Smyth MJ, Trapani JA. Granzymes: exogenous porteinases that induce target cell apoptosis. Immunol Today. 1995;16(4):202–6.

35. Trapani JA, Smyth MJ. Functional significance of the perforin/granzyme cell death pathway. Nat Rev Immunol. 2002;2(10):735–47.

36. Huth T, et al. Characterization of natural killer cell phenotypes in chronic fatigue Syndrome/Myalgic Encephalomyelitis. J Clin Cell Immunol. 2014; 5(223):2.

37. Brenu EW, et al. Role of adaptive and innate immune cells in chronic fatigue syndrome/myalgic encephalomyelitis. Int Immunol. 2013;26(4). https://doi.org/10.1093/intimm/dxt068.

38. Brenu EW, et al. Immunological abnormalities as potential biomarkers in chronic fatigue syndrome/myalgic encephalomyelitis. J Transl Med. 2011; 9(1):81.

39. Klimas NG, et al. Immunologic abnormalities in chronic fatigue syndrome. J Clin Microbiol. 1990;28(6):1403–10.

40. Huth TK, et al. Natural killer cell cytotoxic activity: measurement of the apoptotic inducing mechanisms. Clin Exp Med Sci. 2013;1:373–86.

41. Merkt W, Lorenz H-M, Watzl C. Rituximab induces phenotypical and functional changes of NK cells in a non-malignant experimental setting. Arthritis research & therapy. 2016;18(1):206.

42. Bradley A, Ford B, Bansal A. Altered functional B cell subset populations in patients with chronic fatigue syndrome compared to healthy controls. Clinical & Experimental Immunology. 2013;172(1):73–80.

43. Robertson M, et al. Lymphocyte subset differences in patients with chronic fatigue syndrome, multiple sclerosis and major depression. Clinical & Experimental Immunology. 2005;141(2):326–32.

44. Ramos S, et al. Characterisation of B cell Subsets and Receptors in Chronic Fatigue Syndrome Patients. Journal of Clinical and Cell Immunol. 2015;6(1): 1000288-1-1000288-5.

45. Fluge Ø, et al. Benefit from B-lymphocyte depletion using the anti-CD20 antibody rituximab in chronic fatigue syndrome. A double-blind and placebo-controlled study. PLoS One. 2011;6(10):e26358.

46. Fluge Ø, Mella O. Clinical impact of B-cell depletion with the anti-CD20 antibody rituximab in chronic fatigue syndrome: a preliminary case series. BMC Neurol. 2009;9(1):28.

47. Fluge Ø, et al. B-lymphocyte depletion in myalgic encephalopathy/chronic fatigue syndrome. an open-label phase II study with rituximab maintenance treatment. PLoS One. 2015;10(7):e0129898.

48. Hatjiharissi E, et al. Increased natural killer cell expression of CD16, augmented binding and ADCC activity to rituximab among individuals expressing the FcγRIIIa-158 V/V and V/F polymorphism. Blood. 2007;110(7):2561–4.

49. Veeramani S, et al. Rituximab infusion induces NK activation in lymphoma patients with the high-affinity CD16 polymorphism. Blood. 2011;118(12):3347–9.

50. Capuano C, et al. Anti-CD20 therapy acts via FcγRIIIA to diminish responsiveness of human natural killer cells. Cancer Res. 2015;75(19):4097–108.

51. Lunde S, et al. Serum BAFF and APRIL levels, T-lymphocyte subsets, and immunoglobulins after B-cell depletion using the monoclonal anti-CD20 antibody rituximab in myalgic encephalopathy/chronic fatigue syndrome. PLoS One. 2016;11(8):e0161226.

52. Aubry J-P, et al. Annexin V used for measuring apoptosis in the early events of cellular cytotoxicity. Cytometry. 1999;37(3):197–204.

53. Huth TK, Staines D, Marshall-Gradisnik S. ERK1/2, MEK1/2 and p38 downstream signalling molecules impaired in CD56 dim CD16+ and CD56 bright CD16 dim/– natural killer cells in Chronic Fatigue Syndrome/Myalgic Encephalomyelitis patients. J Transl Med. 2016;14(1):97.

54. Alter G, Malenfant JM, Altfeld M. CD107a as a functional marker for the identification of natural killer cell activity. J Immunol Methods. 2004;294(1):15–22.

55. Flieger D, et al. A novel non-radioactive cellular cytotoxicity test based on the differential assessment of living and killed target and effector cells. J Immunol Methods. 1995;180(1):1–13.

56. Ewen C, Kane K, Bleackley R. A quarter century of granzymes. Cell Death Differ. 2012;19(1):28.

57. McLaughlin P, et al. Rituximab chimeric anti-CD20 monoclonal antibody therapy for relapsed indolent lymphoma: half of patients respond to a four-dose treatment program. J Clin Oncol. 1998;16(8):2825–33.

58. Hertl M, et al. Recommendations for the use of rituximab (anti-CD20 antibody) in the treatment of autoimmune bullous skin diseases. JDDG: Journal der Deutschen Dermatologischen Gesellschaft. 2008;6(5):366–73.

59. Fischer L, et al. The anti-lymphoma effect of antibody-mediated immunotherapy is based on an increased degranulation of peripheral blood natural killer (NK) cells. Exp Hematol. 2006;34(6):753–9.

60. Cox MC, et al. Tumor-associated and immunochemotherapy-dependent long-term alterations of the peripheral blood NK cell compartment in DLBCL patients. Oncoimmunology. 2015;4(3):e990773.

17

An inhibitor of 11-β hydroxysteroid dehydrogenase type 1 (PF915275) alleviates nonylphenol-induced hyperadrenalism and adiposity in rat and human cells

Ling-Ling Chang[1]*[†], Wan-Song Alfred Wun[2] and Paulus S. Wang[3,4,5,6†]

Abstract

Background: Nonylphenol (NP) is an environmental endocrine-disrupting chemical (EDC) detected in human cord blood and milk. NP exposure in developmental periods results in hyperadrenalism and increasing 11β-hydroxysteroid dehydrogenase I (11β-HSD1) activity in an adult rat model. Alleviating 11β-HSD1 activity is therefore a logical and common way to treat hyperadrenalism. PF915275 (PF; 4'-cyano-biphenyl-4-sulfonic acid (6-amino-pyridin-2-yl)-amide) is a selective inhibitor for 11β-HSD1. This study aimed to determine whether PF915275 could alleviate the hyperadrenalism induced by NP. In addition to a rat model, the effects of NP and PF915275 were measured in human preadipocytes.

Methods: For the in vivo rat model, female adult rats exposed to NP during the developmental period were divided into two treatment groups, with one receiving oral DMSO solution and the other receiving PF915275 once per day for 4 weeks. After the final treatment, the rats from each group were sacrificed for analysis. For the in vitro human model, human preadipocytes received 2 regimens of NP treatment. One treatment regimen occurred before differentiation (to mimic the sensitive developmental period; P exposure), and the other included continuous exposure from preadipocytes to fully differentiated adipocytes (to mimic the growing and adult periods, respectively; C exposure). Protein and RNA were extracted from rat tissues and the preadipocytes for western blot and real-time PCR analysis.

Results: In the rat model, PF915275 alleviated NP-induced effects by interfering with adipogenesis pathways, including enhancing PPARα expression, decreasing PPARγ expression, and reducing both 11β-HSD1 protein and mRNA expression levels. Additionally, PF915275 reduced the effects of the adrenal corticoid synthesis pathway by reducing StAR expression and 11β-hydroxylase and aldosterone synthase activities. With short-term exposure, NP enhanced *PPARγ* and *FASN* mRNA expression levels and reduced PPARα expression, whereas PF915275 alleviated these effects. With C exposure, the NP-induced accumulation of intracellular lipids was reduced by PF915275 treatment, which was mediated by decreased PPARγ mRNA and protein expression levels and increased PPARα protein expression.

Conclusions: The effects of NP and PF915275 treatment in both rat and human cell models are similar. Rats may be an appropriate model to study the effects of NP in humans, especially during the developmental period.

Keywords: NP, PF915275, 11β-HSD1, Hyperadrenalism, Adipogenesis

* Correspondence: llchiang@ulive.pccu.edu.tw
[†]Ling-Ling Chang and Paulus S. Wang contributed equally to this work.
[1]Department of Chemical and Materials Engineering, Chinese Culture University, Shih-Lin, Taipei 11114, Taiwan, Republic of China
Full list of author information is available at the end of the article

Background

Man-made chemicals, such as bisphenol A (BPA), dichlorodiphenyl-trichloroethane (DDT), diethylstilbestrol (DES), and nonylphenol (NP), are produced with the intention of benefiting humans. However, these chemicals can also have negative impacts on the environment, wildlife, and public health. These chemicals are categorized as endocrine disruptors (ENDRs) because they mainly target endocrine pathways (i.e., estrogen or corticoids) and can interfere or disrupt physiological endocrine regulation. The incidence of metabolic syndromes has been suggested to correspond with the number of synthetic chemicals produced, especially ENDRs [1]. The pandemic metabolic syndromes, such as obesity, diabetes, and hypertension, are global public health issues [2, 3]. Experts predict that the burden of pandemic metabolic syndromes will continue to worsen worldwide [4]. The health care costs associated with pandemic chronic metabolic syndromes may collapse the global health care system and must therefore be considered an urgent problem [4].

Over the past decade, 11β-hydroxysteroid dehydrogenase type 1 (11β-HSD1) has been reported to be one of the main factors responsible for metabolic syndromes [5]. Since 11β-HSD1 can amplify local glucocorticoids, it is correlated with the cause of obesity and insulin resistance behavior [6, 7]. Theoretically, 11β-HSD1 inhibitors can alleviate or even prevent some metabolic syndromes. Diabetes and hypertension are the common syndromes associated with metabolic diseases and are also frequently observed in ENDR-induced hyperadrenalism (commonly known as Cushing's syndrome). Some encouraging and promising results have been found using 11β-HSD1 inhibitors as therapeutic agents, particularly for metabolic-related diseases [8–10]. Therefore, 11β-HSD1 inhibition appears to be a potential strategy to treat ENDR-induced hyperadrenalism.

In previous experiments [11], rats were supplied with NP-contaminated water during pregnancy (in utero) and lactation (neonatal) to mimic environmental contamination. The female pups showed elevated plasma corticosterone and aldosterone concentrations when they developed into adults. In addition, 11β-HSD1 activities and protein expression and aldosterone synthase activities were increased in the liver and adrenal tissues [11]. Since intracellular 11β-HSD1 regenerates active glucocorticoids (e.g., cortisol in humans and corticosterone in rodents) from inactive 11-keto forms in adipose, liver, and brain tissues, it will strengthen local cellular glucocorticoid action. Central obesity has been suggested to be due to amplified glucocorticoids in adipose tissue mediated by 11β-HSD1 [6, 12–14]. By using a transgenic mouse model, 11β-HSD1 overexpression resulted in visceral obesity, insulin-resistant diabetes, and hyperlipidemia [13]. However, the symptoms of insulin resistance,

hyperglycemia, and dyslipidemia were not observed in 11β-HSD1-knockout mice [15].

These results seem to suggest that 11β-HSD1 inhibition is a potential therapeutic target for treating metabolic syndromes. In this study, we explore whether PF915275 (PF; 4′-cyano-biphenyl-4-sulfonic acid (6-amino-pyridin-2-yl)-amide), a selective inhibitor of 11β-HSD1 [16], can suppress ENDR-induced (i.e., NP-induced) hyperadrenalism and excess 11β-HSD1 activity. Since visceral obesity and hyperlipidemia are evident in 11β-HSD1-overexpressing mice [13], lipid metabolism is an essential aspect in studying 11β-HSD1 inhibition or activation. Researchers have shown that PPAR (peroxisome proliferator-activated receptor) ligands are highly associated with lipid metabolism. PPARs are a family of nuclear receptors, and specific PPAR ligands can activate certain types of PPARs. For example, PPAR type alpha (PPARα) ligand, i.e., fibrates, can activate transcription factors to enhance fatty acid oxidation. PPAR type gamma (PPARγ) ligand, i.e., thiazolidinediones, can reduce blood triglyceride and sugar levels and enhance lipogenesis via fatty acid synthesis. In this study, we explore the impacts of NP and PF on lipid metabolism through the PPAR system.

Demonstration of the therapeutic effectiveness of PF in a rat model (female adult rats exposed to NP during the developmental period to mimic environmental contamination received PF via oral gavage in this in vivo study) would offer hope for treating Cushing's syndrome in humans. The first step was to verify whether NP increases adipogenesis in human adipose cells using in vitro methods. If an adipogenic effect is observed, then the 11β-HSD1 inhibitor requires verification by examining, for example, whether PF can alleviate or prevent this impact. Positive results from this study can serve as a basis for the development of clinical trials for endocrine-disrupting chemical (EDC)-induced metabolic syndrome.

Methods

Materials

NP was purchased from Fluka (Buchs, Switzerland) and dissolved in methanol to produce a 0.425 M stock solution. PF was purchased from Tocris Cookson Ltd. (Bristol, UK). The other chemicals were purchased from Sigma Chemical Co. (St. Louis, MO, USA). [^{3}H]-Aldosterone and [^{3}H]-corticosterone were purchased from Amersham Life Science Limited (Buckinghamshire, UK). Dr. D. M. Stocco (Department of Cell Biology and Biochemistry, Texas Tech University Health Sciences Center, Lubbock, TX, USA) generously provided the anti-steroidogenic acute regulatory (StAR) antibody. Anti-11β-hydroxysteroid dehydrogenase I (11β-HSD1), anti-fatty acid synthase (FASN), anti-proliferator-activated receptor α (PPARα), anti-proliferator-activated receptor γ (PPARγ), and anti-vinculin (Vinculin) antibodies were purchased from Abcam plc. (Cambridge, UK), GeneTex Inc. (San Antonio, TX, USA), Cayman Chemical (Ann Arbor, MI, USA), Cayman Chemical (Ann Arbor, MI, USA), and GeneTex Inc. (San Antonio, TX, USA), respectively. Anti-mouse and anti-rabbit IgG peroxidase-conjugated secondary antibodies were purchased from ICN Pharmaceuticals, Inc. (Aurora, OH, USA). Human preadipocytes were purchased from Cell Applications (San Diego, CA, USA). Preadipocyte medium (PAM) and preadipocyte differentiation medium (PADM) were purchased from ScienCell™ Research Laboratories (Carlsbad, CA, USA). A Lipid Oil Red O staining kit was purchased from BioVision Inc. (Milpitas, CA, USA).

Animal treatment
Animals
Pregnant female Sprague-Dawley rats weighing 250–300 g were provided by the Animal Center of National Yang-Ming University. The pregnant female rats were divided into two groups, including NP mother (drinking NP-containing water (NP concentration 2 µg/ml) during the gestation and lactation periods) and vehicle control mother (drinking regular water). They were housed individually throughout their pregnancy until delivery, which occurred on days 20–22. The female pups of the NP group (mother drinking NP-containing water), the female pups of the vehicle control group (mother drinking regular water) and their mothers were housed in a temperature-controlled room (22 ± 1 °C) in the Animal Center of National Yang-Ming University with photoperiods of 14 h (light):10 h (dark) as previously described [17]. The lights were switched on at 6:30 a.m. and food and water were provided ad libitum. The number of female offspring from the same mother was 4–5 per cage. The female offspring of the NP group were randomly divided into an NP and an NP + PF group at 10 weeks of age. In the NP + PF group, the rats were given PF (4′-cyano-biphenyl-4-sulfonic acid (6-amino-pyridin-2-yl)-amide) at 0.36 mg/kg/ml (PF dissolved in DMSO solution) by oral gavage once per day, and the same amount of DMSO solution was administered orally to the vehicle and NP groups [17]. The treatment began at 10 weeks of age and lasted for 4 weeks. The adult rats (14 weeks old) were anesthetized with 100 mg/kg ketamine by intraperitoneal injection (ketamine dissolved in saline) and then sacrificed on the day after the last oral gavage. The sacrifice was implemented by the method of rapid decapitation. The procedures and precautions for sacrifice were the same as previously described [17]. In brief, the sacrifice began at 7:00 am to avoid adrenal rhythm variations, and sacrifice was sequentially performed in the vehicle group, NP group and NP + PF group. The process was repeated until all the rats were sacrificed. Blood and tissue collection from one rat

required 10–15 min, and approximately 3–3.5 h were required to complete sample collection. Trunk blood was collected and plasma samples were separated and stored at – 20 °C until analysis. The liver, adipose tissue, and adrenal glands were immediately dissected and stored at – 80 °C. The rat carcasses were handled by the Animal Center of National Yang-Ming University.

All animal protocols used in this study were approved by the Institutional Animal Care and Use Committee of the National Yang-Ming University. All animals received humane care in compliance with the Principles of Laboratory Animal Care and the Guide for the Care and Use of Laboratory Animals, published by the National Science Council, Taiwan, R.O.C.

Enzyme activity assays
The oxidoreductase activity assay for 11β-HSD1 was performed by measuring corticosterone produced from 11-dehydrocorticosterne [17–19]. Specific activities were expressed as nanograms of corticosterone formed per hour per gram of protein.

The 11β-hydroxylase activity of the adrenal cortex was measured from the corticosterone produced from deoxycorticosterone treatment [20]. Specific activities were expressed as nanograms of corticosterone formed per hour per microgram of adrenal cortex protein, while the aldosterone measurements after corticosterone treatment [20] represented the aldosterone synthase activity of the adrenal capsule, which was expressed as the amount of aldosterone (usually in nanograms) formed per hour per microgram of adrenal capsule protein.

Corticosterone and aldosterone RIA
Corticosterone or aldosterone in plasma was extracted using diethyl ether as previously described [20]. After the diethyl ether evaporated, assay buffer was added to dissolve the corticosterone or aldosterone. RIA can be used to determine both the concentration of corticosterone [21] and the concentration of aldosterone [22] in the plasma or in media. The plasma corticosterone levels were measured by RIA using antiserum (PSW#4–9), the sensitivity of the corticosterone RIA was 5 pg/tube, and the intra- and inter-assay coefficients of variation were 3.3% ($n = 5$) and 9.2% ($n = 4$), respectively. Additionally, an RIA using JJC-088 antiserum was used to measure plasma aldosterone levels. The sensitivity of the aldosterone RIA was 4 pg/tube, and the intra- and inter-assay coefficients of variation were 3.9% ($n = 5$) and 8.2% ($n = 4$), respectively.

Cell culture and treatment
Cell culture
Human preadipocytes were purchased from Cell Applications (San Diego, CA, USA), maintained in preadipocyte medium (PAM, ScienCell™ Research Laboratories, Carlsbad,

CA, USA) and incubated at 37 °C in 5% CO_2. For differentiation, human preadipocytes were seeded into plates or dishes (48,000 cells/cm^2 in PAM) for 2 days, and then the preadipocytes were incubated with preadipocyte differentiation medium (PADM, ScienCell™ Research Laboratories, Carlsbad, CA, USA) for 6 days by changing the medium every 3 days in the presence or absence of NP or PF at different concentrations. After differentiation, the cells were harvested for the tests described below.

Preadipocyte proliferation

Human preadipocytes were seeded at 4.5×10^3 cells/well in a 96-well plate. The cells were incubated in PAM in the presence of NP or PF for 24 and 72 h. After incubation, the cells were treated with 20 µl of MTT (dissolved in PBS (pH 7.4)) assay reagents (5 mg/ml) for 4 h, and the resulting purple formazan crystals were solubilized in 150 µl of DMSO. The absorbance was measured at 570 nm on a Sunrise™ microplate reader (Tecan Trading AG, Switzerland). The percentages of viable cells were calculated in the NP- or PF-treated groups relative to the control cells (cells incubated with PAM for 24 h).

Cell viability

To assess cell viability after NP or PF treatment, human preadipocytes were seeded onto 96-well plates at a density of 4.5×10^3 cells/well and differentiated with PADM in the presence of NP or PF for 6 days. After incubation, cell viability was quantitatively assessed using the MTT assay. The percentages of viable cells were calculated in the NP- or PF-treated groups relative to that in the control group (cells differentiated with PADM alone for 6 days).

Oil red O staining

To assess lipid accumulation with NP or PF treatment, human preadipocytes were seeded onto 24-well plates at a density of 4.5×10^4 cells/well and differentiated with PADM in the presence of NP or PF for 6 days. The formation of lipid droplets in adipocytes was observed with a Lipid Oil Red O staining kit (BioVision Inc., Milpitas, CA, USA) according to the manufacturer's protocol. To measure lipid accumulation in adipocytes, the cells were washed with 60% isopropanol 3 times, and the completely dried cells were shaken with 100% isopropanol for 5 min. The dissolved lipid was quantified by measuring the absorbance at 492 nm. The results were expressed as the lipid accumulation relative to that in the control cells (cells differentiated with PADM only for 6 days).

Tissue and cell protein extraction

Frozen liver, adrenal, and adipose tissue samples or human preadipocytes were lysed in homogenizing buffer (containing 65 mM Tris-base, 154 mM sodium chloride, 1% NP-40, 6 mM sodium deoxycholate, 1 mM ethylenediaminetetraacetic acid (EDTA), 1 mM phenylmethylsulfonyl fluoride (PMSF), 5 mg/l aprotinin, 5 mg/l leupeptin, 5 mg/l pepstatin, 1 mM sodium orthovanadate, 1 mM sodium fluoride, and 1% proteinase inhibitor cocktail (pH 7.4) for the liver, adipose tissues and human preadipocytes, and containing 1.5% N-lauroylsarcosine sodium, 2.5 mM Tris-base, 1 mM EDTA, 0.68% PMSF, and 2% proteinase inhibitor cocktail (pH 7.8) for the adrenal tissue, the adrenal capsule, and the adrenal cortex) for 30 min on ice. The obtained homogenates were centrifuged at $13,000 \times g$ for 30 min at 4 °C, and the supernatants were sampled. The protein concentration was evaluated using the Bradford assay [23] with bovine serum albumin (BSA) as the standard.

Western blot analysis

The levels of 11β-HSD1 (for liver and adipose tissues), PPARα (for liver, adipose tissues, adrenal tissue, and human preadipocytes), PPARγ (for adipose tissue and human preadipocytes), FASN (for human preadipocytes) and StAR (for adrenal tissue) protein expressions were determined by western blot analysis [24]. For western blotting, samples containing equal amounts of protein (liver protein (100 µg), adipose protein (200 µg), adrenal protein (100 µg), or human preadipocyte protein (50 µg)) were loaded on a 6 or 10% acrylamide sodium dodecyl sulfate-polyacrylamide gel for electrophoresis (SDS-PAGE). After electrophoresis, the relevant proteins were detected on blots by specific antibodies, and signals were developed using enhanced chemiluminescence (ECL western blotting detection reagents, Amersham Pharmacia Biotech, Buckinghamshire, UK) and the Luminescent Image Analyzer Las-4000 (Fuji-Film, Stamford, CT, USA). Additionally, the MultiGauge program (Fuji-Film) was used to quantify proteins, and the protein signals were normalized against the glyceraldehyde-3-phosphate dehydrogenase (GAPDH) or vinculin protein signal.

RNA extraction and quantitative real-time PCR

Total RNA from the liver and human preadipocytes was extracted using TRIzol reagent (Molecular Research Center, Inc., Cincinnati, OH, USA). The concentration of RNA was measured by the OD260, and the purity of RNA was evaluated by measuring the ratio of A260/A280 (selecting values above 1.8) with the aid of a Nanodrop (Thermo Scientific, Waltham, MA, USA). cDNA was synthesized with a cDNA synthesis kit (Bioman Scientific Co., Ltd., Taipei, Taiwan). Real-time PCR reactions were performed with a SYBR Green PCR Master Mix kit (Applied Biosystems, Inc., Foster City, CA, USA) and 50 ng of cDNA in an ABI real-time PCR detection system. Relative mRNA expression was determined by the $2^{-\triangle\triangle Ct}$ method normalized to *GAPDH* or *18S rRNA*, which were used as housekeeping genes. Additionally, the vehicle values were normalized to a group average of 1.0. PCR product purities were verified by melting curve analysis. The primers were synthesized by Tri-I Biotech Inc. (Taipei, Taiwan) (the sequences for the primers are shown in Table 1).

Statistical analysis

The results are expressed as the mean ± S.E.M. Comparisons across a variety of treatments were performed using one-way ANOVA followed by post hoc analysis of Fisher's least significant difference (LSD) or Dunnett's post hoc analysis. Values of $p < 0.05$ were considered statistically significant.

Results

PF suppresses NP-induced hyperadrenalism and adipogenesis

Plasma levels of steroid hormones

Developmental exposure to NP significantly increased plasma corticosterone concentrations in female offspring ($p < 0.01$, Fig. 1a), and PF significantly decreased the corticosterone concentrations in the NP + PF group compared with those in the NP group ($p < 0.05$, Fig. 1a).

The plasma aldosterone concentrations also significantly increased in the NP group ($p < 0.05$, Fig. 1b) compared with those in the vehicle group. PF appeared to reduce the plasma aldosterone concentrations, although not significantly, compared with those in the NP group ($p < 0.1$, Fig. 1b).

Liver

Developmental exposure to NP significantly increased 11β-HSD1 activity in the liver ($p < 0.05$, Fig. 2a), and treatment with PF significantly decreased 11β-HSD1 activity in the liver ($p < 0.01$, Fig. 2a) compared with that in the NP group. The 11β-HSD1 and PPARα protein levels in the liver were determined by western blot analysis (Fig. 2b, c). The 11β-HSD1-to-GAPDH protein ratio was significantly increased in the NP group ($p < 0.05$, Fig. 2b) compared with that in the vehicle group but significantly decreased in the NP + PF group ($p < 0.05$, Fig. 2b) compared to that the NP group. The PPARα-to-GAPDH protein ratio was not significantly different among the vehicle, NP, and NP

+ PF groups (Fig. 2c). The 11β-HSD1 and PPARα mRNA levels in the liver were determined by real-time PCR (Fig. 2d, e). NP exposure during the developmental period did not significantly affect the mRNA expression of 11β-HSD1 and PPARα in the liver compared to that in the vehicle group (Fig. 2d, e). Oral administration of PF in the NP + PF group significantly decreased the mRNA expression of 11β-HSD1 ($p < 0.05$, Fig. 2d) in the liver compared with that in the NP group.

Adipose tissue

NP exposure decreased PPARα protein expression ($p < 0.05$, Fig. 3b) but did not affect PPARγ protein expression (Fig. 3a). PF treatment in the NP + PF group significantly increased PPARα protein expression ($p < 0.01$, Fig. 3b) but decreased PPARγ protein expression ($p < 0.01$, Fig. 3a) compared with that in either the vehicle or NP group. The 11β-HSD1-to-GAPDH protein ratio was not significantly different among the vehicle, NP, and NP + PF groups (Fig. 3c).

Adrenal glands

NP exposure significantly increased aldosterone synthase activity in the adrenal capsule ($p < 0.05$, Fig. 4b). In the NP + PF group, PF significantly decreased 11β-hydroxylase activity in the adrenal cortex ($p < 0.05$, Fig. 4a) and decreased aldosterone synthase activity in the adrenal capsule ($p < 0.05$, Fig. 4b) compared with the activity levels in the NP group. The levels of StAR and PPARα proteins in the adrenal tissues were determined by western blot analysis (Fig. 4c, d). NP exposure apparently increased StAR protein expression, although not significantly, (Fig. 4c), whereas PF significantly decreased StAR protein expression ($p < 0.01$, Fig. 4c) compared with the expression levels in the NP group. NP exposure appeared to decrease PPARα protein expression, although not significantly (Fig. 4d), compared with that in the vehicle group, while PF significantly increased PPARα protein expression ($p < 0.05$, Fig. 4d) compared with that in the NP group.

Table 1 Real-time PCR primers

Gene	Sequence (5′ to 3′ forward)	Sequence (5′ to 3′ reverse)
11β-HSD1	CCTCCCCGTCCTGGTGCTCT	TGCTCCGAGTTCAAGGCAGCG
GAPDH	TGTGAACGGATTTGGCCGTA;	GATGGTGATGGGTTTCCCGT
PPARα	GCTCTGAACATTGGCGTTCG	TCAGTCTTGGCTCGCCTCTA
(h) FASN	CGCGT GGCCGGCTACTCCTAC	CGGCTGCCACACGCTCCTCT
(h) PPARα	CAGAACAAGGAGGCGGAGGTC	TTCAGGTCCAAGTTTGCGAAGC
(h) PPARγ	AGGCGAGGGCGATCTTGACAG	GATGCGGATGGCCACCTCTTT
(h) 18 s rRNA	TGCCATGTCTAAGTACGCACG	TTGATAGGGCAGACGTTCGA

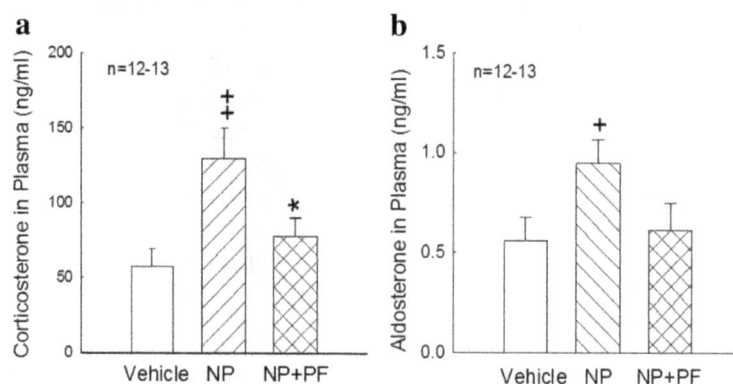

Fig. 1 Corticosterone (**a**) and aldosterone (**b**) concentrations in plasma from vehicle-, NP- and NP + PF-treated female rats (Veh $n = 12$, NP $n = 12$, NP + PF $n = 13$). These concentrations were measured by RIA. The values are presented as the means ± S.E.M. +, ++: $p < 0.05$, 0.01, NP group compared with the vehicle group. *: $p < 0.05$, NP + PF group compared with the NP group

Human preadipocyte culture

Effects of NP and PF on cell proliferation, cell viability and lipid accumulation

Human preadipocytes were grown in PAM supplemented with different concentrations of NP combined with PF for 24 and 72 h. As shown in Fig. 5a, the MTT assay revealed that neither NP nor PF affected preadipocyte proliferation. Human preadipocytes were induced to differentiate in the presence of NP (0–80 μM) combined with PF (0–9 μM) for 6 days. The MTT assay revealed that NP at concentrations of 1–20 μM and PF at concentrations of 4.5 μM did not affect cell viability (Fig. 5b). Therefore, these concentration ranges of NP or PF were selected for further experiments. Human preadipocytes underwent morphological changes from spindle-like features to a round shape and accumulated intracellular lipids after differentiation induction. To examine the accumulation of intracellular lipids, preadipocytes were cultured in PADM for 6 days in the presence of NP (0–20 μM) combined with PF (0–4.5 μM) (Fig. 5c). Lipid accumulation was measured by Oil red O staining. PF at 2 or 4.5 μM decreased lipid accumulation ($p < 0.05$, Fig. 5c). NP at 10 μM increased PF-inhibited lipid accumulation at 1.5 μM PF ($p < 0.05$, Fig. 5c). NP at 20 μM increased PF-inhibited lipid accumulation at 2 μM PF ($p < 0.05$, Fig. 5c). NP alone did not increase lipid accumulation (Fig. 5c), but it increased PF-inhibited lipid accumulation.

Effect of human preadipocyte exposure to NP before differentiation

To elucidate any epigenetic modifications or "memory" effects, human preadipocytes were exposed to NP before differentiation (P exposure). Preadipocytes were seeded into dishes (3.5×10^5 cells in PAM) for 36 h, and then

the medium was changed to PAM in the presence of 20 μM NP for 12 h. After 12 h, preadipocytes were cultured in PADM (without NP) for 6 days in the presence of PF (0, 2 or 4.5 μM). The PPAR pathway and FASN was examined at the mRNA and protein levels.

Priming with NP significantly increased the *PPARγ* and *FASN* ($p < 0.05$, Fig. 6a, c) mRNA expression levels, whereas PF treatment significantly decreased their mRNA expression levels ($p < 0.05$, Fig. 6a, c). In contrast, PF treatment significantly increased *PPARα* mRNA expression ($p < 0.05$, Fig. 6b), and priming with NP significantly decreased PPARα protein expression ($p < 0.01$, Fig. 6e), but PF significantly reversed this phenomenon ($p < 0.05$, Fig. 6e). NP priming enhanced the protein expression of PPARγ and FASN, but not significantly. With the addition of PF, PPARγ and FASN protein expression levels were significantly reduced ($p < 0.05$, Fig. 6d, f). These data suggested that human preadipocytes exposed to NP before differentiation exhibited effects after differentiation. The differentiated adipocytes exhibited memory of exposure to NP and showed increased adipogenesis and decreased lipolysis. Treatment with PF alleviated these effects at the differentiated adipocyte level.

Effects of NP and/or PF on protein and RNA expression after induced adipocyte differentiation

To elucidate the molecular mechanisms by which NP and PF affected adipogenesis after induction into adipocytes, human preadipocytes were seeded into dishes (3.5×10^5 cells in PAM) for 48 h, and the medium was changed to PADM for 6 days in the presence of NP (0 or 20 μM) combined with PF (0, 2 or 4.5 μM). After the induction period, the preadipocytes differentiated into adipocytes. Real-time PCR and western blotting analyses were performed to examine the effects of PF and NP on the expression of adipogenesis-related mRNA and proteins.

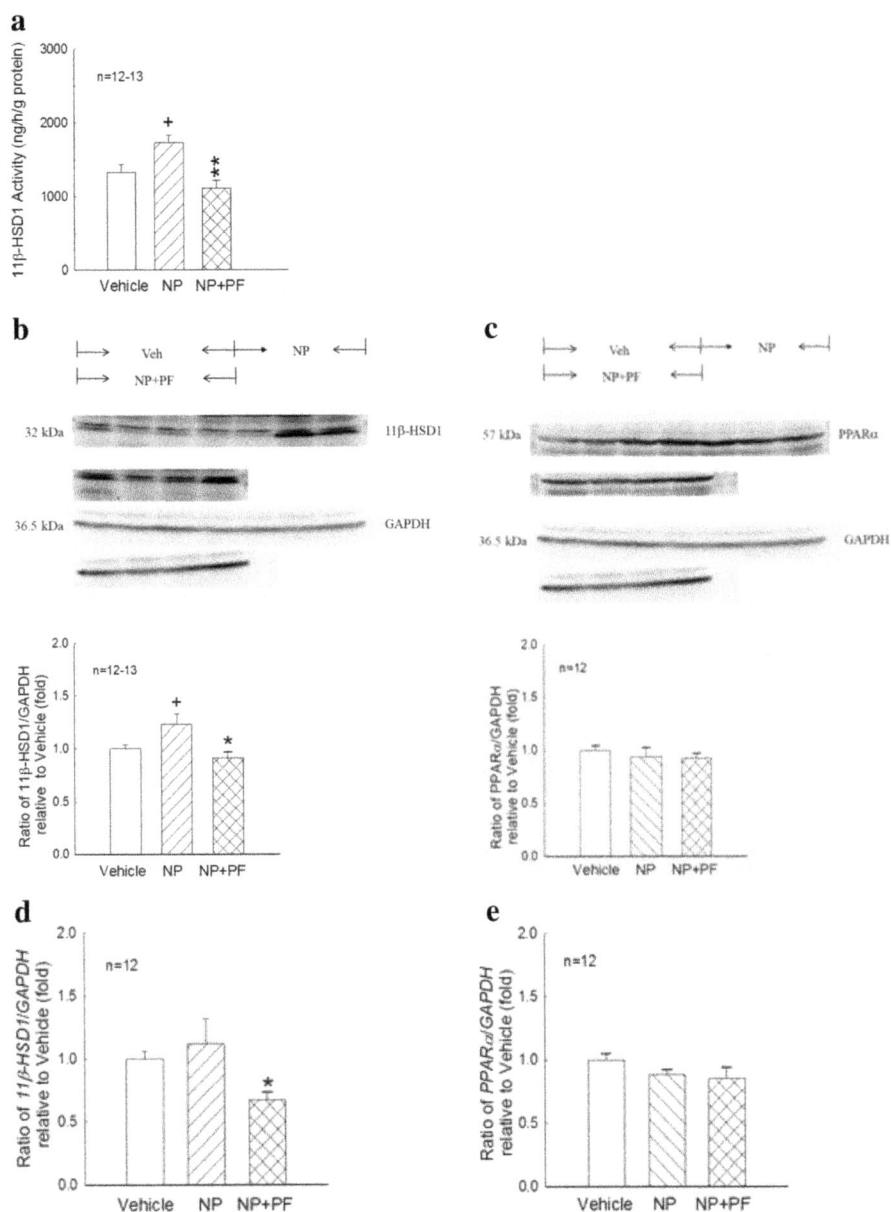

Fig. 2 11β-HSD1 and PPARα activity and expression in the liver from vehicle-, NP- and NP + PF-treated female rats. **a**: The 11β-HSD1 reductase activity was measured in the liver from vehicle-, NP- and NP + PF-treated female rats using 11-dehydrocorticosterone as a substrate in the presence NADPH. Values are shown as the means ± S.E.M. **b** and **c**: Expression of 11β-HSD1 (32 kDa) and PPARα (57 kDa) in livers from vehicle-, NP- and NP + PF-treated female rats were determined by western blot analysis. The representative immunoblot was shown in the upper part, and densitometry for 11β-HSD1 or PPARα normalized to GAPDH was shown in the bottom part. The values are presented as the means ± S.E.M. and are presented as the fold-change compared to the vehicle group. **d** and **e**: The mRNA levels of *11β-HSD1* and *PPARα* in the liver were determined by real-time PCR. The values are presented as the means ± S.E.M. and are presented as the fold-change relative to the vehicle group. +: $p < 0.05$, NP group compared with vehicle group. *, **: $p < 0.05$, 0.01, NP + PF group compared with the NP group

For mRNA expression, adipocytes treated with 20 μM NP had significantly increased *PPARγ* ($p < 0.01$, Fig. 7a) and *FASN* mRNA expression levels ($p < 0.05$, Fig. 7c). Treatment with 4.5 μM PF significantly decreased basal ($p < 0.05$) and NP-induced *PPARγ* mRNA expression ($p < 0.01$, Fig. 7a) and decreased NP-induced *FASN* mRNA expression ($p < 0.05$, Fig. 7c). Adipocytes treated with 20 μM NP had increased PPARγ protein expression ($p < 0.05$, Fig. 7d), while PF reduced PPARγ protein expression ($p < 0.05$, Fig. 7d). PF increased PPARα protein expression, but NP had no significant effect ($p < 0.05$, Fig. 7e). Based on the human preadipocyte model, these data suggested that NP increased lipogenesis via PPARγ and FASN mRNA/protein expression whereas PF counteracted the NP effects.

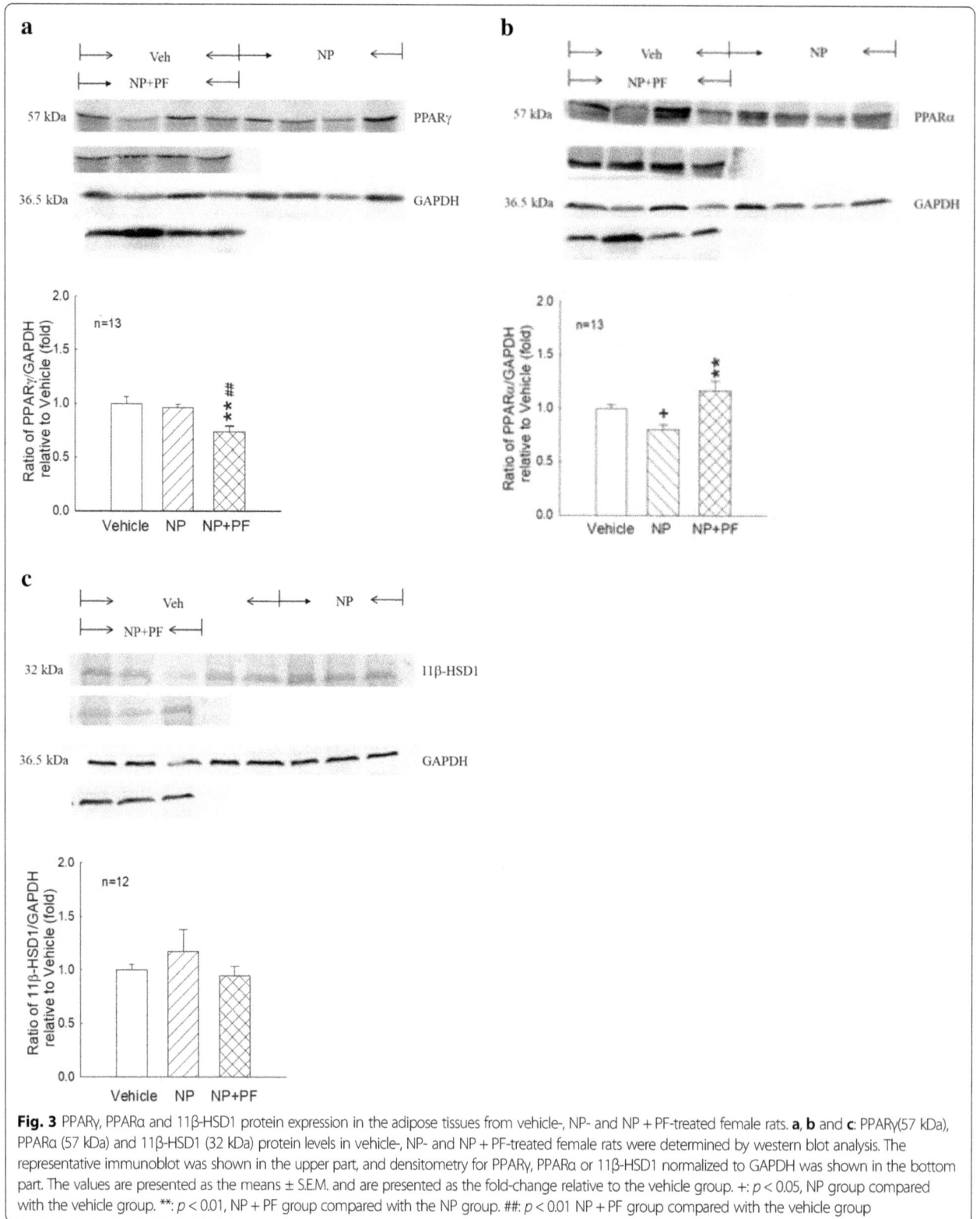

Fig. 3 PPARγ, PPARα and 11β-HSD1 protein expression in the adipose tissues from vehicle-, NP- and NP + PF-treated female rats. a, b and c: PPARγ(57 kDa), PPARα (57 kDa) and 11β-HSD1 (32 kDa) protein levels in vehicle-, NP- and NP + PF-treated female rats were determined by western blot analysis. The representative immunoblot was shown in the upper part, and densitometry for PPARγ, PPARα or 11β-HSD1 normalized to GAPDH was shown in the bottom part. The values are presented as the means ± S.E.M. and are presented as the fold-change relative to the vehicle group. +: $p < 0.05$, NP group compared with the vehicle group. **: $p < 0.01$, NP + PF group compared with the NP group. ##: $p < 0.01$ NP + PF group compared with the vehicle group

Discussion

In this study, water containing NP at a 2 µg/ml concentration mimicked environmentally relevant exposure conditions. Water consumption among female rats during pregnancy and late lactation ranges from approximately 25 ml/day to 100 ml/day. For calculation purposes, NP water consumption was assumed to be 50 ml/day during pregnancy and 100 ml/day during late lactation. Therefore,

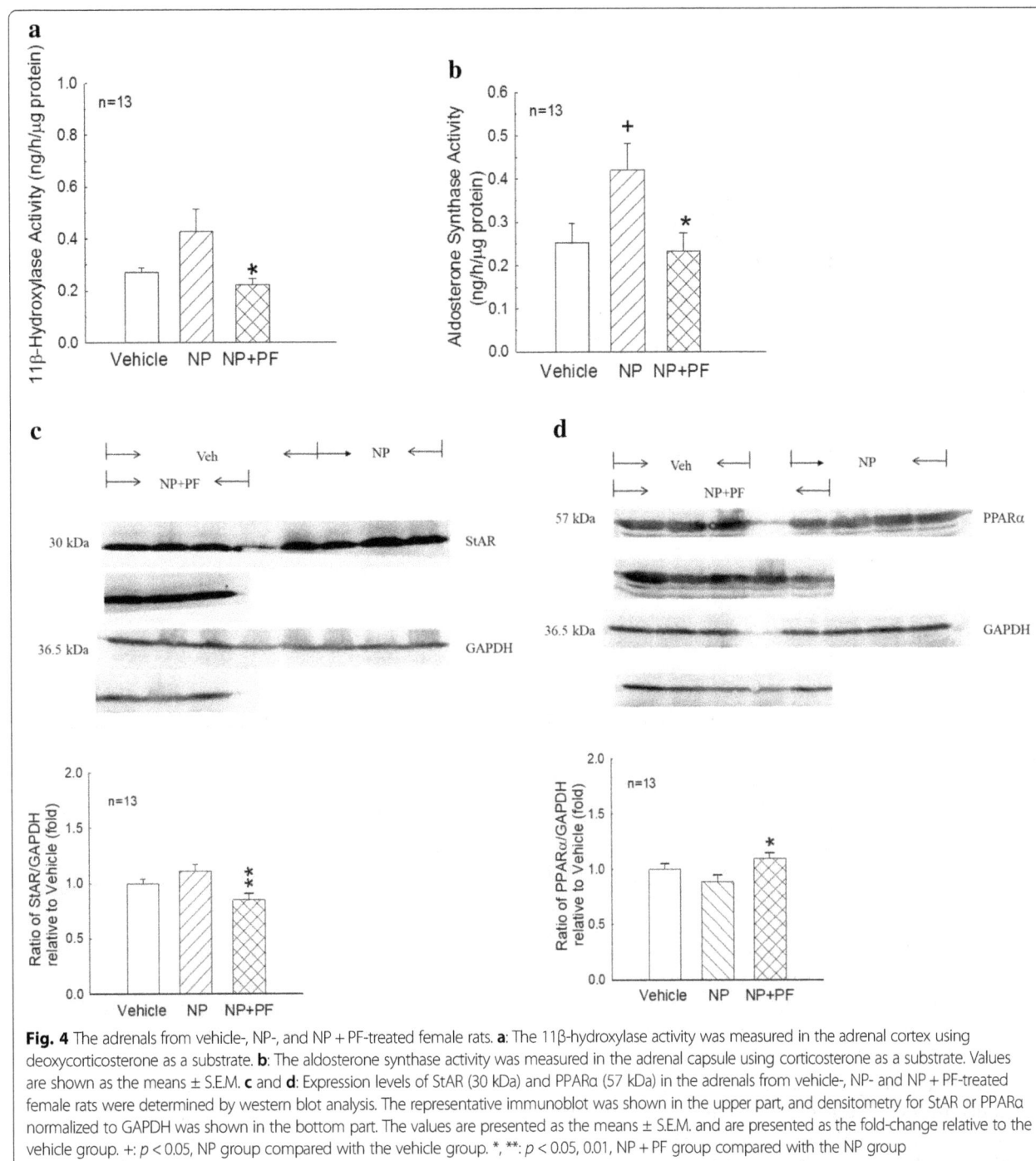

Fig. 4 The adrenals from vehicle-, NP-, and NP + PF-treated female rats. **a**: The 11β-hydroxylase activity was measured in the adrenal cortex using deoxycorticosterone as a substrate. **b**: The aldosterone synthase activity was measured in the adrenal capsule using corticosterone as a substrate. Values are shown as the means ± S.E.M. **c** and **d**: Expression levels of StAR (30 kDa) and PPARα (57 kDa) in the adrenals from vehicle-, NP- and NP + PF-treated female rats were determined by western blot analysis. The representative immunoblot was shown in the upper part, and densitometry for StAR or PPARα normalized to GAPDH was shown in the bottom part. The values are presented as the means ± S.E.M. and are presented as the fold-change relative to the vehicle group. +: $p < 0.05$, NP group compared with the vehicle group. *, **: $p < 0.05$, 0.01, NP + PF group compared with the NP group

the highest daily NP exposure level was estimated to be approximately 400 μg/kg/day during pregnancy and 800 μg/kg/day during late lactation. The examined dose is between the tolerable intake level reported by the Danish Institute of Safety & Toxicity (i.e., 5 μg/kg/day) [25] and the previously reported no-adverse-effects-observed level (i.e., 45–50 mg/kg/day) [26]. The exposure dose used is the lowest amount relative to other dietary exposure levels [27–30]. Courtney et al. [16] proposed that healthy humans could safely

tolerate an oral dose of 0.3 mg/kg/day of PF for 2 weeks and concluded PF was a safe and selective 11β-HSD1 inhibitor. Bhat et al. [31] reported that oral administration of 3 mg/kg of PF could inhibit 11β-HSD1 activity in Cynomolgus monkeys. In this in vivo study, the oral dose of PF was higher and the treatment period was longer than those in the studies of Bhat et al. [31] and Courtney et al. [16] for two reasons: 1) the metabolism of rats is higher than that of humans and monkeys, and 2) the two studies from

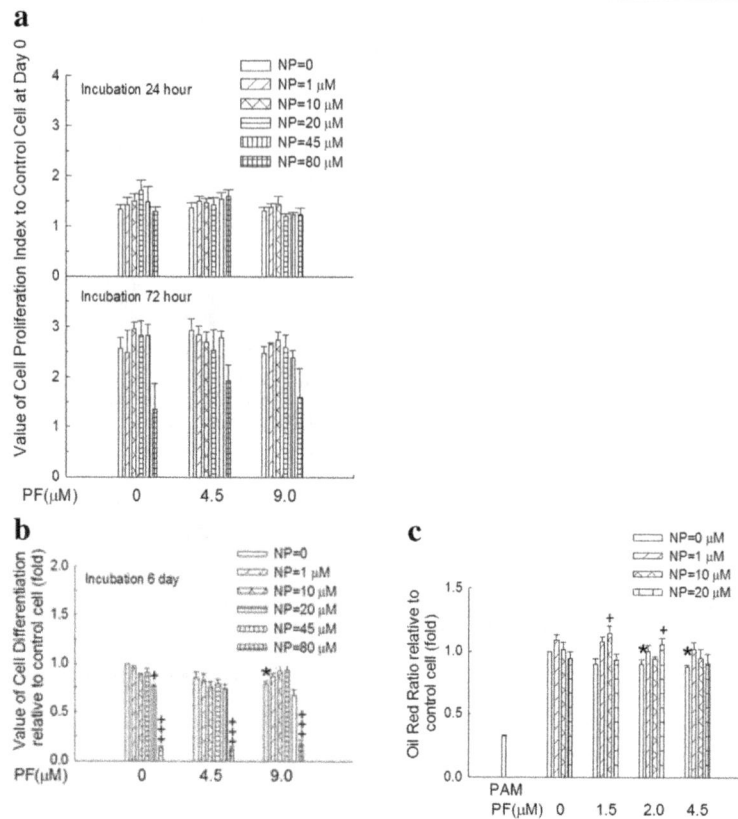

Fig. 5 Effects of NP and PF on cell proliferation, cell viability and lipid accumulation. **a**: Human preadipocytes were seeded onto 96-well plates at a density of 4.5×10^3 cells/well and treated with NP combined with PF for 24 or 72 h. MTT reagent was added to the medium. After 4 h of incubation, the medium was aspirated, and 150 μl DMSO was added to each well. The absorbance was read at 570 nm. **b**: Human preadipocytes were incubated in differentiation medium (PADM) in the presence of NP combined with PF. After 6 days, MTT assay was performed to assess the cell viability. c: Human preadipocytes were incubated in differentiation medium (PADM) in the presence of NP combined with PF for 6 days. Oil Red O staining was performed, and stained lipids were extracted and quantified by measuring absorbance at 492 nm. Values are means of 3 independent experiments, are shown as the mean ± S.E.M, and are presented as the fold-change relative to control cells. a: cells incubated with PAM for 24 h; **b** and **c**: cells differentiated with only PADM for 6 days. +, +++: $p < 0.05$, 0.005, NP effect with the same concentration of PF. *: $p < 0.05$, PF effect with the same concentration of NP

Courtney et al. [16] and Bhat et al. [31] examined the safety and effects of PF in healthy subjects, whereas we examined the effect of PF in affected animals. This study sought to define a therapeutic treatment for rats with induced hyperadrenalism. Other 11β-HSD1 inhibitors are under investigation in therapeutic studies. Wang et al. [32] reported that treating diet-induced obese mice with oral BVT 2733 (a selective 11β-HSD1 inhibitor) at 100 mg/kg/day for 1 week could attenuate obesity and inflammation. Hu et al. [33] also proposed that the lipid profiles of high-fat diet-treated rats could be improved by oral gavage with curcumin (a selective 11β-HSD1 inhibitor) at 200 mg/kg/day for 2 months. As shown in Fig. 5b, a concentration of NP or PF higher than 20 μM or 4.5 μM, respectively, could induce cytotoxicity in human preadipocytes. Therefore, the concentrations of NP and PF used were not greater than 20 μM and 4.5 μM, respectively, in this in vitro study.

Nonylphenol ethoxylate is a non-ionic surfactant with many applications in industrial, agricultural and household products. NP is the degradation product of nonylphenol ethoxylate and an environmental pollutant that drastically disrupts the endocrine system [34]. Most studies regarding its endocrine-disrupting effects have mainly focused on its estrogenic activity [35]. However, our study shows that NP can induce hyperadrenalism both in vitro and in vivo [20, 36, 37]. In addition to the adrenal axis effect, we also observed that local tissues, i.e., adipose tissue, can convert the non-active 11-keto form to an active corticoid through 11β-HSD1. This action does not appear to be under hypothalamo-hypophyseal-adrenal regulation [20]. Increasing cellular 11β-HSD1 activity is associated with obesity and metabolic syndrome [5, 38, 39], which has been identified as an intracellular Cushing's state [40].

Hyperadrenalism was observed in female offspring based on elevated plasma corticosterone levels and decreased sensitivity of the hypothalamic-pituitary-adrenal (HPA) negative feedback system [20]. These observations

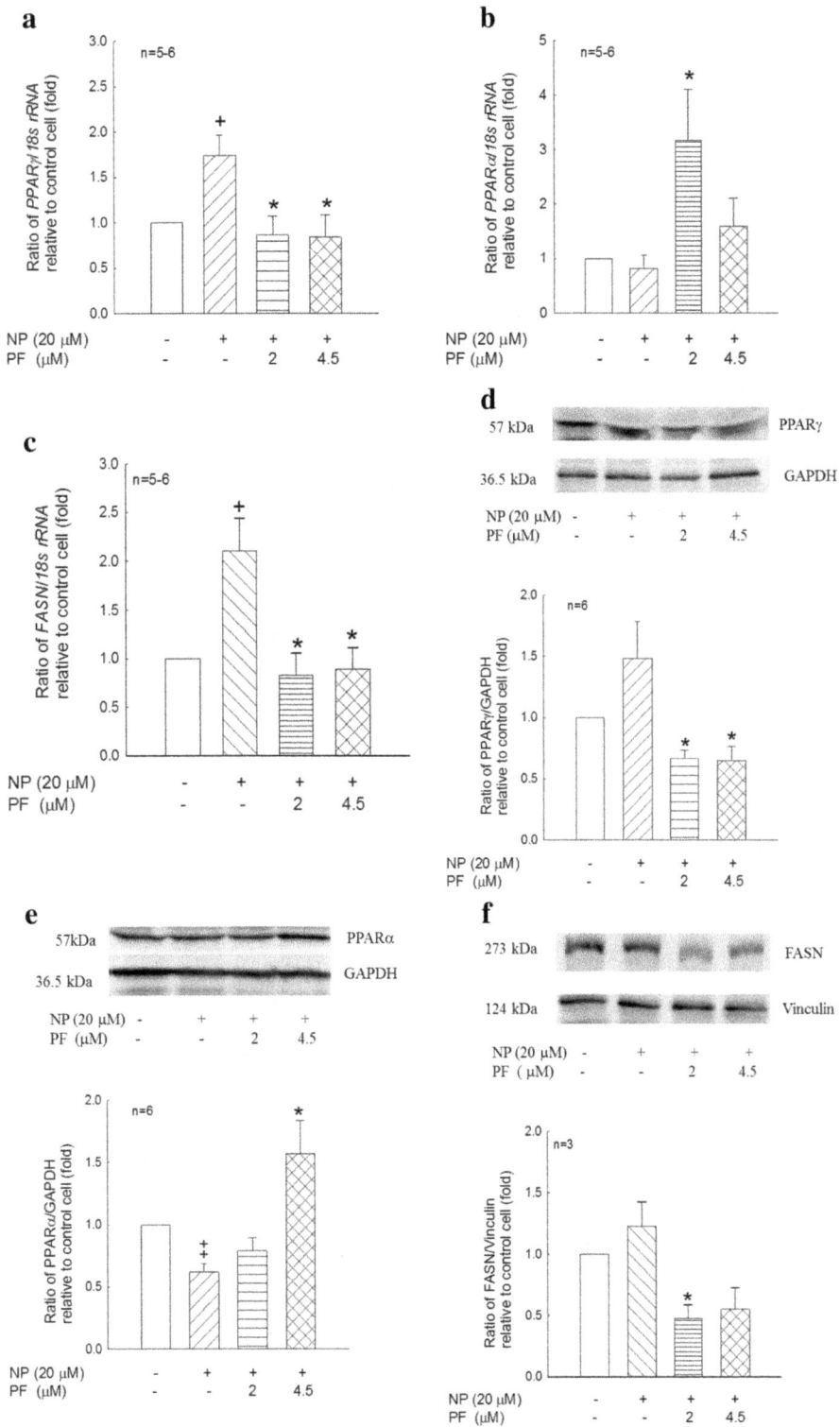

Fig. 6 (See legend on next page.)

(See figure on previous page.)
Fig. 6 Effects of human preadipocyte exposure to NP before differentiation (P exposure) on mRNA and protein expression levels by real-time PCR and western blot analysis. Human preadipocytes were incubated in PAM in the presence of NP (0 or 20 µM) for 12 h. After exposure to NP, the medium was changed to differentiation medium (PADM) in the presence of PF915275 (0, 2 or 4.5 µM). **a, b** and **c**: After 6 days of incubation, *PPARγ, PPARα* and *FASN* mRNA levels in the cells were determined by real-time PCR analysis, and the values were normalized against *18 s rRNA*. **d, e, f**: After 6 days of incubation, PPARγ (57 kDa), PPARα (57 kDa) and FASN (273 kDa) protein levels in the cells were determined by western blot analysis. The representative immunoblot was shown in the upper part, and densitometry for PPARγ, PPARα or FASN normalized to GAPDH (for PPARγ, PPARα) or Vinculin (for FASN) was shown in the bottom part. The values, which are means of independent cultures, are shown as the means ± S.E.M. and are presented as the fold-change relative to control cells (cells were not primed with NP and differentiated with PADM only). +, ++: $p < 0.05$, 0.01, cells with priming with NP and differentiation with PADM compared with control cells. *: $p < 0.05$, cells with priming with NP and differentiation with PADM containing PF compared with cells with priming with NP and differentiation with PADM only

corresponded to a phenomenon of HPA axis activation by prenatal stress or glucocorticoid exposure during pregnancy [39, 41]. We also previously observed that exposure of female pups to NP during the developmental period not only elevated blood corticoid concentrations but also increased 11β-HSD1 protein expression and enzymatic activity in the liver [11]. These findings are consistent with the results in this study. Epigenetic modifications during the sensitive developmental period can induce "fetal origins of adult disease". These epigenetic modifications by DNA methyltransferases can be inherited [42]. NP-induced hyperadrenalism, if left untreated, can impact an individual's health for life. We previously reported [11] that two generations are required for female rats (the F_3 generation recovers compared to the NP-affected F_1 generation) to recover from NP-induced hyperadrenalism. The logical treatment plan for the NP-affected F_1 generation consists of counteracting the increased 11β-HSD1 activity due to its irreversible effects on epigenetic modifications. One potential agent is a selective inhibitor of 11β-HSD1 called PF, which is currently undergoing the initial phase I clinical trial test. Thus far, PF has been shown to be a safe and effective treatment for metabolic syndrome [16, 31, 43]. In this study, oral gavage with PF significantly decreased corticosterone release in plasma (Fig. 1a) and decreased 11β-HSD1 enzyme activity and protein and mRNA expression in the liver (Fig. 2a, b and d). StAR protein can transfer cholesterol from the outer mitochondrial membrane to the inner mitochondrial membrane. Clark et al. [44] purified, cloned and sequenced the StAR protein. In our previous in vivo [11, 20] and in vitro [36] studies, NP did not increase StAR protein expression in the adrenal gland. These findings are consistent with the results in this study (Fig. 4c). Additionally, PF drastically decreased 11β-hydroxylase activity, aldosterone synthase activity and StAR protein expression in the adrenal glands of female rat offspring with developmental exposure to NP (Fig. 4a-c). These results show that PF can alleviate or reduce NP-induced hyperadrenalism in rats.

In vivo, chronic glucocorticoid exposure stimulates both adipogenesis and lipolysis in visceral adipose tissue; adipogenesis increases adipose tissue mass and lipolysis increases circulating free fatty acids and ectopic lipid storage in the

liver and skeletal muscle [45]. Both in vivo and in vitro studies have shown that glucocorticoids stimulate lipolysis via hormone-sensitive lipase [46, 47] and that the resultant free fatty acids may contribute to insulin resistance. Glucocorticoids acting with insulin can regulate lipid homeostasis in human preadipocyte cells [48]. Peroxisome proliferator-activated receptor γ (PPARγ), which is primarily expressed in adipose tissues engaging in adipogenesis, plays an important role in adipocyte differentiation, inflammation, glucose homeostasis and insulin signaling [49]. Octylphenol is another alkylphenol similar to NP. Treatment of C3H10T1/2 cells with octylphenol induces PPARγ expression to inhibit osteoblast differentiation, causing a lineage shift towards adipocytes [50, 51]. Hao et al. [52] showed that NP induced *PPARγ* expression in mouse 3 T3-L1 preadipocytes, and NP increased *PPARγ* expression in mice injected with NP after 24 h. In this study, no significant differences in PPARγ protein expression levels were found between the vehicle and NP groups (Fig. 3a). However, PF treatment significantly decreased the protein expression of PPARγ in adipose tissue (Fig. 3a). In human preadipocytes, P exposure of NP significantly increased *PPARγ* mRNA expression, and PF decreased NP-induced increases in PPARγ mRNA and protein expression to inhibit adipogenesis. These observations may suggest that the effects of NP on human (Fig. 6a) and rodent tissues [52] may be mediated through similar mechanisms at the cellular level. In this in vitro study, P exposure was designed to serve as a model for the human neonatal (not fully differentiated) period. The results showed that preadipocytes had "memory" of NP exposure during the pre-differentiation period, possibly suggesting that P exposure triggered epigenetic modifications or long-term consequences of molecular or biochemical events. The results obtained from human preadipocytes corresponded to the rat model of developmental exposure to NP, which resulted in lifelong hyperadrenalism. This observation supports Barker's hypothesis of the "fetal origins of adult disease" [53]. C exposure was designed as a model to examine the effects of NP exposure during the human adult period. C exposure of NP in human preadipocytes significantly increased PPARγ mRNA and protein

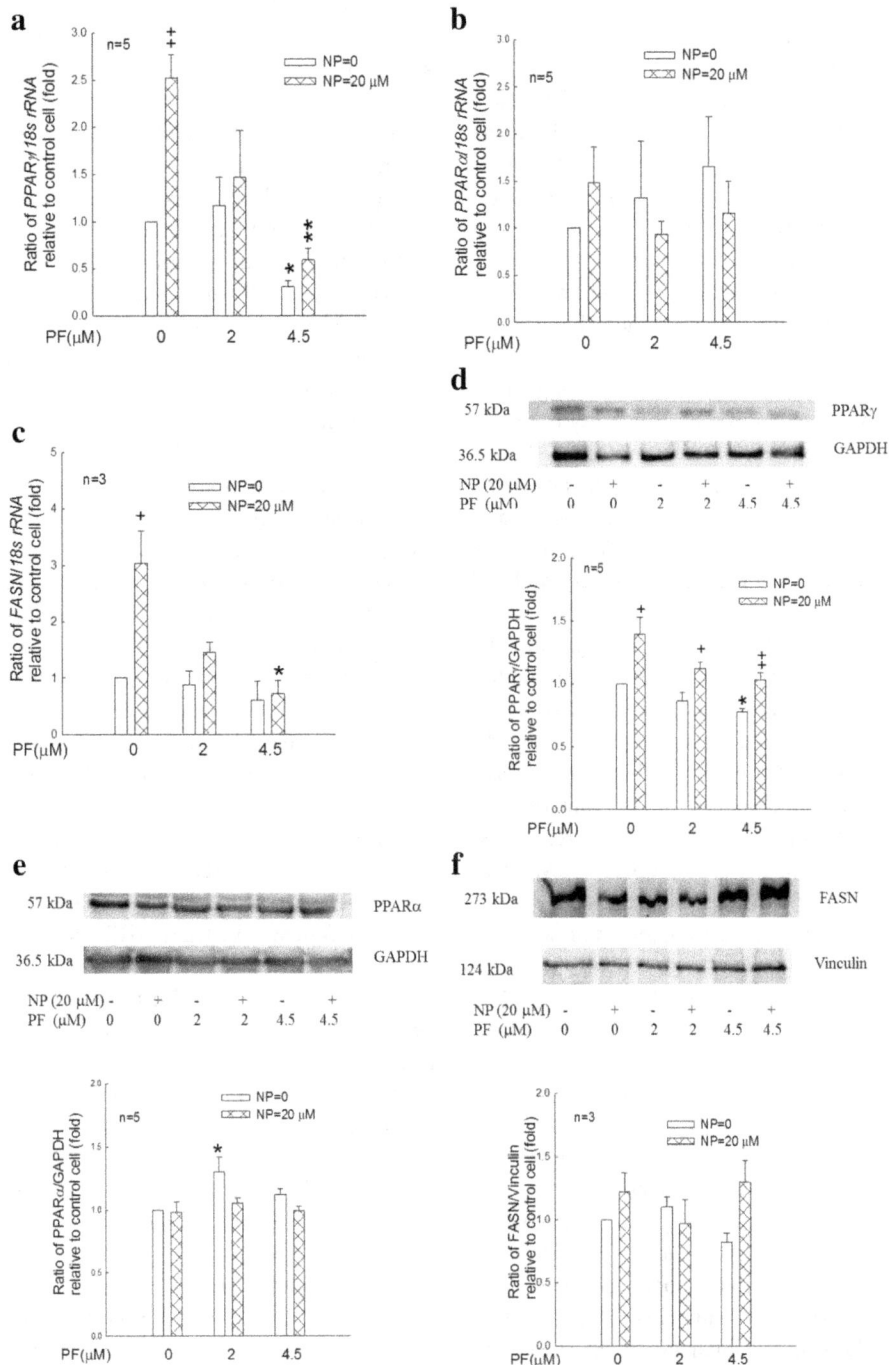

Fig. 7 Effects of NP and PF on mRNA and protein expression levels by real-time PCR and western blot analysis. Human preadipocytes were incubated in differentiation medium (PADM) in the presence of NP (0 or 20 μM) combined with PF915275 (0, 2 or 4.5 μM). **a**, **b** and **c**: After 6 days of incubation, *PPARγ*, *PPARα* and *FASN* mRNA levels in the cells were determined by real-time PCR analysis, and the values were normalized against *18 s rRNA*. **d**, **e** and **f**: After 6 days of incubation, PPARγ (57 kDa), PPARα (57 kDa) and FASN (273 kDa) protein levels in the cells were determined by western blot analysis. The representative immunoblot was shown in the upper part, and densitometry for PPARγ, PPARα or FASN normalized to GAPDH (for PPARγ, PPARα) or Vinculin (for FASN) was shown in the bottom part. The values, which are means of independent cultures, are presented as the means ± S.E.M. and represent the fold-change relative to control cells (cells differentiated with PADM only). +, ++: $p < 0.05$, 0.01, NP effect with the same concentration of PF. *, **: $p < 0.05$, 0.01, PF effect with the same concentration of NP

expression levels, and PF decreased NP-induced PPARγ mRNA and protein expression (Fig. 7a, d). NP exposure appeared to trigger hyperadrenalism [20]. Whether hyperadrenalism induced by NP exposure during the adult stage had "memory" effects was unclear. Nevertheless, both life stages (P exposure and C exposure) showed adipogenic consequences of exposure to NP. These observations support the Baillie-Hamilton theory [1] that environmental ENDRs are partially responsible for pandemic metabolic syndromes. The effects of the 11β-HSD1 inhibitor PF reflect the possibility of treating and alleviating the impacts of environmental pollution.

Fatty acid synthase (FASN) is a key enzyme in lipogenesis. Sprague-Dawley rat pups fed with a high-carbohydrate diet exhibited obesity later in life and overexpressed FASN in the liver and adipose tissue [54]. NP exposure by either the P or C protocol can increase FASN mRNA expression, and PF can inhibit NP-induced FASN mRNA expression (Figs. 6c, 7c). In human cells, preadipocytes accumulated intracellular lipids after the induction of differentiation. NP alone could not increase lipid accumulation (Fig. 5c). The commercial PADM used in this study contains dexamethasone 1 μM with insulin 7.5 μg/ml, and dexamethasone combined with insulin dose-dependently upregulated adipogenesis and fat accumulation in cultured adipocytes [55]; therefore, the NP effect on adipogenic activity was masked by the optimized differentiation medium. PF decreased while NP increased PF-inhibited (PF at 1.5 or 2 μM) lipid accumulation (Fig. 5c). These results indicate that: 1) PF decreases PPARγ mRNA and protein expression and increases PPARα protein (Fig. 7a, d, e); 2) NP increases PPARγ mRNA and protein expression (Fig. 7a, d); and 3) depending on the dose, NP and PF have mutual antagonistic capabilities.

PPARα is a ligand-activated nuclear transcription factor that regulates lipid catabolism and inflammation. Increasing fatty acid oxidation by PPARα activation can lower circulating triglyceride levels, decrease liver and muscle steatosis, and reduce adiposity, which improves insulin sensitivity [56–58]. Morton et al. [15] demonstrated that 11β-HSD1-deficient mice exhibited increased PPARα expression in their livers to increase lipid catabolism, reduce intracellular glucocorticoid concentrations, and increase hepatic insulin sensitivity. In the rat model in this study, developmental exposure to NP significantly decreased the protein expression of PPARα in adipose tissues (Fig. 3b), and PF significantly alleviated NP-inhibited PPARα protein expression in adipose tissues (Fig. 3b) and adrenal glands (Fig. 4d). In human preadipocytes, P exposure to NP significantly decreased PPARα protein expression, and PF alleviated the NP-inhibited PPARα protein expression ($p < 0.05$, Fig. 6e). The results from both the human cell in vitro model and the rat in vivo model indicate that

NP-induced adiposity can be alleviated or prevented by PF administration via increased PPARα protein expression and subsequently increased lipid catabolism. They also show that the rodent model is an adequate model to mimic NP's effects and treatment in human cells. NP did not affect PPARα mRNA expression with either P or C exposure in human preadipocytes (Figs. 6b, 7b), possibly because NP may affect PPARα expression at the translation stage in human preadipocytes.

Bost et al. [59] proposed that transient activation of the MEK/MAPKs signaling pathway is required for the differentiation of preadipocytes. Additionally, the authors demonstrated that wild-type mice had more adipocytes and increased adiposity compared to ERK1$^{-/-}$ mice [60]. Furthermore, the differentiation of preadipocytes isolated from ERK1$^{-/-}$ mice was impaired [60]. PPARγ is expressed after MEK/MAPK activation in preadipocytes [61]. Adipocyte lipolysis is catalyzed by adipose triglyceride lipase and hormone-sensitive lipase, leading to hydrolysis of triglycerides to glycerol and free fatty acids [62]. Hormone-sensitive lipase is considered the rate-limiting enzyme in lipolysis [63], and its activity is mainly driven by phosphorylation of a serine residue through cAMP-dependent protein kinase A (PKA) [64]. This study shows that PF can alleviate NP-induced adipogenesis through the PPAR system; however, the associated mechanism is not clear. We will further explore the mechanisms of NP and PF in adipogenesis through MEK/MAPK, PKA, or other pathways.

We found that developmental exposure to NP results in hyperadrenalism in adulthood in our rat model. However, whether this phenomenon in rats reflects human conditions remains questionable. The most ethical approach would be to examine the effects of NP using in vitro models with human progenitor cells. Adipose tissue is one of the organs affected by NP; therefore, preadipocytes are a logical choice for studying the effects of NP. Priming human preadipocytes with NP for a short period of time (12 h, P exposure) results in decreased PPARα protein expression after 6 days of culture in differentiated adipocytes (Fig. 6e). These results are similar to the results from adipose tissues in the rat in vivo model (Fig. 3b). If human preadipocytes are continuously exposed to NP (C exposure, Fig. 7), the PPARγ and FASN response patterns are very similar between P (Fig. 6) and C exposure. These observations suggest the following 3 considerations. First, short-term NP exposure during critical developmental periods results in long-term consequences. Second, NP exposure results in adiposity. The 3rd consideration is whether the rat model can adequately reflect NP's impact on human cells. Table 2

Table 2 Comparison of NP and PF effect on lipogenic attributes on rat adipose tissue and human preadipocyte

		mRNA			Protein		
		PPARα	PPARγ	FASN	PPARα	PPARγ	FASN
Rat	NP vs. control	n.s.[a]	$p < 0.01$[a] increase	n.s.[a]	$p < 0.05$ decrease	n.s.	n.s.[a]
	NP + PF vs. NP	n.s.[a]	$p < 0.01$[a] decrease	$p < 0.05$[a] decrease	$p < 0.01$ increase	$p < 0.01$ decrease	n.s.[a]
Human	NP vs. control	n.s.	$p < 0.05$ increase	$p < 0.05$ increase	$p < 0.01$ decrease	n.s.	n.s.
	NP + PF vs. NP	$p < 0.05$ increase	$p < 0.05$ decrease	$p < 0.05$ decrease	$p < 0.05$ increase	$p < 0.05$ decrease	$p < 0.05$ decrease

n.s not significant; [a]data from previous report (Chang et al. 2016) [17]

shows a compilation of data from a previous report [17] and from this study. The rat model included rat pups exposed to NP during the developmental period in an in vivo system. The human model included human preadipocytes exposed to NP before differentiation (P exposure) in an in vitro system. Generally, PPARα has lipolysis functions, while PPARγ has lipogenesis functions. The data show a trend of decreasing PPARα expression at the protein level with NP exposure, and PF can antagonize NP's effects in both the rat and human models. NP increased PPARγ mRNA expression but not protein expression, and PF could significantly antagonize NP's effects at both the mRNA and protein levels. This phenomenon is evident in both the rat and human models. NP had no significant effect on FASN mRNA and protein expression levels, whereas PF significantly decreased FASN mRNA expression but not protein expression in the rat model. In the human model, NP increased FASN mRNA and protein expression, although not significantly, at the protein level. PF appeared to decrease NP's effects at both the mRNA and protein levels. The comparison of the effects of NP and PF shows similar responses between the human and rat models. Therefore, rats may serve as an appropriate experimental model for human study.

Conclusions

NP exposure during developmental periods results in hyperadrenalism and adiposity. One of the mechanisms of NP's action is mediated through cellular 11β-HSD1. Inhibition of 11β-HSD1 can alleviate or prevent the impact of NP on not only adrenal gland function but also on the intracellular Cushing's state. NP's mechanism of action appears to also be mediated through the cellular PPAR system. The results from the rat model adequately reflect the impact of NP and PF on human preadipocytes. These observations suggest that rats serve as an adequate experimental model to examine the impact of NP and

possible treatments for humans. Therefore, these results offer hope for the treatment of pandemic Cushing's syndrome, especially ENDR-induced Cushing's syndrome.

Abbreviations
11β-HSD1: 11β-hydroxysteroid dehydrogenase I; BPA: Bisphenol A; DDT: Dichlorodiphenyl-trichloroethane; DES: Diethylstilbestrol; EDC: Endocrine-disrupting chemical; ENDRs: Endocrine disruptors; ERK: Extracellular signal–regulated kinase; FASN: Fatty acid synthase; GAPDH: Glyceraldehyde-3-phosphate dehydrogenase; MAPK: Mitogen-activated protein kinase; NADPH: Nicotinamide adenine dinucleotide phosphate; NP: Nonylphenol; PADM: Preadipocyte differentiation medium; PAM: Preadipocyte medium; PF PF915275: 4'-cyano-biphenyl-4-sulfonic acid (6-amino-pyridin-2-yl)-amide; PKA : Protein kinase A; PPAR : Proliferator-activated receptor; PPARα: Proliferator-activated receptor α; PPARγ: Proliferator-activated receptor γ; RIA : Radioimmunoassay; StAR : Steroidogenic acute regulatory

Acknowledgments
We would like to thank Dr. Douglas M. Stocco (Department of Cell Biology and Biochemistry, Texas Tech University Health Science Center, Lubbock, Texas, USA) for kindly providing the anti-StAR antibody.

Funding
This work was supported by the National Science Council, Taiwan, ROC (NSC102–2221-E-034-013).

Authors' contributions
LLC and WSAW conceived and designed the study. LLC carried out the experiments and assays. LLC and WSAW performed statistical analyses. LLC, WSAW and PSW wrote the paper, contributed to the revision of the manuscript and read and approved the final manuscript.

Competing interests
The authors declare that they have no competing interests.

Author details
[1]Department of Chemical and Materials Engineering, Chinese Culture University, Shih-Lin, Taipei 11114, Taiwan, Republic of China. [2]Fertility Specialists of Houston, Houston, TX 77054, USA. [3]Department of Physiology,

School of Medicine, National Yang-Ming University, Taipei 11221, Taiwan, Republic of China. [4]Department of Medical Research and Education, Taipei Veterans General Hospital, Taipei 11217, Taiwan, Republic of China. [5]Medical Center of Aging Research, China Medical University Hospital, Taichung 40402, Taiwan, Republic of China. [6]Department of Biotechnology, Asia University, Taichung 41354, Taiwan, Republic of China.

References

1. Baillie-Hamilton PF. Chemical toxins: a hypothesis to explain the global obesity epidemic. J Altern Complement Med. 2002;8:185–92.

2. Kearney PM, Whelton M, Reynolds K, Muntner P, Whelton PK, He J. Global burden of hypertension: analysis of worldwide data. Lancet. 2005;365:217–23.

3. Padwal RS, Sharma AM. Prevention of cardiovascular disease: obesity, diabetes and the metabolic syndrome. Can J Cardiol. 2010;26(Suppl C):18C–20C.

4. Centers for Disease Control and Prevention. National Diabetes Statistics Report: estimates of diabetes and its burden in the United States; 2014. Atlanta, GA: US Department of Health and Human Services; 2014.

5. Wamil M, Seckl JR. Inhibition of 11beta-hydroxysteroid dehydrogenase type 1 as a promising therapeutic target. Drug Discov TodayDrug Discov Today. 2007;12:504–20.

6. Rask E, Walker BR, Söderberg S, Livingstone DE, Eliasson M, Johnson O, Andrew R, Olsson T. Tissue-specific changes in peripheral cortisol metabolism in obese women: increased adipose 11beta-hydroxysteroid dehydrogenase type 1 activity. J Clin Endocrinol Metab. 2002;87:3330–6.

7. Tomlinson JW, Walker EA, Bujalska IJ, Draper N, Lavery GG, Cooper MS, Hewison M, Stewart PM. 11beta-hydroxysteroid dehydrogenase type 1: a tissue-specific regulator of glucocorticoid response. Endocr Rev. 2004;25:831–66.

8. Anagnostis P, Katsiki N, Adamidou F, Athyros VG, Karagiannis A, Kita M, Mikhailidis DP. 11beta-hydroxysteroid dehydrogenase type 1 inhibitors: novel agents for the treatment of metabolic syndrome and obesity-related disorders? Metabolism. 2013;62:21–33.

9. Ge R, Huang Y, Liang G, Li X. 11beta-hydroxysteroid dehydrogenase type 1 inhibitors as promising therapeutic drugs for diabetes: status and development. Curr Med Chem. 2010;17:412–22.

10. Wang M. Inhibitors of 11beta-hydroxysteroid dehydrogenase type 1 in antidiabetic therapy. Handb Exp Pharmacol. 2011;203:127–46.

11. Chang LL, Wun AWS, Wang PS. Recovery from developmental nonylphenol exposure is possible for female rats. Chem Biol Interact. 2014;221:52–60.

12. Livingstone DE, Jones GC, Smith K, Jamieson PM, Andrew R, Kenyon CJ, Walker BR. Understanding the role of glucocorticoids in obesity: tissue-specific alterations of corticosterone metabolism in obese Zucker rats. Endocrinology. 2000;141:560–3.

13. Masuzaki H, Paterson J, Shinyama H, Morton NM, Mullins JJ, Seckl JR, Flier JS. A transgenic model of visceral obesity and the metabolic syndrome. Science. 2001;294:2166–70.

14. Rask E, Olsson T, Soderberg S, Andrew R, Livingstone DE, Johnson O, Walker BR. Tissue-specific dysregulation of cortisol metabolism in human obesity. J Clin Endocrinol Metab. 2001;86:1418–21.

15. Morton NM, Holmes MC, Fievet C, Staels B, Tailleux A, Mullins JJ, Seckl JR. Improved lipid and lipoprotein profile, hepatic insulin sensitivity, and glucose tolerance in 11β-hydroxysteroid dehydrogenase type 1 null mice. J Biol Chem. 2001;276:41293–300.

16. Courtney R, Stewart PM, Toh M, Ndongo MN, Calle RA, Hirshberg B. Modulation of 11beta-hydroxysteroid dehydrogenase (11betaHSD) activity biomarkers and pharmacokinetics of PF-00915275, a selective 11betaHSD1 inhibitor. Clin Endocrinol Metab. 2008;93:550–6.

17. Chang LL, Wun WS, Wang PS. Nonylphenol-induced hyperadrenalism can be reversed/alleviated by inhibiting of 11-β hydroxysteroid dehydrogenase type. Environ Toxicol Pharmacol. 2016;44:1–12.

18. Eijken M, Hewison M, Cooper MS, de Jong FH, Chiba H, Stewart PM, Uitterlinden AG, Pols HA, van Leeuwen JP. 11 beta-Hydroxysteroid dehydrogenase expression and glucocorticoid synthesis are directed by a molecular switch during osteoblast differentiation. Mol Endocrinol. 2005;19:621–31.

19. McCormick KL, Wang X, Mick GJ. Evidence that the 11 beta-hydroxysteroid dehydrogenase (11beta-HSD1) is regulated by pentose pathway flux. Studies in rat adipocytes and microsomes. J Biol Chem. 2006;281:341–7.

20. Chang LL, Wun W-SA, Wang PS. In utero and neonatal exposure to nonylphenol develops hyperadrenalism and metabolic syndrome late in life. I. First generation (F1). Toxicology. 2012;301:40–9.

21. Lo MJ, Kau MM, Chen YH, Tsai SC, Chiao YC, Chen JJ, Liaw C, Lu CC, Lee BP, Chen SC, Fang VS, Ho LT, Wang PS. Acute effects of thyroid hormones on the production of adrenal cAMP and corticosterone in male rats. Am J Phys. 1998;274(2 Pt 1):E238–45.

22. Kau MM, Chen JJ, Wang SW, Cho WL, Wang PS. Age-related impairment of aldosterone secretion in zona glomerulosa cells of ovariectomized rats. J Investig Med. 1999;47:425–32.

23. Bradford MM. A rapid and sensitive method for the quantitation of microgram quantities of protein utilizing the principle of protein-dye binding. Anal Biochem. 1976;72:248–54.

24. Lo MJ, Chang LL, Wang PS. Effect of estradiol on corticosterone secretion in ovariectomized rats. J Cell Biochem. 2000;77:560–8.

25. Ademollo N, Ferrara F, Delis M, Fabietti F, Funari E. Nonylphenol and octylphenol in human breast milk. Environ Int. 2008;34:984–7.

26. Cunny HC, Mayes BA, Rosica KA, Trutter JA, Van Miller JP. Subcronic toxicity (90 day) study with Para-nonylphenol in rats. Regul Toxicol Pharmacol. 1997;26:172–8.

27. Ferguson SA, Delclos KB, Newbold RR, Flynn KM. Few effects of multi-generational dietary exposure to genistein or nonylyphenol on sodium solution intake in male and female Sprague-Dawley rats. Neurotoxicol Teratol. 2009;31:143–8.

28. Hossaini A, Dalgaard M, Vinggaard AM, Frandsen H, Larsen J-J. In utero reproductive study in rats exposed to nonylphenol. Reprod Toxicol. 2001;15:537–43.

29. Jie X, Yang W, Lie Y, Hashim JH, Liu X-Y, Fan Q-Y, Yan L. Toxic effect of gestational exposure to nonylphenol on F1 male rats. Birth Defects Res B Dev Reprod Toxicol. 2010;89:418–28.

30. Nagao T, Wada K, Marumo H, Yoshimura S, Ono H. Reproductive effects of nonylphenol in rats after gavage administration: a two generation study. Reprod Toxicol. 2001;15:293–315.

31. Bhat BG, Hosea N, Fanjul A, Herrera J, Chapman J, Thalacker F, Stewart PM, Rejto PA. Demonstration of proof of mechanism and pharmacokinetics and pharmacodynamic relationship with 4'-cyano-biphenyl-4-sulfonic acid (6-amino-pyridin-2-yl)-amide (PF-915275), an inhibitor of 11 -hydroxysteroid dehydrogenase type 1, in cynomolgus monkeys. J Pharmacol Exp Ther. 2008;324:299–305.

32. Wang L, Liu J, Zhang A, Cheng P, Zhang X, Lv S, Wu L, Yu J, Di W, Zha J, Kong X, Qi H, Zhong Y, Ding G. BVT.2733, a selective 11b-hydroxysteroid dehydrogenase type 1 inhibitor, attenuates obesity and inflammation in diet-induced obese mice. PLoS One. 2012;(7):e40056,1–10.

33. Hu G-X, Lin H, Lian Q-Q, Zhou S-H, Guo J, Zhou H-Y, Chu Y, Ge R-S. Curcumin as a potent and selective inhibitor of 11b-Hydroxysteroid dehydrogenase 1: improving lipid profiles in high-fat=diet-treated rats. PLoS One. 2013;8:e49976,1–7.

34. Yang O, Kim HL, Weon JI, Seo YR. Endocrine-disrupting chemicals: review of toxicological mechanisms using molecular pathway analysis. J Cancer Prev. 2015;20:12–24.

35. Kim HR, Kim YS, Yoon JA, Lyu SW, Shin H, Lim HJ, Hong SH, Lee DR, Song H, Barker DJ. Egr1 is rapidly and transiently induced by estrogen and bisphenol a via activation of nuclearestrogen receptor-dependent ERK1/2 pathway in the uterus. Reprod Toxicol. 2014;50:60–7.

36. Chang LL, Wun Alfred WS, Wang PS. Effects and mechanisms of nonylphenol on corticosterone release in rat zona fasciculata-reticularis cells. Toxicol Sci. 2010;118:411–9.

37. Chang LL, Wun Alfred WS, Wang PS. Effects and of nonylphenol on aldosterone release from rat zona glomerulosa cells. Chem Biol Interact. 2012;195:11–7.

38. Bujalska IJ, Gathercole LL, Tomlinson JW, Darimont C, Ermolieff J, Fanjul AN, Rejto PA, Stewart PM. A novel selective 11beta-hydroxysteroid dehydrogenase type 1 inhibitor prevents human adipogenesis. J Endocrinol. 2008;197:297–307.

39. Reynolds RM. Glucocorticoid excess and the development origins of disease: two decades of testing the hypothesis – 2012 Curt Richter award winner. Psychoneuroendocrinology. 2013;38:1–11.

40. Iwasaki Y, Takayasu S, Nishiyama M, Taguchi T, Asai M, Yoshida M, Kambayashi M. Hashimoto K. Is the metabolic syndrome an intracellular Cushing state? Effects of multiple humoral factors on the transcriptional activity of the hepatic glucocorticoid-activating enzyme (11β –HSD1) gene. Mol Cell Endocrinol. 2008;285:10–8.

41. Cottrell EC, Seckl JR. Prenatal stress, glucocorticoids and the programming of adult disease. Front Behav Neurosci. 2009;3:1–9.

42. Bestor TH. The DNA methyltransferases of mammals. Hum Mol Genet. 2000; 9:2395–402.

43. Fotsch C, Wang M. Blockade of glucocorticoid excess at the tissue level: inhibitors of 11beta-hydroxysteroid dehydrogenase type 1 as a therapy for type 2 diabetes. J Med Chem. 2008;51:4851–7.

44. Clark BJ, Wells J, King SR, Stocco DM. The purification, cloning and expression of a novel LH-induced mitochondrial protein in MA-10 mouse Leydig tumor cells: characterization of the steroidogenic acute regulatory protein (StAR). J Biol Chem. 1994;269:28314–22.

45. Campbell JE, Peckett AJ, D'souza AM, Hawke TJ, Riddell MC. Adipogenic and lipolytic effects of chronic glucocorticoid exposure. Am J Physiol Cell Physiol. 2011;300:C198–209.

46. Djurhuus CB, Gravholt CH, Nielsen S, Mengel A, Christiansen JS, Schmitz OE, Møller N. Effects of cortisol on lipolysis and regional interstitial glycerol levels in humans. Am J Physiol Endocrinol Metab. 2002;283:E172–7.

47. Slavin BG, Ong JM, Kern PA. Hormonal regulation of hormone-sensitive lipase activity and mRNA levels in isolated rat adipocytes. J Lipid Res. 1994;35:1535–41.

48. Gathercole LL, Morgan SA, Bujalska IJ, Hauton D, Stewart PM, Tomlinson JW. Regulation of lipogenesis by glucocorticoids and insulin in human adipose tissue. PLoS One. 2011;6:e26223.

49. Kersten S, Desvergne B, Wahli W. Roles of PPARs in health and disease. Nature. 2000;405:421–4.

50. Grün F, Blumberg B. Environmental obesogens: organotins and endocrine disruption via nuclear receptor signaling. Endocrinology. 2006;147(6 Suppl): S50–5.

51. Miyawaki J, Kamei S, Sakayama K, Yamamoto H, Masuno H. 4-tert-Octylphenol regulates the differentiation of C3H10T1/2 cells into osteoblast and adipocyte lineages. Toxicol Sci. 2008;102:82–8.

52. Hao CJ, Cheng XJ, Xia HF, Ma X. The endocrine disruptor 4-nonylphenol promotes adipocyte differentiation and induce obesity in mice. Cell Physiol Biochem. 2012;30:382–94.

53. Barker DJ. The origins of developmental origins theory. J Intern Med. 2007;261:412–7.

54. Hiremagalur BK, Vadlamudi S, Johanning GL, Patel MS. Long-term effects of feeding high carbohydrate diet in pre-weaning period by gastrostomy: a new rat model for obesity. Int J Obes Relat Metab Disord. 1993;17:495–502.

55. Taylor PR, Mi-Jeong L, Kalypso K, Adam G, Susan FK. Depot dependent effects of dexamethasone on gene expression in human omental and abdominal subcutaneous adipose tissues from obese women. PLoS One. 2016;11:e0167337.

56. Berger JP, Akiyama TE, Meinke PT. PPARs: therapeutic targets for metabolic disease. Trends Pharmacol Sci. 2005;26:244–51.

57. Kim H, Haluzik M, Asghar Z, Yau D, Joseph JW, Fernandez AM, Reitman ML, Yakar S, Stannard B, Heron-Milhavet L, Wheeler MB, LeRoith D. Peroxisome proliferator-activated receptor-alpha agonist treatment in a transgenic model of type 2 diabetes reverses the lipotoxic state and improves glucose homeostasis. Diabetes. 2003;52:1770–8.

58. Michalik L, Auwerx J, Berger JP, Chatterjee VK, Glass CK, Gonzalez FJ, Grimaldi PA, Kadowaki T, Lazar MA, O'Rahilly S, Palmer CN, Plutzky J, Reddy JK, Spiegelman BM, Staels B, Wahli W. International Union of Pharmacology. LXI. Peroxisome proliferator-activated receptors. Pharmacol Rev. 2006;58: 726–41.

59. Bost F, Aouadi M, Binetruy B. The role of MAPKs in adipocyte differentiation and obesity. Biochimie. 2005;87:51–6.

60. Bost F, Aouadi M, Caron L, Even P, Belmonte N, Prot M, Dani C, Hofman P, Pages G, Marchand-Brustel YL, Binetruy B. The extracellular signal-regulated kinase isoform ERK1 is specifically required for in vitro and in vivo adipogenesis. Diabetes. 2005;54:402–11.

61. Farmer SR. Transcriptional control of adipocyte formation. Cell Metab. 2006;4:263–73.

62. Zimmermann R, Strauss JG, Haemmerle G, Schoiswohl G, Birner-Gruenberger R, Riederer M, Lass A, Neuberger G, Eisenhaber F, Hermetter A, Zechner R. Fat mobilization in adipose tissue is promoted by adipose triglyceride lipase. Science. 2004;306:1383–6.

63. Carey GB. Mechanisms regulating adipocyte lipolysis. Adv Exp Med Biol. 1998;441:157–70.

64. Londos C, Brasaemle DL, Schultz CJ, Adler-Wailes DC, Levin DM, Kimmel AR, Rondinone CM. On the control of lipolysis in adipocytes. Ann N Y Acad Sci. 1999;892:155–68.

18

Toxicological evaluation of therapeutic and supra-therapeutic doses of Cellgevity® on reproductive function and biochemical indices in Wistar rats

O. Awodele[1*], W. A. Badru[1], A. A. Busari[1], O. E. Kale[1], T. B. Ajayi[1], R. O. Udeh[1] and P. M. Emeka[2]

Abstract

Background: The misconception about dietary supplements being safe has led many into the in-patient wards. Cellgevity® (CGV) is a Max International premiere antioxidant supplement formula used by a large population. This study evaluated the effects of therapeutic and supra-therapeutic doses of CGV on reproductive function and biochemical indices in Wistar rats.

Methods: Seventy-two Wistar rats weighing 130 ± 15.8 g were grouped into two categories (male or female) of six rats per group. Control group received distilled water (10 ml/kg). Others received therapeutic (14.3 mg/kg or 28.6 mg/kg) and supra-therapeutic CGV doses (1000, 2000 or 3000 mg/kg) body weight per oral respectively.

Results: After 60 days, supra-therapeutic doses of CGV reduced sperm motility ($p < 0.05$) by 31.8%, 31.3% and 34.5% respectively and increased ($p < 0.05$) abnormality in sperms by 200%, 241% and 141.3% respectively. CGV altered male (luteinizing, follicle stimulating hormones and testosterone) and female reproductive hormones (luteinizing, follicle stimulating hormones estrogen and progesterone) respectively. Therapeutic doses of CGV elevated reduced glutathione, superoxide dismutase, catalase and glutathione S-transferase, although, this was exceeded by supra-therapeutic doses and more in females than male rats. Supra-therapeutic dose (3000 mg/kg CGV) decreased body weight in both male and female rats by 50% ($F(1.5, 30) = 1.2, p = 0.041$) and 62.7% ($F(2.1, 30) = 0.38, p = 0.038$) respectively in treated rats. Supratherapeutic (3000 mg/kg) dose of CGV increased ($p < 0.05$) creatinine level by 99.1% while serum total protein was reduced ($p < 0.05$) by 60.1% (2000 mg/kg) and 57.2% (3000 mg/kg) respectively in male animals. In Female rats, supra-therapeutic doses of CGV elevated creatinine levels by 72.2% (1000 mg/kg), 60.2% (2000 mg/kg) and 124.8% (3000 mg/kg) respectively and 3000 mg/kg produces elevated serum low density lipoprotein by 34.6% in treated rats. Serum cholesterol, triglycerides, albumin, alkaline phosphatase were unaltered by CGV dosing. Histology shows seminiferous tubules with reduced spermatogenic cells. Also, female rat kidney revealed acute tubular necrosis at highest dose used in this study.

Conclusion: Overall, these data suggest that pro-oxidant potential of the supra-therapeutic CGV doses is evident. Hence, it is necessary that its administration be done with caution using appropriate doses.

Keywords: Cellgevity, Dietary supplements, Therapeutic dose, Supra-therapeutic dose, Toxicological profile, Subchronic toxicity study

* Correspondence: awodeleo@gmail.com; awodeleo@gmail.com
[1]Toxicology Unit, Department of Pharmacology, Therapeutics and Toxicology, College of Medicine, University of Lagos, PMB 12003, Idi-Araba Campus, Lagos, Nigeria
Full list of author information is available at the end of the article

Background

A complementary and alternative and medicine (CAM) practice has been promoting dietary supplements as one of the most easily accessible adjunct therapies acceptable worldwide [1]. This is in commonplace with a general theme underlying a majority of alternative therapies in their emphasis on natural modes of healing. However, certain problems have been reported concerning the consumption of these supplements, which include inappropriate use, excessive intake, and non-disclosure of amount being present in dietary supplements being used by patients resulting in concomitant use of various oversaturated dietary supplements with or without orthodox counterparts [2]. Cellgevity® (CGV) is one of the most widely used glutathione supplement that have been considered to be harmless, nevertheless, this general assumption should not be overlooked. It is marketed so as to salvage for the body glutathione and/or complements its production [3]. RiboCeine which is the active compound in CGV comprises mainly of D-Ribose and L-Cysteine. However, other components that are of scientific interest are; vitamin c, selenium, alpha lipoic, broccolli seed extract, curcumin, resveratrol, grape seed extract, quercetin, milk thistle seed extract, cordyceps, black pepper, aloe leaf. The manufacturer acclaimed ultimate reduced glutathione (GSH) enhancing effects for its use and various antioxidant supplementation studies have revealed a beneficial trend [4, 5]. This is because GSH is an important antioxidant that plays a major role in the biotransformation process in the body [6]. Evidence abounds that levels of GSH in the body decreases naturally with age [7]. Both stressful life style and some artificial components of foods are the popular culprits [8]. Due to some theoretical benefits of maintaining antioxidant defenses status, several approaches to increase systemic and/or tissue-specific glutathione concentrations have been of scientific interests. We now know that thiol-disulfides redox balancing is a major work of GSH in various body cells [9]. However, reduction of reactive oxygen or even nitrogen species by sulfhydryls enhances transcriptional activation, whereas oxidation inhibits activation [10]. Another important role of GSH supplementations are abilities to promote hypoxic apoptosis and improve protein function in a perturbed environment thereby yielding survival pathway [11]. In respect, the diversify roles of GSH supplementations have been well discussed [12]. Denovo alteration in antioxidant levels has been implicated in various diseases including those affecting the central nervous system [13]. The safety of some dietary supplements, such as protein supplements and others, remain a safety concern. The body's ability to absorb nutrients is known to decrease with age and exposure to toxins takes its toll [14]. The aforementioned play a

role in decreasing the Glutathione levels unless steps are taken to offset this process. Previous studies have reported that dietary supplements are now being used to prevent and treat various diseases [15, 16]. However, a number of adverse events have been reported over the past few years with the use of herbs and herbal products [17, 18]. Furthermore, concerns over drug-herbs interactions and irrational drug use (high dose) of CAM have arisen. In this present study, we investigated the toxicological activities of CGV using therapeutic and supra-therapeutic doses following a subchronic administration in Wistar rats.

Methods

Drugs and chemicals

Cellgevity (Riboceine®) was purchased in bulk from a subsidiary of Max international, Ikeja, Lagos state and it was the sole agent administered in this present study. Thiobarbituric acid (TBA), Ellman's reagent (DTNB) and 1-Chloro-2,4,-dinitrobenzene (CDBN) from Sigma (USA) were purchased from Sigma Chemical Company (USA). Reduced glutathione (GSH), Metaphosphoric acid and Trichloroacetic acid (TCA) were purchased from J.I. Baker (USA). Bovine serum albumin fraction V (BSA) was purchased from SRL, India. Rat Follicle Stimulating Hormone (FSH) (Cat. No.: Rshakrfs-010R) and Luteinizing Hormone (LH) ELISA (Rshakrlh-010SR) kits were purchased from (Biovendor, Shibayagi Co., Ltd. (Japan). RAT Testosterone (RTC001R) ELISA was obtained from Biovendor, Laboratorni, medicinaa.sKarasek (Czech Republic). Sodium hydroxide was obtained from MERCK (Germany). All other chemicals and reagents used were of analytical grades. Atomic UV/ Visible Spectrophotometer obtained from JENWAY, Bibby Scientific (Model 7300 and 7305) (USA).

Animals

Adult Wistar rats weighing between 100g and 153 g used in this study were purchased and nursed in the Laboratory Animal Centre of the College of Medicine, University of Lagos, Nigeria. The rats were housed under controlled conditions in the experimental animal handling facility of the College of Medicine, University of Lagos, Nigeria. The experimental animal room had a 12 h light/12 h dark schedule and maintained at a temperature of 22 ± 3 °C throughout the study. Animals were fed with commercially available rat pelleted diet (Livestock Feed Plc., Lagos, Nigeria) and were allowed access to water ad libitum throughout the period of the experiment. The experimental protocols were approved by the Institutional Animal Care and Use Committee, Department of Pharmacology, Therapeutic and Toxicology, College of Medicine, University of Lagos. Animals were certified fit for the experiment by the Institution's Animal Health Officers before the commencement of the study. Beddings were changed on alternate days and the animals were sacrificed in a humane manner at the end of the experiment by cervical dislocation. The investigation conforms to the Guide for the Care and Use of Laboratory Animals published by the U. S. National Institutes of Health (NIH Publication No. 85–23, revised 1996)" for studies involving experimental animals and the procedures as documented by Kilkenny et al. [19] for reporting animal research.

Experimental design and necropsy

Seventy-two (72) Wistar rats of both sexes weighing 130 ± 15.8 g were grouped into two categories (male or female) of six (6) rats per group. Controls groups received distilled water (10 ml/kg). Other groups received therapeutic (14.3 mg/kg or 28.6 mg/kg) and supratherapeutic doses (1000, 2000 or 3000 mg/kg) body weight per oral respectively. Treatments lasted for 60 days. Rats were weighed weekly throughout the course of the experiment. Twenty four hours after the last administration, blood samples were obtained by ocular puncture into either lithium heparin or ethylene diaminetetraacetic acid (EDTA) bottles and animals were subsequently sacrificed by cervical dislocation. The anticoagulated blood samples were centrifuged at 4200 rpm for 5 min to separate the plasma from which all biochemical assays were carried out. The testis and epididymis were all harvested, weighed and homogenized in four volumes of buffer solution (0.1 M, pH 7.4). A portion of each organ was taken out for histology. The remaining was weighed and homogenized for biochemical assays.

Analysis of sperm characteristics and morphology

The testes from each rat were carefully exposed and removed along with its adjoining epididymis. The slides on which the sperm cells were counted were heated to 37 ° C until the time of the analysis. The analysis was carried out at room temperature using one epididymis of each rat. The left testis was separated from the epididymis and the caudal epididymal tissue was removed and placed in a petri dish containing 1 mL normal saline solution. An incision of about 1 mm was made in the caudal epididymis to liberate its spermatozoa into the saline solution. Progressive sperm motility, sperm count, and sperm viability were then examined under the microscope attached to a Celestron® Digital Microscope Imager (Torrance, CA 90503) and viewed under X40 objective as described elsewhere [18]. Epididymal sperm motility was assessed by calculating motile spermatozoa per unit area and was expressed as percentage motility. Epididymal sperm count was done using the improved Neubauerhemocytometer and expressed as million/ml of suspension. The sperm viability was also determined using Eosin/Nigrosin stain. The motile (live) sperm cells

were unstained while the non-motile (dead) sperms absorbed the stain. The stained and unstained sperm cells were counted and an average value for each was recorded from which percentage viability was calculated. Sperm morphology was evaluated by staining the sperm smears on microscope slides with two drops of Walls and Ewa stain after they were air-dried. The slides were examined under the microscope under oil immersion with X 100 objectives.

Assessments of oxidant/antioxidant status

Lipid peroxidation activity was determined by measuring the formation of thiobarbituric acid reactive substances according to the method of Varshney and Kale [20] The method of Beutler et al. [21] was used for the determination of activity of reduced glutathione. While glutathione S-transferase activity was determined according to the method described by Habig et al. [22]. The levels of superoxide dismutase and catalase activities were determined by the method of Misra and Fridovich [23] and Sinha [24] respectively.

Reproductive hormone assessments

Serum concentrations of male reproductive hormones were measured using micro plate enzyme-linked immunosorbent assay (ELISA) and expressed as Units/l. Studies protocols were discussed below.

Rat FSH and LH ELISA

Briefly, in Rat FSH or LH ELISA Kit, biotin-conjugated anti- FSH/anti-LH and standard or sample were incubated in monoclonal anti-FSH antibody-coated wells. After 15 h incubation and wash-ing, HRP (horse radish peroxidase)-conjugated avidin was added, and incubated for 30 min. After washing, HRP-complex remaining in wells was reacted with a chromogenic substrate (TMB) for 20 min, and reaction was stopped by addition of acidic solution, and absorbance of yellow product was measured spectrophotometrically at 450 nm. Triplicates samples of LH/FSH were tested twice on one plate, respectively (Intra-Assay: CV < 8% and inter-assay: CV < 10%). The absorbance is nearly proportional to FSH or LH concentration. FSH or LH concentrations in unknown samples were then extrapolated via given their respected standard curve [25].

Rat testosterone ELISA

A 10 µl of each of sample with new disposable tips into appropriate wells was dispensed in a 100 µl of incubation Buffer into each well. Added was a 50 µl enzyme Conjugate into each well which was incubated for 60 min at room temperature on a microplate mixer. This was discarded and the well rinsed 4 times with diluted washing solution (300 µl per well). Then 200 µl was added of substrate solution to each well and incubated standing for 30 min in the dark. Triplicates samples of testosterone was tested twice on one plate, respectively (Intra-Assay: CV < 15% and inter-assay: CV < 15%). The reaction was stopped by adding 50 μl of stop solution to each well and the absorbance determined for each well at 450 nm [26].

Rat estrogen ELISA

The blank well and or 50 μl of standard in triplicate or sample per well were prepared. Then added was a 50 μl of HRP-conjugate to each well except for the blank. Then 50 μl antibody was added to each well. The solution was thorough mixed, and then incubated for 3 h at 37 °C. Each well was washed with buffer (350 μl), wait 10 s and spin. Following the last wash, remaining wash buffer was aspirated. Plate was inverted and blotted against clean paper towels. A 50 μl of substrate A was added and substrate B to each well, and mixed. Solution was incubated for 15 min at 37 °C. Triplicates samples of estrogen was tested twice on one plate, respectively (Intra-Assay: CV < 8% and inter-assay: CV < 12%). In a dark environment, a 50 μl of stop solution was added to each well. The color change appeared uniform. Determination of the optical den-sity was carried out within 10 min, using a microplate reader set to 450 nm [27].

Rat progesterone ELISA

Rat progesterone ELISA A dispensed 25 μl of each sample with new disposable tips into appropriate wells and added 50 μl of incubation Buffer into each well. Added was a 100 μl enzyme conjugate into each well and incubated for 1 h at 22 ± 2 °C on a microplate mixer. Following a thorough rinsing up to 4 times with diluted wash solution, a 200 μl of substrate solution was added to each well and incubated for 30 min in the dark. Triplicates samples of progesterone was tested twice on one plate, respectively (Intra-Assay: CV < 10% and inter-assay: CV < 10%). This reaction was terminated by the addition of a 50 μl of stop solution to each well. The progesterone level was measured at 450 nm within 15 min [27].

Assessment of biochemical parameters

Plasma alkaline phosphate was carried out according to the method described by Roy [28] to assess liver function. Renal function was assessed by measuring plasma creatinine levels and blood urea nitrogen was assayed following the method of Fossati et al. [29] and Skegg's [30]. Total serum protein concentration was determined according to the principles based on the Biuret reaction. Albumin concentrations were determined according to the principles based on the bromocresol green reaction

[31] respectively. Uric acid levels were determined according to the methods of Fossati et al. [32]. Total plasma cholesterol and Triglyceride concentrations were estimated following the method described by Trinder [33] by using commercial kits obtained from Randox Laboratories Ltd. (Crumlin, UK). High-Density Lipoprotein was estimated according to Warnick and Albers [34] while serum low-density lipoprotein was calculated using Freidewald formula [35].

Statistics

Results were expressed as mean ± standard error of mean (SEM). Differences between groups were determined by one-way analysis of variance (ANOVA) using Statistical Package for Social Sciences (SPSS, 20.0) software for windows. Post hoc testing was performed for intergroup comparisons using the least significant difference (LSD), followed by Dunnett's test, and the two-tailed p-value < 0.05 was considered significant. Figures were obtained using GraphPad Prism 6.

Results
Acute toxicity test

CGV acute toxicity study followed the guidelines according to the OECD Test Guidelines on Acute Oral Toxicity No 420 (OECD, 1992) [36]. An acute intragastric administration of 500, 1000 and 2000 mg/kg doses body weight ($n = 5$ per sex) of CGV in mice did not show physically observed adverse reactions on the fur, skin, subcutaneous swelling, eyes dullness, eyes opacities, colour and consistency of feaces, teeth and breathing abnormalities. However, mice administered 4000 mg/kg of CGV orally demonstrated reduced locomotion, dullness, raised of fur, and tears respectively. In addition, the group administered 4 g/kg had 20% mortality. Thus, 1000, 2000, and 3000 mg/kg were used for supra-therapeutic administration.

Figure 1 results show the effects of therapeutic and supra-therapeutic doses of Cellgevity (Ribceine) on sperm motility, sperm count and morphology abnormality in male rats. Therapeutic doses of CGV neither alter sperm motility nor counts when compared with control distilled water group. In contrast, supra-therapeutic doses of 1000 mg/kg, 2000 mg/kg and 3000 mg/kg reduced sperm motility ($F_{(5.2, 30)} = 1.5$, $p < 0.048$) by 31.8%, 31.3% and 34.5% respectively. Also, 3000 mg/kg CGV reduced sperm counts by 3.7%. CGV administration at 1000 mg/kg, 2000 mg/kg and 3000 mg/kg produce increased ($F_{(1.4, 28)} - 0.48$, $p = 0.001 - 0.002$) abnormality in sperms by 200%, 241% and 141.3% respectively.

Results in Fig. 2 show the effects of therapeutic and supra-therapeutic doses of CGV on male reproductive hormones in rat. CGV showed increased ($F_{(4, 26)} = 0.56$,

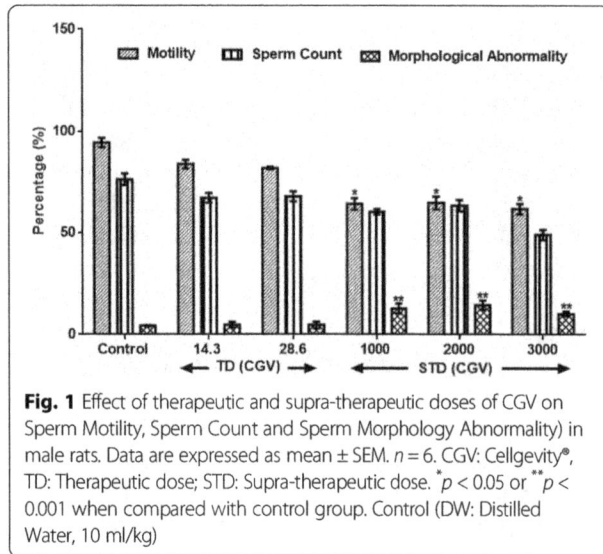

Fig. 1 Effect of therapeutic and supra-therapeutic doses of CGV on Sperm Motility, Sperm Count and Sperm Morphology Abnormality) in male rats. Data are expressed as mean ± SEM. $n = 6$. CGV: Cellgevity®, TD: Therapeutic dose; STD: Supra-therapeutic dose. $^{*}p < 0.05$ or $^{**}p < 0.001$ when compared with control group. Control (DW: Distilled Water, 10 ml/kg)

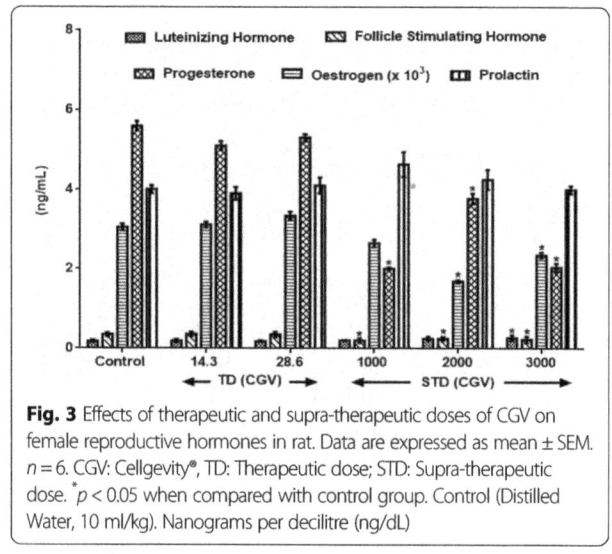

Fig. 3 Effects of therapeutic and supra-therapeutic doses of CGV on female reproductive hormones in rat. Data are expressed as mean ± SEM. $n = 6$. CGV: Cellgevity®, TD: Therapeutic dose; STD: Supra-therapeutic dose. $^{*}p < 0.05$ when compared with control group. Control (Distilled Water, 10 ml/kg). Nanograms per decilitre (ng/dL)

$p = 0.034$) LH at 1000 mg/kg while it shows decreased ($F_{(1.3, 24)} = 0.33$, $p < 0.151$) at higher doses of 2000 and 3000 mg/kg by 51.85% and 7.4% respectively when compared with control. Similarly, FSH was increased at 1000 mg/kg by 15% ($F_{(2, 28)} = 2.6$, $p = 0.135$). Both 2000 mg/kg and 3000 mg/kg of CGV did not alter FSH levels. Also, all the supra-therapeutic doses of CGV used in this study did not significantly alter testosterone levels when compared with control.

Figure 3 results show the effects of therapeutic and supra-therapeutic doses of CGV on female reproductive hormones in rat. An administration of 1000 mg/kg and 2000 mg/kg slightly although insignificantly elevated ($F_{(3.1, 25)} = 31.6$, $p < 0.235$) LH levels when compared

with control, whereas, 3000 mg/kg increased ($F_{(4, 24)} = 0.37$, $p = 0.038$) LH levels by 50%. Also, CGV doses of 1000 mg/kg and 3000 mg/kg decreased ($p < 0.05$) FSH levels by 42.9% and 34.3% respectively when administrated to rats. More so, a dose dependent decrease was obtained in PROG levels following the administration of 1000 mg/kg ($F_{(5.3, 28)} = 6.8$, $p < 13.1\%$), 2000 mg/kg ($F_{(2.2, 27)} = 0.88$, $p = 0.042$; 44.8%) and 3000 mg/kg ($p < 0.05$, 64%) respectively in treated animals. Similar decrease was observed with ESTRL at 1000, 2000 and 3000 mg/kg by 64.3%, 32.7% and 64% respectively. However, there were no changes observed in the PRL level in all rats.

Results in Table 1 show the effects of therapeutic and supra-therapeutic doses of CGV on oxidative stress parameters and antioxidant indices in rat testis. Lipid peroxidation, a biomarker of oxidative stress, measured as malondialdehyde (MDA) was unaltered given the therapeutic doses of CGV (14.3 and 28.6 mg/kg) when compared with control distilled water group as observed in this study. Similarly, given the supra-therapeutic doses of CGV, there was no significant alteration in MDA levels. Both doses of CGV, 14.3 mg/kg and 28.6 mg/kg, increased ($F_{(3, 30)} = 1.6$, $p < 0.061$) GSH (14.5% and 107%), SOD (121.6% and 54.5%), CAT (85.1% and 107.7%) and GST (44.1% and 16.9%) respectively when compared with control distilled water group. CGV at dose of 2000 mg/kg reduced GST activity by 35.1%. Furthermore, given 3000 mg/kg CGV, there was significantly reduced ($F_{(4, 22)} = 0.38$, $p < 0.05$) SOD (34.7%) and GST (44.4%) activities respectively.

Results in Table 2 show the effects of therapeutic and supra-therapeutic doses of CGV on oxidative stress parameters and antioxidant indices in rat ovaries. Lipid peroxidation, a biomarker of oxidative stress, measured

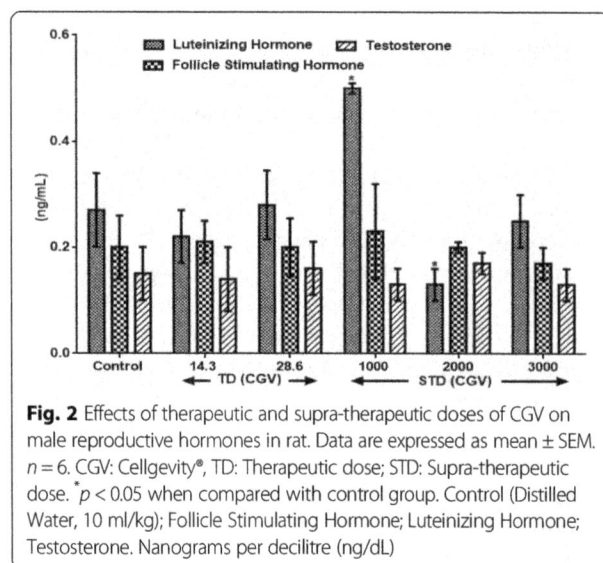

Fig. 2 Effects of therapeutic and supra-therapeutic doses of CGV on male reproductive hormones in rat. Data are expressed as mean ± SEM. $n = 6$. CGV: Cellgevity®, TD: Therapeutic dose; STD: Supra-therapeutic dose. $^{*}p < 0.05$ when compared with control group. Control (Distilled Water, 10 ml/kg); Follicle Stimulating Hormone; Luteinizing Hormone; Testosterone. Nanograms per decilitre (ng/dL)

Table 1 Effects of therapeutic and supra-therapeutic doses of CGV on antioxidant indices in rat testes

Treatment	GSH	SOD	CAT	GST	MDA
Control (DW, 10 ml/kg)	21.27 ± 0.98	1.67 ± 0.14	13.00 ± 0.95	5.4 ± 0.03	1.37 ± 0.02
14.3 mg/kg	24.35 ± 1.98 (− 14.5)	3.70 ± 0.16* (− 121.6)	24.06 ± 1.98*(− 85.1)	7.78 ± 0.52*(44.1)	1.12 ± 0.03 (18.2)
28.6 mg/kg	44.05 ± 1.24** (107.1)	2.58 ± 0.34*(− 54.5)	27.00 ± 1.04*(− 107.7)	6.31 ± 0.04(− 16.9)	1.17 ± 0.01 (14.6)
1000 mg/kg	24.58 ± 1.25 (− 15.6)	1.61 ± 0.33 (3.6)	14.81 ± 0.44 (− 13.9)	4.40 ± 0.09 (18.5)	1.36 ± 0.02 (0.7)
2000 mg/kg	20.48 ± 0.55 (3.7)	1.31 ± 0.02 (21.6)	14.51 ± 0.93(− 11.6)	3.50 ± 0.01*(35.1)	1.45 ± 0.01 (− 5.8)
3000 mg/kg	19.33 ± 0.68 (10)	1.09 ± 0.15* (34.7)	10.78 ± 0.95 (17.1)	3.00 ± 0.04* (44.4)	1.35 ± 0.05 (1.5)

Data are expressed as mean ± SEM. $n = 6$, * $p < 0.05$ or ** $p < 0.001$ when compared with control group. Values in parenthesis represent % change; (−) increase; (+) decrease. Control (Distilled Water, 10 ml/kg); Superoxide dismutase (µmol/mg protein), Catalase (µmol/min/mg protein), GST Glutathione S-transferase (µmol/ml/mg protein), MDA Malondialdehyde (nmol/mg protein), SOD Superoxide dismutase (µmol/mg protein); GSH Reduced glutathione (µmol/mg protein)

Table 2 Effects of therapeutic and supra-therapeutic doses of CGV on antioxidant indices in rat ovaries

Treatment	GSH	SOD	CAT	GST	MDA
Control	21.94 ± 1.77	17.9 ± 0.13	12.47 ± 1.46	6.3 ± 0.05	1.13 ± 0.02
14.3	$59.68 \pm 3.77^{**}$ (−172)	13.21 ± 1.06 (26.2)	$16.48 \pm 2.58^{*}$ (−32.2)	3.95 ± 1.15 (37.3)	1.13 ± 0.22 (0.0)
28.6	$61.72 \pm 5.19^{**}$ (−181.3)	13.78 ± 2.17 (23)	$16.89 \pm 1.04^{*}$ (−35.4)	3.98 ± 1.49 (36.8)	0.93 ± 0.13 (17.7)
1000	18.31 ± 1.00 (16.5)	13.9 ± 0.12 (22.3)	12.91 ± 0.67 (−3.5)	3.7 ± 0.03 (41.3)	$1.5 \pm 0.04^{*}$ (−32.7)
2000	21.62 ± 1.96 (1.5)	12.8 ± 0.12 (28.5)	12.54 ± 0.41 (−0.6)	3.4 ± 0.03 (46.0)	$1.45 \pm 0.04^{*}$ (−28.3)
3000	20.37 ± 1.51 (7.2)	16.0 ± 0.04 (10.6)	13.41 ± 0.47 (−7.5)	4.2 ± 0.01 (33.3)	$1.57 \pm 0.02^{*}$ (−38.9)

Data are expressed as mean ± SEM. $n = 6.$ $^{*}p < 0.05$ or $^{**}p < 0.001$ when compared with control group. Values in parenthesis represent % change; (−) increase; (+) decrease. Control (Distilled Water, 10 ml/kg); Superoxide dismutase; GSH Reduced glutathione (µmol/mg protein), SOD Superoxide dismutase (µmol/mg protein), Catalase (µmol/min/mg protein), GST Glutathione S-transferase (µmol/ml/mg protein), MDA Malondialdehyde (nmol/mg protein)

as malondialdehyde (MDA) was unaltered given the therapeutic doses of CGV (14.3 and 28.6 mg/kg) as observed in this study. However, at supra-therapeutic doses of 1000 mg/kg, 2000 mg/kg and 3000 mg/kg of CGV, an increased MDA of 32.7%, 28.3% and 38.9% were obtained respectively when compared with control animals. Interestingly, therapeutic but not supra-therapeutic doses of CGV improved GSH significantly ($F_{(5.5, 27)} = 0.74$, $p < 0.003$) by 172% and 181.3% respectively. Also, catalase levels given the 14.3 mg/kg, 28.6 mg/kg, 1000 mg/kg, 2000 mg/kg and 3000 mg/kg doses of CGV increased ($F_{(3.4, 30)} = 13.6$, $p < 0.315$) by 32.2%, 35.4%, 3.5%, 0.6% and 7.5% respectively in the treated rats. In contrast, SOD and GST activities were insignificantly decreased ($p > 0.05$) both at the therapeutic as well as supra-therapeutic doses of CGV in rats.

Results in Fig. 4 show the difference in body weight following therapeutic and supra-therapeutic CGV administration in male and female rats. The initial weight of the animals and final weight were compared and expressed as g/kg body weight. An administration of CGV doses of 1000 and 2000 mg/kg produce insignificant decreased ($F_{(2.6, 30)} = 13.1$, $p < 0.217$) body weight in rats of both sexes by 14.9%, 7.7% (male) and 23%, 10.7% (female) when compared with control distilled water group. However, at the maximum supra-therapeutic dose (3000 mg/kg) used in this study, there was decrease ($F_{(4.1, 28)} = 0.47$, $p < 0.05$) in male and female rats by 50% and 62.7% respectively in treated rats.

The effects of therapeutic and supra-therapeutic doses of CGV on serum biochemical indices in male rats were assessed (Table 3). Therapeutic doses of CGV did not cause any change in urea and creatinine levels. However,

3000 mg/kg dose of CGV increased ($F_{(5, 24)} = 0.06$, $p = 0.0036$) creatinine level by 99.1% when compared with control distilled water group. Also, neither serum total cholesterol nor triglycerides was altered following therapeutic and supra-therapeutic doses of CGV in treated rats. Both serum high density lipoprotein and low density lipoprotein remained unchanged in all animals. Alkaline aminotransferase level of treated rats was not significantly different from those of control distilled water group. In addition, serum total protein but not albumin levels was reduced ($F_{(5.6, 26)} = 0.89$, $p < 0.041$) by 60.1% (2000 mg/kg) and 57.2% (3000 mg/kg) respectively.

Results in Table 4 show the effects of therapeutic and supra-therapeutic doses of CGV on serum biochemical indices in Female Rats. The administration of CGV did not alter biochemical parameter levels of serum urea, total cholesterol, high density lipoprotein, alkaline phosphatase, albumin as well as total protein respectively. However, supra-therapeutic doses of CGV elevated ($F_{(3.8, 28)} = 0.12$, $p < 0.045$) creatinine levels by 72.2% (1000 mg/kg), 60.2% (2000 mg/kg) and 124.8% (3000) respectively. Similarly, 3000 mg/kg of CGV increased serum low density lipoprotein by 34.6% in treated rats.

Discussion

The demand for intake of antioxidant food or dietary antioxidant has increase in recent time with the hope to keep body healthy and free from diseases [37]. However, it is a great concern that people often take supplements containing antioxidants irrationally at higher doses than recommended. We reported the hypothesis that CGV which supposedly should provide a maximum antioxidant function by GSH synthesis rates and concentrations as expressed by the manufacturer could act as a pro-oxidant causing oxidative damage in normal humans particularly at the supra therapeutic doses following a subchronic administration in Wistar rats. Halliwell [38] describes antioxidant as any substance whose presence, even at low concentration may delays or inhibits the oxidation of a substrate. Antioxidant therapy exists long time ago and is still in the forefront of preventive medicine [39]. Taking into account the pro and cons of antioxidant enzymes on reproductive function and health, we cannot keep any longer our eyes closed on the potential adverse drug effects that could result from self-indulged overdose. CGV is a dietary supplementation of some key molecules, D-Ribose and L-Cysteine, which would increase intracellular GSH synthesis and concentrations and thus lower oxidative stress. Also, vitamin C, selenium, alpha lipoic, broccolli seed extract, curcumin, resveratrol, grape seed extract, quercetin, milk thistle seed extract, cordyceps, black pepper, aloe leaf are present to complement this effort

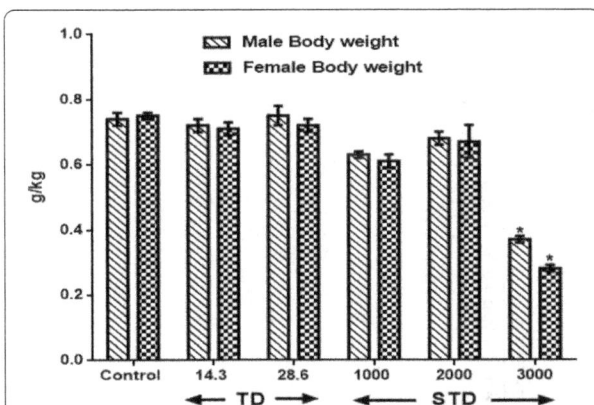

Fig. 4 Effect of therapeutic and supra-therapeutic doses of CGV on Body Weight of male and female rats after a subchronic administration for 60 days. Data are expressed as mean ± SEM. $n = 6$. CGV: Cellgevity®, TD: Therapeutic dose; STD: Supra-therapeutic dose. *$p < 0.05$ or **$p < 0.001$ when compared with control group. Control (Distilled Water, 10 ml/kg)

Table 3 Effects of therapeutic and supra-therapeutic doses of CGV On Serum Biochemical Indices in Male Rats

Treatment/ mg/kg	UREA (mg/l)	CREAT (mmol/l)	CHOL (mmol/l)	TG (mol/l)	HDL (mmol/l)	LDL (mmol/l)	ALP (U/l)	ALB (U/l)	TP (U/l)
Control	10.55 ± 0.86	4.43 ± 0.76	1.64 ± 0.09	0.91 ± 0.16	0.57 ± 0.05	0.35 ± 0.04	18.90 ± 1.82	27.52 ± 1.81	13.71 ± 0.02
14.3	10.10 ± 0.21 (4.3)	4.11 ± 1.04 (7.2)	1.44 ± 0.22 (12.2)	0.89 ± 0.07 (2.1)	0.58 ± 0.02 (−1.8)	0.33 ± 0.05 (5.7)	18.43 ± 2.02 (2.5)	26.25 ± 1.70 (4.6)	12.3 ± 0.47 (10.3)
28.6	10.90 ± 0.25 (3.3)	4.21 ± 1.03 (5.0)	1.38 ± 0.08 (15.9)	0.78 ± 0.11 (14.3)	0.52 ± 0.04 (8.8)	0.32 ± 0.03 (8.6)	18.06 ± 3.93 (4.4)	27.76 ± 2.05 (−0.9)	11.47 ± 0.15 (16.3)
1000	9.58 ± 0.28 (9.2)	3.65 ± 0.99 (17.6)	1.57 ± 0.12 (4.3)	0.76 ± 0.07 (16.5)	0.55 ± 0.02 (3.5)	0.35 ± 0.02 (0)	18.32 ± 3.02 (3.1)	30.55 ± 3.70 (11)	13.3 ± 1.47 (3)
2000	9.50 ± 0.69 (10.0)	4.95 ± 2.13 (−11.7)	1.57 ± 0.18 (4.3)	0.77 ± 0.11 (15.4)	0.59 ± 0.03 (−3.5)	0.37 ± 0.07 (−5.7)	17.66 ± 3.93 (6.6)	28.45 ± 3.05 (−3.4)	5.47 ± 0.25* (60.1)
3000	9.90 ± 0.80 (10.1)	8.82 ± 1.75* (−99.1)	1.61 ± 0.21 (1.8 s)	0.75 ± 0.07 (17.5)	0.56 ± 0.03 (1.8)	0.4 ± 0.08 (−14.3)	18.75 ± 1.8 (0.8)	28.50 ± 3.12 (−3.6)	5.87 ± 1.11* (57.2)

Data are expressed as mean ± SEM. $n = 6$. $^*p < 0.05$ or $^{**}p < 0.001$ when compared with control group. Values in parenthesis represent % change; (−) increase; (+) decrease. Control (Distilled Water, 10 ml/kg). CREA Creatinine, CHOL cholesterol, TG Triglycerides, HDL High density lipoprotein, LDL Low density lipoprotein, ALP Alkaline phosphatase, ALB Albumin, TP total protein

Table 4 Effects of therapeutic and supra-therapeutic doses of CGV On Serum Biochemical Parameters in Female Rats

Treatment/ mg/kg	UREA (mg/dl)	CREA (mmol/l)	CHOL (mmol/l)	TG (mol/l)	HDL (mmol/l)	LDL (mmol/l)	ALP (U/l)	ALB (U/l)	TP (U/l)
Control	9.47 ± 0.52	1.33 ± 0.40	1.31 ± 0.08	0.86 ± 0.06	0.58 ± 0.01	0.26 ± 0.04	16.18 ± 1.59	27.78 ± 1.60	9.72 ± 1.19
14.3	9.55 ± 0.42 (−0.8)	1.29 ± 0.21 (3.0)	1.36 ± 0.09 (−3.8)	0.87 ± 0.02 (−1.1)	0.55 ± 0.02 (5.2)	0.27 ± 0.04 (−3.8)	16.22 ± 1.78 (0.2)	31.03 ± 1.54 (−12.7)	9.93 ± 1.01 (−2.16)
28.6	9.16 ± 0.55 (−0.8)	1.13 ± 1.31 (15)	1.32 ± 0.02 (0.8)	0.77 ± 0.03 (10.5)	0.58 ± 0.03 (0)	0.28 ± 0.02 (−7.7)	16.30 ± 1.29 (−0.7)	30.44 ± 1.63 (−9.6)	10.46 ± 1.22 (−7.6)
1000	9.65 ± 0.32 (−2.17)	2.29 ± 0.27* (72.18)	1.46 ± 0.11 (−11.5)	0.68 ± 0.03 (20.9)	0.56 ± 0.01 (3.4)	0.29 ± 0.03 (−11.5)	16.22 ± 2.80 (−0.2)	33.43 ± 2.54 (20)	10.32 ± 1.21 0
2000	9.25 ± 0.78 (2.3)	2.13 ± 1.32* (60.2)	1.32 ± 0.03 (−0.8)	0.69 ± 0.04 (19.8)	0.59 ± 0.02 (−1.7)	0.27 ± 0.03 (−3.8)	16.30 ± 2.29 (−0.7)	30.25 ± 3.63 (−8.9)	11.36 ± 1.82 (−6.2)
3000	9.90 ± 0.21 (−4.5)	2.99 ± 2.07* (−124.8)	1.57 ± 0.09 (−19.8)	0.72 ± 0.03 (16.3)	0.57 ± 0.01 (1.7)	0.35 ± 0.03* (34.6)	15.42 ± 1.44 (4.7)	29.98 ± 3.02 (−7.9)	11.08 ± 1.25 (−14.0)

Data are expressed as mean ± SEM. n = 6. $^*p < 0.05$ or $^{**}p < 0.001$ when compared with control group. Values in parenthesis represent % change; (−) increase; (+) decrease. Control (Distilled Water, 10 ml/kg). CREA Creatinine, CHOL cholesterol, TG Triglycerides, HDL High density lipoprotein, LDL Low density lipoprotein, ALP Alkaline phosphatase, ALB Albumin, TP total protein

[40]. Glutathione, the most abundant endogenous intracellular antioxidant, plays a central role in antioxidant defenses, and irreversible cell damage supervenes when the cell is unable to maintain intracellular glutathione concentrations [41]. However, reduction in intake of antioxidant substances may increase the chance of oxidative stress which may lead to cell damage [42]. Therefore, intake of such natural antioxidants may give protective effect against free radical induced diseases. Some reports have suggested that concentrations of glutathione decline with aging and in disease conditions [43, 44]. Also, the mechanisms of glutathione deficiency in relation to aging have been documented and have been suggested to be associated with an increased pro-oxidizing shift and elevated oxidative stress [45]. Still, how GSH could act as a pro-oxidant molecule is not well understood.

Vitamin C is vitally needed for cellular collagen [46] and neurotransmitters biosynthesis and plays important antioxidant defense against atherogenic, carcinogenic substance and neurodegeneration [47]. Selenium utilizes glutathione peroxidase to carry out an antioxidant function [48]. Thus, CGV which contains selenium could modulate the functional ability of selenoproteins. Broccoli contains much health promoting phytochemicals including glucosinolates with chemopreventive activity against cancer as well as having antioxidant properties [49]. More so, alpha lipoic acid is present naturally in edible meats, spinach, broccoli, potatoes, yams, carrots, beets, and even yeast [50]. It has a potent thiol-containing antioxidant and may contribute to the development of cardiovascular risk factors [51]. Alpha lipoic acid is actively involved in free radicals turnover, arrest inflammation and promote actions of endothelial relaxing factor in vesicles and endothelium [52]. Curcumin, resveratrol, grape seed extract, quercetin, milk thistle seed extract, cordyceps, black pepper, aloe leaf have been documented for antioxidants [53]. From the results obtained in our study, therapeutic doses of CGV neither alter sperm motility nor counts when compared with control group. However, in contrast, supra-therapeutic administration reduced sperm motility as well as sperm counts. Spermatozoa possess primarily enzymatic antioxidants, with superoxide dismutase being the most predominant [54]. Dietary antioxidants are usually present in the form of vitamins, carotenoids, and flavonoids. Metal-binding proteins such as albumin, ceruloplasmin, metallothionein, transferrin, ferritin, and myoglobin function by inactivating transition metal ions that otherwise would have catalyzed the production of free radicals [55]. In addition, CGV supra-therapeutic indication enhances abnormality of sperm cells and demonstrated such tendency to influence

body hormones as observed in our results. CGV increases luteinizing and follicle stimulating hormones at the lowest supra-therapeutic dose employed in this study, although, this was reversed as the doses increases. This lack of effects due to higher doses of CGV could results from a saturation activity at lower doses, although, we did not assess the neuroendocrine effects of CGV. However, such feedback mechanisms could implicate some unidentifiable regions in the brain playing pro-antioxidant roles to supra-therapeutic dosing which may require further investigations. CGV showed increased LH at 1000 mg/kg while it shows decreased at higher doses of 2000 and 3000 mg/kg by 51.85% and 7.4% respectively when compared with control.

On the other hand, follicle stimulating hormone remained unaltered given a supra-therapeutic CGV administration. Also, all the supra-therapeutic doses of CGV used in this study did not significantly alter testosterone levels in rats. In female animals, increasing the doses of CGV supra-therapeutically could elevate luteinizing hormone level, whereas such an increase of the same would decrease follicle stimulating hormone level as seen in this study. Also, a similar but dose dependent decrease was obtained in progesterone levels following supra-therapeutic dosing of CGV, whereas, a decrease was observed with estrogen while prolactin remains unperturbed compared with control rats. Although, evidences to support the roles of antioxidants on hormonal regulations are available, however, it may require a chronic administration in order to appreciate the modulatory roles of CGV in this process. The effects of therapeutic and supra-therapeutic doses of CGV on oxidative stress parameters and antioxidant indices in rats were assessed. In rats of both sexes, lipid peroxidation, a biomarker of oxidative stress, measured as malondialdehyde (MDA) was unaltered given the therapeutic doses of CGV when compared with control in this study. Similarly, given the supra-therapeutic doses of CGV, there was no alteration in MDA levels. Pro-oxidants are chemical compounds capable of generating potential toxic oxygen species. Although, a normal cell has an appropriate pro-oxidant–antioxidant balance, however, this balance can be shifted which may not favour the antioxidant system or when levels of antioxidants are diminished [45]. These may result in oxidative stress in which molecular signaling is altered. At this point, since supra-therapeutic doses were ineffective to produce oxidative stress, a very high dose of CGV given for a long period of time may be required. There have been positive correlations between total activities of reduced glutathione, catalase, superoxide dismutase and glutathione peroxidase with total content of MDA in seminal plasma from normozoospermic samples [56]. However, antioxidant enzyme activities were modulated by CGV. For instance, in male rats that were administered supra-therapeutic doses, an increased GSH level was obtained in addition to elevated SOD and CAT activities. Highest doses of CGV reduced GST activity in treated rats. However, at supra-therapeutic doses of CGV administration, MDA levels were elevated. In contrast, SOD and GST activities were slightly reduced both at the therapeutic as well as supra-therapeutic doses of CGV in rats. There are studies to show that numerous cellular processes such as gene expression can influence changes in redox balance where moderate reactive oxygen and reactive nitrogen species production can lead to alterations in cellular and extracellular redox state [57]. This can cause alterations that may signal changes in cell functions. There are chances as obtained in our results that CGV could alter reproductive function in experimental animals. Evidences abound of lowered antioxidant levels in infertile patients suggesting their relationship to male infertility [58]. The difference in body weight following of CGV administration in male and female rats was investigated. CGV supra-therapeutic dosing insignificantly decreased body weight in rats compared

with control group. However, at the maximum supra-therapeutic dose used in this study, there was decrease in treated rats of both sexes. A supra-therapeutic 3000 mg/kg dose of CGV increases creatinine level in treated male rats. Also, serum total protein in male animals was reduced (2000 and 3000 mg/kg) in the treated male rats while an elevated low density lipoprotein (3000 mg/kg) was obtained in female animals. However, serum alkaline aminotransferase, total cholesterol triglycerides, albumin, and high density remained unchanged in all animals following therapeutic and supra-therapeutic administrations. CGV administrations seem to modulate biochemical parameters in rats, although, a chronic toxicological administration may be required in order to comments on the possible long term outcome. Histological sections (Figs. 5, 6, 7, 8, 9 and 10) show seminiferous tubules with reduced spermatogenic series with 2000 and 3000 mg/kg respectively (Fig. 5). Also, female rat kidney revealed acute tubular necrosis at highest dose used in this study (Fig. 8). As observed in this study, CGV supra-therapeutic applications could trigger some effects similar to those of pro-oxidants affecting reproductive and antioxidant system. In this current study, we were unable to explore the nueroendocrine effects of supra-therapeutic doses of CGV. More so, direct extrapolation of these findings may be difficult due to physiological differences between rodent and humans.

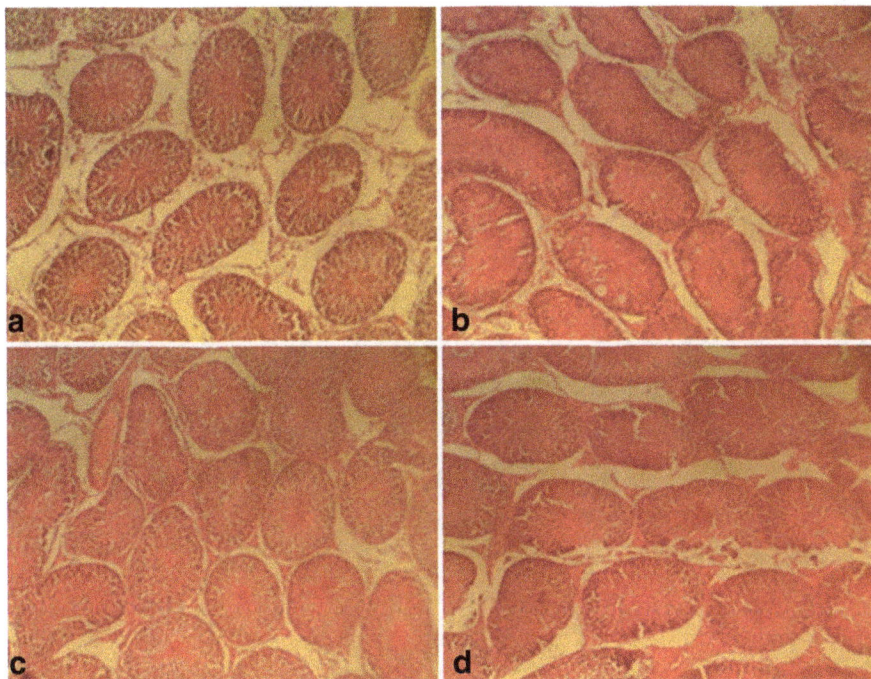

Fig. 5 Male rat testes. Control shows normal testes (distilled water, 10 ml/kg) (**a**), 1000mg/kg CGV shows seminiferous tubules with reduced spermatogenic series (**b**), 2000mg/kg CGV seminiferous tubules with reduced spermatogenic series (**c**), 3000mg/kg CGV seminiferous tubules with reduced spermatogenic series (**d**). (H & E, × 400) (CGV: Cellgevity®)

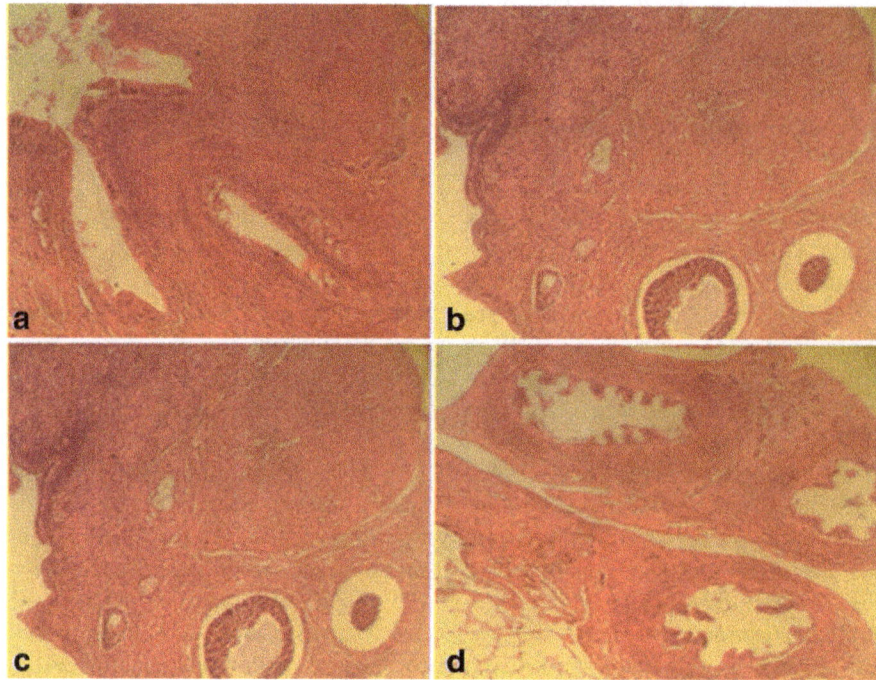

Fig. 6 Female rat ovaries. Control shows normal ovaries (distilled water, 10 ml/kg) (**a**), 1000mg/kg CGV shows normal ovaries (**b**), 2000mg/kg CGV shows normal ovaries (**c**), 3000mg/kg CGV shows normal ovaries (**d**). (H & E, × 400) (CGV: Cellgevity®)

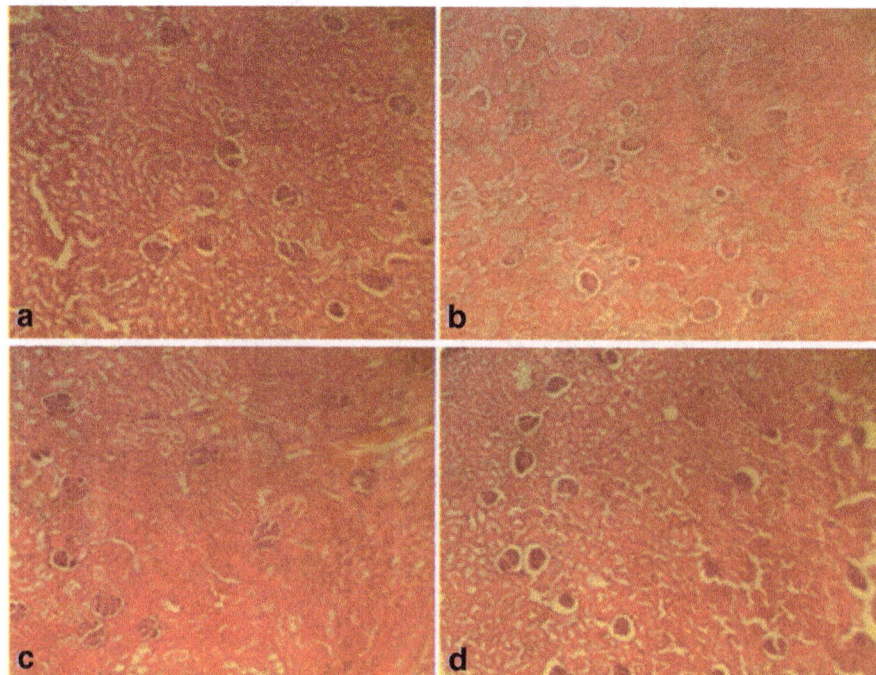

Fig. 7 Male rat kidney. Control shows normal kidney (distilled water, 10 ml/kg) (**a**), 1000mg/kg CGV shows normal kidney (**b**), 2000mg/kg CGV shows normal kidney (**c**), 3000mg/kg CGV shows normal kidney (**d**). (H & E, × 400) (CGV: Cellgevity®)

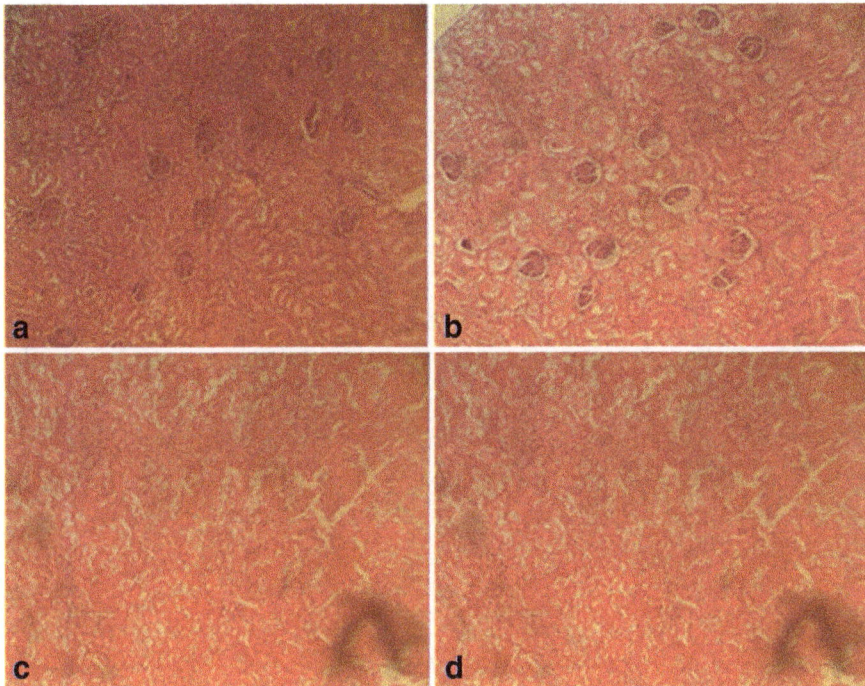

Fig. 8 Female rat kidney. Control shows normal kidney (distilled water, 10 ml/kg) (**a**), 1000mg/kg CGV shows normal kidney (**b**), 2000mg/kg CGV shows normal kidney (**c**), 3000mg/kg CGV shows acute tubular necrosis kidney (**d**). (H & E, × 400) (CGV: Cellgevity®)

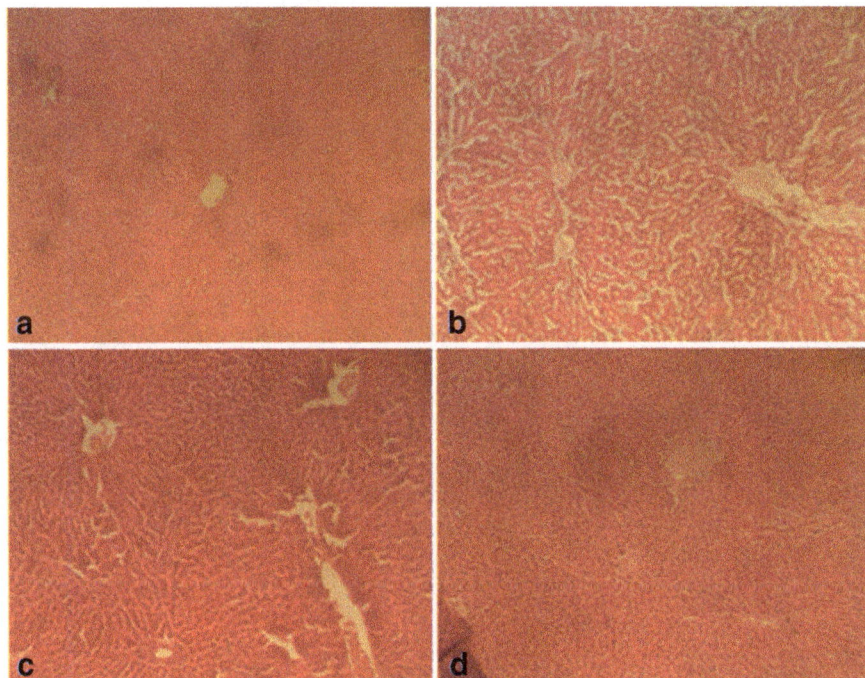

Fig. 9 Male rat liver. Control shows normal liver (distilled water, 10 ml/kg) (**a**), 1000mg/kg CGV shows normal liver (**b**), 2000mg/kg CGV shows normal liver (**c**), 3000mg/kg CGV shows normal liver (**d**). (H & E, × 400) (CGV: Cellgevity®)

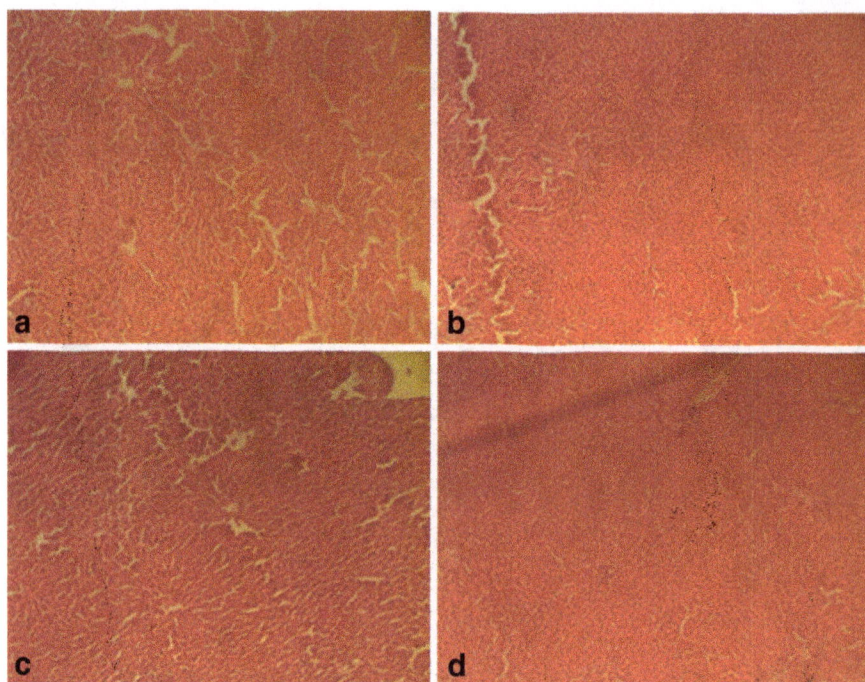

Fig. 10 Female rat liver. Control shows normal liver (distilled water, 10 ml/kg) (**a**), 1000mg/kg CGV shows normal liver (**b**), 2000mg/kg CGV shows normal liver (**c**), 3000mg/kg CGV shows normal liver (**d**). (H & E, × 400) (CGV: Cellgevity®)

Conclusion

Overall, our data further affirmed that CGV is an anti-oxidant supplement at therapeutic doses. However, the effects on reproductive and biochemical parameters at therapeutic doses are relatively safe during a subchronic administration, although, the pro-oxidant potential of the supra-therapeutic CGV doses was evident as observed is this present study. Hence, it is necessary that its administration be done with caution.

Abbreviations
CGV: Cellgevity®; ELISA: Enzyme-linked immunosorbent assay; GSH: Reduced glutathione

Acknowledgements
The technical assistance of Mr. Chijioke M. of the Department of Pharmacology, Therapeutics and Toxicology, College of Medicine, University of Lagos, Nigeria, is gratefully acknowledged.

Funding
This research was self-funded. This research was solely funded by AO, BWA, BAA, KOE, ATB, URO, and EPM respectively.

Authors' contributions
AO designed and coordinated all laboratory experiments. BWA, BAA, KOE, ATB and URO conducted all experiments. AO, BWA, BAA and KOE performed the statistical analysis while AO, BWA, BAA, KOE, ATB, URO and EPM interpreted the results and wrote the manuscript. Additionally, AO, BWA, BAA, KOE, ATB, URO and EPM read and approved the manuscript.

Competing interests
This research received no specific grant from any funding agency in the public, commercial, or not-for-profit sectors. The authors declare that they have no competing interests.

Author details
[1]Toxicology Unit, Department of Pharmacology, Therapeutics and Toxicology, College of Medicine, University of Lagos, PMB 12003, Idi-Araba Campus, Lagos, Nigeria. [2]Department of Pharmaceutical Sciences, College of Pharmacy, King Faisal University Hofuf, Hofuf, Kingdom of Saudi Arabia.

References
1. Cheung CK, Wyman JF, Halcon LL. Use of complementary and alternative therapies in community-dwelling older adults. J Altern Complement Med. 2007;13(9):997–1006.
2. Udo IA, Festus A. Concomitant use of dietary supplements and orthodox medicines among primary care patients due to non-communication with physicians in a tertiary hospital in Uyo. Eur J Biol Med Sci Res. 2016;4(2):1–10.

3. Nagasawa HT, inventor; Max International, Llc, assignee. Method to enhance delivery of glutathione and atp levels in cells. United States patent application US 14/838,274; 2015. p. 27.

4. Pokorný J. Are natural antioxidants better–and safer–than synthetic antioxidants? Eur J Lipid Sci Technol. 2007;109(6):629–42.

5. Finley JW, Kong AN, Hintze KJ, Jeffery EH, Ji LL, Lei XG. Antioxidants in foods: state of the science important to the food industry. J Agric Food Chem. 2011;59(13):6837–46.

6. Kale OE, Akinpelu OB, Bakare AA, Yusuf FO, Gomba R, Araka DC, Ogundare TO, Okolie AC, Adebawo O, Odutola O. Five traditional Nigerian Polyherbal remedies protect against high fructose fed, Streptozotocin-induced type 2 diabetes in male Wistar rats. BMC Complement Altern Med. 2018;18(1):160.

7. Mosley RL, Benner EJ, Kadiu I, Thomas M, Boska MD, Hasan K, Laurie C, Gendelman HE. Neuroinflammation, oxidative stress, and the pathogenesis of Parkinson's disease. Clin Neurosci Res. 2006;6(5):261–81.

8. Tong L, Li K, Zhou Q. The association between air pollutants and morbidity for diabetes and liver diseases modified by sexes, ages, and seasons in Tianjin, China. Environ Sci Pollut Res. 2015;22(2):1215–9.

9. Biswas S, Chida AS, Rahman I. Redox modifications of protein–thiols: emerging roles in cell signaling. Biochem Pharmacol. 2006;71(5):551–64.

10. Ray PD, Huang BW, Tsuji Y. Reactive oxygen species (ROS) homeostasis and redox regulation in cellular signaling. Cell Signal. 2012;24(5):981–90.

11. Dalle-Donne I, Rossi R, Colombo G, Giustarini D, Milzani A. Protein S-glutathionylation: a regulatory device from bacteria to humans. Trends Biochem Sci. 2009;34(2):85–96.

12. Ortega AL, Mena S, Estrela JM. Glutathione in cancer cell death. Cancers. 2011;3(1):1285–310.

13. Mattson MP, Shea TB. Folate and homocysteine metabolism in neural plasticity and neurodegenerative disorders. Trends Neurosci. 2003;26(3):137–46.

14. Dubey S, Shri M, Misra P, Lakhwani D, Bag SK, Asif MH, Trivedi PK, Tripathi RD, Chakrabarty D. Heavy metals induce oxidative stress and genome-wide modulation in transcriptome of rice root. Funct Integr Genomics. 2014;14(2):401–17.

15. Nobili S, Lippi D, Witort E, Donnini M, Bausi L, Mini E, Capaccioli S. Natural compounds for cancer treatment and prevention. Pharmacol Res. 2009;59(6):365–78.

16. Fulda S. Modulation of apoptosis by natural products for cancer therapy. Planta Med. 2010;76(11):1075–9.

17. Calixto JB. Efficacy, safety, quality control, marketing and regulatory guidelines for herbal medicines (phytotherapeutic agents). Braz J Med Biol Res. 2000;33(2):179–89.

18. Kale OE, Awodele O. Safety evaluation of bon-santé cleanser® polyherbal in male Wistar rats. BMC Complement Altern Med. 2016;16(1):188.

19. Kilkenny C, Browne W, Cuthill IC, Emerson M, Altman DG. Animal research: reporting in vivo experiments—the ARRIVE guidelines. J Cereb Blood Flow Metab. 2011;31(4):991.

20. Varshney R, Kale RK. Effects of calmodulin antagonists on radiation-induced lipid peroxidation in microsomes. Int J Radiat Biol. 1990;58(5):733–43.

21. Beutler E. Improved method for determination of blood glutathione. J Lab Clin Med. 1963;61(5):882–8.

22. Habig WH, Pabst MJ, Jakoby WB. Glutathione S-transferases the first enzymatic step in mercapturic acid formation. J Biol Chem. 1974;249(22):7130–9.

23. Misra HP, Fridovich I. The role of superoxide anion in the autoxidation of epinephrine and a simple assay for superoxide dismutase. J Biol Chem. 1972 May 25;247(10):3170–5.

24. Sinha AK. Colorimetric assay of catalase. Anal Biochem. 1972;47(2):389–94.

25. Odell WD, Parlow AF, Cargille CM, Ross GT. Radioimmunoassay for human follicle—stimulating hormone: physiological studies. J Clin Investig. 1968;47(12):2551.

26. Joshi UM, Shah HP, Sudhama SP. A sensitive and specific enzymeimmunoassay for serum testosterone. Steroids. 1979;34(1):35–46.

27. Abraham GE, Swerdloff R, Tulchinsky DA, Odell WD. Radioimmunoassay of plasma progesterone. J Clin Endocrinol Metab 1971;32(5):619–24.

28. Roy AV. Rapid method for determining alkaline phosphatase activity in serum with thymolphthalein monophosphate. Clin Chem. 1970;16(5):431–6.

29. Fossati P, Prencipe L, Berti G. Use of 3, 5-dichloro-2-hydroxybenzenesulfonic acid/4-aminophenazone chromogenic system in direct enzymic assay of uric acid in serum and urine. Clin Chem. 1980;26(2):227–31.

30. Skeggs LT. An automatic method for colorimetric analysis. Am J Clin Pathol. 1957;28:311–22.

31. Doumas BT, Watson WA, Biggs HG. Albumin standards and the measurement of serum albumin with bromcresol green. Clin Chim Acta. 1971;31(1):87–96.

32. Fossati P, Prencipe L, Berti G. Enzymic creatinine assay: a new colorimetric method based on hydrogen peroxide measurement. Clin Chem. 1983;29(8):1494–6.

33. Trinder P. Quantitative determination of triglyceride using GPO-PAP method. Ann Biochem. 1969;6:24–7.

34. Warnick GR, Albers JJ. A comprehensive evaluation of the heparin-manganese precipitation procedure for estimating high density lipoprotein cholesterol. J Lipid Res. 1978;19(1):65–76.

35. Friedewald WT, Levy RI, Fredrickson DS. Estimation of the concentration of low-density lipoprotein cholesterol in plasma, without use of the preparative ultracentrifuge. Clin Chem. 1972;18(6):499–502.

36. OECD. OECD guidelines for testing of chemicals. No 420: Acute Oral Toxicity-fixed Dose Method. Paris: Organisation for Economic Co-operation and Development; 1992.

37. Rajendran P, Nandakumar N, Rengarajan T, Palaniswami R, Gnanadhas EN, Lakshminarasaiah U, Gopas J, Nishigaki I. Antioxidants and human diseases. Clin Chim Acta. 2014;436:332–47.

38. Halliwell B. Reactive oxygen species in living systems: source, biochemistry, and role in human disease. Am J Med. 1991;91(3):S14–22.

39. Bryan NS. Pharmacological therapies, lifestyle choices and nitric oxide deficiency: a perfect storm. Pharmacol Res. 2012;66(6):448–56.

40. Nagasawa HT, Bagley D, Momii S, Nagasawa S. US Patent Application No 14/235; 2012. p. 152.

41. Costa VM, Carvalho F, Bastos ML, Carvalho RA, Carvalho M, Remião F. Contribution of catecholamine reactive intermediates and oxidative stress to the pathologic features of heart diseases. Curr Med Chem. 2010;18(15):2272–314.

42. Valko M, Rhodes C, Moncol J, Izakovic MM, Mazur M. Free radicals, metals and antioxidants in oxidative stress-induced cancer. Chem Biol Interact. 2006;160(1):1–40.

43. Sohal RS, Weindruch R. Oxidative stress, caloric restriction, and aging. Science (New York, NY). 1996;273(5271):59.

44. Dröge W, Schipper HM. Oxidative stress and aberrant signaling in aging and cognitive decline. Aging Cell. 2007;6(3):361–70.

45. Finkel T, Holbrook NJ. Oxidants, oxidative stress and the biology of ageing. Nature. 2000;408(6809):239–47.

46. Al-Gubory KH, Fowler PA, Garrel C. The roles of cellular reactive oxygen species, oxidative stress and antioxidants in pregnancy outcomes. Int J Biochem Cell Biol. 2010;42(10):1634–50.

47. Naidu KA. Vitamin C in human health and disease is still a mystery? An overview. Nutr J. 2003;2(1):7.

48. Burk RF. Selenium, an antioxidant nutrient. Nutr Clin Care. 2002;5(2):75–9.

49. Dillard CJ, German JB. Phytochemicals: nutraceuticals and human health. J Sci Food Agric. 2000;80(12):1744–56.

50. Gorąca A, Huk-Kolega H, Piechota A, Kleniewska P, Ciejka E, Skibska B. Lipoic acid–biological activity and therapeutic potential. Pharmacol Rep. 2011;63(4):849–58.

51. Packer L, Witt EH, Tritschler HJ. Alpha-lipoic acid as a biological antioxidant. Free Radic Biol Med. 1995;19(2):227–50.

52. Valko M, Jomova K, Rhodes CJ, Kuča K, Musílek K. Redox-and non-redox-metal-induced formation of free radicals and their role in human disease. Arch Toxicol. 2016;90(1):1–37.

53. Li Y, Ding Y. Minireview: therapeutic potential of myricetin in diabetes mellitus. Food Sci Human Wellness. 2012;1(1):19–25.

54. Sikka SC. Relative impact of oxidative stress on male reproductive function. Curr Med Chem. 2001;8(7):851–62.

55. Halliwell B. Commentary oxidative stress, nutrition and health. Experimental strategies for optimization of nutritional antioxidant intake in humans. Free Radic Res. 1996;25(1):57–74.

56. Ben Abdallah F, Dammak I, Attia H, Hentati B, Ammar-Keskes L. Lipid peroxidation and antioxidant enzyme activities in infertile men: correlation with semen parameter. J Clin Lab Anal. 2009;23(2):99–104.

57. Seifried HE, Anderson DE, Fisher EI, Milner JA. A review of the interaction among dietary antioxidants and reactive oxygen species. J Nutr Biochem. 2007;18(9):567–79.

58. Pasqualotto FF, Sharma RK, Nelson DR, Thomas AJ, Agarwal A. Relationship between oxidative stress, semen characteristics, and clinical diagnosis in men undergoing infertility investigation. Fertil Steril. 2000;73(3):459–64.

19

Purification, characterization and immunogenicity assessment of glutaminase free L-asparaginase from *Streptomyces brollosae* NEAE-115

Noura El-Ahmady El-Naggar[1]* (iD), Sahar F. Deraz[2], Sara M. El-Ewasy[1] and Ghada M. Suddek[3]

Abstract

Background: L-asparaginase is a potential therapeutic enzyme widely used in the chemotherapy protocols of pediatric and adult patients with acute lymphoblastic leukemia. However, its use has been limited by a high rate of hypersensitivity in the long-term used. Hence, there is a continuing need to search for other L-asparaginase sources capable of producing an enzyme with less adverse effects.

Methods: Production of extracellular L-asparaginase by *Streptomyces brollosae* NEAE-115 was carried out using submerged fermentation. L-asparaginase was purified by ammonium sulphate precipitation and pure enzyme was reached using ion-exchange chromatography, followed by enzyme characterization. Anticancer activity towards Ehrlich Ascites Carcinoma (EAC) cells was investigated in female Swiss albino mice by determination of tumor size and the degree of tumor growth inhibition. The levels of anti-L-asparaginase IgG antibodies in mice sera were measured using ELISA method.

Results: The purified L-asparaginase showed a total activity of 795.152 with specific activity of 76.671 U/mg protein and 7.835 – purification fold. The enzyme purity was confirmed by using SDS–PAGE separation which revealed only one distinctive band with a molecular weight of 67 KDa. The enzyme showed maximum activity at pH 8.5, optimum temperature of 37 °C, incubation time of 50 min and optimum substrate concentration of 7 mM. A Michaelis-Menten constant analysis showed a K_m value of 2.139×10^{-3} M with L-asparagine as substrate and V_{max} of 152.6 $UmL^{-1} min^{-1}$. The half-life time ($T_{1/2}$) was 65.02 min at 50°C, while being 62.65 min at 60°C. Furthermore, mice treated with *Streptomyces brollosae* NEAE-115 L-asparaginase showed higher cytotoxic effect (79% tumor growth inhibition) when compared to commercial L-asparaginase group (67% tumor growth inhibition).

Conclusions: The study reveals the excellent property of this enzyme which makes it highly valuable for development of chemotherapeutic drug.

Keywords: *Streptomyces brollosae* NEAE-115, L-asparaginase, Purification, DEAE Sepharose CL-6B, Characterization, Immunogenicity assessment

* Correspondence: nouraelahmady@yahoo.com
[1]Department of Bioprocess Development, Genetic Engineering and Biotechnology Research Institute, City of Scientific Research and Technological Applications, Alexandria, Egypt
Full list of author information is available at the end of the article

Background

L-asparaginase (EC 3.5.1.1) is the enzyme that catalyzes the hydrolysis of L-asparagine to L-aspartic acid and ammonia. The leukemic cells cannot synthesize L-asparagine due the absence of L-asparagine synthetase [1]. "These cells require huge amount of L-asparagine and rely on the exogenous sources for their proliferation and survival. Thus, intravenously injection of L-asparaginase in cancer patients destroys the exogenous L-asparagine and results in depletion of L-asparagine in the blood. L-asparagine starvation affecting selectively the tumor cells, since they are unable to complete protein synthesis [2]". On the contrary, normal cells are protected from L-asparagine starvation due to their ability to synthesize this amino acid which is essential for both cell survival and protein synthesis [3]. Hence, in combination therapy of children acute lymphoblastic leukemia (ALL), L-asparaginase is considered as the effective drug of choice [4, 5]. In addition, L-asparaginase is significantly used for the treatment of other malignant disorders including lymphosarcoma, acute lymphoblastic leukemia, chronic lymphocytic leukemia, acute myelomonocytic leukemia, acute myelocytic leukemia, Hodgkin disease, melanosarcoma and reticulosarcoma [6].

Currently, two formulations of L-asparaginases are effectively in clinical use for ALL treatments, one from *Erwinia chrysanthemi* and the other from *E. coli*. However, its therapeutic long-term use leads to unpleasant side effects as a result of exerting normal cells toxicity, patient's hypersensitivity and the rapid clearance of the enzyme from the blood stream which limited its administration. Clinical uses indicate that the L-asparaginases toxicity is mainly resulted from enzyme glutaminase activity and bacterial endotoxins in enzyme preparations [7]. Hepatotoxicity is the important adverse effect in the majority of patients [8], L-asparaginase causes a wide spectrum of side effects, such as skin rashes, fever, hepatic dysfunction, leucopoenia, pancreatitis, diabetes, neurological seizures and abnormal coagulation tests that may lead to intracranial thrombosis or haemorrhage [3]. L-asparaginase purification consider as an essential step for its physical and biological characterization. Moreover, for effective therapeutic administration with less adverse effects, L-asparaginase preparation must be free of any contaminants and impurities which also required efficient purification step.

In an attempt to minimize the allergenic reactions caused by impurities, enormous numbers of research groups have achieved production and purification of L-asparaginase [9]. Manivasagan et al. [10] reported that actinomycetes have been recognized to be a good source for L-asparaginase production, in particular *Streptomyces* species which are responsible for providing almost half of the useful drugs of bioactive secondary metabolites, especially antibiotics followed by enzymes and anti cancer agents. Several *Streptomyces* species have been explored for L-asparaginase production such as *Streptomyces parvus* NEAE-95 [11], *Streptomyces olivaceus* NEAE-119 [12] and *Streptomyces gulbargensis* [13]. The aim of the present work is the purification, characterization and immunogenicity assessment of an extracellular L-asparaginase produced under submerged fermentation from *Streptomyces brollosae* NEAE-115.

Methods

Microorganisms and cultural conditions

Soil samples collected from different areas in Egypt "Mansoura city, Damietta city, north western coast of Egypt from New Borg El-Arab to El Saloum, Janaklis (Beheira) and Brollos Lake" and three soil samples collected from Taif in Saudi Arabia were used for the isolation of actinomycetes, mainly *Streptomyces* spp. *Streptomyces brollosae* NEAE-115 was isolated from soil sample collected from Brollos Lake at the Mediterranean coast of Egypt. *Streptomyces* spp. had been isolated from the soil using standard dilution plate method on starch nitrate agar medium containing the following constituents (g/L): Starch, 20; $CaCO_3$, 3; $MgSO_4.7H_2O$, 0.5; KNO_3, 2; NaCl, 0.5; K_2HPO_4, 1; $FeSO_4.7H_2O$, 0.01; agar, 20. The incubation was carried at 30 °C for a period of 7 days. The obtained isolates of *Streptomyces* were purified and stored as spore suspensions in 20% (*v/v*) glycerol at − 20 °C for subsequent investigation.

Screening of L-asparaginase production by plate assay method

According to De Jong [14], an increase in the culture filtrates pH is accompanied by L-asparaginase production. All actinomycetes isolates were tested for their abilities to produce L-asparaginase using plates containing asparagine dextrose salts agar (ADS agar) medium [15]. The constituents of the ADS agar medium were (%): L-asparagine 1.0; K_2HPO_4 0.1; $MgSO_4$ 0.05; dextrose 0.2; agar 1.5, pH was adjusted to 6.8–7. The medium was incorporated with pH indicator (phenol red, 0.009% w/v) prepared in ethanol according to the procedure of Gulati et al. [16]. The actinomycetes isolates were inoculated on ADS agar plates and incubated at 30 °C for 7 days. The formation of a pink zone around the microbial colonies due to change of pH was considered as a positive result for L-asparaginase production . Two control plates were prepared one was uninoculated medium while the other was without dye. The more potent isolate exhibiting L-asparaginase activity was selected for further study.

Inoculum preparation

Three disks (8 mm each) were taken from old stock culture grown on starch nitrate agar medium for 7 days and inoculated into 50 mL of asparagine dextrose salts broth containing (%): L-asparagine 1.0; K_2HPO_4 0.1; dextrose 0.2; $MgSO_4$ 0.05. The inoculated 250 mL

Erlenmeyer flasks were grown at 30 °C and 150 rpm for 48 h and cultured medium was further used for subsequent experiments.

Production of L-asparaginase by submerged fermentation

The production of extracellular L-asparaginase from *Streptomyces brollosae* NEAE-115 was carried using the medium containing (g/L): Dextrose 2, starch 20, L-asparagine 10, KNO_3 1, K_2HPO_4 1, $MgSO_4.7H_2O$ 0.5, NaCl 0.1, pH 7. Fifty mL of the broth medium was dispensed in 250 mL Erlenmeyer conical flask. The inoculated flasks (with inoculum size of 4%, *v/v*) were incubated on a rotary shaker incubator at 150 rpm and 30 °C. After 7 days of incubation time, the broth was centrifuged with cooling centrifuge at 6000×*g* for 30 min at 4 °C and the clear supernatant served as crude enzyme.

Assay of L-asparaginase activity

Extracellular L-asparaginase activity was determined according to the method of Wriston and Yellin [17] using nesslerization to measure the amount of liberated ammonia. The reaction mixture containing 1.5 mL of 0.04 M L-asparagine prepared in 0.05 M Tris-HCl buffer, pH 8.6 and 0.5 mL of the enzyme to make up the total volume to 2 mL. The tubes were incubated at 37 °C for 30 min. The reaction was terminated by the addition of 0.5 mL of 1.5 M trichloroacetic acid (TCA). The blank was run by adding TCA followed by enzyme preparation. To remove the precipitated protein, the reaction contents were centrifuged at 10,000×*g* for 5 min and the filtrate was collected. For quantification of liberated ammonia, 0.5 mL filtrate was diluted to 7 mL with distilled water and 1 mL Nessler's reagent was added to the resulting mixture. The color reaction was allowed to proceed for 20 min before measuring the absorbance at 480 nm using Optizen Pop –UV/Vis spectrophotometer. A coloration of yellow indicates the presence of ammonia. However, a brown precipitate is formed at higher concentrations. The amount of liberated ammonia by the test sample was calculated by comparing the absorbance with a standard curve prepared from solutions of ammonium chloride as the ammonia source. One unit (U) of L-asparaginase is the amount of enzyme which generates 1μmole of ammonia in 1 min at 37 °C and pH 8.6.

Assay of L-glutaminase

L-glutaminase activity was determined using L-glutamine as substrate according to Imada et al. [18] method and the released ammonia was measured by using Nesseler's reagent.

Purification of L-asparaginase from *Streptomyces brollosae* NEAE-115

The crude enzyme extract used in L-asparaginase purification was obtained from production medium centrifuged at 6000×*g* for 30 min and the resulted supernatant was transferred into a conical flask placed in ice cold condition with stirring. Finely powdered ammonium sulfate was added until complete dissolving takes place to give 45% saturation with ammonium sulphate and kept overnight in the refrigerator at 4 °C. The precipitate was collected by centrifugation at 11000×g for 30 min, while the supernatant was brought to 55–85% saturation with ammonium sulphate. Then, the formed precipitates were separately collected by centrifugation and dissolved in 50 mM Tris-HCl buffer pH 8.4. The dialysis of the ammonium sulphate was carried out in a pre-treated dialysis tube. Precipitate formed during dialysis was removed by centrifugation and was discarded. For the present study dialysis tubing (SERVA pro, 44,144, diameter 21 mm × 5 m) was used. After dialysis, the samples were used for protein estimation by the method of Lowry et al. [19] and enzyme was assayed by the direct nesslerization method according to the method of Wriston and Yellin [17] and stored at – 20 °C for further purification. The concentrated enzyme solution was applied to the ion exchange column of DEAE-Sepharose CL-6B (2.7 × 20 cm) that was pre-equilibrated with 50 mM Tris-HCl buffer (pH 8.4). It was eluted with the same buffer containing increased concentration (0.1–0.5 M) of NaCl solution to elute the enzyme at a flow rate of 10 mL per 1 h. Fractions of 2 mL were collected, after fractions dialysis, the samples were subjected to protein estimation [19] and assay of L-asparginase activity [17]. Fractions showing high L-asparaginase activity were collected for further use.

Physicochemical characterization of the purified enzyme

The optimum pH of the purified enzyme was studied over the pH range of 4.5 to 10.5 with L-asparagine as a substrate dissolved in different buffers of 0.05 M: citric acid- Na_2HPO_4 (pH 4.5–7.5), Tris-HCl (pH 8.5) and glycine-NaOH (pH 9.5–10.5). The influence of temperature on L-asparaginase activity was analysed by incubating the assay mixture over the temperature range of 25 to 60 °C in 0.05 M Tris-HCl buffer under assay conditions. The optimum substrate concentration for the enzyme activity was determined by incubating the purified enzyme in the presence of different substrate concentration (1–10 mM). To evaluate the incubation time effect on L-asparginase activity, the reaction mixture was incubated for different times (10, 20, 30, 40, 50, 60, 70 and 80 min). Along the characterization of the enzyme, activity was determined as reported earlier.

Determination of the kinetic parameters K_m and V_{max}

The kinetic parameters, Michaelis–Menten constant (K_m) and maximal velocity (V_{max}) of the purified L-asparaginase were determined with different concentrations of L-asparagine (1–10 mM) as substrate and the data were fitted to a one-phase exponential association nonlinear regression curve using Graph-Pad Prism 5 software (GraphPad Software Inc., San Diego, CA). The enzyme activity was determined by measuring the rate of hydrolysis of L-asparagine under standard assay conditions using the Michaelis–Menten equation:

$$V_0 = \frac{V_{max}[S]}{K_m + [S]} \tag{1}$$

Whereas: initial reaction velocity (V_0), substrate concentration [S], the Michaelis-Menten constant (K_m) and maximal velocity (V_{max}).

Thermal stability of L-asparaginase

The stability of the L-asparaginase to temperature was determined by pre-incubating the reaction mixture (without its substrate) containing buffered enzyme for different time interval (0.0 to 90 min) with different temperatures (40, 50, 60, 70 and 80°C). After the end of the incubation periods, the enzyme was cooled and the residual activities were assayed.

Estimation of deactivation rate constant (k_d) and half-life time ($T_{1/2}$)

The heat inactivation half-life ($T_{1/2}$) of the enzyme and thermal deactivation constant (k_d) of the purified L-asparaginase produced by *Streptomyces brollosae* NEAE-115 were determined by using GraphPad Prism 5 software (GraphPad Software Inc., San Diego, CA). It was assumed that enzyme thermal deactivation is a reaction follows the first order kinetics (single step two-stage theory) [20] as follows:

$$E \rightarrow E_d \tag{2}$$

Where, E is the active enzyme state and E_d is the deactivated state. The first order deactivation can be represented as follows:

$$\frac{dE}{dt} = -K_d[E] \tag{3}$$

Where, K_d is the deactivation rate constant, [E] is concentration of the active enzyme.

Eq. (3) integrated with the initial condition, gives:

$$\ln\left(\frac{E_d}{E}\right) = -K_d t \tag{4}$$

This result is the exponential decay model. Therefore, by plotting log of (E_d/E) against time, the deactivation rate constant value (K_d) is obtained [21].

The half-life of the enzyme activity ($T_{1/2}$) is the time it takes for the activity to reduce to a half of the initial activity value. The half-life time was determined by using the following equation:

$$T_{1/2} = \frac{\ln 2}{k_d} = \frac{0.693}{k_d} \tag{5}$$

Where: K_d is deactivation rate constant.

The deactivation rate constant (K_d) at each temperature was determined from Arrhenius equation as:

$$\ln\left(\frac{k_d}{k_0}\right) = -\left(\frac{E}{RT}\right) \tag{6}$$

Plotting the log of K_d as a function of the inverse of the absolute temperature. The values of the deactivation energy (E) and k_0 (frequency factor, min^{-1}) were obtained from the slope and intercept of the plot of ln (k_d) versus (1/T); respectively. R is the universal gas constant and T is absolute temperature.

Effect of pH on L-asparaginase stability

To study the optimum pH for L-asparaginase stability, the enzyme in absence of its substrate was pre-incubated at room temperature for 0, 6, 12, 18, and 24 h in buffers of various pH values (pH 4.5–10.5). The residual activity was assayed under the standard assay conditions.

Effect of metal ions, inhibitors and surfactants on L-asparaginase activity

The effects of various metal ions, inhibitors and surfactants on L-asparaginase activity were determined by preincubating the enzyme with individual metal ions solutions prior to adding the substrate at a final concentration of 5 mM concentration and inhibitors and surfactants at 1 mM concentration for 30 min [22] at 4 °C. The residual activity of the enzyme was measured under the standard assay conditions. The relative activities were determined by considering 100% activity of the enzyme without the addition of metal ions or inhibitors or surfactants as control.

Molecular weight determination

The purity degree and the mass of the purified L-asparaginase enzyme was determined by sodium dodecyl sulfate polyacrylamide gel electrophoresis (SDS-PAGE) according to the method of Laemmli [23] with a 10% separating acrylamide gel (pH 8.8) and a 5% stacking gel (pH 6.8) containing 0.1% SDS. Gels were stained with coomassie brilliant blue R-250 followed by distaining step with a mixture of methanol- acetic acid and water in the ratio of 4:1:5. Molecular weight of L-asparaginase was determined using standard molecular weight protein marker ranged from 9 to 178 kDa.

Experimental animals

Female Swiss albino mice with body weight of 20–30 g were received from Urology and Nephrology Center of Mansoura University, Mansoura, Egypt, used to compare the cytotoxic effect of L-asparaginase purified from

Streptomyces brollosae NEAE-115 and those commercially available L-asparaginase from *E. coli* (Sigma-Aldrich, Product Number: A3809; CAS Number: 9015-68-3). Animals were housed in a conditioned atmosphere at temperature of 24 ± 1 °C and $55 \pm 5\%$ relative humidity with regular 12 h light/12 h dark cycles and free access to standard laboratory food and water. All experiments have been conducted under the regulations and the ethical guidelines for laboratory animals approved by the Ethical Committee of Faculty of Pharmacy, Mansoura University, Egypt.

Transplantation of tumor

Ehrlich ascites carcinoma cells (EAC) were supplied by the Netherlands Cancer Institute. The cells were maintained in vivo in female Swiss albino mice by serial intraperitoneal transplantation [24] in the laboratory of Faculty of Pharmacy, Mansoura University, Egypt.

In vivo experiment and evaluation of antitumor activity

The 7–10 days old EAC cells were used along experiment. Ascites fluid from tumor-bearing mice was withdrawn using a needle aspiration under aseptic conditions from the peritoneal cavity, and subjected to three times washing with normal saline followed by centrifugation at $67 \times g$. Tryphan blue exclusion test was used for tumor viability determination and haemocytometer was used for cells counting. To get ascitic fluid with a concentration of 5×10^5 viable EAC cells/0.1 mL of tumor cell suspension normal saline was used and was injected into the right thigh of the lower limb of mice to obtain ascitic tumor [25].

The largest tumor diameter and its perpendicular were measured by a digital caliper and used for tumor growth determination [26].

$$\text{Tumor size } (\text{mm}^3) = 0.5 \text{ Xa Xb}^2 \qquad (7)$$

Whereas: largest tumor diameter (a) and its perpendicular (b).

When the primary tumor reached a size of 50–100 mm^3, Swiss albino mice were divided into three groups of six each. Group (1) received normal saline (EAC-bearing control, 5 mL/kg). Group (2) received commercial L-asparaginase. Group (3) received L-asparaginase produced by *Streptomyces brollosae* NEAE-115. L-asparaginase treatments were given five days after the inoculation, two times a week for two weeks. After 24 h of the last dose and then 18 h of fasting, animals of each group were sacrificed by cervical dislocation to determine the antitumor activity of the tested L-asparaginase. Antitumor activity was calculated by the determination of ΔT (change of tumor size in the treatment group) and ΔC (change of tumor size in the control). The degree of

tumor growth inhibition can be obtained from $\Delta T/\Delta C$ X 100 [26].

Immunogenicity assessment

Two groups each of 6 mice received intraperitoneal administration of either commercial L-asparaginase (250 U/kg) or *Streptomyces brollosae* NEAE-115 L-asparaginase (250 U/kg) twice a week for 4 weeks. Levels of specific antibodies (IgG immunoglobulin) against L-asparaginase or commercial product were measured in sera using ELISA method and microplate reader was used at absorbance of 450 nm. The direct enzyme-linked immunosorbent assay (ELISA) was carried out to evaluate the presence of asparaginase–specific IgG antibodies in serum samples by employing horseradish peroxidase–conjugated goat-anti mouse IgG (from Southern Biotech). All ELISA steps were conducted at room temperature, and 2.5% casein (w/v) was utilized as binding and blocking buffer. The assay steps and conditions were as follows: 2 h blocking of asparaginase-coated plates followed by extensive washing using PBS-Tween, incubated with diluted serum samples for 2 h, washed, incubated with detection antibody for 1 h, washed, developed with 3, 3′, 5, 5′-tetramethylbenzidine substrate for 30 min, and quenched with 9.8% (v/v) H_2SO_4 in water. IgG titers were calculated.

Results

Production of the L-asparaginase by *Streptomyces brollosae* NEAE-115 was detected by plate assay. The enzyme production was indicated by color change in the medium from yellow to pink zone surrounding the colony. A broad diameter of the pink zone around the colony indicated that the organism was an efficient producer of L-asparaginase. During shake flasks production of L-asparaginase, the mycelial growth has been formed as large, spherical pellets which may lead to better yield of L-asparaginase than growth as free filaments. The glutaminase activity of L-asparaginase was investigated and the enzyme is free from glutaminase activity.

Purification of L-asparaginase from *Streptomyces brollosae* NEAE-115

Purification of L-asparaginase of *Streptomyces brollosae* NEAE-115 was carried out using crude culture filtrate having a total activity of 30538.87 U, protein content 3120.42 mg and specific activity of 9.786 U/mg protein. The dialysed ammonium sulphate concentrated enzyme had a specific activity of 69.004 U/mg protein with protein content of 158.86 mg and the enzyme recovery was 35.895% with purification fold of 7.051 (Table 1). The dialyzed enzyme obtained after ammonium sulphate precipitation was used to purify the enzyme with DEAE Sepharose CL-6B packed column which resulting 260 fractions with major L-asparaginase peak on the

Table 1 Summary of the purification steps of the L-asparaginase produced by *Streptomyces brollosae* NEAE-115

Purification step	Total protein content (mg)	L-asparaginase activity		Recovery (%)	Purification fold
		Total activity (U)	Specific activity (U/mg protein)		
Culture filtrate	3120.42	30538.87	9.786	100	1
(NH₄)₂SO₄, post dialysis	158.86	10,962	69.004	35.895	7.051
Ion exchange on DEAE Sepharose	10.371	795.152	76.671	7.254	7.835

chromatogram (Fig. 1). The final purification step, DEAE Sepharose CL-6B column, showed a total enzyme activity of 795.152, protein content of 10.371 mg with enzyme specific activity of 76.671 U/mg of protein and the results of all purification steps applied to purify L-asparaginase produced by *Streptomyces brollosae* NEAE-115 are summarized in Table 1.

SDS-PAGE and molecular weight determination
The purity and molecular weight of the purified enzyme was determined by SDS-PAGE according to the method of Laemmli [23] with gel system contained a separating gel of 10% and a stacking gel 5%. After the electrophoresis, protein bands were visualized by staining with coomassie brilliant blue R-250. The resolved electrophoretic bands of the enzyme from different purification steps on the SDS-PAGE showed that the enzyme purity was successfully improved. SDS–PAGE separation of the enzyme preparation showed no detectable contamination and electrophoretic resolved only one distinctive band. By using different molecular markers with known molecular weight ranged from 9 to 178 kDa, the molecular mass of the purified L-asparaginase was estimated. The relative mobility (R_f) value was calculated for the distinctive single band. The calculated R_f value is compared with the different standard proteins of known molecular

weight. Hence the molecular weight for individual band is determined with a molecular mass of 67 kDa (Fig. 2).

Physicochemical properties of the purified L-asparaginase
The purified L-asparginase of *Streptomyces brollosae* NEAE-115 was characterized for its activity at different pH levels, temperatures, substrate concentrations and incubation times.

Effect of pH on L-asparaginase activity
The pH of the reaction played a vital role in most of enzymatic processes. There are number of reports on the enzyme activity at near physiological range. Fig. 3 shows that the purified L-asparaginase was active over a broad pH range of 4.5 to 10.5 with an optimum of 48.462 U/mL at pH 8.5. At higher pH's, the enzyme activity was decreased. The enzyme retains 71.595% activity even at pH 10.5 and 58.919% at pH 5.5.

Incubation time effect on enzyme activity
L-asparaginase activity of *Streptomyces brollosae* NEAE-115 (Fig. 4) was gradually increased with increasing incubation time up to 50 min (L-asparaginase activity of 71.327 U/mL). After which only a slight decrease in L-asparaginase activity was observed.

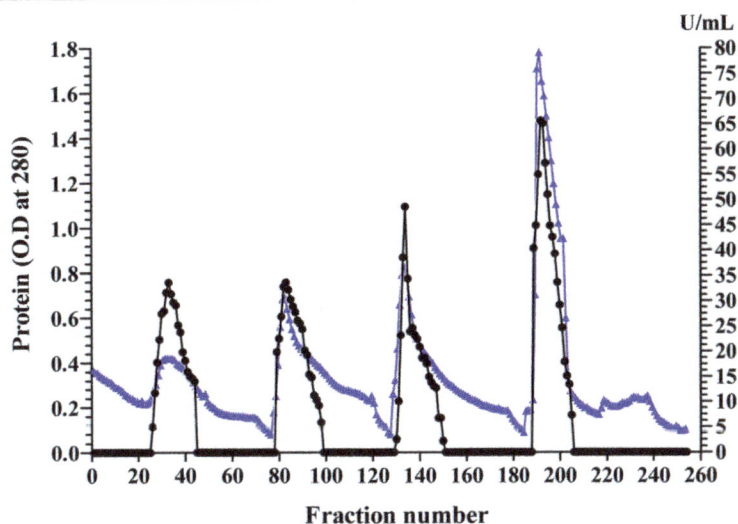

Fig. 1 Purification of L-asparaginase produced by *Streptomyces brollosae* NEAE-115 using ion exchange on DEAE Sepharose. (▲) refer to protein, (●) refer to L-asparaginase activity

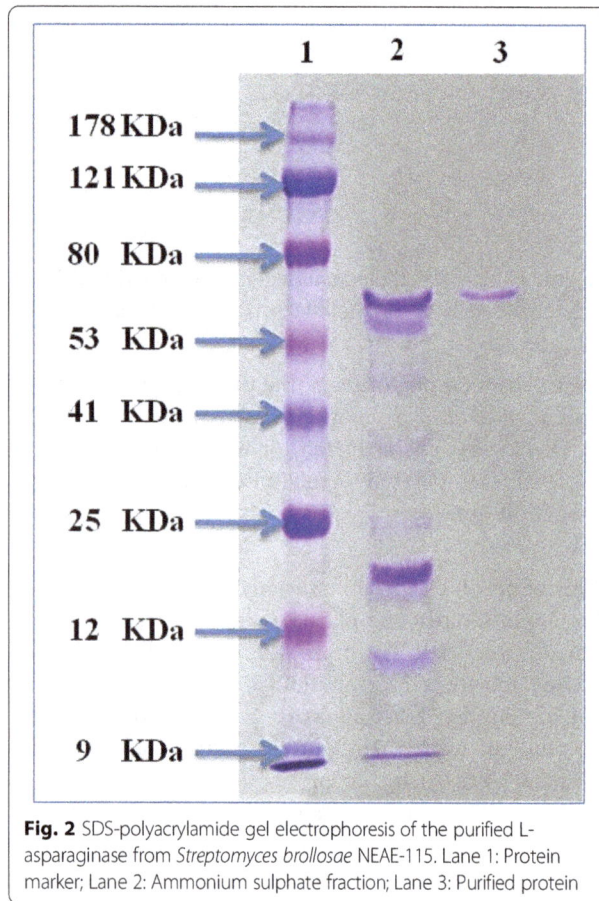

Fig. 2 SDS-polyacrylamide gel electrophoresis of the purified L-asparaginase from *Streptomyces brollosae* NEAE-115. Lane 1: Protein marker; Lane 2: Ammonium sulphate fraction; Lane 3: Purified protein

Temperature effect on L-asparaginase activity

Figure 5 shows that the purified L-asparaginase was active over a wide range of temperature range of 25 to 60 °C with an optimum L-asparaginase activity of 87.81 U/mL at 37 °C and lower L-asparaginase activity observed at higher temperatures.

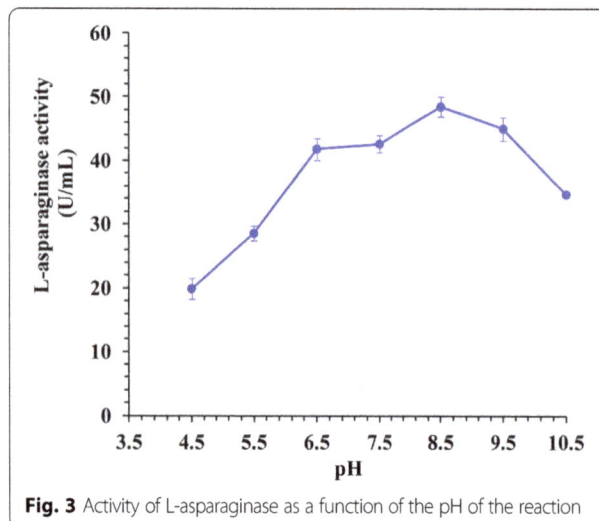

Fig. 3 Activity of L-asparaginase as a function of the pH of the reaction

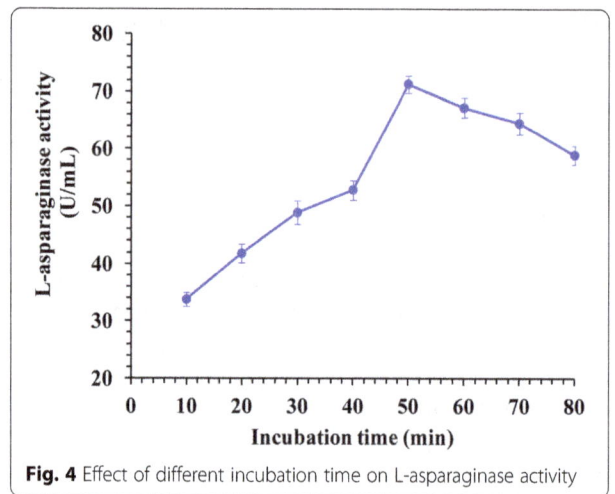

Fig. 4 Effect of different incubation time on L-asparaginase activity

Effect of substrate concentration on the activity of L-asparaginase

The results in Fig. 6 showed the effect of various substrate concentrations ranging from 1 to 10 mM on the activity of L-asparaginase and verified the optimum required substrate concentration that gives the maximum L-asparaginase activity. The obtained results illustrated a gradual enzyme activity increase with increasing of the substrate concentration up to 7 mM demonstrating the optimum substrate concentration for enzyme activity. However, higher substrate concentration (8 to 10 mM) resulted in decreasing of enzyme activity. Activation of asparagine hydrolysis was investigated in terms of change in values of kinetic constants (K_m and V_{max}). The K_m and V_{max} values were calculated through Michaelis-Menten plot by plotting the relation between different substrate concentrations [S] versus enzyme activity (V), using enzyme kinetic template of Graph-Pad Prism 4 software. Michaelis-Menten plot showed in Fig. 7 illustrated the K_m and V_{max} values for L-asparaginase

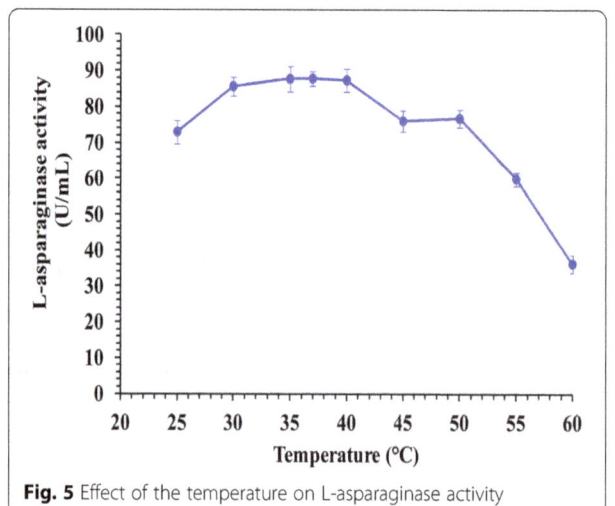

Fig. 5 Effect of the temperature on L-asparaginase activity

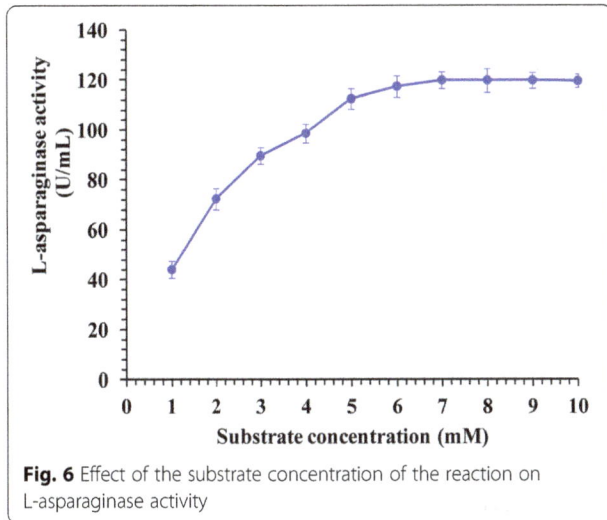

Fig. 6 Effect of the substrate concentration of the reaction on L-asparaginase activity

and longer incubation time of 50 °C and 80 °C for 90 min led to observed rapid decrease in L-asparaginase activity with residual activity of 31.84 and 7.69%; respectively.

On the other hand, to reveal heat inactivation half-life time ($T_{1/2}$) of the enzyme at the used temperatures and heat deactivation constant (k_d), the linear regression of the obtained results was performed using Graph-Pad Prism software by fitting the data points to first order equation according to Eqs. (4) and (5) and their values were listed in Table 2. The stability of L-asparaginase was expressed as a percentage of residual activity compared to the initial activity of the un-treated enzyme activity which considered as a control (100%). The enzyme half life time ($T_{1/2}$) of L-asparaginase was found to be 65.02 min at 50°C and 62.65 min at 60°C. However, enzyme activity destruction was recorded at 80 °C with low half-life time (49.60 min).

enzyme. The plot gave K_m value of 2.139×10^{-3} M and V_{max} of 152.6 UmL^{-1} min^{-1} for the hydrolysis of L-asparagine by L-asparaginase from *Streptomyces brollosae* NEAE-115 and K_m value of 1.76×10^{-4} M and V_{max} of 121.7 UmL^{-1} min^{-1} for the hydrolysis of L-asparagine by commercially available L-asparaginase from *E. coli* (Sigma-Aldrich, Product Number: A3809; CAS Number: 9015–68-3).

Thermal stability

The temperature impact on L-asparaginase stability was studied and the maximum L-asparaginase stability was recorded at 40 °C (Fig. 8) with retained enzyme activity of 97.44% from initial activity after incubation time of 20 min. However, enzyme exposure to higher temperature

pH stability

The purified L-asparaginase was more stable in alkaline pH than the acidic one; it retains 92.81% activity at pH 8.5 even after incubation for 6 h and 61.64% activity after 24 h (Fig. 9). Moreover, the enzyme retains about 84.22% of its activity after 6 h at the pH 9.5. At pH 4.5 the enzyme retained 64.80% activity after 6 h and the residual activity was 20.47% after 24 h. Half life time values in hours ($T_{1/2}$) based on pH studies of L-asparaginase produced by *Streptomyces brollosae* NEAE-115 are represented in Table 3. The enzyme half life time of L-asparaginase was found to be 33.135 h at pH 8.5 and 28.506 h at pH 9.5. However, enzyme activity destruction was recorded at pH 4.5 with low half-life time (15.888 h).

Effect of metal ions, inhibitors and surfactants on L-asparaginase activity

The effect of various metal ions, inhibitors and surfactants on the enzyme activity is represented in Fig. 10. The purified L-asparaginase from *Streptomyces brollosae* NEAE-115 was not significantly affected by the presence of metal ions (Na^+, K^+, Fe^{2+}) and β-mercaptoethanol. It is evident from the Fig. 10 that the enzyme activity enhanced considerably in the presence of Mg^{2+} (111.81%) and was maximal in the presence of Mn^{2+}, Co^{2+} and Tween 80 by 145.15, 143.04 and 121.52%; respectively (acted as activators for L-asparaginase activity). However, a slight decrease, around 14.8 and 16%, in L-asparaginase activity was observed in the presence of Zn^{2+} and Ca^{2+}; respectively. Moreover, the presence of EDTA and urea acted as inhibitors of L-asparaginase activity reducing its activity by 37.55 and 57.8%; respectively. The presence of Ni^{2+}, Hg^{2+}, Ba^{2+} and Cu^{2+} acted as a potent inhibitor, reducing about 74.68, 59.5, 56.4 and 49.8%; respectively of the L-asparaginase activity. The presence of sodium azide

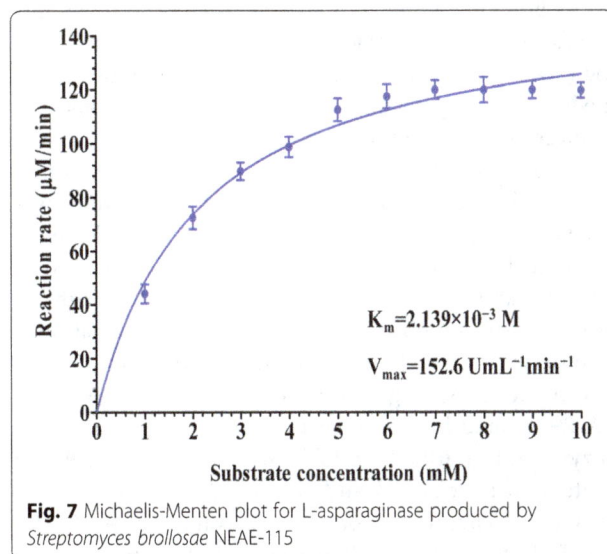

Fig. 7 Michaelis-Menten plot for L-asparaginase produced by *Streptomyces brollosae* NEAE-115

$K_m = 2.139 \times 10^{-3}$ M

$V_{max} = 152.6$ $UmL^{-1}min^{-1}$

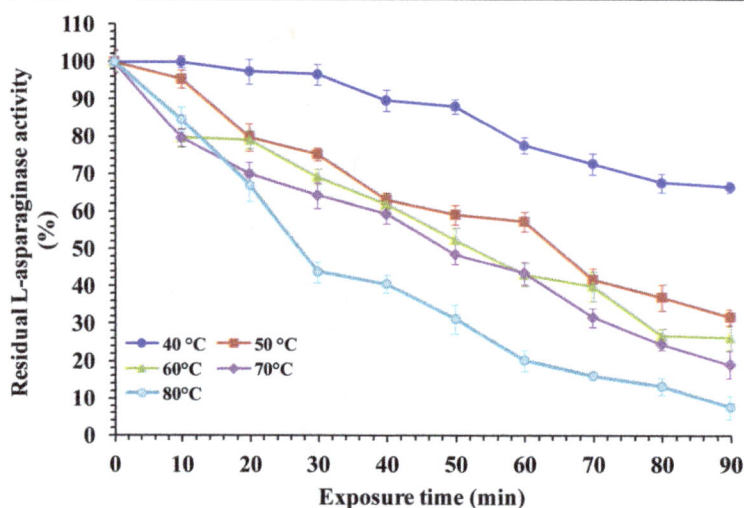

Fig. 8 Thermal stability of L-asparaginase as a function of the time of the reaction

also acted as an inhibitor, reducing about 45.15% of the L-asparaginase activity.

Antitumor activity of purified L-asparaginase and immunogenicity assessment

Treatment with commercial L-asparaginase significantly decreased the relative tumor size compared to the control group, showing 33% tumor growth (i.e. 67% tumor growth inhibition). While mice treated with *Streptomyces brollosae* NEAE-115 L-asparaginase showed 79% tumor growth inhibition showing a significantly higher cytotoxic effect when compared to commercial L-asparaginase group (Table 4). One of the most important limitation of L-asparaginase as anticancer drug is that the allergic reactions exhibited by immune system of the patients receiving the medication of L-asparaginase. Characterization of the immunogenicity profile of L-asparaginase in mice and the levels of specific antibodies (IgG immunoglobulin) against L-asparaginase was measured in sera using ELISA method. Therapeutic efficacy and evaluation of anti-L-asparaginase IgG antibody concentrations in mice receiving *Streptomyces brollosae* NEAE-115 L-asparaginase preparations was carried out simultaneously with the commercial L-asparaginase in

order to evaluate the superiority of the new product. There was a gradual increase in L-asparaginase IgG titre in both commercial L-asparaginase or *Streptomyces brollosae* NEAE-115 L-asparaginase-inoculated mice (Fig. 11). However significant anti-asparaginase IgG titer was observed in commercial L-asparaginase group when compared to the other group of mice inoculated by *Streptomyces brollosae* NEAE-115 L-asparaginase due to the highly immunogenic nature of the commercial asparaginase. The results demonstrated that the immunogenicity of the *Streptomyces brollosae* NEAE-115 L-asparaginase was remarkably reduced.

Discussion

In the current study, L-asparaginase produced by *Streptomyces brollosae* NEAE-115 was detected by forming pink zone surrounding the colony. The pink zone resulted from the breakdown of amide bond in asparagine in the growth medium by L-asparaginase to aspartate and ammonia that changed the color of phenol red to pink [27].

The produced enzyme was partially purified by ammonium sulphate precipitation and pure enzyme was reached using ion-exchange chromatography. Recently L-asparaginase enzyme from strains *Streptomyces noursei* [28] and *Streptomyces gulbergenesis* [13] with an overall purification of 98.23 and 82.12 fold in final purification were carried out successfully. Sahu et al. [27] extracted the L-asparaginase from the actinomycete strain LA-29 isolated from the gut contents of the fish and the enzyme was purified 18-fold and from which 1.9% of protein was recovered and showed the specific activity of about 13.57 IU/mg of protein. Narayana et al. [29] and El-Bessoumy et al. [30] reported 99.3 and 106 fold

Table 2 Half life time ($T_{1/2}$) and heat deactivation constant (k_d) of L-asparaginase produced by *Streptomyces brollosae* NEAE-115

Temperature (°C)	Half life time (min)	k_d (min)	R^2 value
40	116.50	0.006	0.94
50	65.02	0.011	0.98
60	62.65	0.011	0.97
70	59.91	0.012	0.97
80	49.60	0.014	0.93

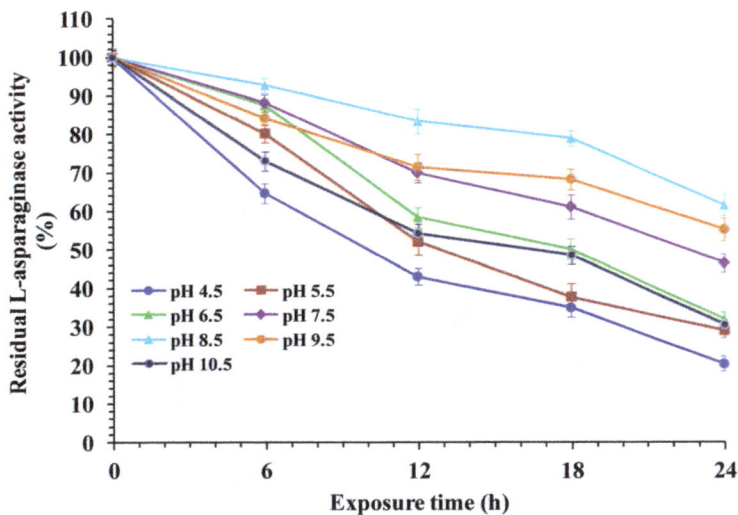

Fig. 9 pH stability of L-asparaginase at different times of the reaction

purification of L-asparaginase from *Streptomyces albidoflavus* and *Pseudomonas aeroginosa* 50,071; respectively, by CM Sephedex C-50 column chromatography.

SDS–PAGE separation revealed only one distinctive band of the enzyme preparation, no detectable contamination. L-asparaginase was therefore a homogenous protein. The molecular weight for the individual band is determined with a molecular mass of 67 kDa. The molecular weight of the L-asparaginase was found to be varied according to the source of enzyme. Purified L-asparaginase from *Bacillus* sp. [31], *Streptomyces gulbargensis* [13], *Streptomyces albidoflavus* [29], *Streptomyces* PDK2 [32], and *Streptomyces noursei* [28] exhibited a molecular weight of 45, 85, 112, 140 kDa and 102 kDa; respectively.

The amidases enzymes such as L-asparaginase are generally stable and active at neutral and alkaline pH, whereas, earlier reporters showed optimum amidase activity at pH ranging from 5.0 to 9.0 [33]. The optimum pH 8.5 was also reported for L-asparaginase purified from *Streptomyces* sp. PDK7 [32]. However, the optimal L-asparaginase activity from *Streptomyces gulbargensis*

Table 3 Half life time values in hours ($T_{1/2}$) based on pH studies of L-asparaginase produced by *Streptomyces brollosae* NEAE-115

pH	$T_{1/2}$ (h)	P-value	R^2 value
4.5	15.888	0.0077	0.9321
5.5	16.276	0.0029	0.9644
6.5	17.289	0.0017	0.9740
7.5	22.422	0.0003	0.9921
8.5	33.135	0.0039	0.9563
9.5	28.506	0.003	0.9634
10.5	18.355	0.0039	0.9564

was reported at pH 9.0 [13]. Narayana et al. [29] have reported the maximum L-asparaginase at pH 7.5 by *Streptomyces albidoflavus*. Khamna et al. [34] have also reported maximum L-asparaginase activity at pH 7.0 using *Streptomyces* sp.

The L-asparaginase activity of *Streptomyces brollosae* NEAE-115 was gradually increased with increasing incubation time up to 50 min. However, longer time of incubation with substrate resulted in reduction of L-asparaginase activity which may due to the product inhibition. The purified L-asparaginase from *Streptomyces noursei* showed maximum activity at 35 min of incubation time [28]. In addition, L-asparaginase purified from *Pseudomonas aeruginosa* 50,071 reached its maximum activity at 30 min [30].

L-asparaginase was active over a wide range of temperature from 25 to 60 °C with an optimum L-asparaginase activity of 87.81 U/mL at pH 37 °C and lower L-asparaginase activities observed at higher temperatures. Similarly, Siddalingeshwara and Lingappa [35] recorded optimum temperature 37 °C for maximum enzyme activity from *Aspergillus terreus* KLS2. This property of enzyme makes it most suitable for complete elimination of asparagine from the body when tumor patient treated with L-asparaginase. Comparable results were reported for the maximum activity of purified L-asparaginase from *Streptomyces gulbargensis* at 40 °C [13].

Michaelis-Menten plot gave a K_m value of 2.139×10^{-3} M with L-asparagine as substrate and V_{max} of 152.6 UmL^{-1} min^{-1} for the hydrolysis of L-asparagine by L-asparaginase from *Streptomyces brollosae* NEAE-115 and K_m value of 1.76×10^{-4} M and V_{max} of 121.7 UmL^{-1} min^{-1} for the hydrolysis of L-asparagine by commercially available L-asparaginase from *E. coli* (Sigma-Aldrich,

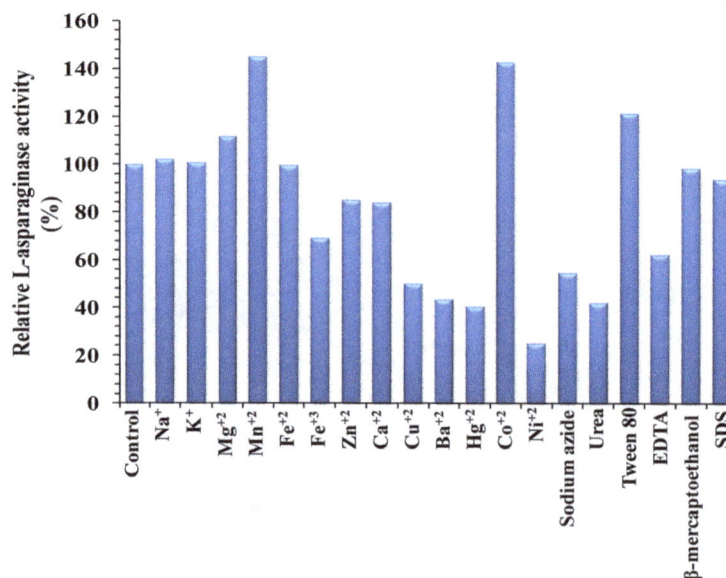

Fig. 10 Effect of metal ions, inhibitors and surfactants on L-asparaginase activity

Product Number: A3809; CAS Number: 9015–68-3). Senthil Kumar and Selvam [36] have reported the apparent K_m and V_{max} of 5.98×10^{-2} M and 3.547 IU/µg; respectively in *Streptomyces radiopugnans* MS. Table 5 summerize the biochemical properties of some microbial L-asparaginases [13, 21, 22, 29, 30, 36–48].

L-asparaginase of different microbial sources has different K_m value which defined as the half maximal velocity of the enzymatic reaction as a function of substrate concentrations and stating the filling of half of the enzyme active sites in the tested sample in the steady state. Therefore, K_m values illustrate the affinity of the enzyme for its substrate [49]. In consequence, lower and higher K_m values mean stronger binding ability and lower enzyme affinity to its substrate; respectively. However, the kinetic constants of the enzymes in terms of K_m and V_{max} can be affected by many factors, including, enzyme type, enzyme different forms (crude, modified or purified), enzyme source, used conditions (temperature, pH, etc.), substrate type and the used procedure of assay [50]. The rate of an enzyme-catalyzed reaction increases with the increasing of the substrate concentration beyond a certain level called maximal velocity rate (V_{max});

at V_{max} increase in substrate concentration does not cause any increase in reaction rate as there is no more enzyme available for reacting with substrate. The maximal rate, V_{max}, reveals the number of substrate molecules converted into product by the enzyme per unit of time when the catalytic sites on the enzyme are fully saturated with its substrate [51].

According to the data reported under this investigation, the maximum thermal stability behavior of L-asparaginase was at 40 °C. An earlier study demonstrated by Senthil Kumar and Selvam [36], the pre incubation at 40 °C for 60 min of the purified L-asparaginase from *Streptomyces radiopugnans* MS1 resulted in no significant loss of enzyme activity. Similar results were recorded with many other microorganisms such as *Streptomyces noursei* [28], *Pseudomonas stutzeri* MB 405 [38] and *E. carotovora* [52]. "Enzyme stability and thermal deactivation are considered the major constraints in rapid development of biotechnology process. In addition, it considered a very important tool used in enzyme selection for industrial uses".

The purified L-asparaginase was more stable in alkaline pH and similar findings were reported for L-asparaginase

Table 4 Effect of L-asparaginase on tumor size in mice after treatment

Treatment	Tumor size (mm³)		ΔT/ΔC (%)	% Inhibition
	Day 0	Day 14		
Control	69.0 ± 2.2	585.0 ± 40.8	100	0
Commercial L-asparaginase	67.0 ± 4.5	$240.7 \pm 9.4^*$	33	67
Streptomyces brollosae NEAE-115 L-asparaginase	77.6 ± 3.7	$188.3 \pm 8.33\$$	21	79

Data are expressed as mean ± SEM, $n = 6$
* Significantly different from control group using One-Way ANOVA followed by Tukey-Kramer multiple comparisons test ($P < 0.05$). $ Significantly different from commercial L-asparaginase-treated group using One-Way ANOVA followed by Tukey-Kramer multiple comparisons test ($P < 0.05$). Mann-Whitney U test, *$P < 0.05$

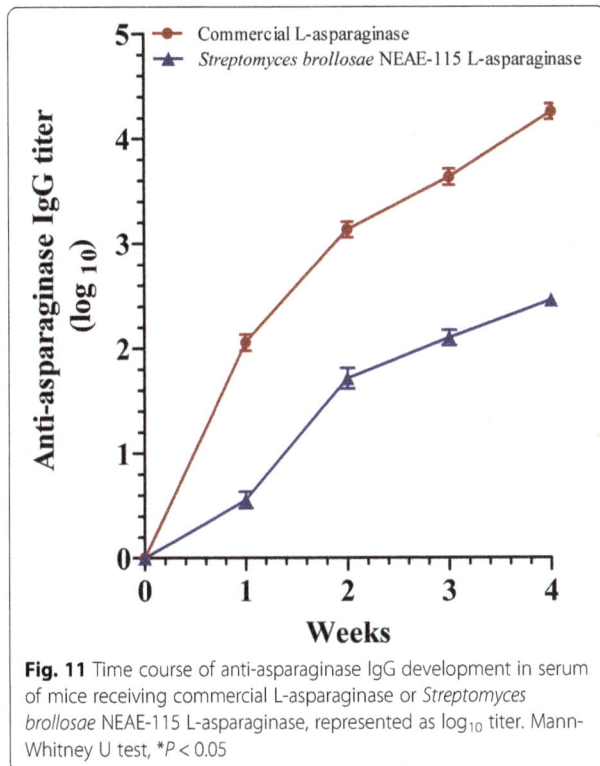

Fig. 11 Time course of anti-asparaginase IgG development in serum of mice receiving commercial L-asparaginase or *Streptomyces brollosae* NEAE-115 L-asparaginase, represented as $\log_{10}$ titer. Mann-Whitney U test, *P < 0.05

extracted from *Pseudomonas stutzeri* MB–405 which is maximally stable at pH range from 7.5 to 9.5 [38] .

Among the different metal ions tested Mn^{2+} enhanced the L-asparaginase activity by 18% as reported by earlier workers on *Fusarium culmorum* ASP-87 and *Mucor*

hiemalis [22, 53]. Husain et al. [37] reported that the monovalent cations such as Na^+ and K^+ enhanced the activity of *Enterobacter cloacae* L-asparaginase. K^+ acted also as enhancer on *Pectobacterium carotovorum* asparaginase [54]. Radha et al. [21] reported that the activity of *Vibrio cholerae* L-asparaginase was enhanced in presence of Ca^{2+} to 130%. Also, Meghavarnam and Janakiraman [22] reported that the non ionic surfactant tween 80 was found to enhance the activity of the enzyme by 16%. Senthil Kumar and Selvam [36] reported that the EDTA acts as an inducer in *Streptomyces radiopugnans* MS1. EDTA as metal chelator agent had no effect on *P. carotovorum* asparaginase [54]. However, L-asparaginase was completely inhibited by EDTA as reported by Borkotaky and Bezbaruah [55]. Whereas, EDTA inhibited the activity of fungal L-asparaginase from *Trichoderma viride* by 88% [56]. Also, the L-asparaginase activity of *Fusarium Culmorum* ASP-87 was inhibited by EDTA, SDS and Cu^{2+} [22]. Husain et al. [37] reported that the divalent and trivalent cations, Ca^{2+}, Mg^{2+}, Zn^{2+}, Mn^{2+}, and Fe^{3+} inhibited the enzyme activity. Radha et al. [21] reported that the activity of *Vibrio cholerae* L-asparaginase was inhibited by divalent cations Ni^{2+}, Mg^{2+}, Fe^{2+}, Mn^{2+}, Zn^{2+} and the complete loss in the activity was perceived in the presence Cu^{2+}. Whereas, Archana and Raja [57] reported that Cu^{2+} inhibited the activity of L-asparaginase produced by *Aspergillus nidulans* by 84%. Kumar et al. [54] reported that Hg^{2+} inhibited the L-asparaginase activity produced by *Pectobacterium carotovorum* by 80%. However, L-asparaginase was completely inhibited by Fe^{2+} and Ni^{2+} [58] and Cu^{2+} and Zn^{2+} [59]. While, Husain et al. [37]

Table 5 Biochemical properties of some microbial L-asparaginases

Microbial source	pH optima	Temperature optima (°C)	K_m (M)	V_{max}	Specific activity (U/mg protein)	Molecular weight (kDa)	References
Streptomyces albidoflavus	7.5	35	–	–	437	112	[29]
Streptomyces gulbargensis	9	40	–	–	2053	85	[13]
Streptomyces radiopugnans MS	6	40	5.98×10^{-2}	3.547 IU/µg	5035.28	133.25	[36]
Enterobacter cloacae	7–8	35–40	1.58×10^{-3}	2.22 IU/µg	105.07	52	[37]
Pseudomonas aeruginosa	9	37	0.147×10^{-3}	35.7 IU	1900	160	[30]
Vibrio cholerae	7	37	1.1×10^{-3}	1006 µM/min	648.9	132	[21]
Pseudomonas stutzeri	9	37	1.45×10^{-4}	–	732.3	34	[38]
Pseudomonas fluorescens	8–9		4.1×10^{-4}	–	500	70	[39]
Azotobacter vinelandii	8.6	48	1.1×10^{-4}		2.47	84	[40]
E. coli	7–8	37	3.5×10^{-3}	–	150–250	139	[41–43]
Erwinia aroideae	8.2	45	2.8×10^{-3}	–	–	155	[44]
Corynebacterium glutamicum	7	40	2.5×10^{-3}		2020	80	[45]
Bacillus coagulans	8.8–9.7	55	5×10^{-3}	5.83×10^{-5} M/h	10.9	84	[46]
Bacillus licheniformis	6–10	40	1.4×10^{-5}	4.03 IU	697.09	134.8	[47]
Aspergillus oryzae CCT 3940	8	50	0.66×10^{-3}	313 IU/mL	91	115	[48]
Fusarium culmorum ASP-87	8	45	3.57×10^{-3}	0.5 µmol/mL/min	16.66	90	[22]

reported that the asparaginase activity did not detected when enzyme was incubated with metal ions viz. Cd^{2+}, Ni^{2+} and Hg^{2+}. Other metal ions like Ca^{2+} and Mg^{2+} did not have much effect on enzyme activity [22] and β-mercaptoethanol did not have any effect on fungal L-asparaginase activity from *Trichoderma viride* [56].

Mn^{2+}, Co^{2+} and Mg^{2+} ions increase the enzyme activity suggests that these metals ions can serve as co-factors, which can help to activate the enzymatic reaction. Mg^{2+} was thought to be the activating metal; Mg^{2+} may activate the substrate, bound directly to the enzyme-substrate complex. Mg^{2+} locks the enzyme-substrate complex in place and then rapidly causes release of the reaction products [60]. This corresponds to fast dissociation rates for the enzyme-product complex rendering more favorable substrate binding sites. Metal ions play a crucial role in maintaining the active configuration of the enzymes at elevated temperatures by protecting them against thermal denaturation [61]. It was reported that the divalent cations Mn^{2+} and Mg^{2+} increased the thermal stability of *Bacillus* alkaline proteases [62]. Whereas, the monovalent cations, Na^+ were found to enhanced asparaginase activity, indicates that the enzyme might contain Na^+ ions [37]. Thakur et al. [53] found that Mn^{2+} enhanced L-asparaginase activity and concluded that L-asparaginase is in general a metal-activated enzyme. Tween 80 was found to enhance the activity of the enzyme by 21.52%. Surfactants appear to increase quick and direct contact of enzymes with substrate sites [63]. McAllister et al. [64] reported that Tween 80 increased the stability and substrate binding capacity of enzymes under in vitro conditions.

One of the most important limitation of L-asparaginase as anticancer drug is that the allergic reactions exhibited by immune system of the patients receiving the medication of L-asparaginase. The patient immune system reacts in many different ways against the drug such as, the development of high titers of serum IgG antibodies which in the majority of cases interfere with the therapeutic effect of the enzyme [65]. Drug's immunogenicity is fundamental obstacle which limits the therapy with foreign proteins in humans. A real immunological tolerance that would require antigen specific T-cell mediated immunosuppression is difficult to achieve. One way to overcome this problem for a limited time is to switch to another preparation [66].

Conclusions

This study is clearly revealed that soils can be considered as a rich source of L-asparaginase producing actinomycetes. *Streptomyces brollosae* NEAE-115 isolated from Egypt soil has the ability to produce a significant amount of L-asparaginase. A pure and efficient enzyme activity of L-asparaginase could be obtained using only two purification steps. The excellent characteristics of this enzyme like high catalytic activity over a wide range of

temperature and pH, high substrate specificity, maximum activity at body temperature and its considerable thermal and pH stabilities, makes it highly valuable to be exploited as a potent anticancer agent. Furthermore, mice treated with *Streptomyces brollosae* NEAE-115 L-asparaginase showed 79% tumor growth inhibition with higher cytotoxic effect when compared to commercial L-asparaginase group. The current investigation concluded the isolated *Streptomyces brollosae* NEAE-115 used in this study could be a valuable potential source for L-asparaginase.

Abbreviations
ELISA: Enzyme-linked immunosorbent assay; IgG: Immunoglobulin G; KDa: kilodalton; K_m: Michaelis–Menten constant; SDS–PAGE: Sodium dodecyl sulfate–polyacrylamide gel electrophoresis; $T_{1/2}$: Half-life time; V_{max}: Maximal velocity

Acknowledgments
The authors gratefully acknowledge the Science and Technology Development Fund (STDF), Egypt, for their financial support of this paper which is a part of the Grant No. 4943.

Funding
The Science and Technology Development Fund (STDF), Egypt.

Authors' contributions
NEE proposed the research concept, designed the experiments, providing necessary tools for experiments, experimental instructions, conducted most of the experiments, analyzed and interpreted the data, wrote the manuscript and final approval of the manuscript. SFD contributed in the purification step using DEAE Sepharose CL-6B column, contributed to revision of this part of the manuscript. SME performed the experiments and contributed substantially to acquisition of data and drafting the manuscript. GMS contributed substantially to conception and design, acquisition, analysis and interpretation of data, conducted and wrote the part of antitumor activity and immunogenicity assessment. All authors agreed to be accountable for all aspects of the work in ensuring that questions related to the accuracy or integrity of any part of the work are appropriately investigated and resolved. All authors read and approved the manuscript to be published.

Competing interests
The authors declare that they have no competing interests.

Author details
[1]Department of Bioprocess Development, Genetic Engineering and Biotechnology Research Institute, City of Scientific Research and Technological Applications, Alexandria, Egypt. [2]Department of Protein Research Genetic Engineering and Biotechnology Research Institute, City of Scientific Research and Technological Applications, Alexandria, Egypt. [3]Department of Pharmacology and Toxicology, Faculty of Pharmacy, Mansoura University, Mansoura, Egypt.

References

1. Savitri AN, Azmi W. Microbial L-asparaginase: A potent antitumour enzyme. Indian J Biotechnol. 2003;2:184–94.

2. Narta UK, Kanwar SS, Azmi W. Pharmacological and clinical evaluation of L-aspaprginase in the treatment of leukemia. Crit Rev Oncol Hematol. 2007;61: 208–21.

3. Duval M, Suciu S, Ferster A, Rialland X, Nelken B, Lutz P, Benoit Y, Robert A, Manel AM, Vilmer E. Comparison of Escherichia coli–asparaginase with Erwinia-asparaginase in the treatment of childhood lymphoid malignancies: results of a randomized European Organisation for Research and Treatment of Cancer-Children's leukemia group phase 3 trial. Blood. 2002;99:2734–9.

4. Ambi Rani S, Sundaram L, Vasantha P.B. A study on in vitro antioxidant and anticancer activity of L-asparaginase. J Pharm Res. 2011;5:1463–66.

5. El-Naggar NE, El-Ewasy SM, El-Shweihy NM. Microbial L-asparaginase as a potential therapeutic agent for the treatment of acute lymphoblastic leukemia: the pros and cons. Int J Pharmacol. 2014;10:182–99.

6. Verma N, Kumar K, Kaur G, Anand S. E. coli K-12 asparaginase-based asparagine biosensor for leukemia. Artif Cells Blood Substit Immobil Biotechnol. 2007;35:449–56.

7. Kotzia GA, Labrou NE. Cloning, expression and characterisation of Erwinia carotovora L-asparaginase. J Biotechnol. 2005;119:309–23.

8. Ohnuma T, Holland JF, Freeman A, Sinks LF. Biochemical and pharmacological studies with L-asparaginase in man. Cancer Res. 1970;30:2297–305.

9. El-Naggar NE, Diras SF, Soliman HM, El-Deeb NM, El-Ewasy SM. Purification, characterization, cytotoxicity and anticancer activities of L-asparaginase, anti-colon cancer protein, from the newly isolated alkaliphilic Streptomyces fradiae NEAE-82. Sci Rep. 2016;6:32926.

10. Manivasagan P, Venkatesan J, Sivakumar K, Kim SK. Marine actinobacterial metabolites: current status and future perspectives. Microbiol Res. 2013;168:311–32.

11. El-Naggar NE. Extracellular production of the oncolytic enzyme, L-asparaginase, by newly isolated Streptomyces sp. strain NEAE-95 as potential microbial cell factories: Optimization of culture conditions using response surface methodology. Curr Pharm Biotechnol. 2015;16:162–78.

12. El-Naggar NE, Moawad H, El-Shweihy NM, El-Ewasy SM. Optimization of culture conditions for production of the anti-leukemic glutaminase free L-asparaginase by newly isolated Streptomyces olivaceus NEAE-119 using response surface methodology. Biomed Res Int. 2015;627031. https://doi.org/10.1155/2015/627031.

13. Amena S, Vishalakshi N, Prabhakar M, Dayanand A, Lingappa K. Production, purification and characterization of L-asparaginase from Streptomyces gulbargensis. Brazil J Microbiol. 2010;41:173–8.

14. De Jong PJ. L-asparaginase production by Streptomyces griseus. Appl Microbial. 1972;23:1163–4.

15. Saxena RK, Sinha U. L-asparaginase and glutaminase activities in culture filtrates of Aspergillus nidulans. Curr Sci. 1981;50:218–9.

16. Gulati R, Saxena R, Gupta R. A rapid plate assay for screening L-asparaginase producing microorganisms. Lett Appl Microbiol. 1997;24:23–6.

17. Wriston J, Yellin T. L-asparaginase: a review. Adv Enzymol Relat Areas Mol Biol. 1973;39:185–248.

18. Imada A, Igarasi S, Nakahama K. Isona. M. Asparaginase and glutaminase activities of microorganisms. J Gen Microbiol. 1973;76:85–99.

19. Lowry OH, Rosebrough NJ, Farr AL, Randall RJ. Protein measurement with the Folin phenol reagent. J Biol Chem. 1951;193:265–75.

20. Sadana A. Biocatalysis: fundamentals of enzyme Deactvation kinetics. Englewood Cliffs: Prentice-Hall, Inc.; 1995.

21. Radha R, Arumugam N, Gummadi SN. Glutaminase free L-asparaginase from Vibrio cholerae: heterologous expression, purification and biochemical characterization. Int J Biol Macromol. 2018;4(111):129–38.

22. Meghavarnam AK, Janakiraman S. Purification and characterization of therapeutic enzyme L-asparaginase from a tropical soil fungal isolate Fusarium culmorum ASP-87. MOJ Proteomics Bioinform. 2015;2(6):1–6.

23. Laemmli UK. Cleavage of structural proteins during the assembly of the head of bacteriophage T4. Nature. 1970;227:680–5.

24. Gothoskar SV, Ranadive KJ. Anticancer screening of SAN-AB; an extract of marking nut, semecarpus anacardium. Indian J Exp Biol. 1971;9:372–5.

25. Raja Naresh RA, Ndupa N, Uma DP. Effect of macrophage activation on niosome encapsulated bleomycin in tumor-bearing mice. Ind J Pharamcol. 1996;28:175–80.

26. Schirner M, Hoffmann J, Menrad A, Schneider MR. Antiangiogenic chemotherapeutic agents: characterization in comparison to their tumor growth inhibition in human renal cell carcinoma models. Clin Cancer Res. 1998;4:1331–6.

27. Sahu MK, Poorani E, Sivakumar K, Thangaradjou T, Kannan L. Partial purification and anti-leukemic activity of L-asparaginase enzyme of the actinomycete strain LA-29 isolated from the estuarine fish. Mugil cephalus (Linn). J Environ Biol. 2007;28:645–50.

28. Dharmaraj S. Study of L-asparaginase production by Streptomyces noursei MTCC 10469, isolated from marine sponge Callyspongia diffusa. Iran J Biotechnol. 2011;9:102–8.

29. Narayana K, Kumar K, Vijayalakshmi M. L-asparaginase production by Streptomyces albidoflavus. Indian J Microbiol. 2008;48:331–6.

30. El-Bessoumy AA, Sarhan M, Mansour J. Production, isolation, and purification of L-asparaginase from Pseudomonas aeruginosa 50071 using solid-state fermentation. J Biochem Mol Biol. 2004;37:387–93.

31. Moorthy V, Ramalingam A, Sumantha A, Shankaranaya RT. Production, purification and characterisation of extracellular L-asparaginase from a soil isolate of Bacillus sp. Af J Microbiol Res. 2010;4:1862–7.

32. Dhevagi P, Poorani E. Isolation of L-asparaginase producing actinomycetes from marine sediments. Int J Curr Res Aca Rev. 2016;4:88–97.

33. Ohshima M, Yamamoto T, Soda K. Further characterization of glutaminase isozymes from Pseudomonas aeruginosa. Agri Biol Chem. 1976;40:2251–6.

34. Khamna S, Yokota A, Lumyong S. L-asparaginase production by actinomycetes isolated from some Thai medicinal plant rhizosphere soils. Int J Integ Biol. 2009;6:1–22.

35. Siddalingeshwara KG, Lingappa K. Production and characterization of L-asparaginase- a tumour inhibitor. Int J Pharm Tech Res. 2011;3:314–9.

36. Senthil Kumar M, Selvam K. Isolation and purification of high efficiency L-asparaginase by quantitative preparative continuous elution SDS PAGE electrophoresis. J Microbial Biochem Technol. 2011;3:073–83.

37. Husain I, Sharma A, Kumar S, Malik F. Purification and characterization of glutaminase free asparaginase from Enterobacter cloacae: In-Vitro evaluation of cytotoxic potential against human myeloid leukemia HL-60 cells. PLoS One. 2016;11(2):e0148877.

38. Manna S, Sinha A, Sadhukhan R, Chakrabarty S. Purification, characterization and antitumor activity of L-asparaginase isolated from Pseudomonas stutzeri MB-405. Curr Microbiol. 1995;30:291–8.

39. Nilolaev AI, Sokolov NN, Kozlov EA, Kutsman ME. Isolation and properties of a homogeneous L-asparaginase preparation from Pseudomonas fluorescens AG. Biokhimiia. 1975;40:984–9.

40. Gaffar SA, Shethna YI. Purification and some biological properties of asparaginase from Azotobacter vinelandii. Appl Environ Microbiol. 1977;33:508–14.

41. Cedar H, Schwartz JH. Localization of the two L-asparaginases in anaerobically grown Escherichia coli. J Biol Chem. 1967;242:3753–4.

42. Whelan BA, Wriston JC. Purification and properties of asparaginase from Escherichia coli B. Biochemist. 1969;8:2386–93.

43. Willis RC, Woolfolk CA. Asparagine utilization in Escherichia coli. J Bacteriol. 1974;118:231–41.

44. Tiwari N, Dua RD. Purification and preliminary characterization of L-asparaginase from Erwinia aroideae NRRL B-138. Indian J Biochem Biophys. 1996;33:371–6.

45. Mesas JM, Gil JA, Martín JF. Characterization and partial purification of L-asparaginase from Corynebacterium glutamicum. J Gen Microbiol. 1990;136:515–9.

46. Law AS, Wriston JC Jr. Purification and properties of Bacillus coagulans L-asparaginase. Arch Biochem Biophys. 1971;147:744–52.

47. Mahajan RV, Kumar V, Rajendran V, Saran S, Ghosh PC, Saxena RK. Purification and characterization of a novel and robust L-asparaginase having low-glutaminase activity from Bacillus licheniformis: In vitro evaluation of anti-cancerous properties. PLoS One. 2014;9(6):e99037.

48. Dias FFG, Ruiz ALTG, Della Torre A, Sato HH. Purification, characterization and anti-proliferative activity of L-asparaginase from Aspergillus oryzae CCT 3940 with no glutaminase activity. Asian Pac J Trop Biomed. 2016;6:785–94.

49. Wulff G. Enzyme-like catalysis by molecularly imprinted polymers. Chem Reviews. 2002;102:1–28.

50. Copeland RA. Enzymes, A practical introduction to structure, mechanism and data analysis. 2nd ed. New York; Wiley-VCH; 2000.

51. Bisswanger H.. Enzyme kinetics. Principles and Methods. 2nd ed. Wiley–VCH Verlag GmbH & Co.: Weinheim;2008.

52. Maladkar NK, Singh VK, Naik SR. Fermentative production and isolation of L-asparaginase from Erwinia carotovora, EC-113. Hindustan Antibiot Bull. 1992; 35:77–86.

53. Thakur M, Lincoln L, Niyonzima FN, Sunil S. Isolation, purification and characterization of fungal extracellular L-asapraginase from *Mucor hiemalis*. J Biocat Biotrans. 2013;2:1–9.
54. Kumar S, Venkata Dasu V, Pakshirajan K. Purification and characterization of glutaminase-free L-asparaginase from *Pectobacterium carotovorum* MTCC 1428. Bioresour Technol. 2011;102(2):2077–82.
55. Borkotaky B, Bezbaruah R. Production and properties of asparaginase from a new *Erwinia* sp. Folia Microbiol. 2002;47:473–6.
56. Lincoln L, Francois N, Niyonzima Sunil SM. Purification and properties of a fungal L-asparaginase from *Trichoderma viride* pers: SF GREY. J Microbiol Biotechnol Food Sci. 2015;4(4):310–6.
57. Archana Rani J, Raja RP. Production, purification and characterization of L-asparaginase from *Aspergillus nidulans* by solid substrate fermentation. Eur J Biotechnol Bio. 2014;2(4):51–8.
58. Raha SK, Roy SK, Dey SK, Chakrabarty SL. Purification and properties of an L-asparaginase from *Cylindrocarpon obtusisporum* MB-10. J Biochem Int. 1990; 21:987–1000.
59. Selvakumar N, Vanajakumar and Natarajan R. Partial purification, characterization and antitumor properties of L-asparaginase (antileukemic agent) from a marine Vibrio. Bioactive compounds from marine organisms, Indo-US symposium 1989, edited by Thompson MF, Sarojini R and Nagabhushanam R. 1991;289–300.
60. Knape MJ, Ahuja GL, Bertinetti D, Burghardt NCG, Zimmermann B, Taylor SS, Herberg FW. Divalent metal ions Mg^{2+} and Ca^{2+} have distinct effects on protein kinase a activity and regulation. ACS Chem Biol. 2015;10(10):2303–15.
61. Kumar CG, Takagi H. Microbial alkaline proteases: from a bioindustrial viewpoint. Biotechnol Adv. 1999;17:561–94.
62. Moradian F, Khajeh K, Naderi-Manesh H, Sadeghizadeh M. Isolation, purification and characterization of a surfactants, laundry detergents and organic solvents-resistant alkaline protease from *Bacillus* sp. HR-08. Appl Biochem Biotechnol. 2009;159:33–45.
63. Castanon M, Wilke CR. Effect of the surfactant tween 80 on enzymatic hydrolysis of newspaper. Biotechno Bioengi Techno. 1981;23:1365–72.
64. McAllister TA, Stanford K, Bae HD, Treacher R, Hristov AN, Baah J, Shelford JA, Cheng KJ. Effect of a surfactant and exogenous enzymes on digestibility of feed and on growth performance and carcass traits of lambs. Canadian J Anim Sci. 2000;80:35–44.
65. Usman A. Seeking efficacy in L-asparaginase to combat acute lymphoblastic leukemia (ALL): a review. Afr J Pharm Pharm. 2015;9:793–805.
66. Neeta Asthana S, Azmi W. Microbial L-asparginase: A potent antitumor enzyme. Indian J Biotechnol. 2003;2:184–94.

20

Survivability of hospitalized chronic kidney disease (CKD) patients with moderate to severe estimated glomerular filtration rate (eGFR) after experiencing adverse drug reactions (ADRs) in a public healthcare center: a retrospective 3 year study

Monica Danial[1,2]* iD, Mohamed Azmi Hassali[1], Loke Meng Ong[2] and Amer Hayat Khan[3]

Abstract

Background: Accurate identification and routine preventive practices are crucial steps in lessening the incidence of medications and patients related adverse drug reactions (ADRs).

Methods: Three years retrospective study was conducted among chronic kidney disease (CKD) patients at multi-wards in a tertiary healthcare center. Data collected included demographic characteristics, physical examination results, comorbid conditions, laboratory tests and medications taken. Only medication prescribed during the hospital stay were considered in this study.

Results: From this study only one ADR incident was definitely preventable and majority of other ADRs (88.3%) were possibly preventable. Type of renal replacement therapy ($p = 0.023$) and stages of renal function ($p = 0.002$) were significantly associated with survivability of the hospitalized CKD patients after ADRs. Highest percentage of mortality based on categories were 50–59 years (20.0%), male (16.3%), Indian ethnicity (23.7%), obese (15.0%), smoking (17.1%), consumes alcohol (17.4%), conservative management of renal disease (19.5%) and renal function of < 15 mL/min/1.73m². Overall survivability using Kaplan-Meier analysis reported a significant difference of 18-day survival rate between patients undergoing hemodialysis and patients conservatively managing their renal disease. The 18 days survival rate of patients undergoing hemodialysis, peritoneal dialysis and conservative management were 94.9%, 91.7% and 75.1% respectively. Eighteen days survival rate of patients with renal functions of 30–59 mL/min/1.73m², 15–29 mL/min/1.73m² and < 15 mL/min/1.73m² were 87.4%, 69.8% and 88.6% respectively. Similarly, Cox regression analysis revealed that renal replacement therapy was the only factor significantly contributed to ADRs related mortality. CKD patients whom conservatively managed renal disease or/and with renal function of < 15 mL/min/1.73m² had 5.61 and 5.33 higher mortality risk respectively.

(Continued on next page)

* Correspondence: monicadanial83@gmail.com; monica@crc.moh.gov.my
[1]Discipline of Social and Administrative Pharmacy, School of Pharmaceutical Sciences, Universiti Sains Malaysia, 11800 Minden, Penang, Malaysia
[2]Clinical Research Center (CRC) Penang General Hospital, 10990 Jalan Residensi, Pulau Pinang, Malaysia
Full list of author information is available at the end of the article

(Continued from previous page)

Conclusion: Majority of the reported ADRs were possibly preventable. Renal replacement therapy and/or renal function were significant risk factors for mortality due to ADRs among hospitalized CKD patients stages 3 to 5. Clinician engagement, intensive resources and regular updates aided with online monitoring technology are needed for enhancing care and prevention of ADRs among CKD patients.

Keywords: Chronic kidney disease (CKD), Adverse drug reactions (ADRs), Preventable, Survival rate, Conservative management

Background

Human body is an intricate system where myriad of biological interactions entangles into a network. Minor disruption in the network by a drug can cause diverse reactions including adverse drug reactions (ADRs). ADRs are caused by the drug interaction with undesired targets within our body [1]. In addition, complex underlying disease states of the human body also influences the drug-drug interaction thus contributing to ADRs. Moreover, factors like increase in the number and type of marketed drugs, increase in aging population, immunological factors (gender and pregnancy), pharmacokinetics differences, polypharmacy and urbanization [1–3] elevates the risk of ADRs. The most commonly reported ADRs causing drugs were NSAIDs, aspirin, anti-neoplastic, anti-psychotics, diuretics and anti-arrhythmic [4]. Tan et al. [1] reviewed, that the top drug-induced toxicities were hepatotoxicity (21%), nephrotoxicity (7%), cardiotoxicity (7%), torsade (21%) and rhabdomyolysis (7%). Each drug prescription carries its own risks for causing ADRs, ranging the full spectrum of severity from cosmetic to severe morbidity and mortality due to patients specific reasons [5].

Clinically significant medications and patients related to ADRs were usually predicted and mostly preventable with few not preventable ADRs [6–8]. Moreover, some of the newly introduced drugs' side effects were not fully documented hence would possibly exert severe deleterious impact during usage [9]. In recent years, it was reviewed and reported that all drugs cause side effects, however the impact and severity vary and ranges from mild (for example: mild itching or mild headache) to severe (for example: severe rash, damage to vital organs, primarily the liver and kidneys and possibly even death). Therefore, precise diagnosis of ADRs is crucial to reduce preventable ADRs, which however remains a challenge among clinicians [7].

Causality assessment methods are primarily used in evaluating the medication related causality of ADRs [10, 11]. These methods traditionally utilize three approaches such as expert judgement, probabilistic method and algorithm method. More recent approaches are genetic algorithm, Liverpool algorithm and pediatric algorithm [12]. Severity is used for quantification of discomfort grades. Hatwig and colleague

[13] developed a scale for assessing the severity of ADRs. Classification on severity are mild (slightly bothersome; relieved with symptomatic treatment), moderate (bothersome, interferes with activities; only partially relieved with symptomatic treatment) and severe (prevents regular activities; not relieved with symptomatic treatment) [14–16]. ADRs preventability are determined by ADRs types which ranges from type A till type D. Type A or Type 1 (augmented) reactions results from an exaggeration of a drug's normal pharmacological actions when common therapeutic dose administered. Type A is usually dose dependent. Type B or Type 2 (bizarre) are ADRs that occurs as novel response not expected from known pharmacological action [17]. Type C (chronic) ADRs includes adaptive changes, rebound phenomena and other long-term effects. Type D (delayed) reactions are carcinogenesis, affecting reproduction such as impaired fertility and adverse effects on the foetus during early or later stages of pregnancy and drug availability in breast milk [16].

Chronic kidney disease (CKD) is a major health burden that amplifies the risk for adverse events [18, 19]. CKD is independently associated with increased adverse risks including kidney failure, cardiovascular events and all-cause mortality [19, 20]. An eight-year (1999–2006) retrospective study conducted in the United States revealed that there were more than 2 million deaths which were attributed as ADR-related deaths [3]. Additionally, Pirmohamed et al. [21] reported high incidence of in-hospital ADRs which was about 14.7%. Therefore it is beneficial to evaluate patients risk factors for ADRs individually. For minimization of ADRs events, understanding and knowledge on prescribed drug metabolization mechanisms, magnitude and probable ADRs is essentially to be equipped by the healthcare professionals. Thus, these will establish safe medication prescription practices which stresses cautious consideration of the benefits and risks of concomitant medications [22]. Therefore, this study aimed to assess the causality, severity and preventability of ADRs among hospitalized CKD patients with estimated glomerular filtration rate (eGFR) value of < 60 ml/min/1.73m^2. Additionally, risk factors for mortality due to ADRs were also evaluated.

Methods

Study design and participants

This a 3 years retrospective observational study conducted in Penang General Hospital. It is the seconds largest General Hospital in Malaysia. A total of 1070 medical records of patients experienced ADRs from various wards for the duration of 3 years (January 1, 2014 till December 31, 2016) were screened. CKD patients stages 3–5 (eGFR< 60 ml/min/1.73m^2) with stable serum creatinine (sCr) values during the initial days of admission and experienced ADRs during hospitalization were the primary inclusion criteria of this study. The sCr value obtained during the first day of admission were used to estimate the glomerular filtration rate (GFR). Additional inclusion criteria were patient aged ≥18 years old and admitted for more than 24 h. Medical records which were dubious and incomplete and ward admission due to ADRs or acute kidney injury (AKI) were excluded from this study. Only 160 patients were selected after subsequent screening and identification of records that met the inclusion and exclusion criteria. From the total number of the patient records finally selected, 132 patients survived and 28 patients did not survive ADRs during hospitalization. Prior to study commencement, ethical approval was obtained from Medical Research & Ethics Committee (MREC), Ministry of Health Malaysia (MOH). Study approval number: NMRR-15-1810-28,375(IIR).

Estimation of renal function

For each patient, the sCr value was measured at admission using the standardized GFR method in the hospital laboratory department. The eGFR was then calculated from serum creatinine value using the chronic kidney disease epidemiology collaboration (CKD-EPI) equation [23]. Stages of CKD included in this study were 3A eGFR 45–59 mL/min/1.73 m^2, 3B eGFR 30–44 mL/min/1.73 m^2, 4 eGFR 15–29 mL/min/1.73 m^2 and 5 eGFR < 15 mL/min/1.73 m^2. Based on the type of renal replacement therapy, patients with end stage renal disease (ESRD) were divided into hemodialysis, peritoneal dialysis and patients not undergoing any type of dialysis (will be termed as 'conservative management or conservatively managed renal disease' in subsequent sections).

Data collection

For each patient, data was collected retrospectively from the patients' medical records using a standardized form. Data collected included (a) demographic characteristics such as age and sex; (b) physical examination results such as blood pressure and weight (c) comorbid conditions such as diabetes, hypertension, vascular disease, heart failure, atrial fibrillation and anemia (d) laboratory tests such as serum and biochemical parameters and (e) medications taken before admission, during hospitalization and medications prescribed at discharge. Only medications prescribed during the hospitalization were considered in this study.

Identifications of ADRs

The primary outcome of this study was to determine the incidence and patterns of ADRs among hospitalized CKD patients stages 3 to 5. Identification of adverse drug reaction (ADR) event was done using a 3-step identification process (trigger list/ physician order, confirmation by an independent reviewer and assessment of causality, severity and preventability of identified ADRs by experienced pharmacist). In this study, ADRs was defined according to Edwards and Aronson [24]. Suspected ADRs were then classified based on the system developed by Rawlin and Thompson [25]. For each suspected ADR, information collected were (a) date start and end of ADR (b) the probable ADRs causative drugs, administered dosage and frequency (c) physical examination and laboratory results (d) reported adverse outcomes such as dizziness and rash. The beginning of the ADR was the date of the clinical or biological diagnosis of the ADR. The end of the ADR was the date of normalization of the effect which was obtained from the ADR reporting form and justified with the date of laboratory examination with normal results or the disappearance of clinical symptoms reported by physicians and pharmacist. If the end date of ADR and the date of the patient demise was reported on the same day therefore the cause of death is regarded as due to ADRs. The ADRs lasted from 1 day to several weeks. Major drug classes that attributed to ADRs were anti-infective, anti-hypertensive, analgesic, statins and anti-diabetic. Furthermore, anti-infectives contributed to highest number of mortality in this study (Danial M, Hassali AMA, Ong LM and Khan AH. Direct cost associated with adverse drug reactions among hospitalized chronic kidney patients in a public healthcare facility: A retrospective 3 year study, submitted).

Assessment of causality, preventability and severity of ADRs

Assessment of ADRs were done based on causality, severity and preventability. The drug related causality was assessed by using Naranjo algorithm [26]. Only definite and probable ADRs were considered for further assessment. The severity of ADRs were then scored using Hartwig and Siegel [13] scale into mild, moderate or severe. Preventability of ADRs were determined using Hallas et al. [27] criteria into definitely preventable, possibly preventable and non-preventable. The overall incidence of ADRs were defined as the total number of patients who suffered ADRs during hospitalization in relation to the total number of patients admitted to various wards during the 3-year study period.

Statistical analysis

For the purpose of descriptive analysis, baseline characteristics of patients with ADRs were analyzed using either chi-square test for categorical variables and t-test or Mann-Whitney test, depending on the skewness of data, for continuously distributed variables. The Cox regression analysis was used to estimate of the relative risk of having an ADR during hospital stay in relation to stages of renal function (stages 3 to 5) or for ESRD in relation to the three types of renal replacement therapy (hemodialysis, peritoneal dialysis and conservative management). The Cox regression model is the most frequently used model for analyzing time-to-event data [28]. In this case, the time from hospital admission to day on which the ADR occurred was considered as the time to event and the outcome of the model is either survival or death. The advantage of using Cox regression model is the ability to censor patients who fail to reach the study end-point [29]. In this case, patients who survived of an ADR during the hospitalization were censored. The hazard ratio is the probability that a patient survived the event or the outcome to a certain time point [29]. The hazard ratio survival of the ADR event was reported graphically using the Kaplan-Meier estimates, plotting the log-minus survival function over time. The log-rank test was used to investigate the association with the outcome. All analysis was performed using SPSS (version 22; SPSS Inc., Chicago, IL). Two-sided p-values of less than 0.05 were considered statistically significant.

Results

Baseline characteristics of patients

Baseline characteristic of patients were similar as reported in (Danial M, Hassali AMA, Ong LM and Khan AH. Direct cost associated with adverse drug reactions among hospitalized chronic kidney patients in a public healthcare facility: A retrospective 3 year study, submitted). CKD patients were grouped into survived ($n = 132$) and whom did not survive after ADRs ($n = 28$) event during hospitalization. Majority of the study patients were Chinese; male; aged ≥60 years; with eGFR value of < 15 mL/min/ 1.73m^2 and conservatively managed the renal disease (Table 1). Furthermore, the CKD patients were reported to have comorbidities primarily such as diabetes, dyslipidaemia and hypertension. Additionally, it was reported that they consumed ≥23 of total number of medications (Danial M, Hassali AMA, Ong LM and Khan AH: Development of a mortality score to assess risk of adverse drug reactions among hospitalized patients with moderate to severe chronic kidney disease, submitted).

Causality assessment of ADRs

Based on Naranjo scale there were 25 (15.6%) definite, 78 (48.8%) probable, 56 (35.0%) possible and 1(0.6%) doubtful ADRs respectively (Fig. 1). Cumulatively, the

Table 1 Demographic characteristics of the study participants ($n = 160$)

Characteristics	n (%)	Survived ($n = 132$)	Died ($n = 28$)
Demographics			
Age			
≤ 49 years	41 (25.6)	34 (21.3)	7(4.4)
50–59 years	40 (25.0)	32(20.0)	8(5.0)
≥ 60 years	79 (49.4)	66(41.3)	13(8.1)
Gender			
Male	92 (57.5)	77(48.1)	15(9.4)
Female	68 (42.5)	55(34.4)	13(8.1)
Ethnicity			
Malay	52 (32.5)	44(27.5)	8(5.0)
Chinese	68 (42.5)	57(35.6)	11(6.9)
Indian	36 (25.0)	27(18.1)	9(5.6)
Currently or previously smoking	41 (25.6)	34(21.3)	7(4.4)
Currently or previously consumed alcohol	23(14.4)	19(11.9)	4(2.5)
Renal Replacement Therapy			
Haemodialysis	61 (38.1)	52(32.5)	9(5.6)
Peritoneal dialysis	12 (7.5)	10(6.3)	2(1.3)
Conservative management	87 (54.4)	70(43.8)	17(10.6)
Renal Function			
30–59 mL/min/1.73m^2	49 (30.6)	46(28.7)	3(1.9)
15–29 mL/min/1.73m^2	29 (18.1)	22(13.8)	7(4.4)
< 15 mL/min/1.73m^2	82 (51.2)	64(40.0)	18(11.3)

definite and probable ADRs accounted for 103 (64.4%) of the total ADRs. Subsequently, type A accounted for 89 (86.4%) ADRs as per the Rawlin and Thompson classification system. Preventability assessment using Hallas et al. [27] criteria indicated that only one ADR incident was definitely preventable, 91 (88.3%) were possibly preventable and 11 (10.7%) of incidence were non-preventable. Cumulatively, preventable ADRs were about 92 (89.3%) (Table 2). Severity assessment using modified Hartwig and Siegel scale categorized 14 (13.6%) severe, 61 (59.2%) moderate and 28 (27.2%) mild ADRs (Table 3).

Logistic regression

Categories that were more prone for mortality after ADR events were patients aged 50–59 years (20.0%); male (16.3%), Indian ethnicity (23.7%); obese (15.0%); with current or past history of smoking (17.1%); with current or past history of alcohol consumption (17.4%); conservatively managed renal disease (19.5%) and with renal function of < 15 mL/min/1.73m^2 (Table 4). The multiple logistic regression values indicated that the age category of 50–59 years had 2.05 (95% CI 0.57–7.34)

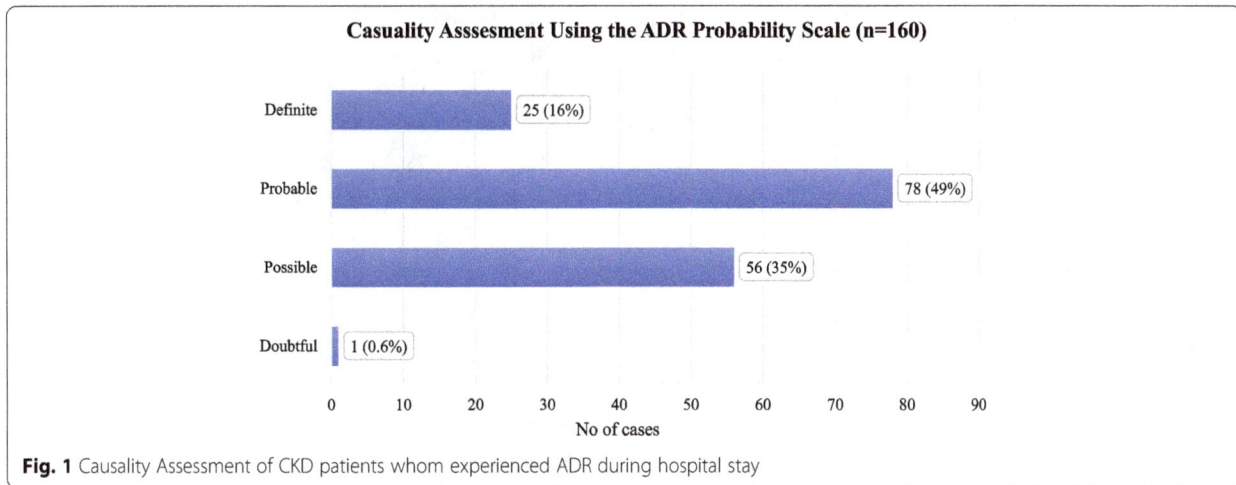

Fig. 1 Causality Assessment of CKD patients whom experienced ADR during hospital stay

higher rates of not surviving ADRs compared to age categories of ≤49 years and ≥60 years old. Additionally, males had higher mortality rate than females. Indian ethnicity had 2.59 (95% CI 0.77–8.72) higher death rates compared to Malay and Chinese ethnicity. Lowest mortality rate was reported in Chinese ethnicity (OR: 0.70; 95% CI 0.20–2.44). BMI category obese (OR: 1.34; 95% CI 0.18–9.71) had higher rates of mortality compared to overweight, normal and underweight after ADRs. CKD patients with current or past history of smoking and alcohol consumption had higher death rates with OR: 1.19 (95% CI 0.32–4.47) and OR: 1.06 (95% CI 0.21–5.46) respectively. Furthermore, patients whom conservatively managed their renal disease had higher death rate (OR: 5.90; 95% CI 1.63–21.34) compared to those undergoing peritoneal dialysis and hemodialysis. Similarly, CKD patients with renal function of < 15 mL/min/1.73m^2 recorded highest mortality rate (OR: 22.37; 95% CI 3.99–125.31) in its category. Overall, types of renal replacement therapy ($p = 0.023$) and renal function ($p = 0.002$) were significant factors that influenced the survivability of the hospitalized CKD patients after ADRs.

Table 2 Classification and preventability assessment of the ADRs

Assessments of ADRs	No.*	(%)
Classification of ADR based on;		
[a]Type A	89	86.4
[a]Type B	14	13.6
[b]Definitely preventable	1	1
[b]Possibly preventable	91	88.3
[b]Non-preventable	11	10.7

Abbreviations: ADR, adverse drug reaction
*The total number of definite or probable ADRs, $n = 103$
[a] Type A and Type B ADR are classified based on Rawlin and Thompson (1991)
[b] Definitely preventable, Possibly preventable and Non-preventable are classified based on Hallas et al. [27]

Kaplan-Meier overall survivability

The Kaplan-Meier overall survivability analysis performed indicated 85.0% survival for the duration of 18 days (Fig. 2). The Kaplan-Meier survival analysis revealed the differences in survival after ADRs among patients with different renal replacement therapy. Eighteen days survival rates of patients undergoing hemodialysis, peritoneal dialysis and conservative management were 94.9%, 91.7% and 75.1% respectively. However, no survival differences were observed in categories of age, gender, ethnicity, BMI, smoking status, alcohol consumption status and renal function. Eighteen days survival rates of age groups ≤49 years,

Table 3 Severity assessment of the ADRs

Level	Description	Scale	No.*	(%)
1	An ADR occurs but requires no change in treatment with the suspected drug.	Mild	7	6.8
2	The ADR requires that the suspected drug be withheld, discontinued or otherwise changed. No changed antidote or other treatment is required, and there is no increase in length of stay.	Mild	21	20.4
3	The ADR requires that the suspected drug be withheld, discontinued or otherwise changed, and/or an antidote or other treatment is required, and there is no increase in length of stay.	Moderate	31	30.1
4	a) Any level 3 ADR that increases length of stay by at least one day, or (b) The ADR is the reason for admission	Moderate	30	29.1
5	Any level 4 ADR that requires intensive medical care.	Severe	13	12.6
6	The adverse reaction causes permanent harm to the patient.	Severe	0	0
7a	The adverse reaction indirectly linked to the death of patient.	Severe	1	1.0
7b	The adverse reaction directly linked to the death of patient.	Severe	0	0

Abbreviations: ADR, adverse drug reaction
*The total number of definite or probable ADRs, $n = 103$

Table 4 Factors associated with survivability after ADR events using simple logistic and multiple regression

Variables	Survived N(%)	Died N(%)	Crude OR	(95% CI)	p -value[a]	Adj. OR	(95% CI)	p -value[b]
Age category								
≤ 49 years	34 (82.9%)	7 (17.1%)	1.00(ref.)		0.888	1.00(ref.)		0.490
50–59 years	32 (80.0%)	8 (20.0%)	1.21	(0.40, 3.73)	0.735	2.05	(0.57,7.34)	
≥ 60 years	66 (83.5%)	13 (16.5%)	0.96	(0.35, 2.62)	0.931	1.14	(0.35, 3.66)	
Gender								
Male	77 (83.7%)	15 (16.3%)	1.00(ref.)		0.644	1.00(ref.)		0.829
Female	55 (80.9%)	13 (19.1%)	1.21	(0.54,2.75)		0.88	(0.28,2.75)	
Ethnicity								
Malay	44 (84.6%)	8 (15.4%)	1.00(ref.)		0.544	1.00(ref.)		0.108
Chinese	57 (83.8%)	11 (16.2%)	1.06	(0.39,2.86)	0.906	0.70	(0.20, 2.44)	
Indian	29 (76.3%)	9 (23.7%)	1.71	(0.59,4.93)	0.324	2.59	(0.77,8.72)	
BMI category								
Underweight	14 (82.4%)	3 (17.6%)	1.00(ref.)		0.917	1.00(ref.)		0.825
Normal	58 (84.1%)	11 (15.9%)	0.89	(0.22,3.60)	0.865	0.82	(0.17, 4.05)	
Overweight	43 (79.6%)	11 (20.4%)	1.19	(0.29,4.90)	0.806	1.33	(0.27, 6.56)	
Obese	17 (85.0%)	3 (15.0%)	0.82	(0.14,4.74)	0.828	1.34	(0.18, 9.71)	
Smoking								
No	98 (82.4%)	21 (17.6%)	1.00(ref.)		0.934	1.00(ref.)		0.800
Yes	34 (82.9%)	7 (17.1%)	0.96	(0.38,2.46)		1.19	(0.32, 4.47)	
Alcohol consumption								
No	113 (82.5%)	24 (17.5%)	1.00(ref.)		0.988	1.00(ref.)		0.943
Yes	19 (82.6%)	4 (17.4%)	0.99	(0.31, 3.18)		1.06	(0.21, 5.46)	
Renal replacement therapy								
Hemodialysis	52 (85.2%)	9 (14.8%)	1.00(ref.)		0.751	1.00(ref.)		0.023*
Peritoneal dialysis	10 (83.3%)	2 (16.7%)	1.16	(0.22,6.17)	0.866	1.21	(0.21, 6.940)	
Conservative management	70 (80.5%)	17 (19.5%)	1.40	(0.58,3.40)	0.453	5.90	(1.63,21.34)	
Renal function								
30–59 mL/min/1.73m^2	46 (93.9%)	3 (6.1%)	1.00(ref.)		0.062	1.00(ref.)		0.002*
15–29 mL/min/1.73m^2	22 (75.9%)	7 (24.1%)	4.88	(1.15,20.69)	0.032	8.90	(1.76, 44.94)	
< 15 mL/min/1.73m^2	64 (78.0%)	18 (22.0%)	4.31	(1.20,15.51)	0.025	22.37	(3.99,125.31)	

Note: [a]Simple Logistic Regression;
[b]Multiple Logistic Regression;
Crude OR = Crude Odds Ratio;
Adj. OR = Adjusted Odds Ratio;
95% CI = 95% confidence interval
*p value< 0.05

50–59 years and ≥ 60 years were 86.2%, 85.6% and 84.2% respectively. Eighteen days survival rates based on gender were 84.7% male and 85.5% female. Eighteen days survival rates based on ethnic groups were 86.1% Malay, 80.0% Chinese and 94.7% Indian. Eighteen days survival rate of patients based on BMI categories were 63.0% underweight, 92.0% normal, 73.0% overweight and 93.8% obese. Eighteen days survival rate of patients based smoking status were 84.5% non-smokers and 86.6% smokers. Eighteen days survival rate of patients-based alcohol consumption were 84.5% no and 87.7% yes. Eighteen days survival rate of patients with

renal functions of 30–59 mL/min/1.73m^2, 15–29 mL/min/1.73m^2 and < 15 mL/min/1.73m^2 were 87.4%, 69.8% and 88.6% respectively (Table 5).

Cox regression

The Cox regression analysis revealed that only renal replacement therapy contributed significantly to mortality associated with ADRs among CKD patients. Factors such as age, gender, ethnicity, BMI, smoking status, alcohol consumption status and renal function were not significantly linked to mortality due to ADRs among CKD patients

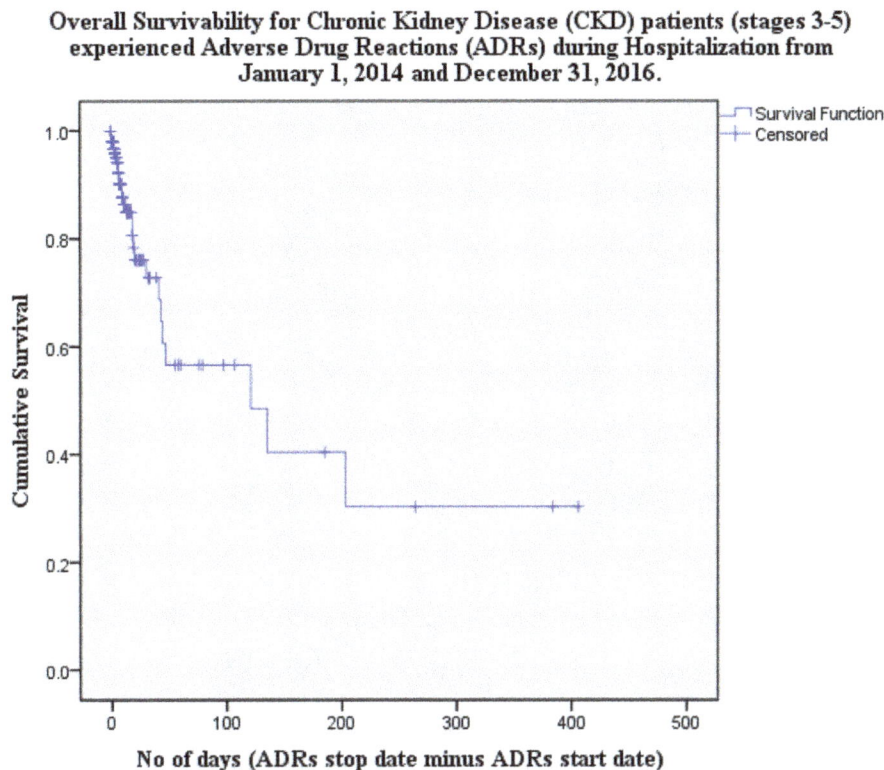

Fig. 2 Overall Survivability for Chronic Kidney Disease (CKD) patients (stages 3–5) experienced Adverse Drug Reactions (ADRs) during Hospitalization from January 1, 2014 and December 31, 2016

(Table 6). CKD patients whom were conservatively managing their renal disease had 5.61 more risk of dying compared to those whom were undergoing hemodialysis. Additionally, lowest risk of mortality (0.61) were observed in patients undergoing peritoneal dialysis. In terms of renal function, CKD patients with renal function of < 15 mL/min/1.73m^2 had 5.33 higher risk of mortality compared to patients with renal function of 30–59 mL/min/1.73m^2 and 2.91 higher risk of mortality compared to patients with renal function of 30–59 mL/min/1.73m^2.

Hazard ratio

Age group of 50–59 years old had higher risk of dying (HR: 1.08) compared to ≤49 years and ≥ 60 years old. Additionally, male had higher risk of dying (HR: 1.00) compared to females. Indian patients (HR: 1.05) had higher mortality risk compared to Malay and Chinese patients. Overweight patients had higher risk of dying (HR: 1.47) compared to underweight, normal and obese CKD patients. Non-smokers (HR: 1.00) and patients with current or past history alcohol consumption (HR: 1.01) had higher mortality risk after ADRs during hospitalization compared their respective group categories.

Discussions

Identification of ADRs among CKD patients will be useful in clinical practice as to implement appropriate care aimed at reducing the number of ADRs. Survival estimation studies are vital for the prediction of impending disease burden, redirection in approaches of disease screening and planning of clinical trials both intervention and observational studies, thus paving ways for more successful understanding among public, healthcare providers and policy makers [30].

Based on our study, in Penang General Hospital yearly about 13.5% of hospitalized CKD patients stages 3 to 5 experienced ADRs. Our findings were similar with meta-analysis study conducted by Lazarou et al. [31] where they reported that 10.9% of patients experienced ADRs of all severities as inpatients and another study by Davies et al. [32], which estimated that between 10 and 20% of patients experienced ADRs during hospitalization. Moreover, from our study about 88% of ADRs were possibly preventable. Similar results were reported by Chan et al. [33], where it was reported that 50% of ADR were preventable. Preventable ADRs were commonly associated with prescription of diuretics, antiplatelet, anticoagulant, antidiabetic and NSAIDs drugs to the patients [34, 35].

Severity assessment using the Hartwig and Siegal indicated that nearly 27% of ADRs scored mild and nearly 60% of ADRs scored at level 3 or below on the Hartwig scale. This indicated that remedial action was performed to treat the ADRs as reported in the patients' medical

Table 5 Survivability of the CKD patients after ADR event

Variables	Number of Patients	Number of Events	Survivalibility (%)						Comparison	p-value[a]
	n	n	3 days	6 days	9 days	12 days	15 days	18 days		
Overall Survivalibility	160	28	96.7	94.2	87.7	86.4	86.4	85.0		
Age category										0.927
≤ 49 years	41	7	95.1	95.1	95.1	91.3	86.2	86.2		
50–59 years	40	8	97.1	97.1	97.1	85.6	85.6	85.6		
≥ 60 years	79	13	97.3	92.5	84.2	84.2	84.2	84.2		
Gender										0.787
Male	92	15	96.6	96.6	91.3	84.7	84.7	84.7		
Female	68	13	96.9	91.1	88.7	88.7	85.5	85.5		
Ethnicity										0.796
Malay	52	8	97.8	97.8	97.8	90.4	86.1	86.1		
Chinese	68	11	96.8	90.6	80.0	80.0	80.0	80.0		
Indian	38	9	94.7	94.7	94.7	94.7	94.7	94.7		
BMI category										0.206
Underweight	17	3	93.3	93.3	84.0	84.0	63.0	63.0		
Normal	69	11	94.0	92.0	92.0	92.0	92.0	92.0		
Overweight	54	11	100.0	94.7	85.3	77.9	73.0	73.0		
Obese	20	3	100.0	100.0	100.0	93.8	93.8	93.8		
Smoking										0.943
No	119	21	97.3	95.2	89.9	86.5	84.5	84.5		
Yes	41	7	95.1	91.2	91.2	86.6	86.6	86.6		
Alcohol consumption										0.647
No	137	24	96.9	94.0	87.7	86.2	84.5	84.5		
Yes	23	4	95.7	95.7	95.7	87.7	87.7	87.7		
Renal replacement therapy										0.050
a. Hemodialysis	61	9	100.0	100.0	97.8	94.9	94.9	94.9	a vs b	0.874
b. Peritoneal dialysis	12	2	91.7	91.7	91.7	91.7	91.7	91.7	a vs c	0.019
c. Conservative management	87	17	95.2	90.1	83.6	78.4	75.1	75.1	b vs c	0.293
Renal function										0.347
30–59 mL/min/1.73m^2	49	3	100.0	100.0	100.0	87.4	87.4	87.4		
15–29 mL/min/1.73m^2	29	7	93.0	93.0	82.6	76.7	69.8	69.8		
< 15 mL/min/1.73m^2	82	18	96.2	92.0	88.6	88.6	88.6	88.6		

Note: [a]survival analysis using Kaplan-Meier

records. The reported remedial action was either discontinuation of the suspected drug alone and/or treating with the corrective drug. The outcome of the remedial action resulted in additional laboratory investigations, extra procedures, increment in days of hospitalization, admission to intensive care unit and/or death.

Least number of survivors were from age group of ≥60 years (84.2%) using Kaplan-Meier analysis. It has been reported that death is anticipated after an ADR among patients aged more than 55 years [31, 35]. It is attributable to the presence of high levels of albuminuria with impaired level of eGFR among the older adults [30, 36].

In addition, in this study males were more susceptible to mortality due to ADRs compared to female. The Kaplan-Meier survival analysis revealed that the lowest survival experience for male CKD patients to be 84.7%. Inker et al. [30], indicated that the differences between gender may be attributable to faster progression to ESRD in male compared to female, inaccuracies in estimating equations or lower levels of normal GFR in women [37, 38]. For example,

Table 6 Cox regression of the CKD patients after ADR event

Variables	Cencored		Events		Adj. HR	(95% CI)	p -value[c]
	n	(%)	n	(%)			
Age category							0.934
≤ 49 years	34	82.9	7	25.0	1.00	(ref.)	
50–59 years	32	80.0	8	28.6	1.08	(0.34,3.39)	
≥ 60 years	66	83.5	13	46.4	0.89	(0.31,2.58)	
Gender							0.504
Male	77	83.7	15	53.6	1.00	(ref.)	
Female	55	80.9	13	46.4	0.69	(0.23,2.08)	
Ethnicity							0.997
Malay	44	84.6	8	28.6	1.00	(ref.)	
Chinese	57	83.8	11	39.3	1.02	(0.33,3.11)	
Indian	29	76.3	9	32.1	1.05	(0.33,3.35)	
BMI category							0.434
Underweight	14	82.4	3	10.7	1.00	(ref.)	
Normal	58	84.1	11	39.3	0.94	(0.21,4.25)	
Overweight	43	79.6	11	39.3	1.47	(0.32,6.75)	
Obese	17	85.0	3	10.7	0.42	(0.06,2.83)	
Smoking							0.886
No	98	82.4	21	75.0	1.00	(ref.)	
Yes	34	82.9	7	25.0	0.91	(0.24,3.37)	
Alcohol consumption							0.987
No	113	82.5	24	85.7	1.00	(ref.)	
Yes	19	82.6	4	14.3	1.01	(0.20,5.03)	
Renal replacement therapy							0.003
Hemodialysis	52	85.2	9	32.1	1.00	(ref.)	
Peritoneal dialysis	10	83.3	2	7.1	0.61	(0.11,3.39)	
Conservative management	70	80.5	17	60.7	5.61	(1.94,16.20)	
Renal function							0.089
30–59 mL/min/1.73m^2	46	93.9	3	10.7	1.00	(ref.)	
15–29 mL/min/1.73m^2	22	75.9	7	25.0	2.91	(0.65,12.96)	
< 15 mL/min/1.73m^2	64	82.5	18	64.3	5.33	(1.18,24.07)	

Fan et al. [39] reported that the CKD-EPI equation has slight but non-significant overestimation of GFR in women compared with men. Furthermore, gender differences may also due to immunological and hormonal physiology which influences pharmacodynamics and pharmacokinetics responses, particularly in relation to cardiac and psychotropic medications [40].

In this study, significant positive association were found between renal function and survivability after ADR events ($r = 0.02$, $p < 0.05$). Patients whom conservatively managed renal disease (19.5%) and patients with renal function of < 15 mL/min/1.73m^2 were at the highest risk of mortality. Metabolic changes among advanced CKD patients have been associated with impaired physical function, which includes reduced muscle function, grip strength and cognition [41]. Furthermore, poorer degree of CKD is associated with higher frequency of the frailty syndrome and higher risk of functional decline over time [42–44].

Safe drug dosage is specifically influenced and associated with individual factors like physical parameters including age and weight; presence of comorbidities; physiological status including renal and hepatic function; current medications usage and previously reported history of allergies [45]. Age influences drug pharmacokinetics and pharmacodynamics activities [46]. Older age influences the rapid accumulation of total body fat and inversely reduces lean muscle mass and water volume. Thus, it impairs the dissemination of many drugs for example benzodiazepines, antipsychotics and opioids [47]. Additionally, reduced water availability rises toxicity levels. This condition results in lengthening of drug elimination half-life which in turn causes undesirable drug side effect such as drowsiness, falls and unwanted dosage build-up [47].

Likewise, aging causes impairment of GFR like decrease in renal size, nephron function and assimilations which are accountable for comorbidities such as hypertension, diabetes and heart failure [48]. Therefore, estimation of GFR is vital when up-taking renally eliminated drugs like dabigatran and metformin as safe dosage needed to be prescribed as to lessen the risk of an ADR [48]. It also have been reported that aging causes decline in liver mass and perfusion, which can adversely affect drugs with high hepatic extraction ratio such as diltiazem, opiates and warfarin [49]. These drugs systemic bioavailability surges with higher accumulation in serum coupled with enhanced adverse drug effect [47].

Pharmacovigilance of ADRs includes detection, assessment, understanding and prevention of adverse effects or any other drug-related problem with the aim of enhancing medication safety and patient care [50]. Likewise, E-pharmacovigilance will be a resourceful tool in drug safety for potentially predicting an ADR likelihood by utilizing previously obtained information such as laboratory investigations [51]. Moreover, drug safety can be established by adopting programmed electronic methods which can render information on past errors of medication and/or dosage and potential medication interactions. Beneficial attributes of electronic prescribing methods have been applauded by a recent systematic review where it was reported to reduce medical errors and adverse drug effects [47, 52].

Study strengths and limitations

The strength of the current study lies in identifying the ADR event using the 3-step identification process. The study population included all ADR events recorded for 3 years continuously from multiple wards, representing all clinical specialties commonly found in most acute hospitals. Furthermore, the age distribution of our study population was comparable to figures for all in-patient admissions from other literatures. Thus, this study produces highly reliable results that represents the real-world practices. However, the study limitations were firstly, it was conducted in one hospital and there is likely to be variation between different hospitals because of differences in the local population characteristics and the specialties within the hospitals. Secondly, since this study was performed in one hospital, it may limit the generalizability of the results. Finally, survival risks for specific stages may be overestimated because it was derived using only one measurement of GFR.

Conclusions

Conclusively, from this study only one ADR incident was definitely preventable and majority of other ADRs were possibly preventable. Renal replacement therapy and/or renal function were significant risk factors for mortality due to ADRs among hospitalized CKD patients stages 3 to 5. There is a need to develop a high-reliability assessment tool which can meticulously establish suitable diagnostic criteria for ADRs with universal acceptance to improvise the fundamental aspect of drug safety and evades the impending ADRs.

Abbreviations
ADRs: Adverse drug reactions; CKD: Chronic kidney disease; CKD-EPI: Chronic kidney disease epidemiology collaboration; eGFR: estimated glomerulus filtration; ESRD: end stage renal disease; GFR: Glomerular filtration rate

Acknowledgements
We would like to thank the Director General of Health Malaysia for the permission to publish this article.

Funding
The study was not funded in whole or in part by any research grant or funding body.

Authors' contributions
DM, OLM & HMA: made substantial contributions to conception and design, acquisition of data, analysis and interpretation of data. DM, HMA & KAH: been involved in drafting the manuscript or revising it critically for important intellectual content. DM, HMA, OLM & KAH: given final approval of the version to be published. DM, HMA, OLM & KAH: agreed to be accountable for all aspects of the work in ensuring the accuracy or integrity of this study. (Danial M: DM; Hassali MA: HMA; Ong LM: OLM; Khan AH: KAH). All authors read and approved the final manuscript.

Competing interests
The authors declare that they have no competing interests..

Author details
[1]Discipline of Social and Administrative Pharmacy, School of Pharmaceutical Sciences, Universiti Sains Malaysia, 11800 Minden, Penang, Malaysia. [2]Clinical Research Center (CRC) Penang General Hospital, 10990 Jalan Residensi, Pulau Pinang, Malaysia. [3]Discipline of Clinical Pharmacy, School of Pharmaceutical Sciences, Universiti Sains Malaysia, 11800 Minden, Penang, Malaysia.

References

1. Tan Y, Hu Y, Liu X, Yin Z, Chen XW and Liu M. Improving drug safety: From adverse drug reaction knowledge discovery to clinical implementation. *Methods* (San Diego, Calif). 2016.

2. Hinson JA, Roberts DW, James LP. Mechanisms of acetaminophen-induced liver necrosis. Adverse Drug Reactions. Berlin, Heidelberg: Springer; 2010. p. 369–405.

3. Shepherd G, Mohorn P, Yacoub K, May DW. Adverse drug reaction deaths reported in United States vital statistics, 1999-2006. Ann Pharmacother. 2012;46:169–75.

4. Alexopoulou A, Dourakis SP, Mantzoukis D, et al. Adverse drug reactions as a cause of hospital admissions: a 6-month experience in a single center in Greece. Eur J Int Med. 2008;19:505–10.

5. Pirmohamed M, Breckenridge AM, Kitteringham NR, Park BK. Adverse drug reactions. BMJ. 1998;316(7140):1295–8. https://doi.org/10.1136/bmj.316.7140.1295

6. Khan LM, Al-Harthi SE, Saadah OI. Adverse drug reactions in hospitalized pediatric patients of Saudi Arabian University hospital and impact of pharmacovigilance in reporting ADR. Saudi Pharmaceutical J. 2013;21:261–6.

7. Macedo AF, Marques CF, Ribeiro CF, Teixeira F. Causality assessment of adverse drug reactions: comparison of the results obtained from published decisional algorithms and from the evaluations of an expert panel. Pharmacoepidemiol Drug Saf. 2005;14:885–90.

8. Alshammari TM. Drug safety: the concept, inception and its importance in patients' health. Saudi Pharmaceutical J. 2016;24:405–12.

9. Hilmer SN, McLachlan AJ, Le Couteur DG. Clinical pharmacology in the geriatric patient. Fundam Clin Pharmacol. 2007;21:217–30.

10. Arimone Y, Begaud B, Miremont-Salame G, et al. Agreement of expert judgment in causality assessment of adverse drug reactions. Eur J Clin Pharmacol. 2005;61:169–73.

11. Macedo AF, Marques FB, Ribeiro CF, Teixeira F. Causality assessment of adverse drug reactions: comparison of the results obtained from published decisional algorithms and from the evaluations of an expert panel, according to different levels of imputability. J Clin Pharm Ther. 2003;28:137–43.

12. Khan LM, Al-Harthi SE, Osman AMM, Sattar MAAA, Ali AS. Dilemmas of the causality assessment tools in the diagnosis of adverse drug reactions. Saudi Pharmaceutical J. 2016;24:485–93.

13. Hartwig SC, Siegel J, Schneider PJ. Preventability and severity assessment in reporting adverse drug reactions. Am J Hosp Pharm. 1992;49:2229–32.

14. Hartwig SC, Denger SD, Schneider PJ. Severity-indexed, incident report-based medication error-reporting program. Am J Hosp Pharm. 1991;48:2611–6.

15. Schimmel EM. The Hazards of Hospitalization. Ann Intern Med. 1964;60:100–10.

16. Aronson J. Stephens' detection of new adverse drug reactions, 5th edn. Br J Clin Pharmacol. 2004;58(2):227. https://doi.org/10.1111/j.1365-2125.2004.02121.x.

17. Rawlins MD and Thompson JW. Pathogenesis of adverse drug reactions. In: (ed.) DD, (ed.). In Textbook of Adverse Reactions 1977, p. 44.

18. Matsushita K, Mahmoodi BK, Woodward M, et al. Comparison of risk prediction using the CKD-EPI equation and the MDRD study equation for estimated glomerular filtration rate. JAMA. 2012;307:1941–51.

19. Tangri N, Kitsios GD, Inker LA, et al. Risk prediction models for patients with chronic kidney disease: a systematic review. Ann Intern Med. 2013;158:596–603.

20. Rigatto C, Sood MM, Tangri N. Risk prediction in chronic kidney disease: pitfalls and caveats. Curr Opin Nephrol Hypertens. 2012;21:612–8.

21. Pirmohamed M, James S, Meakin S, et al. Adverse drug reactions as cause of admission to hospital: prospective analysis of 18 820 patients. BMJ (Clinical research ed). 2004;329:15–9.

22. Wiggins BS, Saseen JJ, Page RL 2nd, Reed BN, Sneed K, Kostis JB, Lanfear D, Virani S, Morris PB; on behalf of the American Heart Association Clinical Pharmacology Committee of the Council on Clinical Cardiology; Council on Hypertension; Council on Quality of Care and Outcomes Research; and Council on Functional Genomics and Translational Biology. Recommendations for management of clinically significant drug-drug interactions with statins and select agents used in patients with cardiovascular disease: a scientific statement from the American Heart Association. Circulation. 2016;134:e468–e495. https://doi.org/10.1161/CIR.0000000000000456.

23. Levey AS, Stevens LA, Schmid CH, et al. A new equation to estimate glomerular filtration rate. Ann Intern Med. 2009;150:604–12.

24. Edwards IR, Aronson JK. Adverse drug reactions: definitions, diagnosis, and management. Lancet (London, England). 2000;356:1255–9.

25. Rawlins MD, Thompson JW. Mechanisms of adverse drug reactions. In: Davies DM, editor. Textbook of Adverse Drug Reactions. Oxford: Oxford University Press; 1991. p. 18–45.

26. Naranjo CA, Busto U, Sellers EM, et al. A method for estimating the probability of adverse drug reactions. Clin Pharmacol Ther. 1981;30:239–45.

27. Hallas J, Harvald B, Gram LF, et al. Drug related hospital admissions: the role of definitions and intensity of data collection, and the possibility of prevention. J Intern Med. 1990;228:83–90.

28. Cox DR. Regression Models and Life-tables. J R Stat Soc Ser B Methodol. 1972;34:187–220.

29. Cox DR, Oakes D. Analysis of Survival Data. 1st ed. London: Chapman and Hall; 1984, p. 212.

30. Inker LA, Tighiouart H, Aspelund T, et al. Lifetime risk of stage 3-5 CKD in a community-based sample in Iceland. Clin J Am Soc Nephrol. 2015; 10:1575–84.

31. Lazarou J, Pomeranz BH, Corey PN. Incidence of adverse drug reactions in hospitalized patients: a meta-analysis of prospective studies. JAMA. 1998; 279:1200–5.

32. Davies EC, Green CF, Taylor S, Williamson PR, Mottram DR, Pirmohamed M. Adverse drug reactions in hospital in-patients: a prospective analysis of 3695 patient-episodes. PLoS One. 2009;4:e4439.

33. Chan M, Nicklason F, Vial JH. Adverse drug events as a cause of hospital admission in the elderly. Intern Med J. 2001;31:199–205.

34. Howard RL, Avery AJ, Slavenburg S, et al. Which drugs cause preventable admissions to hospital? A systematic review. Br J Clin Pharmacol. 2007;63:136–47.

35. Budnitz DS, Lovegrove MC, Shehab N, Richards CL. Emergency hospitalizations for adverse drug events in older Americans. N Engl J Med. 2011;365:2002–12.

36. Hallan SI, Matsushita K, Sang Y, et al. Age and association of kidney measures with mortality and end-stage renal disease. JAMA. 2012;308:2349–60.

37. Grams ME, Chow EK, Segev DL, Coresh J. Lifetime incidence of CKD stages 3-5 in the United States. Am J Kidney Dis. 2013;62:245–52.

38. Kvasz M, Allen IE, Gordon MJ, et al. Adverse drug reactions in hospitalized patients: a critique of a meta-analysis. MedGenMed. 2000;2:E3.

39. Fan L, Levey AS, Gudnason V, et al. Comparing GFR estimating equations using cystatin C and creatinine in elderly individuals. J Am Soc Nephrol. 2015;26:1982–9.

40. Soldin OP, Chung SH, Mattison DR. Sex differences in drug disposition. J Biomed Biotechnol. 2011;2011:187103.

41. Doyle EM, Sloan JM, Goodbrand JA, et al. Association between kidney function, rehabilitation outcome, and survival in older patients discharged from inpatient rehabilitation. Am J Kidney Dis. 2015;66:768–74.

42. Walker SR, Gill K, Macdonald K, et al. Association of frailty and physical function in patients with non-dialysis CKD: a systematic review. BMC Nephrol. 2013;14:228.

43. Bowling CB, Sawyer P, Campbell RC, Ahmed A, Allman RM. Impact of chronic kidney disease on activities of daily living in community-dwelling older adults. J Gerontol A Biol Sci Med Sci. 2011;66(6):689–94. https://doi.org/10.1093/gerona/glr043

44. Fried LF, Lee JS, Shlipak M, Chertow GM, Green C, Ding J, Harris T, Newman AB. Chronic kidney disease and functional limitation in older people: health, aging and body composition study. J Am Geriatr Soc. 2006;54(5):750–56. https://doi.org/10.1111/j.1532-5415.2006.00727.x

45. Ageno W, Gallus AS, Wittkowsky A, Crowther M, Hylek EM, Palareti G. Oral anticoagulant therapy: antithrombotic therapy and prevention of thrombosis, 9th ed: American College of Chest Physicians Evidence-Based Clinical Practice Guidelines. Chest. 2012;141:e44S–88S.

46. Mangoni AA, Jackson SHD. Age-related changes in pharmacokinetics and pharmacodynamics: basic principles and practical applications. Br J Clin Pharmacol. 2004;57:6–14.

47. Lavan AH, Gallagher P. Predicting risk of adverse drug reactions in older adults. Therapeutic Advances in Drug Safety. 2016;7:11–22.

48. Gottdiener JS, Arnold AM, Aurigemma GP, et al. Predictors of congestive heart failure in the elderly: the cardiovascular health study. J Am Coll Cardiol. 2000;35:1628–37.

49. Woodhouse KW, Wynne HA. Age-related changes in liver size and hepatic blood flow. Clin Pharmacokinet. 1988;15:287–94.

21

Adverse clinical outcomes associated with double dose clopidogrel compared to the other antiplatelet regimens in patients with coronary artery disease

Xiaojun Zhuo[1†], Bi Zhuo[2†], Shenyu Ouyang[1], Pei Niu[1] and Mou Xiao[1*] ⓘD

Abstract

Background: Recently, several newer antiplatelet treatment strategies have been used in patients with coronary artery disease (CAD). Apart from the dual antiplatelet therapy (DAPT) consisting of aspirin and clopidogrel, double dose clopidogrel (DDC), triple antiplatelet therapy (TAPT) consisting of aspirin, clopidogrel and cilostazol and other newer antiplatelet agents have shown to be effective in different ways. In this analysis, we aimed to systematically compare the adverse clinical outcomes and the bleeding events which were observed when DDC was compared to the other antiplatelet regimens in patients with CAD.

Methods: English publications comparing DDC with other antiplatelet regimens were searched from MEDLARS/ MEDLINE, EMBASE, www.ClinicalTrials.gov and Google Scholar. Adverse cardiovascular outcomes and bleeding events were the study endpoints. Statistical analysis was carried out by the RevMan 5.3 software whereby odds ratios (OR) with 95% confidence intervals (CIs) were calculated.

Results: A total number of 23,065 participants were included. Results of this analysis showed major adverse cardiac events (MACEs), all-cause mortality, cardiac death, stroke, stent thrombosis, revascularization and myocardial infarction (MI) to have been similarly manifested in patients who were treated with DDC versus the control group with OR: 0.98, 95% CI: 0.78–1.22; $p = 0.83$, OR: 0.95, 95% CI: 0.77–1.17; $p = 0.62$, OR: 0.97, 95% CI: 0.79–1.20; $p = 0.81$, OR: 0.98, 95% CI: 0.65–1.48; $p = 0.94$, OR: 0.84, 95% CI: 0.40–1.75; $p = 0.64$, OR: 0.88, 95% CI: 0.52–1.49; $p = 0.63$, and OR: 0.89, 95% CI: 0.65–1.21; $p = 0.45$ respectively. Any minor and major bleedings were also similarly manifested. When DDC was compared to DAPT, no significant difference was observed in any bleeding event with OR: 1.58, 95% CI: 0.86–2.91; $p = 0.14$. Even when DDC was compared with either ticagrelor or prasugrel or TAPT, still no significant difference was observed in terms of bleeding outcomes.

Conclusions: In patients with CAD, adverse clinical outcomes were not significantly different when DDC was compared to the other antiplatelet regimens. In addition, bleeding events were also similarly manifested when DDC was compared to DAPT, TAPT or ticagrelor/prasugrel.

Keywords: Double dose clopidogrel, Dual antiplatelet therapy, Ticagrelor, Prasugrel, Triple antiplatelet therapy, Coronary artery disease, Percutaneous coronary intervention

* Correspondence: xiaomou2018@163.com
†Xiaojun Zhuo and Bi Zhuo contributed equally to this work.
[1]Department of Cardiology, Affiliated Changsha Hospital of Hunan Normal University, The Fourth Hospital of Changsha, Changsha 410006, Hunan, People's Republic of China
Full list of author information is available at the end of the article

Background

Coronary artery disease (CAD) is one among the most common non-communicable diseases affecting a large number of the elderly population around the globe [1]. As a measure of secondary prevention, several antiplatelet treatment strategies have been set up based upon the degree and type of intervention which was carried out. In patients with stable CAD where intervention was not required, a single antiplatelet agent was sufficient [2]. For those patients with acute coronary syndrome (ACS) or those patients undergoing percutaneous coronary intervention (PCI) with drug eluting stents (DES), dual antiplatelet therapy (DAPT) consisting of aspirin and clopidogrel has been the mainstay of treatment [3].

However, clopidogrel hyporesponsiveness [4] and platelet hyper-reactivity [5] have recently been observed in several subgroups of patients. Therefore, to overcome this problem, several new antiplatelet treatment strategies have been developed: Double dose clopidogrel (DDC) [6], triple antiplatelet therapy (TAPT) consisting of aspirin, clopidogrel and cilostazol [7] and other newer potential antiplatelet agents such as ticagrelor and prasugrel have been used [8].

Nevertheless, controversies have been observed with the use of DDC. Results of the CURRENT OASIS 7 Trial which was published in the New England Journal of Medicine showed no benefit of DDC in patients with ACS. However, a subgroup analysis of the same data (CURRENT OASIS 7) which was published in The Lancet indicated a beneficial effect of DDC in ACS patients following coronary stenting. However, DDC has never systematically been compared with the other antiplatelet agents.

In this analysis, we aimed to systematically compare the adverse clinical outcomes and the bleeding events which were observed with DDC versus the other antiplatelet regimens in patients with CAD.

Methods

Searched databases and searched strategies

MEDLARS or MEDLINE (Medical Literature Analysis and Retrieval System Online), EMBASE, www.Clinical-Trials.gov and Google Scholar were the online electronic databases which were searched for relevant English publications comparing DDC with other antiplatelet regimens in patients with CAD.

The following searched terms were used to retrieve publications:

- Double dose clopidogrel and coronary artery disease;
- Double dose clopidogrel and percutaneous coronary intervention;
- Double dose clopidogrel and acute coronary syndrome;
- Double dose clopidogrel and acute myocardial infarction;
- Double dose clopidogrel and dual antiplatelet therapy;
- Double dose clopidogrel and triple antiplatelet therapy;
- Double dose clopidogrel and cilostazol;
- Double dose clopidogrel and prasugrel;
- Double dose clopidogrel and ticagrelor;
- Double dose clopidogrel and antiplatelet agents.

The term 'double dose' was also replaced by the term 'high dose' in this search process.

Inclusion and exclusion criteria

Studies were included in this analysis if:

- They compared double dose clopidogrel versus other antiplatelet agents in patients with CAD/PCI;
- They reported adverse clinical outcomes and bleeding events as their endpoints.

Studies were excluded from this analysis if:

- They were review articles, meta-analyses, case studies or letters to editors;
- They did not compare DDC with other antiplatelet agents;
- They did not report adverse clinical outcomes or bleeding events as their clinical endpoints; Instead, they only reported platelet activities;
- They were duplicated studies.

Definitions, outcomes and follow-ups

DAPT: Dual antiplatelet therapy consisted of Aspirin and Clopidogrel;

TAPT: Triple antiplatelet therapy consisted of Aspirin, Clopidogrel and Cilostazol;

DDC: Double dose clopidogrel consisted twice the normal standard dose of clopidogrel given daily; that is, 150 mg clopidogrel.

The following outcomes were assessed:

- Major adverse cardiac events (MACEs) consisting of mortality, myocardial infarction (MI), repeated revascularization, or stroke;
- All-cause mortality;
- Cardiac death;
- MI;
- Stroke;
- Stent thrombosis;
  Revascularization (target vessel revascularization or target lesion revascularization);
- Any bleeding event consisting of any type of bleeding which was reported;
- Any minor bleeding consisting of any minor type of bleeding or minimal bleeding;

– Any major bleeding consisting of any type of major bleeding or serious bleeding.

The follow-up time period varied from study to study. The outcomes which were reported as well as the follow-up time periods have been listed in Table 1.

Data extraction, quality assessment and statistical analysis
Following the search of publications by the PRISMA guideline [9], and after selection of the most suitable articles which were relevant to this analysis, data extraction was carried out by five independent reviewers. The following data were extracted:

The type of study, the number of participants assigned to the DDC group and the control group respectively, the time period when the participants were enrolled, the type of participants, the baseline features, the cardiovascular and bleeding outcomes which were reported, the total number of events in each subgroups, the follow-up time periods and the methodological quality of the trials.

Any disagreement which followed was resolved by consensus.

The methodological quality of the trials was assessed in accordance to the Cochrane Collaboration [10].

Statistical analysis was carried out by the RevMan 5.3 software whereby odds ratios (OR) with 95% confidence intervals (CIs) were calculated.

Heterogeneity was assessed by the (1) Q statistic test whereby a p value less than 0.05 was considered statistically significant and (2) the I^2 statistic test whereby a low heterogeneity was denoted by a low I^2 value and a high heterogeneity was represented by an increased value of I^2.

Concerning the statistical models which were used, a fixed effects model was used if I^2 was less than 50% whereas a random effects model was used if I^2 was greater than 50%.

Sensitivity analysis was carried out by a method of exclusion whereby each trial was excluded one by one and a new analysis was carried out each time to be compared with the main results for any significant difference.

Since this analysis did not include a large volume of studies, publication bias was best assessed through funnel plots which were obtained from the RevMan software.

Results
Searched outcomes
After a careful search, a total number of 1514 publications were obtained. Following an assessment of the titles and abstracts, 1398 articles were eliminated since they were not related to this research topic.

Table 1 Outcomes and follow-up periods

Studies	Outcomes reported	Follow-up periods	DDC versus control group
CURRENT OASIS 7 [11]	CV death, MI, or stroke (MACE); CV death, MI, stroke, total mortality, TIMI major bleeding, minor bleeding, fatal bleeding, intracranial bleeding	30 days	DDC versus SDAPT
ACCEL AMI [12]	Minor bleeding	30 days	DDC versus SDAPT
OPTIMUS2007 [13]	Bleeding complications	30 days	DDC versus SDAPT
CREATIVE [14]	MACE, all-cause death, cardiac death, MI, TVR, stroke, ST, major bleeding	18 months	DDC versus SDAPT
Chen2017 [15]	MACE, in-stent thrombosis, TVR, MI, cardiac death, bleeding events, mild bleeding, severe bleeding	12 months	DDC versus SDAPT
Khatri2013 [16]	Composite efficacy outcomes, any bleeding event	23 months	DDC versus prasugrel
OPTIMUS3 [17]	Major and minor TIMI defined bleeding, adverse drug events	7 days	DDC versus prasugrel
PRINCIPLE TIMI 44 [18]	TIMI major and minor bleeding, minor bleeding, hemorrhagic adverse events, MI	2 weeks	DDC versus prasugrel
Tailor2014 [19]	MACE, MI, ST, CV death, stroke	1 month and 571 days	DDC versus prasugrel
Chen2017 [15]	MACE, in-stent thrombosis, TVR, MI, cardiac death, bleeding events, mild bleeding, severe bleeding	12 months	DDC versus ticagrelor
Wu2017 [20]	MACE, minimal bleeding, minor bleeding	30 days	DDC versus ticagrelor
ACCEL AMI [12]	Minor bleeding	30 days	DDC versus TAPT
ACCEL DM [21]	Bleeding event	30 days	DDC versus TAPT
CREATIVE [14]	MACE, all-cause death, cardiac death, MI, TVR, stroke, ST, major bleeding	18 months	DDC versus TAPT
Ha2013 [22]	MACE	1 month	DDC versus TAPT
HOST ASSURE [23]	MACE, cardiac death, MI, stroke, ST, all-cause death, TLR, TVR, PLATO minor bleeding	30 days	DDC versus TAPT
Jeong2009 [24]	MACE, major and minor bleeding	30 days	DDC versus TAPT

Abbreviations: TAPT: triple antiplatelet therapy consisting of aspirin, clopidogrel and cilostazol, DDC: double dose clopidogrel, SDAPT: standard dual antiplatelet therapy, CV: cardiovascular, MI: myocardial infarction, ST: stent thrombosis, MACE: major adverse cardiac events, TIMI: thrombolysis in myocardial infarction, TVR: target vessel revascularization, TLR: target lesion revascularization

One hundred and sixteen (116) full text articles were assessed for eligibility. Further elimination were carried out for the following reasons:

Meta-analysis (3), review of literature (5), case studies (3), letter to editors (4), did not compare DDC with other antiplatelet agents (32), did not report relevant adverse outcomes (25), and duplicated studies (30).

Finally only 14 studies [11–24] were considered relevant for this analysis as shown in Fig. 1.

General features of the studies

The general features have been listed in Table 2.

A total number of 23,065 participants were included in this analysis whereby 11,217 were assigned to the DDC group and 11,848 participants were assigned to the control group. In detail, the number of participants were assigned as followed: DDC (9019 participants) versus standard dual antiplatelet therapy (9172 participants), DDC (2355 participants) versus TAPT (2356 participants), and DDC (282 participants) versus ticagrelor/prasugrel (320 participants). Eleven studies were randomized trials whereas the other three studies were observational cohorts. The time period of patients' enrollment varied from years 2006 to 2015 as shown in Table 2.

Patients with stable CAD, ACS, diabetes mellitus and those undergoing PCI were included in this analysis.

Baseline features of the studies

The baseline characteristics have been reported in Table 3. Majority of the participants were of male gender with a mean age ranging from 58.1 to 64.9 years. Hypertension, dyslipidemia and diabetes mellitus among the patients varied from 26.0 to 100% as shown in Table 3. According to the baseline features, no significant difference was observed between the two groups of participants.

Adverse cardiovascular outcomes associated with double dose clopidogrel versus the control group

When the adverse cardiovascular outcomes were compared, MACEs, all-cause mortality, cardiac death, stroke, stent thrombosis, revascularization and MI were similarly manifested in patients who were treated with DDC versus the control group with OR: 0.98, 95% CI: 0.78–1.22; $p = 0.83$, OR: 0.95, 95% CI: 0.77–1.17; $p = 0.62$, OR: 0.97, 95% CI: 0.79–1.20; $p = 0.81$, OR: 0.98, 95% CI: 0.65–1.48; $p = 0.94$, OR: 0.84, 95% CI: 0.40–1.75; $p = 0.64$, OR: 0.88, 95% CI: 0.52–1.49; $p = 0.63$, and OR: 0.89, 95% CI: 0.65–1.21; $p = 0.45$ respectively as shown in Fig. 2.

Bleeding associated with double dose clopidogrel versus the control group

The outcome 'any bleeding event' was not significantly different with DDC versus the control group with OR: 1.09, 95% CI: 0.84–1.42; $p = 0.50$. In addition, any minor bleeding

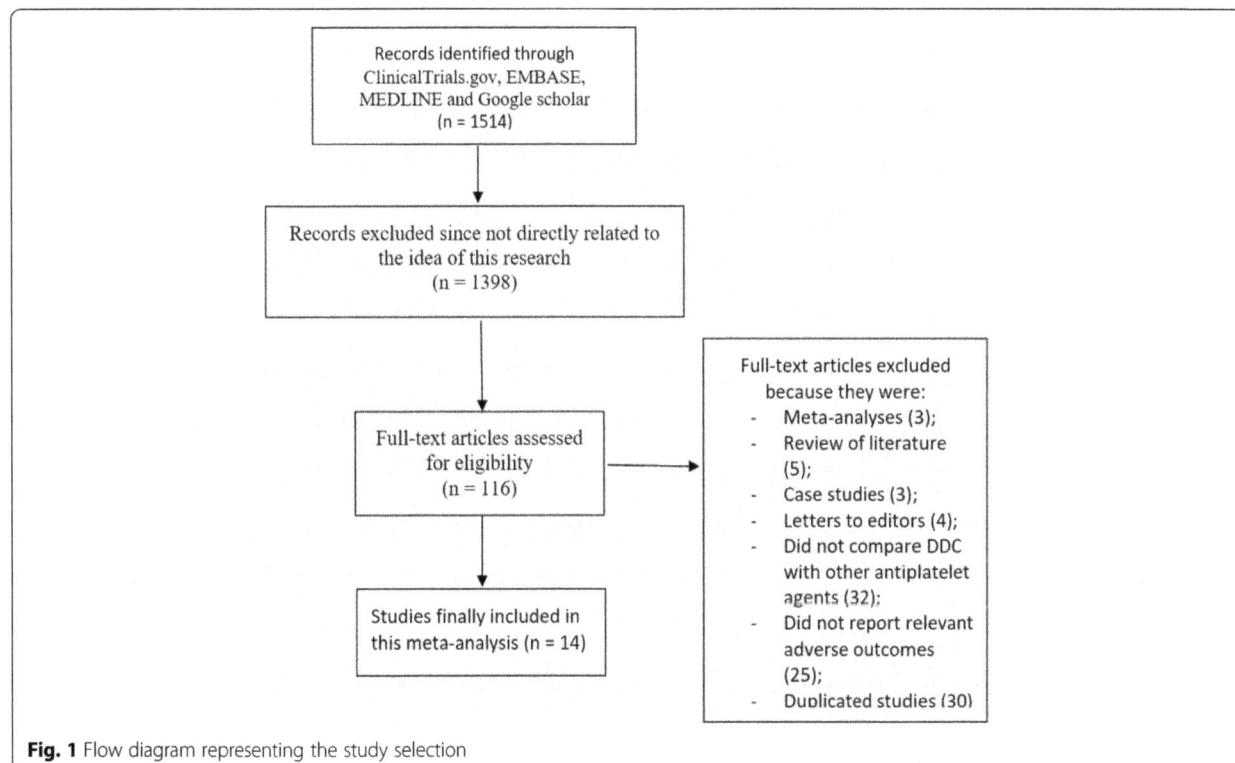

Fig. 1 Flow diagram representing the study selection

Table 2 General features of the studies

Studies	No of patients in the DDC group (n)	No of patients in control group (n)	Year of patients' enrollment	Type of study	Type of participants
CURRENT OASIS 7	8560	8703	2006–2009	RCT	ACS + PCI
OPTIMUS2007	20	20	–	Pilot study	DM + CAD
Khatri2013	26	64	2009–2010	Retrospective study	CAD
OPTIMUS3	35	34	2008–2009	RCT	DM + CAD
PRINCIPLE TIMI 44	99	102	–	RCT	Any CAD with planned PCI
Tailor2014	52	54	2010–2012	RCT	CAD + ACS
Chen2017	50	57 + 46	2012–2014	OC	CAD
Wu2017	20	20	2014–2015	RCT	CAD with planned PCI
ACCEL AMI	30	30 + 30	–	RCT	AMI
ACCEL DM	39	41	–	RCT	DM + AMI undergoing PCI
CREATIVE	359	362 + 355	2012–2015	RCT	CAD + PCI
Ha2013	21	21	–	RCT	DM + PCI
HOST ASSURE	1876	1879	2010–2011	RCT	CAD + PCI
Jeong2009	30	30	–	RCT	CAD + PCI
Total number of patients (n)	11,217	11,848			

Abbreviations: ACS: acute coronary syndrome, PCI: percutaneous coronary intervention, DM: diabetes mellitus, CAD: coronary artery disease, AMI: acute myocardial infarction, RCT: randomized controlled trials, OC: observational studies; DDC: double dose clopidogrel

and any major bleeding were also similarly manifested with OR: 0.62, 95% CI: 0.34–1.12; $p = 0.11$ and OR: 1.41, 95% CI: 0.96–2.07; $p = 0.08$ respectively as shown in Fig. 3.

Bleeding events were further analyzed whereby DDC was compared individually with different antiplatelet regimens.

Bleeding associated with double dose clopidogrel versus standard dual anti-platelet therapy

When DDC was compared with the standard dual anti-platelet therapy (Aspirin and clopidogrel), no significant

difference was observed in any bleeding event with OR: 1.58, 95% CI: 0.86–2.91; $p = 0.14$ as shown in Fig. 4.

Bleeding associated with double dose clopidogrel versus ticagrelor or prasugrel

When DDC was compared with either ticagrelor or prasugrel, still no significant difference was observed in any bleeding events and any minor bleeding with OR: 0.67, 95% CI: 0.39–1.14; $p = 0.14$ and OR: 0.46, 95% CI: 0.20–1.08; $p = 0.07$ respectively as shown in Fig. 5.

Table 3 Baseline features of the studies

Studies	Age (years) DDC/C	Males (%) DDC/C	HBP (%) DDC/C	DS (%) DDC/C	DM (%) DDC/C	CS (%) DDC/C
CURRENT OASIS 7	61.2/61.2	76.0/74.9	59.4/58.8	40.3/40.3	22.3/22.2	37.5/36.6
OPTIMUS2007	64.0/59.0	60.0/70.0	90.0/95.0	90.0/95.0	100/100	15.0/20.0
Khatri2013	64.0/62.0	100/8.00	81.0/91.0	100/97.0	73.0/61.0	69.0/61.0
OPTIMUS3	61.3/61.3	68.6/68.6	94.3/94.3	94.3/94.3	100/100	20.0/20.0
PRINCIPLE TIMI 44	63.8/64.0	77.8/71.6	77.8/85.3	86.9/90.2	29.3/32.4	16.2/17.6
Tailor2014	63.0/63.0	82.7/74.1	82.7/74.1	88.5/83.3	34.6/29.6	67.3/77.8
Chen2017	59.8/60.8	62.0/59.6	56.0/56.1	26.0/28.1	30.0/31.6	38.0/35.1
Wu2017	62.7/60.4	70.0/75.0	70.0/50.0	60.0/80.0	30.0/45.0	30.0/55.0
ACCEL AMI	61.1/62.7	76.7/71.7	36.7/46.7	46.7/36.7	20.0/21.7	73.3/61.7
ACCEL DM	62.0/64.0	66.7/70.7	64.1/75.6	33.3/34.1	100/100	43.6/41.5
CREATIVE	58.1/58.5	61.0/59.3	61.0/65.8	68.5/64.5	32.0/33.8	38.2/36.5
Ha2013	62.3/64.9	71.4/67.7	76.1/71.4	42.5/33.3	100/100	23.8/23.8
HOST ASSURE	63.7/62.8	67.0/69.8	68.6/66.8	62.7/64.2	31.3/31.8	30.8/32.8
Jeong2009	63.0/63.0	66.7/66.7	50.0/53.3	20.0/20.0	16.7/30.0	60.0/36.7

Abbreviations: DDC: double dose clopidogrel, C: control group, HBP: high blood pressure, DS: dyslipidemia, DM: diabetes mellitus, CS: current smoker

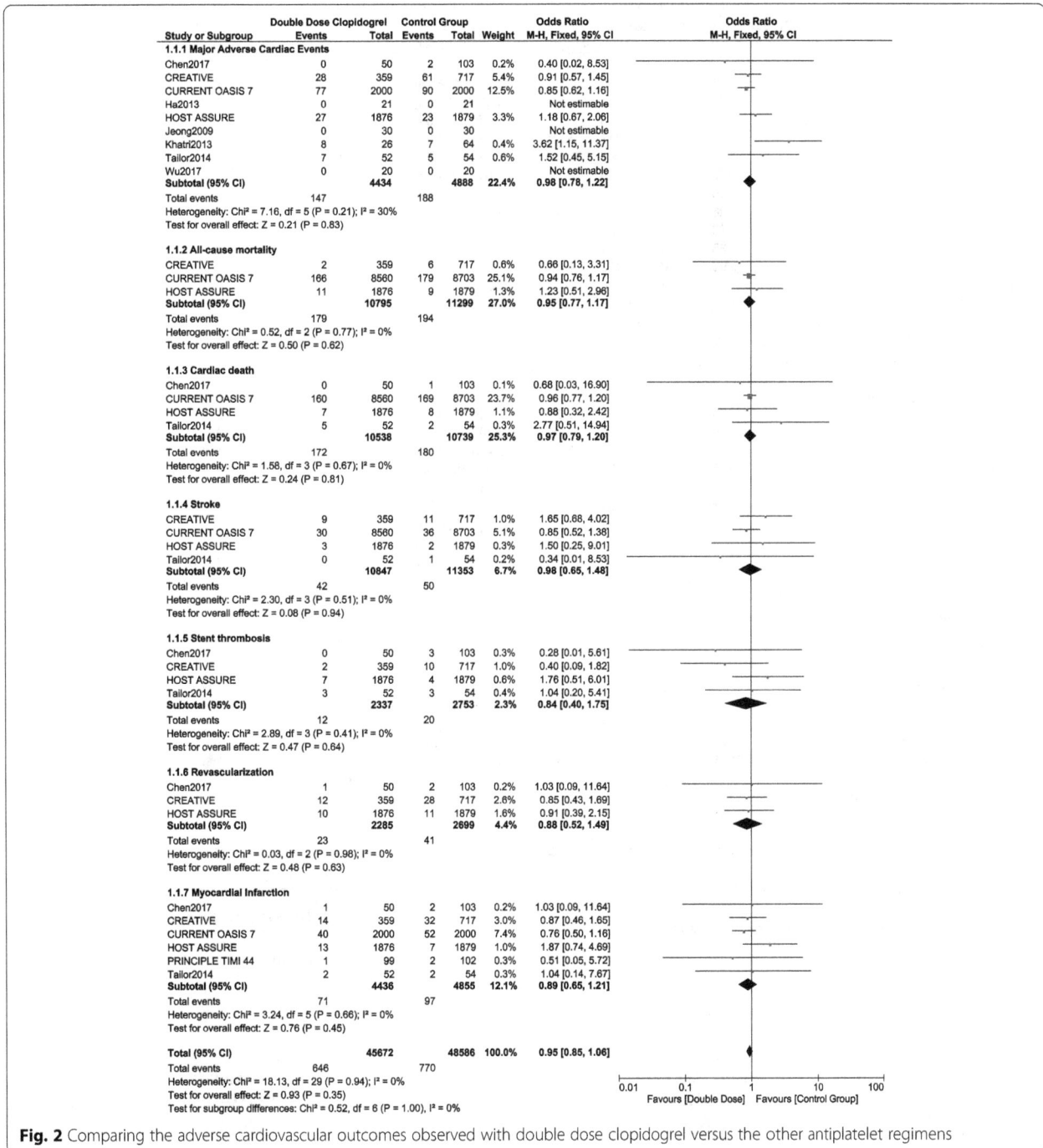

Fig. 2 Comparing the adverse cardiovascular outcomes observed with double dose clopidogrel versus the other antiplatelet regimens

Bleeding associated with double dose clopidogrel versus triple therapy (aspirin, clopidogrel and cilostazol)

When DDC was compared with TAPT, any bleeding event and any minor bleeding were not significantly different with OR: 0.87, 95% CI: 0.48–1.58; $p = 0.65$ and OR: 0.59, 95% CI: 0.25–1.38; $p = 0.22$ respectively as shown in Fig. 6.

Sensitivity analyzes showed consistent results accordingly. A low evidence of publication bias was observed which was visually assessed through funnel plots (Figs. 7 and 8) which were directly obtained through RevMan.

Discussion

This is the first analysis to systematically compare DDC versus the other antiplatelet agents. The current results showed that adverse clinical outcomes were not significantly different with DDC versus the other antiplatelet regimens. In addition, bleeding events (including major and minor bleeding) were also similarly manifested.

Results of the Adjunctive Cilostazol Versus High Maintenance Dose Clopidogrel in Patients With AMI (ACCEL-AMI) Study showed that TAPT demonstrated

Study or Subgroup	Double Dose Clopidogrel Events	Total	Control Group Events	Total	Weight	Odds Ratio M-H, Fixed, 95% CI	Odds Ratio M-H, Fixed, 95% CI
1.2.1 Any bleeding event							
ACCEL AMI	0	30	2	60	0.9%	0.38 [0.02, 8.25]	
ACCEL DM	2	39	1	41	0.5%	2.16 [0.19, 24.85]	
Chen2017	5	50	12	103	3.9%	0.84 [0.28, 2.54]	
CREATIVE	12	359	16	717	5.8%	1.52 [0.71, 3.24]	
CURRENT OASIS 7	69	2000	51	2000	27.5%	1.37 [0.95, 1.97]	
HOST ASSURE	6	1876	12	1879	6.7%	0.50 [0.19, 1.33]	
Jeong2009	0	30	0	30		Not estimable	
Khatri2013	3	26	7	64	2.0%	1.06 [0.25, 4.47]	
OPTIMUS2007	0	20	0	20		Not estimable	
OPTIMUS3	0	35	0	34		Not estimable	
PRINCIPLE TIMI 44	14	99	19	102	9.0%	0.72 [0.34, 1.53]	
Wu2017	4	20	6	20	2.7%	0.58 [0.14, 2.50]	
Subtotal (95% CI)		**4584**		**5070**	**59.0%**	**1.09 [0.84, 1.42]**	
Total events	115		126				
Heterogeneity: Chi² = 7.43, df = 8 (P = 0.49); I² = 0%							
Test for overall effect: Z = 0.67 (P = 0.50)							
1.2.2 Any minor bleeding							
ACCEL AMI	0	30	2	60	0.9%	0.38 [0.02, 8.25]	
ACCEL DM	2	39	1	41	0.5%	2.16 [0.19, 24.85]	
Chen2017	5	50	12	103	3.9%	0.84 [0.28, 2.54]	
HOST ASSURE	6	1876	12	1879	6.7%	0.50 [0.19, 1.33]	
Jeong2009	0	30	0	30		Not estimable	
OPTIMUS3	0	35	0	34		Not estimable	
PRINCIPLE TIMI 44	0	99	2	102	1.4%	0.20 [0.01, 4.26]	
Wu2017	4	20	6	20	2.7%	0.58 [0.14, 2.50]	
Subtotal (95% CI)		**2179**		**2269**	**16.1%**	**0.62 [0.34, 1.12]**	
Total events	17		35				
Heterogeneity: Chi² = 2.11, df = 5 (P = 0.83); I² = 0%							
Test for overall effect: Z = 1.58 (P = 0.11)							
1.2.3 Any major bleeding							
CREATIVE	12	359	16	717	5.8%	1.52 [0.71, 3.24]	
CURRENT OASIS 7	48	2000	35	2000	19.1%	1.38 [0.89, 2.14]	
Jeong2009	0	30	0	30		Not estimable	
OPTIMUS3	0	35	0	34		Not estimable	
PRINCIPLE TIMI 44	0	99	0	102		Not estimable	
Subtotal (95% CI)		**2523**		**2883**	**24.9%**	**1.41 [0.96, 2.07]**	
Total events	60		51				
Heterogeneity: Chi² = 0.04, df = 1 (P = 0.84); I² = 0%							
Test for overall effect: Z = 1.77 (P = 0.08)							
Total (95% CI)		**9286**		**10222**	**100.0%**	**1.10 [0.90, 1.34]**	
Total events	192		212				
Heterogeneity: Chi² = 14.51, df = 16 (P = 0.56); I² = 0%							
Test for overall effect: Z = 0.89 (P = 0.37)							
Test for subgroup differences: Chi² = 5.24, df = 2 (P = 0.07), I² = 61.8%							

Scale: 0.01 — 0.1 — 1 — 10 — 100
Favours [Double Dose]   Favours [Control Group]

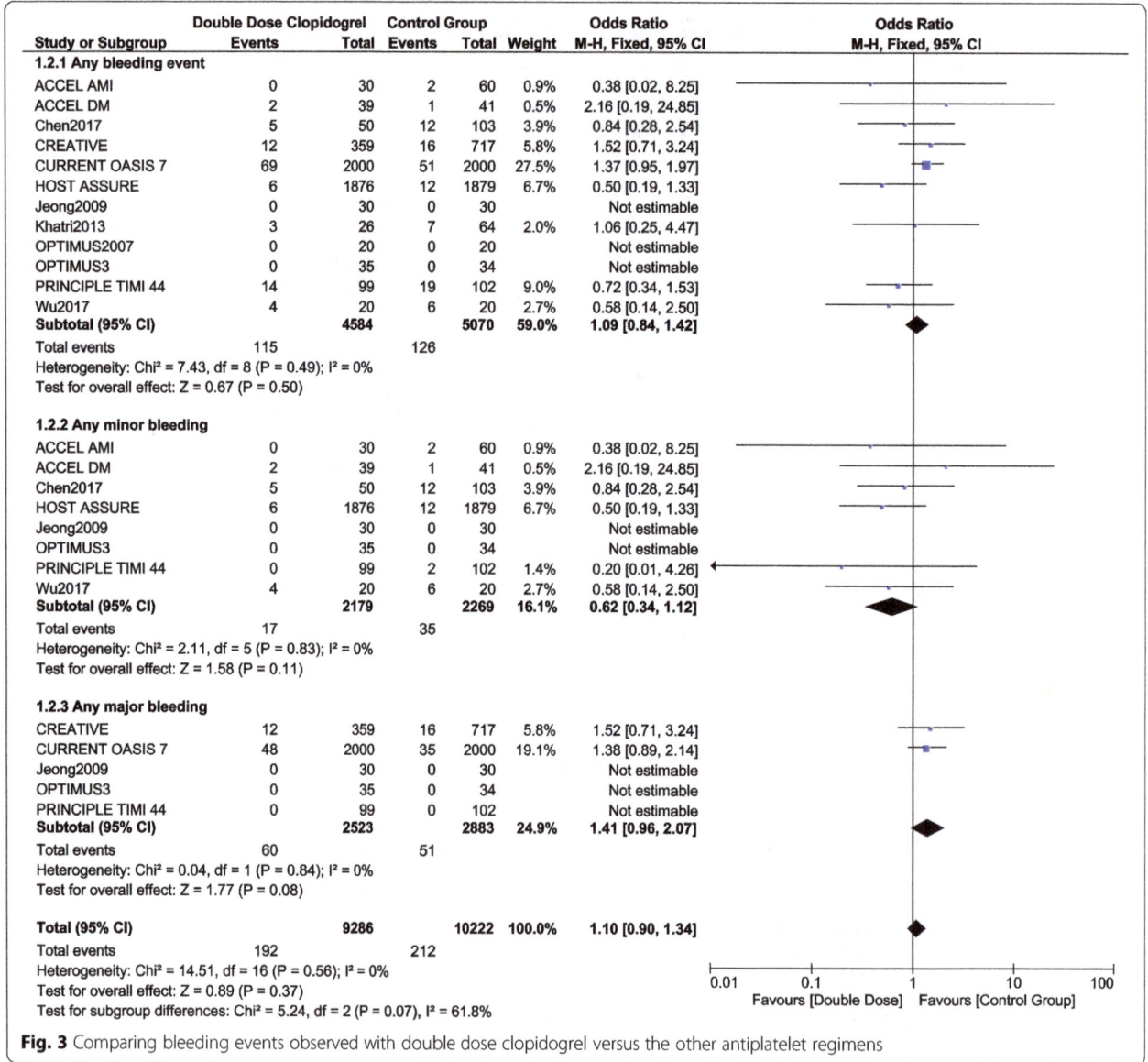

Fig. 3 Comparing bleeding events observed with double dose clopidogrel versus the other antiplatelet regimens

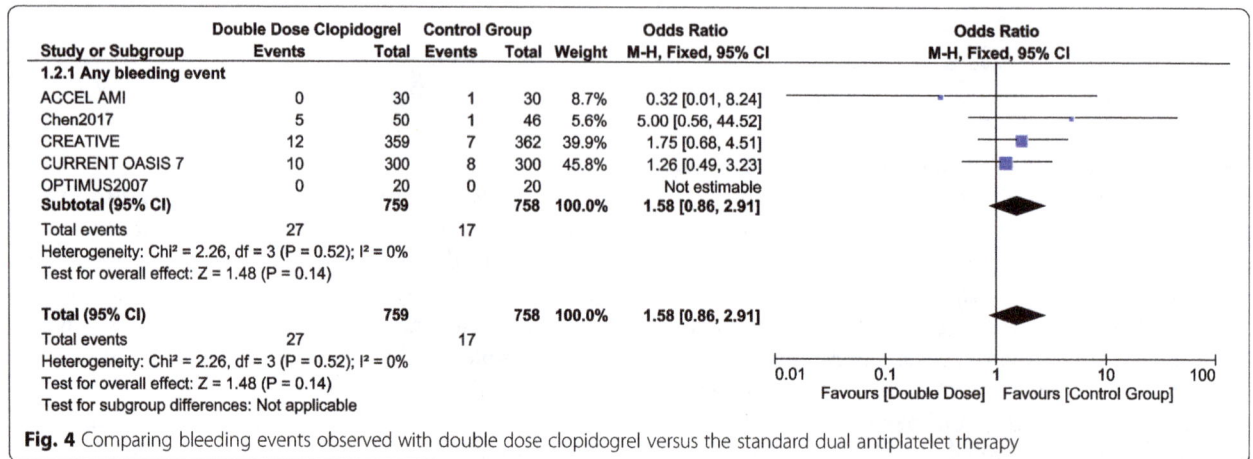

Study or Subgroup	Double Dose Clopidogrel Events	Total	Control Group Events	Total	Weight	Odds Ratio M-H, Fixed, 95% CI	Odds Ratio M-H, Fixed, 95% CI
1.2.1 Any bleeding event							
ACCEL AMI	0	30	1	30	8.7%	0.32 [0.01, 8.24]	
Chen2017	5	50	1	46	5.6%	5.00 [0.56, 44.52]	
CREATIVE	12	359	7	362	39.9%	1.75 [0.68, 4.51]	
CURRENT OASIS 7	10	300	8	300	45.8%	1.26 [0.49, 3.23]	
OPTIMUS2007	0	20	0	20		Not estimable	
Subtotal (95% CI)		**759**		**758**	**100.0%**	**1.58 [0.86, 2.91]**	
Total events	27		17				
Heterogeneity: Chi² = 2.26, df = 3 (P = 0.52); I² = 0%							
Test for overall effect: Z = 1.48 (P = 0.14)							
Total (95% CI)		**759**		**758**	**100.0%**	**1.58 [0.86, 2.91]**	
Total events	27		17				
Heterogeneity: Chi² = 2.26, df = 3 (P = 0.52); I² = 0%							
Test for overall effect: Z = 1.48 (P = 0.14)							
Test for subgroup differences: Not applicable							

Scale: 0.01 — 0.1 — 1 — 10 — 100
Favours [Double Dose]   Favours [Control Group]

Fig. 4 Comparing bleeding events observed with double dose clopidogrel versus the standard dual antiplatelet therapy

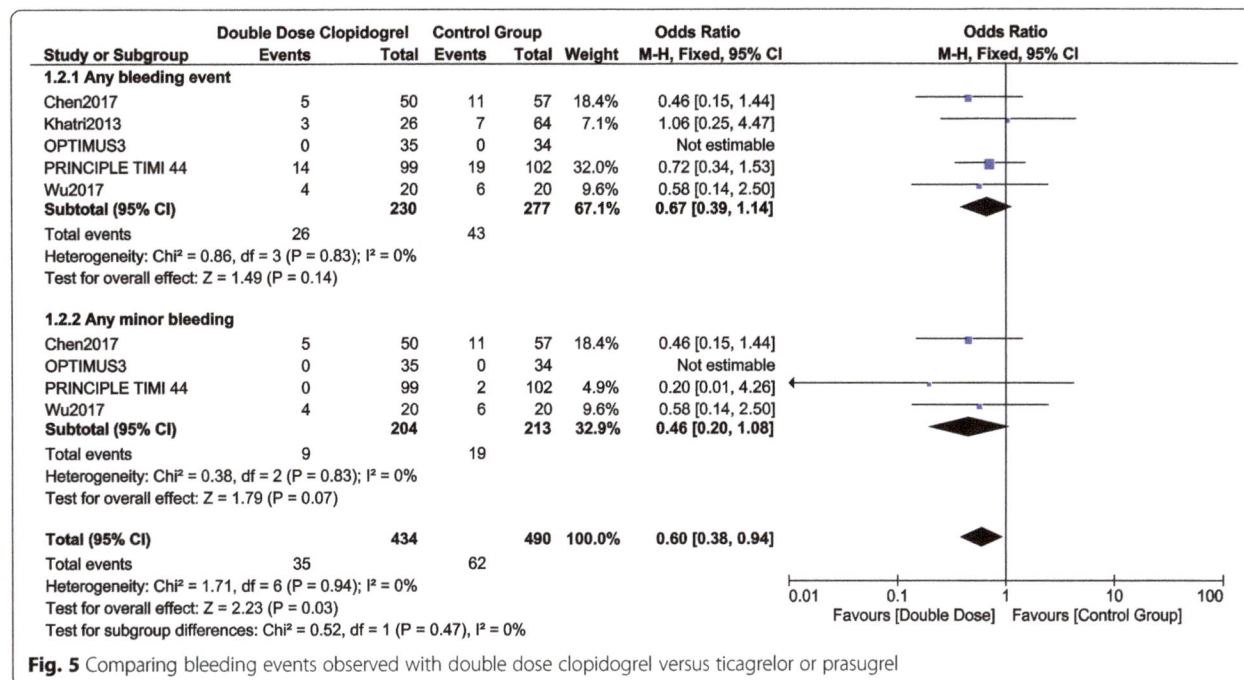

Study or Subgroup	Double Dose Clopidogrel Events	Total	Control Group Events	Total	Weight	Odds Ratio M-H, Fixed, 95% CI
1.2.1 Any bleeding event						
Chen2017	5	50	11	57	18.4%	0.46 [0.15, 1.44]
Khatri2013	3	26	7	64	7.1%	1.06 [0.25, 4.47]
OPTIMUS3	0	35	0	34		Not estimable
PRINCIPLE TIMI 44	14	99	19	102	32.0%	0.72 [0.34, 1.53]
Wu2017	4	20	6	20	9.6%	0.58 [0.14, 2.50]
Subtotal (95% CI)		230		277	67.1%	0.67 [0.39, 1.14]
Total events	26		43			
Heterogeneity: Chi² = 0.86, df = 3 (P = 0.83); I² = 0%						
Test for overall effect: Z = 1.49 (P = 0.14)						
1.2.2 Any minor bleeding						
Chen2017	5	50	11	57	18.4%	0.46 [0.15, 1.44]
OPTIMUS3	0	35	0	34		Not estimable
PRINCIPLE TIMI 44	0	99	2	102	4.9%	0.20 [0.01, 4.26]
Wu2017	4	20	6	20	9.6%	0.58 [0.14, 2.50]
Subtotal (95% CI)		204		213	32.9%	0.46 [0.20, 1.08]
Total events	9		19			
Heterogeneity: Chi² = 0.38, df = 2 (P = 0.83); I² = 0%						
Test for overall effect: Z = 1.79 (P = 0.07)						
Total (95% CI)		434		490	100.0%	0.60 [0.38, 0.94]
Total events	35		62			
Heterogeneity: Chi² = 1.71, df = 6 (P = 0.94); I² = 0%						
Test for overall effect: Z = 2.23 (P = 0.03)						
Test for subgroup differences: Chi² = 0.52, df = 1 (P = 0.47), I² = 0%						

Fig. 5 Comparing bleeding events observed with double dose clopidogrel versus ticagrelor or prasugrel

greater platelet inhibition compared to DDC [12]. However, no major cardiovascular or bleeding outcomes were observed in any of the groups supporting the results of this current analysis. The Adjunctive Cilostazol versus double-dose ClopidogrEL in Diabetes Mellitus study (ACCEL-DM) also showed that when cilostazol was added to DAPT, the new regimen showed greater platelet inhibition in comparison to

DDC [21]. However, no major bleeding was observed in any of the two groups.

Similarly, in the Gauging Responsiveness with A Verify-Now assay-Impact on Thrombosis And Safety (GRAVITAS) randomized study [25], whereby a total number of 2214 patients were assigned to DDC and standard clopidogrel dose, the former did not decrease the incidence of adverse cardiac

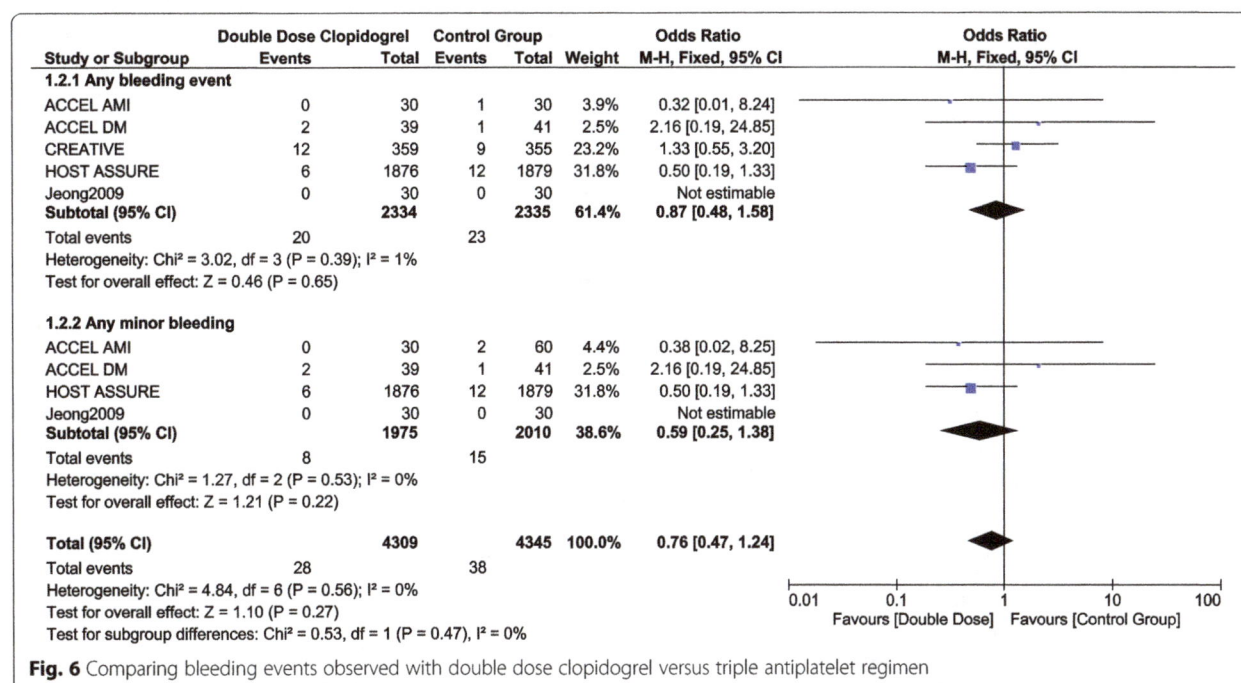

Study or Subgroup	Double Dose Clopidogrel Events	Total	Control Group Events	Total	Weight	Odds Ratio M-H, Fixed, 95% CI
1.2.1 Any bleeding event						
ACCEL AMI	0	30	1	30	3.9%	0.32 [0.01, 8.24]
ACCEL DM	2	39	1	41	2.5%	2.16 [0.19, 24.85]
CREATIVE	12	359	9	355	23.2%	1.33 [0.55, 3.20]
HOST ASSURE	6	1876	12	1879	31.8%	0.50 [0.19, 1.33]
Jeong2009	0	30	0	30		Not estimable
Subtotal (95% CI)		2334		2335	61.4%	0.87 [0.48, 1.58]
Total events	20		23			
Heterogeneity: Chi² = 3.02, df = 3 (P = 0.39); I² = 1%						
Test for overall effect: Z = 0.46 (P = 0.65)						
1.2.2 Any minor bleeding						
ACCEL AMI	0	30	2	60	4.4%	0.38 [0.02, 8.25]
ACCEL DM	2	39	1	41	2.5%	2.16 [0.19, 24.85]
HOST ASSURE	6	1876	12	1879	31.8%	0.50 [0.19, 1.33]
Jeong2009	0	30	0	30		Not estimable
Subtotal (95% CI)		1975		2010	38.6%	0.59 [0.25, 1.38]
Total events	8		15			
Heterogeneity: Chi² = 1.27, df = 2 (P = 0.53); I² = 0%						
Test for overall effect: Z = 1.21 (P = 0.22)						
Total (95% CI)		4309		4345	100.0%	0.76 [0.47, 1.24]
Total events	28		38			
Heterogeneity: Chi² = 4.84, df = 6 (P = 0.56); I² = 0%						
Test for overall effect: Z = 1.10 (P = 0.27)						
Test for subgroup differences: Chi² = 0.53, df = 1 (P = 0.47), I² = 0%						

Fig. 6 Comparing bleeding events observed with double dose clopidogrel versus triple antiplatelet regimen

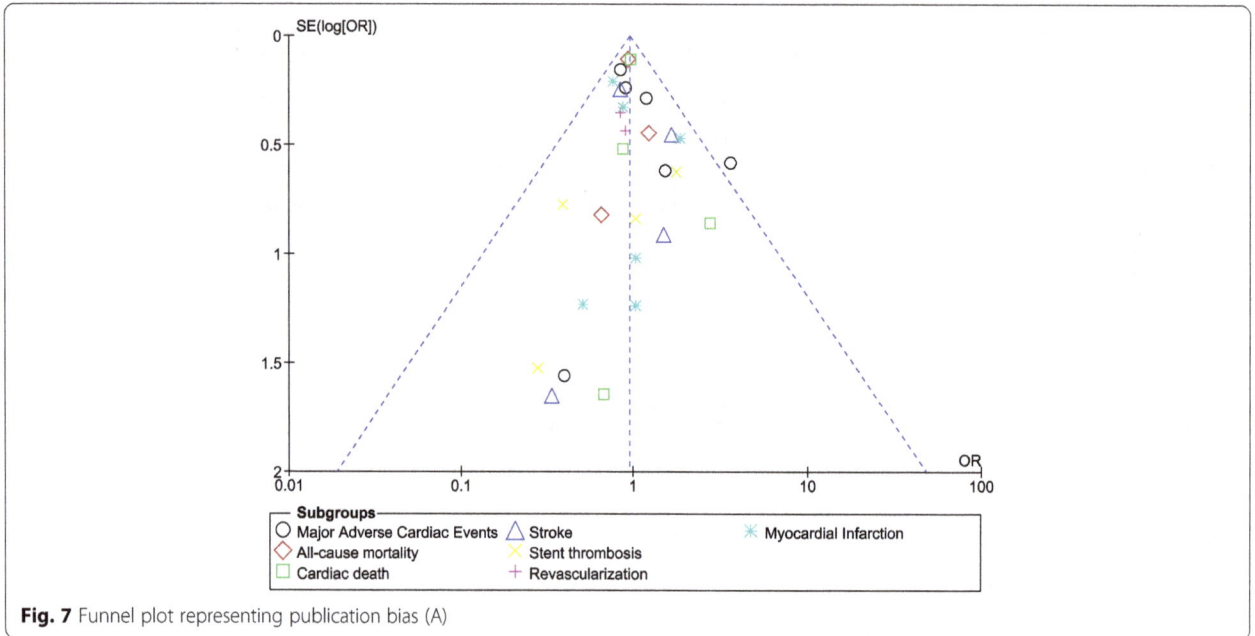

Fig. 7 Funnel plot representing publication bias (A)

outcomes in those patients who underwent PCI. Severe or moderate bleeding were also not significantly different.

Results of the Clopidogrel Response Evaluation and AnTi-platelet InterVEntion in High Thrombotic Risk PCI Patients (CREATIVE) Trial which compared DDC with that of the standard DAPT or cilostazol associated TAPT showed the latter to significantly improved outcomes [14]. However, no significant difference was observed when DDC was compared to the standard DAPT.

In contrast, in the CURRENT OASIS 7 randomized trial, where DDC (whereby 8560 patients were assigned to) was compared with the standard DAPT (where 8703 patients were assigned to) in patients with acute coronary syndrome,

the former significantly improved cardiovascular outcomes and stent thrombosis [11]. In addition, major bleeding was significantly higher with DDC during a follow-up time period of 30 days. However, it should be noted that in the CURRENT OASIS 7, the patients were also exposed to a low versus a high dosage of aspirin in addition to the DDC. However, in this current analysis, most of the studies included patients who did not receive a high dosage of aspirin.

Nevertheless, other studies have shown an impact of the CYP2C19 variant to also have interacted with platelet reactivity. For example, the Accelerated Platelet Inhibition by a Double Dose of Clopidogrel According to Gene Polymorphism study showed that among post-PCI

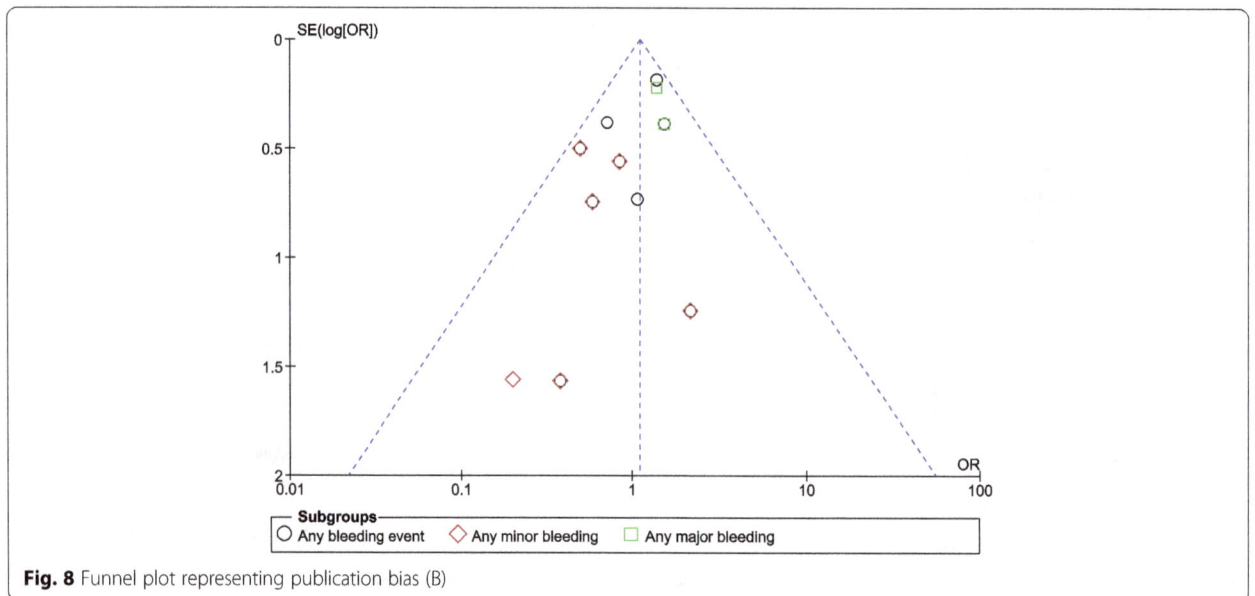

Fig. 8 Funnel plot representing publication bias (B)

treated patients who received DDC, carriage of CYP2C19 variant was associated with a high platelet reactivity which might have shown that DDC was non-inferior to the standard DAPT or TAPT [26]. However, the RESET GENE Trial showed this high treatment platelet reactivity to be completely abolished by prasugrel [27].

In addition, the Atorvastatin and Clopidogrel High Dose in stable patients with residual high platelet activity (ACHIDO) study showed that a high dose of atorvastatin significantly improved the pharmacodynamics effect of DDC [28], which was ignored in this current study.

Novelty

This analysis is new because it is the first research paper to systematically compare DDC with the other antiplatelet regimens in patients with coronary artery disease. In addition, this is an important piece of information which might contribute to the literature of cardiovascular diseases. DDC was compared with the standard dual antiplatelet regimen, the triple antiplatelet regimen, and newer antiplatelet drugs such as prasugrel and ticagrelor which might represent a new feature. Moreover, a low level of heterogeneity was reported among almost all the subgroups, which might further contribute to the novelty of this analysis.

Limitations

Limitations were as followed: Several trials consisted of a very small number of participants which might have been affected by larger trials. However, the proportion of participants were adjusted in larger trials to compensate for the small number of participants in other studies in order to have a final fair result. Different studies had different follow up time periods, and this might have influenced the final outcomes following statistical analysis. In addition, a few of the original studies were pilot studies whereby crossing over of clopidogrel and the control group was reported. This could have influenced the results to a minor extent. Moreover, major and minor bleedings were not reported when a few antiplatelet agents were compared with DDC since data concerning major and minor bleeding were missing in the original papers or they were reported in only one study and a comparison would have not been possible. At last, patients with different stages of coronary disease or intervention were combined and assessed: following PCI, patients with stable coronary artery disease, patients with AMI and other ACS were all together systematically analyzed.

Conclusions

In patients with CAD, adverse clinical outcomes were not significantly different when DDC was compared to the other antiplatelet regimens. In addition, bleeding events were also similarly manifested when DDC was compared to DAPT, TAPT or ticagrelor/prasugrel. Larger upcoming trials should be able to confirm this hypothesis.

Abbreviations

CAD: Coronary artery disease; DAPT: Dual antiplatelet therapy; DDC: Double dose clopidogrel; PCI: Percutaneous coronary intervention; TAPT: Triple antiplatelet therapy

Funding

There was no external funding for this research.

Authors' contributions

XZ, BZ, SO, PN and MX were responsible for the conception and design, acquisition of data, analysis and interpretation of data, drafting the initial manuscript and revising it critically for important intellectual content. XZ and BZ wrote the final manuscript. All authors have read and approved the manuscript as it is.

Competing interests

The authors declare that they have no competing interests.

Author details

[1]Department of Cardiology, Affiliated Changsha Hospital of Hunan Normal University, The Fourth Hospital of Changsha, Changsha 410006, Hunan, People's Republic of China. [2]Department of Pharmacology, People's Hospital of Laibin, Laibin 546100, Guangxi, People's Republic of China.

References

1. Mahmood SS, Levy D, Vasan RS, Wang TJ. The Framingham heart study and the epidemiology of cardiovascular disease: a historical perspective. Lancet. 2014;383(9921):999–1008.
2. Knight CJ. Antiplatelet treatment in stable coronary artery disease. Heart. 2003;89(10):1273–8.
3. Degrauwe S, Pilgrim T, Aminian A, Noble S, Meier P, Iglesias JF. Dual antiplatelet therapy for secondary prevention of coronary artery disease. Open Heart. 2017;4(2):e000651.
4. Lee GY, Hahn JY, Lee SY, Kim HJ, Kim JH, Lee SY, Song YB, Choi SH, Choi JH, Gwon HC. Adjunctive cilostazol versus high maintenance dose of clopidogrel in patients with hyporesponsiveness to chronic clopidogrel therapy. Yonsei Med J. 2013;54(1):34–40.
5. Montalescot G, Rangé G, Silvain J, Bonnet JL, Boueri Z, Barthélémy O, Cayla G, Belle L, Van Belle E, Cuisset T, Elhadad S, Pouillot C, Henry P, Motreff P, Carrié D, Rousseau H, Aubry P, Monségu J, Sabouret P, O'Connor SA, Abtan J, Kerneis M, Saint-Etienne C, Beygui F, Vicaut E, Collet JP, ARCTIC Investigators. High on-treatment platelet reactivity as a risk factor for secondary prevention after coronary stent revascularization: A landmark analysis of the ARCTIC study. Circulation. 2014;129(21):2136–43.
6. Chen S, Zhang Y, Wang L, Geng Y, Gu J, Hao Q, Wang H, Qi P. Effects of dual-dose Clopidogrel, Clopidogrel combined with Tongxinluo capsule, and Ticagrelor on patients with coronary heart disease and CYP2C19*2 Gene mutation after percutaneous coronary interventions (PCI). Med Sci Monit. 2017;23:3824–30.
7. Bundhun PK, Qin T, Chen MH. Comparing the effectiveness and safety between triple antiplatelet therapy and dual antiplatelet therapy in type 2 diabetes mellitus patients after coronary stents implantation: a systematic review and meta-analysis of randomized controlled trials. BMC Cardiovasc Disord. 2015;15:118.
8. Schulz S, Angiolillo DJ, Antoniucci D, Bernlochner I, Hamm C, Jaitner J, Laugwitz KL, Mayer K, von Merzljak B, Morath T, Neumann FJ, Richardt G, Ruf J, Schömig G, Schühlen H, Schunkert H, Kastrati A; Intracoronary Stenting and Antithrombotic Regimen: Rapid Early Action for Coronary Treatment (ISAR-REACT) 5 Trial Investigators. Randomized comparison of ticagrelor versus prasugrel in patients with acute coronary syndrome and planned invasive strategy–design and rationale of the iNtracoronary

Stenting and Antithrombotic Regimen: Rapid Early Action for Coronary Treatment (ISAR-REACT) 5 trial. J Cardiovasc Transl Res. 2014;7(1):91–100.

9. Liberati A, Altman DG, Tetzlaff J, et al. The PRISMA statement for reporting systematic reviews and meta-analyses of studies that evaluate healthcareinterventions: explanation and elaboration. BMJ. 2009;339:b2700.

10. Higgins JP, Thompson SG, Deeks JJ, et al. Measuring inconsistency in meta-analyses. BMJ. 2003;327:557–60.

11. Mehta SR, Tanguay JF, Eikelboom JW, Jolly SS, Joyner CD, Granger CB, Faxon DP, Rupprecht HJ, Budaj A, Avezum A, Widimsky P, Steg PG, Bassand JP, Montalescot G, Macaya C, Di Pasquale G, Niemela K, Ajani AE, White HD, Chrolavicius S, Gao P, Fox KA, Yusuf S, CURRENT-OASIS 7 trial investigators. Double-dose versus standard-dose clopidogrel and high-dose versus low-dose aspirin in individuals undergoing percutaneous coronary intervention for acute coronary syndromes (CURRENT-OASIS 7): a randomised factorial trial. Lancet. 2010;376(9748):1233–43.

12. Jeong YH, Hwang JY, Kim IS, Park Y, Hwang SJ, Lee SW, Kwak CH, Park SW. Adding cilostazol to dual antiplatelet therapy achieves greater platelet inhibition than highmaintenance dose clopidogrel in patients with acute myocardial infarction: results of the adjunctive cilostazol versus high maintenance dose clopidogrel in patients with AMI (ACCEL-AMI) study. Circ Cardiovasc Interv. 2010;3(1):17–26.

13. Angiolillo DJ, Shoemaker SB, Desai B, Yuan H, Charlton RK, Bernardo E, Zenni MM, Guzman LA, Bass TA, Costa MA. Randomized comparison of a high clopidogrel maintenance dose in patients with diabetes mellitus and coronary artery disease: results of the optimizing antiplatelet therapy in diabetes mellitus (OPTIMUS) study. Circulation. 2007;115(6):708–16.

14. Tang YD, Wang W, Yang M, Zhang K, Chen J, Qiao S, Yan H, Wu Y, Huang X, Xu B, Gao R, Yang Y, CREATIVE Investigators. Randomized comparisons of double-dose Clopidogrel or adjunctive Cilostazol versus StandardDual antiplatelet in patients with high posttreatment platelet reactivity: results of the CREATIVE trial. Circulation. 2018;137(21):2231–45.

15. Chen S, Zhang Y, Wang L, Geng Y, Gu J, Hao Q, Wang H, Qi P. Effects of dual-dose Clopidogrel, Clopidogrel combined with Tongxinluo capsule, and Ticagreloron patients with coronary heart disease and CYP2C19*2 Gene mutation after PercutaneousCoronary interventions (PCI). Med Sci Monit. 2017;23:3824–30.

16. Khatri S, Pierce T. Comparing prasugrel to twice daily clopidogrel post percutaneous coronary intervention in a veterans affairs population. Am J Health Syst Pharm. 2015;72(17 Suppl 2):S98–S103.

17. Angiolillo DJ, Badimon JJ, Saucedo JF, Frelinger AL, Michelson AD, Jakubowski JA, Zhu B, Ojeh CK, Baker BA, Effron MB. A pharmacodynamic comparison of prasugrel vs. high-dose clopidogrel in patients with type 2diabetes mellitus and coronary artery disease: results of the optimizing anti-platelet therapy in diabetes MellitUS (OPTIMUS)-3 trial. Eur Heart J. 2011;32(7):838–46.

18. Wiviott SD, Trenk D, Frelinger AL, O'Donoghue M, Neumann FJ, Michelson AD, Angiolillo DJ, Hod H, Montalescot G, Miller DL, Jakubowski JA, Cairns R, Murphy SA, McCabe CH, Antman EM, Braunwald E, PRINCIPLE-TIMI 44 Investigators. Prasugrel compared with high loading- and maintenance-dose clopidogrel in patients with planned percutaneous coronary intervention: the Prasugrel in Comparison to Clopidogrel for Inhibition of Platelet Activation and Aggregation-Thrombolysis in Myocardial Infarction 44 trial. Circulation. 2007;116(25):2923–32.

19. Dridi NP, Johansson PI, Clemmensen P, Stissing T, Radu MD, Qayyum A, Pedersen F, Helqvist S, Saunamäki K, Kelbæk H, Jørgensen E, Engstrøm T, Holmvang L. Prasugrel or double-dose clopidogrel to overcome clopidogrel low-response--the TAILOR(thrombocytes and IndividuaLization of ORal antiplatelet therapy in percutaneous coronaryintervention) randomized trial. Platelets. 2014;25(7):506–12.

20. Wu X, Liu G, Lu J, Zheng XX, Cui JG, Zhao XY, Huang XH. Administration of Ticagrelor and Double-Dose Clopidogrel Based on platelet ReactivityDetermined by VerifyNow-P2Y12 for Chinese subjects after elective PCI. Int Heart J. 2017;58(2):167–73.

21. Jeong YH, Tantry US, Park Y, Kwon TJ, Park JR, Hwang SJ, Bliden KP, Koh EH, Kwak CH, Hwang JY, Kim S, Gurbel PA. Pharmacodynamic effect of cilostazol plus standard clopidogrel versus double-dose clopidogrelin patients with type 2 diabetes undergoing percutaneous coronary intervention. Diabetes Care. 2012;35(11):2194–7.

22. Ha SJ, Kim SJ, Hwang SJ, Woo JS, Kim W, Kim WS, Kim KS, Kim MK. Effect of cilostazol addition or clopidogrel doubling on platelet function profiles in diabeticpatients undergoing a percutaneous coronary intervention. Coron Artery Dis. 2013;24(8):690–7.

23. Park KW, Kang SH, Park JJ, Yang HM, Kang HJ, Koo BK, Park BE, Cha KS, Rhew JY, Jeon HK, Shin ES, Oh JH, Jeong MH, Kim S, Hwang KK, Yoon JH, Lee SY, Park TH, Moon KW, Kwon HM, Chae IH, Kim HS. Adjunctive cilostazol versus double-dose clopidogrel after drug-eluting stent implantation: the HOST-ASSURE randomized trial (Harmonizing Optimal Strategy for Treatment of Coronary Artery Stenosis-Safety & Effectiveness of Drug-Eluting Stents & Anti-platelet Regimen). JACC Cardiovasc Interv. 2013;6(9):932–42.

24. Jeong YH, Lee SW, Choi BR, Kim IS, Seo MK, Kwak CH, Hwang JY, Park SW. Randomized comparison of adjunctive cilostazol versus high maintenance dose clopidogrel in patients with high post-treatment platelet reactivity: results of the ACCEL-RESISTANCE (adjunctive Cilostazol versus high maintenance dose Clopidogrel in patients with ClopidogrelResistance) randomized study. J Am Coll Cardiol. 2009;53(13):1101–9.

25. Price MJ, Berger PB, Teirstein PS, Tanguay JF, Angiolillo DJ, Spriggs D, Puri S, Robbins M, Garratt KN, Bertrand OF, Stillabower ME, Aragon JR, Kandzari DE, Stinis CT, Lee MS, Manoukian SV, Cannon CP, Schork NJ, Topol EJ, GRAVITAS Investigators. Standard- vs high-dose clopidogrel based on platelet function testing after percutaneous coronary intervention: the GRAVITAS randomized trial. JAMA. 2011;305(11):1097–105.

26. Jeong YH, Kim IS, Park Y, Kang MK, Koh JS, Hwang SJ, Kwak CH, Hwang JY. Carriage of cytochrome 2C19 polymorphism is associated with risk of high post-treatmentplatelet reactivity on high maintenance-dose clopidogrel of 150 mg/day: results of the ACCEL-DOUBLE (accelerated platelet inhibition by a double dose of Clopidogrel according to Gene polymorphism) study. JACC Cardiovasc Interv. 2010;3(7):731–41.

27. Sardella G, Calcagno S, Mancone M, Palmirotta R, Lucisano L, Canali E, Stio RE, Pennacchi M, Di Roma A, Benedetti G, Guadagni F, Biondi-Zoccai G, Fedele F. Pharmacodynamic effect of switching therapy in patients with high on-treatment plateletreactivity and genotype variation with high clopidogrel dose versus prasugrel: the RESET GENE trial. Circ Cardiovasc Interv. 2012;5(5):698–704.

28. Leoncini M, Toso A, Maioli M, Angiolillo DJ, Giusti B, Marcucci R, Abbate R, Bellandi F. High-dose atorvastatin on the pharmacodynamic effects of double-dose clopidogrel in patientsundergoing percutaneous coronary interventions: the ACHIDO (atorvastatin and Clopidogrel HIgh DOse in stable patients with residual high platelet activity) study. JACC Cardiovasc Interv. 2013;6(2):169–79.

22

The impact of vancomycin trough concentrations on outcomes in non-deep seated infections: a retrospective cohort study

Michael Wan[1], Sandra A. N. Walker[1,2,3,4]* (iD), Elaine Martin[7], Marion Elligsen[1], Lesley Palmay[1] and Jerome A. Leis[3,4,5,6]

Abstract

Background: Guidelines recommending vancomycin trough concentrations > 10 mg/L in non-deep seated infections are based on expert opinion. The objective of this study was to evaluate patients with non-deep seated infections treated with short-course vancomycin to determine whether there were differences in outcomes with trough concentrations of ≤10 mg/L (low) versus > 10 mg/L (high).

Methods: A retrospective cohort study of patients hospitalized between March 10, 2010 and December 31, 2015 who received ≤14 days of vancomycin to treat a non-deep seated infection and had at least one steady state trough concentration was completed. Patient data for the low versus high trough cohorts were compared using appropriate statistical tests and binary logistic regression was used to identify factors associated with clinical outcome.

Results: Of 2098 patients screened, 103 (5%) met inclusion criteria. Baseline characteristics between cohorts were not different. Clinical cure was not different between the low (42/48 [88%]) and high trough (48/55 [87%]) cohorts (p > 0.99) and vancomycin trough concentration was not associated with clinical outcome (p = 0.973). More patients in the high trough group had dosing changes (7/48 [15%] vs. 22/55 [40%], p = 0.0046), with approximately three times more dose adjustments per patient (0.17 vs. 0.55, p = 0.0193). No signal for increased vancomycin resistance associated with vancomycin troughs was identified.

Conclusions:: No difference in clinical or microbiological outcomes based on vancomycin trough concentrations were observed in patients with non-deep seated infections treated with vancomycin for ≤14 days. Targeting higher vancomycin trough concentrations of > 10 mg/L may be associated with increased workload with no corresponding benefit in clinical or microbiological outcomes in these patients.

Keywords: Vancomycin, Non-deep seated infections, Trough concentrations, Levels, Therapeutic drug monitoring, Outcomes

* Correspondence: sandra.walker@sunnybrook.ca
[1]Department of Pharmacy, Sunnybrook Health Sciences Centre, 2075 Bayview Avenue, Toronto, ON M4N 3M5, Canada
[2]Leslie Dan Faculty of Pharmacy, University of Toronto, 144 College Street, Toronto, ON M5S 3M2, Canada
Full list of author information is available at the end of the article

Background

Vancomycin was discovered over 60 years ago; however, it was not until the early 1980s that its clinical use sharply increased in response to a rise in the worldwide prevalence of methicillin-resistant *Staphylococcus aureus* (MRSA) [1]. Unfortunately, controversy regarding the optimal dosing and pharmacokinetic/pharmacodynamic targets continues to plague the use of vancomycin [2]. Current guidelines recommend targeting vancomycin serum trough concentrations of 15–20 mg/L for complicated infections (e.g. endocarditis, osteomyelitis, pneumonia, meningitis, etc.), and suggest maintaining a trough of > 10 mg/L for all patients (including those with non-deep seated infections with a planned duration of ≤14 days) to avoid development of resistance to vancomycin (Quality and Grade of Evidence for each recommendation in the 2009 IDSA guidelines was IIIB) [3–5].

The emergence of vancomycin resistance has not been observed in patients treated with short term vancomycin (≤14 days) for the management of non-deep seated infections (e.g. bacteremia when endocarditis or other non-cardiac seeding [e.g. bone or brain] has been ruled out; uncomplicated skin and soft tissue infections; and urinary tract infections in the absence of anatomic abnormalities, renal stones, or renal abscess).

Clinical evidence to support the need to maintain vancomycin serum trough concentrations above 10 mg/L for management of non-deep seated infections is lacking and the practice of targeting higher trough concentrations has obvious downsides. This practice increases the complexity of the dosing and monitoring of vancomycin, results in additional blood draws from the patient, increases the workload for the clinical team, and may therefore, increase the risk of medical error and harm to the patient. We hypothesize that there is no difference in clinical or microbiological outcomes associated with vancomycin trough concentrations of ≤10 mg/L versus > 10 mg/L when vancomycin is used in the setting of non-deep seated infections for a period of ≤14 days.

The primary objective of this study was to evaluate patients with non-deep seated infections who were treated with vancomycin for a period of ≤14 days to determine whether there were differences in clinical outcome with serum trough concentrations of vancomycin of ≤10 mg/L versus > 10 mg/L. The secondary objectives of this study were to identify factors which may affect clinical outcome, evaluate safety outcomes (kidney injury), assess workload based on dose adjustment(s), and identify changes in microbial resistance during the vancomycin treatment course.

Methods
Study design

A retrospective chart review of eligible patients was conducted. Patients were identified for eligibility using the Stewardship Program Integrating Resource Information Technology (SPIRIT) database of our Antimicrobial Stewardship Program [6]. A SPIRIT query generated a list of inpatients at SHSC between March 12th, 2010 and December 31st, 2015, inclusive, with at least one steady state vancomycin trough concentration. Hospital charts for the patients identified by this query were retrieved from Health Data Resources (HDR) and reviewed to confirm patient eligibility for this study.

Patient eligibility

Adult inpatients (aged ≥18 years) were eligible for study inclusion if they were admitted to SHSC between March 12th, 2010 and December 31st, 2015, received a minimum of 48 h and a maximum of 14 days of vancomycin for a presumed or confirmed non-deep seated infection (defined below) associated with any bacteria for which vancomycin may be indicated, and for whom at least one steady state vancomycin trough concentration was available. A steady state vancomycin trough concentration was defined as a level obtained at the earliest prior to the 3rd dose for ≥ every 12 h dosing, and prior to the 4th dose for ≤ every 8 h dosing; or a random vancomycin concentration obtained at least 24 h after vancomycin initiation in patients receiving continuous infusion. An exception was made for inclusion of patients receiving a maximum of 15 days of vancomycin, if the treating physician's intent was to treat for 14 days. Patients were eligible for inclusion if their infection-related diagnosis was:

- Uncomplicated skin and soft tissue infections (SSTI): folliculitis, carbuncle(s), surgical site infections, wound infections, non-suppurative cellulitis or erysipelas;
- Urinary tract infections (UTI) in the absence of anatomic abnormalities, renal abscess, or renal stones;
- Bacteremia without any evidence of seeding to heart, bone/joint, brain, or lungs; or
- Coagulase negative *Staphylococci* (CNST) line-related infections (excluding tunnel infection or vascular graft infections).

If patients received more than one course of vancomycin during their hospital stay, only data from their first vancomycin course was included, with documentation of any subsequent courses of vancomycin within 14 days of vancomycin discontinuation or patient readmission within 30 days of completion of their initial vancomycin treatment course. Subsequent vancomycin treatment courses and patient readmission were considered markers of potential relapsing infection (clinical failure) with a risk of development of a vancomycin resistant bacterial isolate. Patients were excluded if there was a presumed or documented diagnosis of abscess at any site, endocarditis, meningitis, osteomyelitis, joint infection, febrile neutropenia, pneumonia, or sinusitis; were switched to an alternate antibiotic on day 2 or 3 of vancomycin due to culture and sensitivity results; received antibiotics for no documented infection (e.g. prophylactic antibiotics); received renal replacement therapy; or if vancomycin was discontinued as a result of a patient care plan that was changed to palliative.

Data collection and definitions

Required patient clinical and laboratory data were extracted from the hospital's electronic databases (SPIRIT, electronic patient records [EPR/Sunnycare]) and patient medical records (HDR/Sovera) and entered into a Microsoft Excel workbook. Patients were stratified to vancomycin low or high trough cohorts based on their final documented vancomycin steady-state trough concentration (≤ 10 mg/L or > 10 mg/L, respectively). The primary outcome of this study was clinical cure, defined as all of the following:

- Resolution of all presenting signs and symptoms of infection within ≤ 14 days therapy with vancomycin; whereby patients could be discharged home on a short course of vancomycin (total duration ≤ 14 days) with documentation of improvement during hospital stay;
- Maintained resolution of all presenting signs and symptoms of infection for 14 days following vancomycin discontinuation;
- No additional course of antibiotics within 14 days with the same indication as initial vancomycin treatment course;
- No documentation of hospital readmission requiring antibiotic therapy within 30 days of completion of their initial vancomycin treatment course.

Secondary outcomes:

- Identification of clinical, demographic or microbiological factors associated with clinical cure;
- Kidney injury outcomes as per RIFLE (Risk, Injury, Failure, Loss of kidney function, and End-stage kidney disease) criteria [7];
- Workload based on number of dose adjustment(s) during the vancomycin course; and
- Development of microbiological resistance during the vancomycin treatment course or within 30 days of completion of the initial vancomycin treatment course.

Severity of illness was measured with the Acute Physiology and Chronic Health Evaluation (APACHE) II score for intensive care unit (ICU) patients and Pitt Bacteremia score for ward patients [8, 9]. As there are no other validated measures of severity of illness in hospital ward patients, the Pitt Bacteremia score was used in these patients, recognizing that the Pitt Bacteremia score has only been validated in patients with bacteremia. Hospital location (ICU versus ward) at time of vancomycin initiation was identified and ICU patients included those with admission or transfer to a critical care bed within 48 h of vancomycin initiation. Concomitant antibiotics were defined as any antibiotic whose administration overlapped that of vancomycin by at least 48 h and was administered for at least 48 h. The time required for each vancomycin dose adjustment was estimated from typical nursing, physician, pharmacist and pharmacy technician practices at our institution (Appendix).

Sample size calculation

The literature was reviewed to provide an estimate of the vancomycin treatment failure rate in non-deep seated infections. Although three studies provided a treatment failure rate in SSTIs (ranging from 12 to 38% for all organisms; and 17–35% for MRSA only), the SSTIs included in these studies were complicated skin and soft tissue infections (cSSTIs) that involved deep soft tissue or required significant surgical intervention (infected ulcers, burns, and major abscesses) [10–12]. No reliable treatment failure estimates were available for UTIs or isolated uncomplicated bacteremia associated with bacteria for which vancomycin may be used. Since only patients with non-deep seated infection(s) were eligible for this study, the treatment failure rates were predicted to be lower than those reported in the literature for cSSTIs.

Based on the only available published literature, we estimated our rate of treatment failure to be between 10 and 25%; 10% being a hypothesized estimate, and 25% being the midpoint of treatment failure rates observed in the literature for cSSTIs. Thus, using a standard sample size equation for dichotomous data, 93 to 348 patients per group (based upon treatment failure rates of 10 to 25% in the high trough cohort) would be required to detect a minimal difference in failure (Δ) of 10 percentage points between patients with a trough of ≤ 10 mg/L versus > 10 mg/L (2-tailed, $p = 0.05$, power = 0.80).

Statistics & data analysis

Comparison of the study cohorts for interval, nominal and ordinal data were analyzed using GraphPad InStat (version 3.05, 32-bit for Win95/NT; GraphPad Software Inc., La Jolla, California). Nominal data were expressed as total number (proportion) of patients; and low trough and high trough groups were compared using the Fisher Exact test (odds ratio, 95% confidence interval and *p*-value). Interval data were expressed as mean ± standard deviation (and range) and the Kolmogorov Smirov test was used to evaluate the data for normality. If interval data passed the test for normality and standard deviations were not significantly different then a two-sided unpaired t-test was used to compare the study cohorts. If interval data were normally distributed, but standard deviations between groups were significantly different then the cohorts were compared using the two-sided un-paired t-test with Welch correction. If interval data did not pass the test for normality then a two tailed Mann-Whitney test was used. A *p*-value of < 0.05 was considered as statistically significant.

A Pearson's Correlation matrix (univariable analysis) (SPSS version 13.0 for Windows, created September 1, 2004) was completed to identify patient clinical, microbiological, laboratory and vancomycin dosing related parameters (independent variables) associated with clinical cure (dependent variable). Patient related parameters that were evaluated by univariable analysis as independent variables were: sex, age, hospital location, length of stay at vancomycin initiation, comorbidities, immunosuppressive medications, nephrotoxic medications, severity of illness, baseline serum creatinine, final serum creatinine, serum creatinine change, risk of renal injury, kidney injury, Gram positive bacterial species identified in culture, and infectious diagnosis for which vancomycin was prescribed. Vancomycin dosing related factors that were evaluated by univariable analysis were initial dose, final dose, initial steady state vancomycin trough, final steady state vancomycin trough, and high versus low trough cohort. Any independent variables that were available for > 20% of patients and had a *p* value < 0.05 with Pearson's Correlation were maintained in the multivariable analysis of binary logistic regression (SPSS version 13.0 for Windows, created September 1, 2004) to identify the existence of a statistically significant model (*p* < 0.05) in which all independent variables remaining in the model had an odds ratio of > 1.

Results

A total of 2098 patients on vancomycin during the study period were identified from the SPIRIT database query for screening, and 103 (5%) met inclusion criteria for the study (Low trough cohort: *n* = 48, High trough cohort: *n* = 55) (Fig. 1). Of the 1995 excluded patients, the most common reason for exclusion was the presence of a deep-seated infection (1134 patients). The two groups were well-balanced in terms of baseline demographic, clinical and microbiological factors (Table 1).

There was no significant difference in clinical cure (88% vs. 87%, OR 1.02, 95% CI 0.32–3.28, *p* > 0.99) or survival (100% vs. 98%, OR 2.67, 95% CI 0.11–67.13, *p* > 0.99) between the low trough and high trough groups (Table 2). One patient passed away in the high trough group for a reason unrelated to infection. Two patients in the high trough group (4%) and no patients in the low trough group (0%) were re-admitted within 30 days for the same indication as the original course of vanco-mycin. The 95% confidence intervals around clinical cure in the low trough versus high trough cohorts were 78–97% versus 78–96%, which completely overlap to support the finding of no significant difference in clinical cure. To detect a minimum difference in treatment failure of 1%, a sample size of 17,370 patients per group would be required. To detect a minimum difference in treatment failure of 0.5%, a sample size of 68,850 patients per group would be required. A Monte Carlo Simulation (Oracle Crystal Ball, build 11.1.4100 on 12/23/2014, 32-bit) (MCS) of 1 million iterations, using a binomial distribution, with the study observed probability of cure (Low trough = 0.88, High trough = 0.87), was conducted to determine the probability that clinical cure could theoretically be ≥10% better in the high trough cohort compared to the low trough cohort. This probability was determined to be 3%.

The average final steady state vancomycin troughs were 7.38 ± 1.95 mg/L and 16.56 ± 6.56 mg/L in the low and high trough groups, respectively, and the median duration of therapy in both groups was 7 ± 3 days. Although the median total daily dose between groups was similar (2 g per day in both groups), patients in the high trough group were more likely to receive 3 or more grams of vancomycin per day (*p* = 0.04) and had a significant increase from initial to final vancomycin troughs (*p* = 0.0009). Patients in the high trough group had more vancomycin dosing changes (*p* = 0.02), which in turn translated to a three-fold higher investment of health care worker time related to vancomycin therapy per patient in the high trough group (p = 0.02) (Table 2). Renal function outcomes were similar between the two groups, with no significant difference in change in serum creatinine (*p* = 0.13) and number of patients at risk for kidney injury (*p* = 0.12). However, it is noteworthy that while no patient in the low trough group was at risk for kidney injury, 4 patients in the high trough group were at risk for kidney injury (Table 2).

Univariable analysis identified five independent variables that were significantly associated with clinical outcome; however, none of these variables remained significant with multivariable analysis (Table 3). Notably, low/high trough categorization was not significantly associated with clinical outcome in patients with a non-deep seated infection with univariable analysis. The patient to variable ratio for the multivariable analysis was 21:1.

Discussion

This retrospective study evaluated whether differences in clinical cure exist when targeting trough concentrations

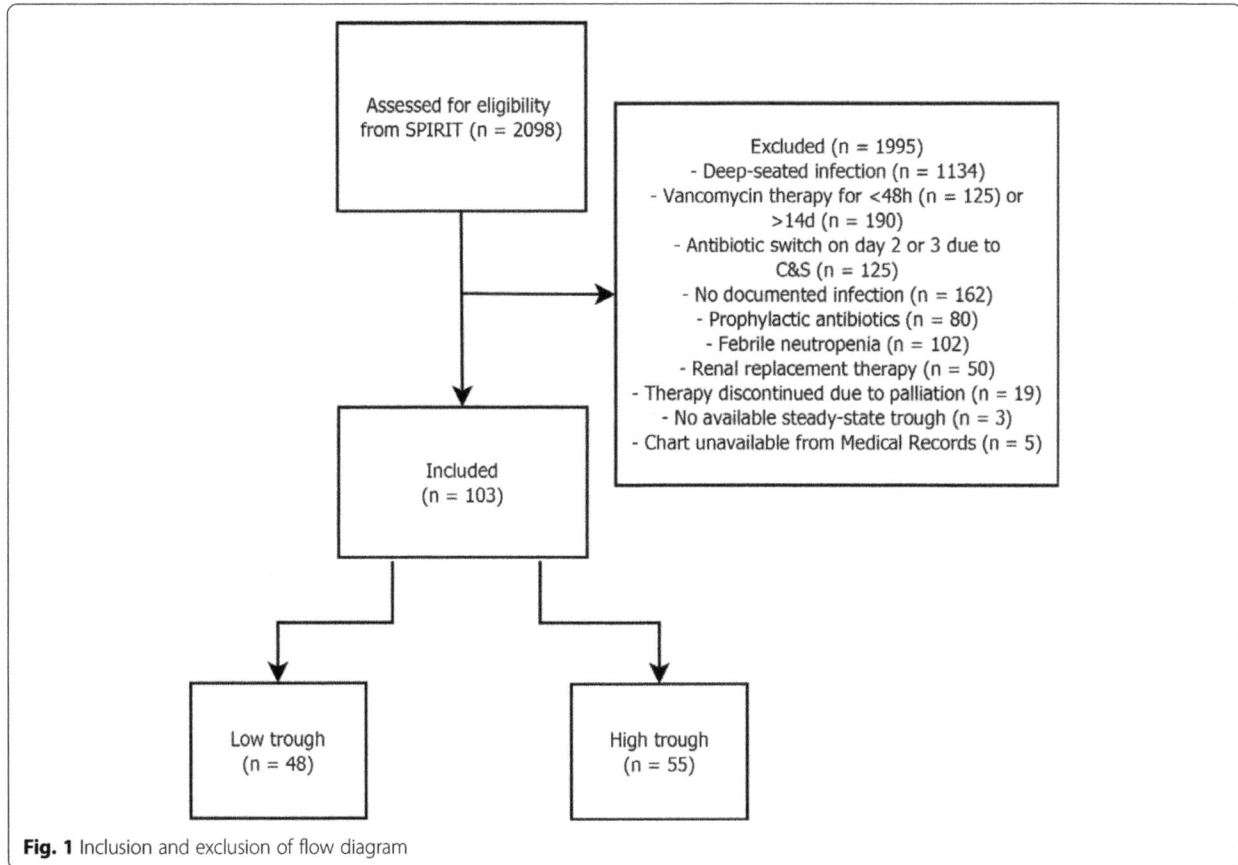

Fig. 1 Inclusion and exclusion of flow diagram

≤10 mg/L versus > 10 mg/L in patients with non-deep seated infections treated with vancomycin for ≤14 days; and, to the best of our knowledge, is the first study to do so. Although limited by a small sample size, the study enrollment reflects the entire population of patients with non-deep seated infections treated with vancomycin at our hospital between March 12th, 2010 and December 31st, 2015, inclusive. Strict eligibility criteria for study entry were used and the cohorts were well balanced for all baseline characteristics. We did not measure any difference in clinical cure with higher vancomycin trough concentrations and there was no signal for selection of resistant Gram positive bacteria in patients with a non-deep seated infection receiving ≤14 days of vancomycin. However, there was a three-fold increase in healthcare personnel workload, which introduces unnecessary complexity (increased pharmacist, pharmacy technician, nursing and physician time involvement, additional blood work, and risk of medication error with more frequent dose adjustments).

In current infectious diseases guidelines, the rationale for maintaining trough concentrations above 10 mg/L is to prevent the development of resistance; emergence of vancomycin resistance in patients treated with ≤14 days of vancomycin has never been reported in the literature [3–5].

We did not observe the emergence of any resistance to vancomycin in our study, and no patients with low vancomycin levels (< 10 mg/L) required re-admission for recurrent infection; this is a reassuring finding, since one reason for recurrent infection may be the emergence of vancomycin resistance. Vancomycin resistance in *Staphylococcus aureus* with low vancomycin levels for ≤14 days has only been observed in vitro with purposeful selection; and clinically in patients who received prolonged vancomycin exposure (6–18 weeks) [2, 13–23]. No association between vancomycin trough concentrations and emergence of vancomycin resistance has been observed for any other bacteria (e.g. CNST, *Enterococci*, other Gram positive organisms) for which vancomycin may be indicated.

As a single-center, retrospective analysis, our study has several limitations. To maximize our sample size, we screened all potential patients since the inception of our Antimicrobial Stewardship database until study closing. Despite our efforts, our final sample size was only sufficient to detect a difference of 25% points between the two groups for our primary outcome; we set a difference of 10% between the two groups as being clinically important to identify in our sample size calculation, and observed a difference of less than 1% (non-rounded clinical cure rates in low versus high trough cohorts 87.5% vs. 87.3%) between

Table 1 Patient Characteristics (N = 103)

	Low Trough (N = 48)	High Trough (N = 55)	Odds Ratio	95% Confidence Interval	p-value
Gender (Male)	27 (56%)	28 (51%)	1.24	0.57–2.70	0.69
Age on Admission (Years), mean ± SD (Range)	59 ± 19 (21–91)	67 ± 21 (19–96)			0.06
Hospital Location at Vancomycin Initiation (Ward)	38 (79%)	44 (80%)	0.95	0.36–2.48	> 0.99
Length of Stay at the time of Vancomycin Initiation (Days),median[a](Range)	2(0–70)	2(0–187)			0.89
Any Comorbidity[b]	19 (40%)	25 (45%)	0.79	0.36–1.72	0.56
• Congestive Heart Failure	3 (6%)	8 (15%)	0.39	0.098–1.57	0.21
• Chronic Obstructive Pulmonary Disease	2 (4%)	7 (13%)	0.30	0.06–1.51	0.17
• Diabetes Mellitus	7 (15%)	10 (18%)	0.77	0.27–2.21	0.79
• Immunosuppression due to disease or drug[c]	8 (17%)	6 (11%)	1.63	0.52–5.10	0.57
APACHE II[d], mean ± SD (ICU patients)	17 ± 6 (11–25)	23 ± 11 (6–41)			0.32
Critically Ill Ward Patients (Pitt Bacteremia Score ≥ 4)	1 (2%)	4 (7%)	0.27	0.03–2.52	0.37
Baseline Creatinine (mmol/L)	77 ± 32 (23–185)	83 ± 45 (18–254)			0.42
Use of Concomitant Nephrotoxins[e]	35 (73%)	36 (65%)	1.42	0.61–3.31	0.52
• # of Concomitant Nephrotoxins[a] (median)	1 (0–3)	1 (0–4)			0.49
Use of Concomitant Antibiotics[f]	21 (44%)	17 (31%)	1.74	0.78–3.90	0.22
• Same Indication as Vancomycin[g]	18 (86%)	14 (82%)	1.29	0.22–7.37	> 0.99
Included Infections					
• All SSTIs	31 (65%)	32 (58%)	1.31	0.59–2.91	0.55
o Cellulitis	25 (52%)	22 (40%)	1.63	0.75–3.57	0.24
o Wound/Surgical Site Infection	6 (12%)	10 (18%)	0.64	0.21–1.92	0.59
• All UTIs	11 (23%)	7 (13%)	2.04	0.72–5.77	0.20
o MRSA UTI	2 (4%)	1 (2%)	2.35	0.21–26.75	0.60
o Enteroccocal UTI	9 (19%)	6 (11%)	1.88	0.62–5.75	0.28
• All Bacteremias	4 (8%)	10 (18%)	0.41	0.12–1.40	0.16
o CNST Bacteremia[h]	3 (6%)	8 (15%)	0.39	0.10–1.57	0.21
• Any Positive CNST in Blood	5 (10%)	14 (25%)	0.34	0.11–1.03	0.07
Microbiology					
• Patients With Positive Non-Screening Cultures for Resistant Gram positive isolates[i]	10 (21%)	22 (40%)	0.39	0.16–0.95	0.054
o Patients with MRSA Clinical Culture	2 (4%)	5 (9%)	0.43	0.08–2.35	0.44
o Patients with CNST Clinical Culture	8 (17%)	17 (31%)	0.45	0.17–1.16	0.11
• MRSA-colonized Patients	2 (4%)	8 (15%)	0.26	0.05–1.27	0.10
• VRE-colonized Patients	1 (2%)	0	3.50	0.14–88.15	0.47

ACEI Angiotensin converting enzyme inhibitor, AIDS Acquired immune deficiency syndrome, *APACHE* Acute Physiology and Chronic Health Evaluation, *ARB* Angiotensin II receptor blocker, *ASA* Acetylsalicylic acid, *HCTZ* Hydrochlorothiazide, *CNST* Coagulase-negative *Staphylococci*, *HIV* Human immunodeficiency virus, *ICU* Intensive Care Unit, *NSAID* Nonsteroidal anti-inflammatory drug, *PPI* Proton pump inhibitor, *SD* Standard deviation, *SSTI* Skin and soft tissue infection, *TNF-α* Tumor necrosis factor alpha, *UTI* Urinary tract infection, *VRE* Vancomycin-resistant *Enterococci*
[a]For non-normally distributed data, the median with range was reported
[b]Patients may have had more than 1 comorbidity, thus totals for specific comorbidities sum to a value greater than the number of patients with any comorbidity
[c]Disease: HIV/AIDS, asplenia, hematological malignancies, transplantation. Drug: Corticosteroids (prednisone > 5 mg/day, chemotherapy, TNF-α inhibitors, transplant medications)
[d]Arterial blood gases were not available for all ICU patients and APACHE II scoring could not be completed for these patients; reported values are based on 6 patients in low trough cohort and 7 patients in high trough cohort
[e]NSAIDs, ACEIs, ARBs, cyclosporine, tacrolimus, acyclovir, aminoglycosides, amphotericin, colistin, indinavir, adefovir, cidofovir, tenofovir, chemotherapy (e.g. carmustine, semustine, cisplatin, methotrexate, mitomycin), foscarnet, contrast dye, zoledronate, loop diuretics, HCTZ, triamterene, hydralazine, interferons, PPIs, sulfonamides, lithium, aristocholic acid, acetaminophen at > 1 g/day for > 2 years, ASA at > 1 g/day for > 2 years)
[f]Concomitant antibiotic defined as: ≥48 h overlap with vancomycin and administered for ≥48 h
[g]Denominator for percentage calculations is the number of patients (n) on concomitant antibiotics (i.e. low trough n = 18; high trough n = 14)
[h]Defined as ≥2 positive blood cultures on the same day
[i]Methicillin Resistant *Staphylococcus aureus*, Coagulase-negative *Staphylococci*, or Vancomycin Resistant *Enterococci* cultured from 3 days prior to initiation or during vancomycin course of therapy and includes a single positive culture for CNST

Table 2 Results (N = 103)

	Low Trough (N = 48)	High Trough (N = 55)	Odds Ratio	95% Confidence Interval	p-value
Clinical Outcomes					
• Clinical Cure (Primary Outcome)	42 (88%)	48 (87%)	1.02	0.32–3.28	> 0.99
• Survival	48 (100%)	54 (98%)	2.67	0.11–67.13	> 0.99
• Readmission within 30 days for same indication as original course of vancomycin	0 (0%)	2 (4%)	0.22	0.01–4.71	0.50
Microbiological Outcome					
• Patients With Positive Non-Screening Cultures for Resistant Gram positive Isolates[a] identified up to 2 weeks after discontinuation of vancomycin	0	0	–	–	–
Vancomycin Use and Dosing					
• Final Total Daily Dose, median[b] (mg) (Range)	2000 (500–3000)	2000 (666–4500)			0.46
• Number of Patients With Daily Dose ≥3 g/day[c]	4 (8%)	14 (25%)	0.27	0.08–0.88	0.04
• Initial Steady State Trough (mg/L)[d]	7.13 ± 2.24	12.20 ± 5.30			<0.0001[e]
• Final Steady State Trough (mg/L)[d]	7.38 ± 1.95	16.56 ± 6.56[f]			< 0.0001[f]
• Duration of Vancomycin Therapy (days)[g]	7 ± 3	7 ± 3			0.73
• # Patients Requiring Dose Adjustment	7 (15%)	22 (40%)	0.26	0.10–0.67	0.005
• # of Dose Adjustments Per Patient[b]	0.17 ± 0.43	0.55 ± 0.79			0.02[f]
• Time Estimate for Dose Adjustments Per Patient (minutes)[b]	9 ± 23	29 ± 42			0.02[f]
Renal Function Outcomes					
• Final Serum Creatinine (mmol/L)	71 ± 28	83 ± 46			0.11[e]
• % Change in Serum Creatinine	−5 ± 18	3 ± 30			0.13[e]
• At Risk for Kidney Injury[h]	0 (0%)	4 (7%)	0.12	0.01–2.25	0.12

[a]Methicillin Resistant *Staphylococcus aureus*, Coagulase-negative *Staphylococci*, or Vancomycin Resistant *Enterococci*
[b]For non-normally distributed data, the median was reported rather than the mean ± standard deviation, with the exception of: # of Dose Adjustments Per Patient, and Time Estimate for Dose Adjustment Per Patient
[c]No patients in the low trough group and 2 patients in the high trough group received ≥4 g vancomycin per day
[d]Initial vs. Final steady state trough concentration comparisons within groups: Low trough p-value = 0.5607 (equal SD, unpaired t-test); High trough p-value = 0.0009 (unequal SD, unpaired t-test Welch Corrected)
[e]Unequal SD, unpaired t-test Welch Corrected
[f]Did not pass test for normality, two tailed Mann-Whitney U test used
[g]Patients were included if the intent was to treat for ≤14 days (2 patients in the high trough group were treated for 15 days)
[h]≥50% increase from baseline serum creatinine as per RIFLE Criteria [5]

the cohorts. To be adequately powered for a difference in treatment failure of 1% or 0.5%, a sample size of 17,370 or 68,850 patients per cohort, respectively, would be necessary. Since a difference of 1% in treatment failure would not be considered clinically important in non-deep seated bacterial infections, this point illustrates the futility for the need to increase the sample size of our study and minimizes any argument that insufficient sample size may have biased against seeing a difference in clinical outcomes between the low and high trough cohorts. To further address the risk of a type II error, we conducted a MCS of 1 million iterations, using a binomial distribution, with the study

Table 3 Univariable and Multivariable Analyses to Identify Factors Associated with Clinical Outcome

Independent Variables	Univariable (Pearson's Correlation)		Multivariable (Binary Logistic Regression)	
	Correlation	P-value	Odds Ratio	P-value
Low/High Trough Categorization	−0.003	0.973	–	–
Length of Stay at Vancomycin Initiation	−0.259	0.008	0.988	0.554
Heart Failure	−0.247	0.012	2.513	0.319
Pitt Bacteremia Score ≥ 4	−0.322	0.001	4.22	0.256
% Change in Serum Creatinine	−0.201	0.042	3.139	0.538
At Risk for Kidney Injury	−0.378	< 0.0001	23.606	0.163

observed probability of cure (Low trough = 0.88, High trough = 0.87) and found only a 3% probability that clinical cure in the high trough cohort could theoretically be ≥10% better than the low trough cohort. This result further supports the validity of the study findings that clinical cure was not significantly different between cohorts. Patients that were treated with vancomycin for less than 48 h were excluded to minimize the risk of including patients in whom infection was not considered by the physician. Although this exclusion may introduce selection bias due to early mortality, early death attributable to infection would not be anticipated with non-deep seated infections.

Due to the retrospective nature of this study, unidentified confounding factors may exist, and we made assumptions in the definition of steady state levels, as well as the definition of clinical cure and failure. We were unable to calculate the APACHE II score for all ICU patients, as not all patients had arterial blood gases available; we also extrapolated the use of the Pitt Bacteremia score to all hospital ward patients, as there are no other validated measures of severity of illness in this patient population. However, it is reassuring that both groups were well-balanced for all identified demographic, clinical and microbiological factors, including the number of patients with concomitant antibiotics, as well as the number of patients with concomitant antibiotics for the same indication as vancomycin. Only 5% of patients on vancomycin were eligible for study inclusion, primarily because most patients had deep-seated infections. Therefore, the non-deep seated infection patient population may constitute a small portion of those patients placed on vancomycin, but nevertheless, avoidance of unnecessary increases in vancomycin dosing to provide higher trough concentrations in these patients is an important quality improvement initiative to potentially reduce medication errors associated with frequent dose changes.

Conclusions

To our knowledge, this is the first study to evaluate clinical and microbiological outcomes associated with trough concentrations in patients with non-deep seated infections treated with short course vancomycin. Our results show an increase in workload with no corresponding clinical benefit, and no signal for increased risk of resistance with vancomycin trough concentrations ≤10 mg/L for short term therapy (≤ 14 days) in non-deep seated infections.

Appendix
Time Estimate for Vancomycin Dose Adjustment

- Ordering vancomycin levels: 5 min
- Checking vancomycin level in Electronic Medical Record: 1 min

- Verify correct timing of dosing and levels in Medication Administration Record: 10 min
- Pharmacokinetic calculations: 10 min
- Contact physician for recommendation, obtain telephone order, write telephone order and inform nurse of new medication order: 10 min
- Pharmacist order entry: 2 min
- Preparation of new vancomycin minibag by pharmacy technician: 10 min
- Delivery of new vancomycin minibag to floor: 5 min

Total: 53 min.

Abbreviations
ACEI: Angiotensin converting enzyme inhibitor; AIDS: Acquired immune deficiency syndrome; APACHE: Acute Physiology and Chronic Health Evaluation; ARB: Angiotensin II receptor blocker; ASA: Acetylsalicylic acid; CNST: Coagulase-negative *Staphylococci*; cSSTI: Complicated skin and soft tissue infection; EPR: Electronic Patient Record; HCTZ: Hydrochlorothiazide; HDR: Health Data Records; HIV: Human immunodeficiency virus; ICU: Intensive Care Unit; MCS: Monte Carlo Simulation; MRSA: Methicillin-resistant *Staphylococcus aureus*; NSAID: Nonsteroidal anti-inflammatory drug; PPI: Proton pump inhibitor; RIFLE: Risk, Injury, Failure, Loss of kidney function, and End-stage kidney disease; SD: Standard deviation; SHSC: Sunnybrook Health Sciences Centre; SPIRIT: Stewardship Program Integrating Resource Information Technology; SSTI: Skin and soft tissue infection; TNF-α: Tumor necrosis factor alpha; UTI: Urinary tract infection; VRE: Vancomycin-resistant *Enterococci*

Funding
This research received no specific grant from any funding agency in the public, commercial or not-for-profit sectors.

Authors' contributions
SW conceived the project idea, was the project supervisor and is the senior investigator. SW, MW, EM, ME, LP and JA contributed to the design of the study and manuscript development. SW, MW and ME were responsible for development of the data collection tool. MW, EM and ME completed the data collection. SW along with MW and EM analyzed the results. All authors read and approved the final manuscript.

Competing interests
The authors declare that they have no competing interests.

Author details
[1]Department of Pharmacy, Sunnybrook Health Sciences Centre, 2075 Bayview Avenue, Toronto, ON M4N 3M5, Canada. [2]Leslie Dan Faculty of Pharmacy, University of Toronto, 144 College Street, Toronto, ON M5S 3M2, Canada. [3]Division of Infectious Diseases, Sunnybrook Health Sciences Centre, 2075 Bayview Avenue, Toronto, ON M4N 3M5, Canada. [4]Sunnybrook Research Institute, Sunnybrook Health Sciences Centre, 2075 Bayview Avenue, Toronto, ON M4N 3M5, Canada. [5]Department of Medicine, Sunnybrook Health Sciences Centre, 2075 Bayview Avenue, Toronto, ON M4N 3M5, Canada. [6]Faculty of Medicine, University of Toronto, 1 King's College Circle, Toronto, ON M5S 1A8, Canada. [7]Present address: Elaine Martin, Trillium Health Partners, 100 Queensway W, Mississauga, ON L5B 1B8, Canada.

References

1. Levine DP. Vancomycin: a history. Clin Infect Dis. 2006;42:S5–12.
2. Rybak MJ. The pharmacokinetic and pharmacodynamics properties of vancomycin. Clin Infect Dis. 2006;42:S35–9.
3. Rybak MJ, Lomaestro BM, Rotschafer JC, Moellering RC, Craig WA, Billeter M, et al. Therapeutic monitoring of vancomycin in adults summary of consensus recommendations from the American Society of Health-System Pharmacists, the Infectious Diseases Society of America, and the Society of Infectious Diseases Pharmacists. Pharmacotherapy. 2009;29:1275–9.
4. Matsumoto K, Takesue Y, Ohmagari N, Mochizuki T, Mikamo H, Seki M, et al. Practice guidelines for therapeutic drug monitoring of vancomycin: a consensus review of the Japanese Society of Chemotherapy and the Japanese Society of Therapeutic Drug Monitoring. J Infect Chemother. 2013; 19:365–80.
5. Ye Z, Chen Y, Chen K, Zhang X, Du G, He B, et al. Therapeutic drug monitoring of vancomycin: a guideline of the division of therapeutic drug monitoring, Chinese pharmacological society. J Antimicrob Chemother. 2016;71:3020–5.
6. Elligsen M, Walker SA, Simor AE, Daneman N. Prospective audit and feedback of antimicrobial stewardship in critical care: program implementation, experience, and challenges. Can J Hosp Pharm. 2012;65: 31–6.
7. Bellomo R, Ronco C, Kellum J, Mehta R, Palevsky P. Acute dialysis quality initiative workgroup. Acute renal failure - definition, outcome measures, animal models, fluid therapy and information technology needs: the second international consensus conference of the acute dialysis quality initiative (ADQI) group. Crit Care. 2004;8:R204–12.
8. Knaus WA, Draper EA, Wagner DP, Zimmerman JE. APACHE II: a severity of disease classification system. Crit Care Med. 1985;13:818–29.
9. Feldman C, Alanee S, Yu VL, Richards GA, Ortgvist A, Rello J, et al. Severity of illness scoring systems in patients with bacteraemic pneumococcal pneumonia: implications for the intensive care unit care. Clin Microbiol Infect. 2009;15:850–7.
10. Weigelt J, Itani K, Stevens D, Lau W, Dryden M, Knirsch C, et al. Linezolid versus vancomycin in treatment of complicated skin and soft tissue infections. Antimicrob Agents Chemother. 2005;49:2260–6.
11. Stevens DL, Herr D, Lampiris H, Hunt JL, Batts DH, Hafkin B. Linezolid versus vancomycin for the treatment of methicillin-resistant *Staphylococcus aureus* infections. Clin Infect Dis. 2002;34:1481–90.
12. Itani KM, Dryden MS, Bhattacharyya H, Kunkel MJ, Baruch AM, Weigelt JA. Efficacy and safety of linezolid versus vancomycin for the treatment of complicated skin and soft-tissue infections proven to be caused by methicillin-resistant *Staphylococcus aureus*. Am J Surg. 2010;199:804–16.
13. Sakoulas G, Eliopoulos GM, Moellering RC, Novick RP, Venkataraman L, Wennersten C, et al. *Staphylococcus aureus* accessory gene regulator (agr) group II: is there a relationship to the development of intermediate-level glycopeptide resistance? J Infect Dis. 2003;187:929–38.
14. Rose W, Rybak M, Tsuji B, Kaatz G, Sakoulas G. Correlation of vancomycin and daptomycin susceptibility in *Staphylococcus aureus* in reference to accessory gene regulator (agr) polymorphism and function. J Antimicrob Chemother. 2007;59:1190–3.
15. Tsuji BT, Rybak MJ, Lau KL, Sakoulas G. Evaluation of accessory gene regulator (agr) group and function in the proclivity towards vancomycin intermediate resistance in *Staphylococcus aureus*. Antimicrob Agents Chemother. 2007;51:1089–91.
16. Zelenitsky S, Alkurdi N, Weber Z, Ariano R, Zhanel G. Preferential emergence of reduced vancomycin susceptibility in health care-associated methicillin-resistant *Staphylococcus aureus* isolates during continuous-infusion vancomycin therapy in an in vitro dynamic model. Antimicrob Agents Chemother. 2011;55:3627–30.
17. Charles PG, Ward PB, Johnson PD, Howden BP, Grayson ML. Clinical features associated with bacteremia due to heterogeneous vancomycin intermediate *Staphylococcus aureus*. Clin Infect Dis. 2004;38:448–51.
18. Centers for Disease Control and Prevention. Reduced susceptibility of *Staphylococcus aureus* to vancomycin--Japan. 1996 MMWR Morb Mortal Wkly Rep. 1997;46:624–6.
19. Centers for Disease Control and Prevention. *Staphylococcus aureus* with reduced susceptibility to vancomycin--United States, 1997. MMWR Morb Mortal Wkly Rep. 1997;46:765–6.
20. Centers for Disease Control and Prevention. Update: *Staphylococcus aureus* with reduced susceptibility to vancomycin--United States, 1997. MMWR Morb Mortal Wkly Rep. 1997;46:813–5.
21. Smith TL, Pearson ML, Wilcox KR, Cruz C, Lancaster MV, Robinson-Dunn B, et al. Emergence of vancomycin resistance in *Staphylococcus aureus*. N Engl J Med. 1999;340:493–501.
22. Hageman JC, Pegues DA, Jepson C, Bell RL, Guinan M, Ward KW, et al. Vancomycin-intermediate *Staphylococcus aureus* in a home health-care patient. Emerg Infect Dis. 2001;7:1023–5.
23. Fridkin SK, Hageman J, McDougal LK, Jarvis WR, Perl TM, Tenover FC, et al. Epidemiological and microbiological characterization of infections caused by *Staphylococcus aureus* with reduced susceptibility to vancomycin, United States, 1997-2001. Clin Infect Dis. 2003;36:429–39.

23

Variability of efavirenz plasma concentrations among pediatric HIV patients treated with efavirenz based combination antiretroviral therapy in Dar es Salaam, Tanzania

Selemani Saidi Sungi[1], Eliford Ngaimisi[2], Nzovu Ulenga[3], Philip Sasi[4] and Sabina Mugusi[4]* (iD)

Abstract

Background: Children are subject to varying drug pharmacokinetics which influence plasma drug levels, and hence treatment outcomes especially for drugs like efavirenz whose plasma concentrations are directly related to treatment outcomes. This study is aimed at determining plasma efavirenz concentrations among Tanzanian pediatric HIV-1 patients on efavirenz-based combination antiretroviral therapy (cART) and relating it to clinical, immunological and virologic treatment responses.

Methods: A cross sectional study involving pediatric HIV patients aged 5–15 years on efavirenz-based cART for ≥ 6 months were recruited in Dar es Salaam. Data on demographics, cART regimens, efavirenz dose and time of the last dose were collected using structured questionnaires and checklists. Venous blood samples were drawn at 10–19 h post-dosing for efavirenz plasma analysis.

Results: A total of 145 children with a mean ± SD age of 10.83 ± 2.75 years, on cART for a mean ± SD of 3.7 ± 2. 56 years were recruited. Median [IQR] efavirenz concentration was 2.56 [IQR = 1.5–4.6] μg/mL with wide inter-patient variability (CV 111%). Poor virologic response was observed in 70.8%, 20.8% and 15.9% of patients with efavirenz levels < 1 μg/mL, 1–4 μg/mL and > 4 μg/mL respectively. Patients with efavirenz levels of < 1 μg/mL were 11 times more likely to have detectable viral loads. Immunologically, 31.8% of children who had low levels (< 1 μg/mL) of efavirenz had a CD4 count of < 350 cells/μL.

Conclusion: Wide inter-individual variability in efavirenz plasma concentrations is seen among Tanzanian children in routine clinical practice with many being outside the recommended therapeutic range. Virologic failure is very high in children with sub-therapeutic levels. Concentrations outside the therapeutic window suggest the need for dose adjustment on the basis of therapeutic drug monitoring to optimize treatment.

Keywords: cART, Efavirenz, Variability, Tanzania

* Correspondence: sabina.mugusi@gmail.com
[4]Department of Clinical Pharmacology, School of Medicine, Muhimbili University of Health and Allied Sciences (MUHAS), Dar es Salaam, Tanzania
Full list of author information is available at the end of the article

Background

Combination antiretroviral therapy (cART) has revolutionized the lives of HIV-1infected adults and children across the world contributing to the continual decrease of new infections [1]. With adequate resources, management of pediatric HIV infection using cART has shown substantial clinical benefits and improved quality of life such as improvement in immunologic status, sustained virologic suppression and enhancement of survival. Such favorable responses are similar to those observed in adults, however, these benefits are observed when optimal plasma drug concentrations of cART drugs are attained and maintained [2].

Treatment for HIV-1 infections in Tanzania involves the use of a combination of antiretroviral drugs commonly with two Nucleoside Reverse Transcriptase Inhibitors (NRTI) and one Non-Nucleoside Reverse Transcriptase Inhibitor (NNRTI) [3]. The National AIDS Control Program (NACP) guidelines currently recommend protease inhibitor (PI)-based regimens for all pediatric HIV patients previously exposed to nevirapine (an NNRTI) during prevention of mother to child transmission. The recommended regimen for the under-three-years-old pediatric patients now is abacavir, lamivudine and lopinavir/ritonavir (a protease inhibitor - based cART) [3]. After reaching three years of age the protease inhibitor is replaced by an NNRTI particularly efavirenz.

The use of efavirenz-based regimens among pediatric patients aged at least three years and above is an advantage in resource-constrained settings because efavirenz has fewer drug interactions compared to protease inhibitors and appears to be better tolerated with less risk of leading to severe adverse effects than nevirapine [4–7]. This has led to better treatment outcomes compared to nevirapine making it a better NNRTI option, with recommendations from the world health organization (WHO) to make efavirenz the NNRTI of choice in first line treatment of HIV-1 infections [4, 5, 8]. More recent research has shown the safety of prolonged cART use among HIV-infected children and suggest that suppressive NNRTI-based regimens can be associated with lower levels of systemic inflammation [9]. Efavirenz is a key drug in the treatment of HIV infection among pediatric patients aged three years and above in Tanzania [3].

Efavirenz is available in both liquid and solid formulations (suspension and tablet/capsule). For patients older than three years efavirenz dosing is in accordance with weight bands starting with children weighing at least 10Kg [3]. Both inter and intra-individual variability in pharmacokinetics of efavirenz leads to variability in efavirenz steady state plasma concentrations. Concentrations above 4 µg/mL are normally associated with increased central nervous system (CNS) adverse effects such as insomnia, frequent nightmares and hallucinations, whereas efavirenz plasma concentrations below 1 µg/mL result into more frequent treatment failures [10] . Some of the factors associated with efavirenz pharmacokinetic variability include; host genetic factors, body weight, gender, ethnicity, drug interactions and binding to plasma proteins [8, 11–13]. The appropriate use of cART in pediatric patients requires careful considerations of individual drugs' disposition kinetics, as well as the impact on the drugs' pharmacokinetics and pharmacodynamics occurring during developmental changes as a child grows [14].

These variations in pharmacokinetic parameters lead to unpredictable responses to treatment in pediatric patients [15]. Therefore, even with the use of pediatric fixed-dose combination antiretroviral tablets, treatment outcome may still be suboptimal in a considerable proportion of patients [16]. This variability may lead to sub-therapeutic or supra-therapeutic concentrations of efavirenz in pediatric patients which is a major threat to the long-term success of antiretroviral treatment. Resulting sub-therapeutic concentrations may be associated with lack of potency in suppressing viral replication leading to an increased chance of developing mutations, subsequently resistance, and hence treatment failure [13]. Supra-therapeutic concentrations increase the risk for toxicity, poor adherence and eventual treatment failure as well.

Treatment failures among pediatric patients on efavirenz-based cART are still observed in our settings as evidenced by pediatric patients being switched to alternative first line regimens or to the more complex and costly second-line regimens. This may be associated with children not achieving therapeutic efavirenz concentrations which leads to inadequate suppression of viral replication and hence treatment failure. Resistance and eventual treatment failure is of great concern because of fewer first line alternative options in our settings as well as the high cost of second line regimens (which are complex and may not be available in our settings) [17]. This is particularly important for children who will be in need of cART for their whole lives.

Methods

Study sites and study design

This was a cross sectional study conducted at six HIV clinics namely; Muhimbili National Hospital (MNH), Temeke Municipal Hospital, Infectious Diseases Centre (IDC), Mwananyamala Hospital, Mbagala Rangi Tatu Hospital and Sinza Palestina Hospital in Dar es Salaam, Tanzania. The study recruited HIV-positive pediatric patients (aged 3-15 years) attending HIV care and treatment centers (CTC) who were using efavirenz-based cART for at least six months. Pediatric patients with diarrhea, vomiting, those with renal or liver disease were excluded from the study. Pediatric patients using medicines with known potential interactions with efavirenz such as rifampicin, fluconazole and ketoconazole were also excluded from the study.

Data collection and laboratory analysis

The sample size for this study was calculated based on methods for establishing reference intervals and on previous studies with children of similar age groups which found that 29% and 28% of children had sub and supra-therapeutic EFV plasma concentrations respectively [12, 18, 19]. Taking this into account therefore a sample size of 150 children was proposed with a relative precision of 10% and a confidence interval (CI) of 95%. The children were recruited using consecutive sampling method until a desired sample size was obtained. Interviews were conducted with the aid of structured questionnaires. The interviews extracted data such as demographics, the time efavirenz dose was last taken, data on missed dose(s) in the previous three days, adverse effects and if any over the counter medicine(s) had been taken in the past seven days. A standardized checklist was used to extract more data from patients' CTC files. Data extracted included weight, WHO clinical stage, current clinical signs and symptoms, cART regimen in use, efavirenz dose in use, previous cART regimen used, last viral load measured and last CD4 cell counts. Clinical examinations were conducted by the attending clinicians, and data on this and prescription information was extracted from the CTC files.

For clinical responses, we were observing; current clinical signs and symptoms, frequency of opportunistic infections, weight, growth/development progress of a child, mid upper arm circumference (MUAC) and WHO clinical staging; weight for age(WAZ) and height for age(HAZ) ≥ -2 z-score were used to define good clinical outcomes [20, 21]. Weight-for-age and height-for-age were calculated using weight and height for age WHO calculator. Body mass index (BMI) for age percentiles were also calculated using the age-and-sex-specific percentile for BMI using the Centers for Disease Control calculator for children and teens aged 2-19 years [22]. Virologic response was determined using HIV-1 RNA levels (viral load) measurements where a positive response was considered if a child's viral load was below the cutoff point of 400 copies/mL [10] . With immunological response the focus was on the CD4 cell count/percentage; a CD4 cell count of above the cutoff point of 350 cells/mm^3 was considered as a positive immunological response as recommended by the NACP guideline for children aged five years and above, and CD4 cell count of 25% or 750cells/mm^3 for those below five years of age [3].

Blood sampling was done between 12 and 19 h post-dosing (after the interview). This would help to get the relevant information on mid-dosing interval plasma levels because of the long half-life of efavirenz [10]. Venous blood samples were taken for estimation of efavirenz mid-dosing interval plasma concentrations, viral load and CD4 cell count.

Blood samples for viral load and efavirenz plasma concentration analysis was collected in two sterile ethylene diamine tetra-acetic acid tubes and centrifuged within 6 h of sample collection [23]. Centrifugation was at 100% $(5100 \times 1000$ U/minute) for 10 min using Benchtop centrifuge w/6-Well Fixed Angle Rotor model EBA 3S (Hettich Universal, Germany) and later stored at -80 °C. The viral load measurements were done using Roche Molecular Diagnostic's COBAS,® TaqMan® Analyzer. The plasma efavirenz levels were analyzed using a validated reverse phase High Performance Liquid Chromatography (HPLC) with ultraviolet detection at Muhimbili University of Health and Allied Sciences (MUHAS) - Swedish International Development Cooperation Agency (Sida) Bioanalytical Laboratory. The individual steady state mid-dosing interval plasma concentration of efavirenz of each child in the study was obtained, the concentrations were checked to see whether they lie within manufacturers' recommended or published intervals of between 1 and 4 μg/mL [10].

The chromatographic analysis using the HPLC System consisted of auto sampler (SIL-20A, 20 MPa Max Pressure, Shimadzu), UV-detector (SPD-20AV, Shimadzu) and pump (LC-20AT, Shimadzu) with a degasser (DGU-2A3, Shimadzu) and the analytical column was Zorbax Extend C18 (150 × 4.6 mm I.D, 5 μm particle size; Agilent Technologies, Netherlands). Detection wavelength and flow rate were set at 275 nm and 0.8 mL/minute respectively. Carbamazepine was used as the internal standard whereas efavirenz was used as the reference standard. Mobile phase consisted of 25 mM of triethylamine –in-water – acetonitrile mixture (65:35, v/v). Method validation of the efavirenz assay was done and both inter-day and intra-day accuracy and precision fulfilled the FDA's acceptance criteria of being within ±15% for bioanalytical methods [24].

Statistical analysis

The collected data was entered in SPSS computer statistical package version 21(Copyright 2007, SPSS Inc.; Chicago, IL, USA), followed by data coding, checking and cleaning. Data entry was done twice to ensure appropriate data consistency and quality. Inter-individual pharmacokinetic variability was evaluated using percentage of coefficient of variation (CV %) calculated as a ratio of standard deviation to the mean plasma efavirenz concentration multiplied by 100. Continuous variables were compared using Student's t-test, while categorical variables were compared using chi-square test. The predicting value of efavirenz plasma concentrations for cART responses (virologic, immunologic and clinical) and CNS adverse effects were determined using univariate and multivariate logistic regression analysis. Variables in univariate analysis with a $p < 0.2$ was included in multivariate analysis to assure that all pertinent and potentially predictive variables are studied. Pearson correlation test was used to analyze the correlation between treatment responses and efavirenz plasma concentration and duration of efavirenz use. A p-value of less than 5% ($p < 0.05$) was considered to be statistically significant.

Results

A total of 327 children were screened from the clinic attendance registers, whereby 151 children were approached at MNH [10], IDC (44), Temeke Hospital [25], Mwananyamala Hospital [26], Mbagala Rangi Tatu Hospital [27] and Sinza Palestina Hospital [5]. Of these 151 children approached, 6 could not be included into the study for various reasons (the parents of five children refused consent, and phlebotomists could not take a blood sample from one). The study thus involved 145 pediatric HIV patients aged between 5 and 15 years with mean ± SD age of 10.83 ± 2.75 years weighing between 13 and 58Kg (mean ± SD weight of 28.30 ± 8.66Kg), with more males (58.6%) compared to females. A total of 43.4% of the children included in the study were orphaned (having lost one parent or both). The most frequent NRTIs used in combination with efavirenz were zidovudine and lamivudine (in 86.2% of children).

At the time of sample collection 44 (30.3%) of the study participants were using cART concomitantly with other drugs (21.4% cotrimoxazole, 2.1% artemether lumefantrine, and 2.8% amoxycillin). None of the patients reported to be taking any traditional medicine (natural health products) and none were on isoniazid preventive therapy (IPT). Using the mid upper arm circumference to evaluate the patients' nutritional status, 64.6% of the patients had normal nutrition status, whereas 32.6% and 2.8% had moderate and severe malnutrition respectively. Anthropometric weight-for-age Z-scores (WAZ) showed a high proportion of children who were severely undernourished (14.5%) and moderately undernourished (22.1%), with 63.4% having a normal weight. The height-for-age scores showed that 35.1% of the children had varying degrees of stunting (26.2% moderately stunted and 8.9% severely stunted). Using the BMI-for-age percentiles a relatively large proportion of children (31.7%) fell below the 5th percentile indicating underweight among these children. Among the underweight, 54.3% were below the 1st percentile indicating wasting.

The median CD4 T-cell count of the patients was 763 (Interquartile range [IQR] = 498–1069) cells/μL with most of the children (84.8%) having CD4 cell counts of above 350 cells/μL. Virological assessment revealed that

27.7% of patients had detectable viral loads of over 400 copies/mL despite having used cART for a mean ± SD duration of 3.7 ± 2.56 years. All patients had good self-reported adherence to their cART therefore good adherence statuses had been recorded in their CTC-2 cards. Table 1 describes these sociodemographic and clinical characteristics of the children involved in the study.

Mid-interval steady state Efavirenz plasma concentration
The median time for sample collection for mid-interval efavirenz plasma concentration was 15.6 [IQR = 14.5–17.2] hours. The overall median mid-interval steady state efavirenz plasma concentration was found to be 2.56 [IQR = 1.5–4.6] μg/mL for all the patients. There was no significant difference in efavirenz plasma concentrations for patients whose sampling times were 12 ± 2 and 17 ± 2 h post-dosing (median 2.69 [IQR = 21.7–4.4] versus 2.39 [IQR = 1.4–5.1] hours respectively). Results based on the mean ± SD plasma efavirenz concentration of 4.41 ± 4.89 μg/mL, the calculated coefficient of variation was found to be 111% for inter-patient variability of efavirenz plasma concentration.

Only 53.1% of the children were within the recommended efavirenz plasma concentration levels of 1–4 μg/mL with 16.6% having concentrations below 1 μg/mL. Table 1 summarizes the sociodemographic characteristics of the patients based on the recommended plasma efavirenz concentrations cutoff points of < 1 μg/mL, 1–4 μg/mL and > 4 μg/mL. Majority of male participants (61.2%) had efavirenz concentrations between 1 and 4 μg/mL compared to female participants, however this was not statistically significant (X^2 ($N = 145$) = 5.48, $p = 0.064$). The 5–10 years age group had a significantly larger number of patients (65.1%) with plasma efavirenz concentrations within the 1–4 μg/mL interval compared to those aged 11–15 (43.9%), whereas those aged 11–15 had significantly more children with efavirenz concentrations below 1 μg/ml compared with children aged 5–10 years (20.7% versus 11.1%) (X^2 (N = 145) = 6.57, $p = 0.037$). It was found that 55.3% of the participants with CD4 T-cell counts greater than the cutoff point of 350 cells/μL (good immunological response) had efavirenz plasma concentrations between 1 and 4 μg/mL, whereas 30.9% of the patients with CD4 below 350 cells/μL had plasma efavirenz levels < 1 μg/mL. Efavirenz plasma concentrations of > 1 μg/mL was found to be associated with good immunological response (OR = 3.1 {95% CI: 0.86–8.95}, $p = 0.051$).

The study found that a statistically significant association ($p < 0.001$) exists between efavirenz plasma concentrations and viral load. Of the 105 participants with good virologic response (viral load < 400 copies/mL) 58.1% had therapeutic efavirenz plasma concentrations (1–4 μg/mL) while 35.2% were found to have efavirenz plasma concentrations above 4 μg/mL. Efavirenz plasma

Table 1 Sociodemographic characteristics of patients based on the efavirenz plasma concentrations' recommended cutoff points

Participant variable		Efavirenz concentration			
		< 1 μg/mL n (%)	1 - 4 μg/mL n (%)	> 4 μg/mL n (%)	p value
Sex	Male	11(12.9%)	52(61.2%)	22(25.9%)	0.064
	Females	13(21.7%)	25(41.7%)	22(36.7%)	
Age group (years)	5–10	7(11.1%)	41(65.1%)	15(23.8%)	0.037
	11–15	17(20.7%)	36(43.9%)	29(35.4%)	
Orphan status	Not orphaned	11 (13.4%)	53 (64.6%)	18 (22.0%)	0.006
	Orphaned	13 (20.6%)	24 (38.1%)	26 (41.3%)	
BMI-for-age percentiles	<5th percentile	5 (10.9%)	18 (39.1%)	23 (50.0%)	0.011
	5-85th percentile	19 (19.4%)	58 (59.2%)	21 (21.4%)	
	>85th percentile	0	1 (100%)	0	
Weight for age (WAZ)	Normal weight	15(16.3%)	53(57.6%)	24(26.1%)	0.341
	Moderately undernourished	6(18.8%)	12(37.5%)	14(43.8%)	
	Severely undernourished	3(14.3%)	12(57.1%)	6(28.6%)	
Height for age (HAZ)	Normal height	17(18.1%)	49(52.1%)	28(29.8%)	0.906
	Moderately stunted	5(13.2%)	20(52.6%)	13(34.2%)	
	Severely stunted	2(15.2%)	8(61.5%)	3(23.1%)	
MUAC	Normal nutrition	16(17.2%)	54(58.1%)	23(24.7%)	0.690
	Moderate malnutrition	6(12.8%)	21(44.7%)	20(42.6%)	
	Severe malnutrition	2(50.0%)	2(50.0%)	0(0.0%)	
CD4 cell count (cells/μL)	> 350 cells	17 (13.8%)	68(55.3%)	38(30.9%)	0.108
	< 350 cells	7(31.8%)	9(40.9%)	6(27.3%)	
Viral load (copies/mL)	< 400 copies	7(6.7%)	61(58.1%)	37(35.2%)	0.000
	400–1000 copies	1(33.3%)	1(33.3%)	1(33.3%)	
	> 1000 copies	16(43.2%)	15(40.5%)	6(16.2%)	
Concurrent Medication	No	15 (14.9%)	51 (50.5%)	35 (34.7%)	0.218
	Yes	9 (20.5%)	26 (59.1%)	9 (20.5%)	

Key: BMI Body Mass Index, *WAZ* Weight for age Z-scores, *HAZ* Height for age Z-scores, *MUAC* Mid Upper Arm Circumference

concentration of > 1 μg/mL was therefore found to be associated with virologic success (OR = 9.5{95% CI: 3.6–25.1}, $p < 0.01$). Virologic failure was found to be 70% among those with sub-therapeutic levels compared to only 20.5% and 15.6% in the therapeutic and supra-therapeutic levels. Figure 1 shows the relation between efavirenz concentrations and the virological, immunological and clinical outcomes.

Univariate and multivariate analysis was done with the inclusion of relevant factors in predicting outcomes associated with efavirenz levels below the recommended plasma concentrations of < 1 μg/mL (Table 2). It was found that CD4 cell counts, viral load levels, sex and child age group were some of the risk factors associated with very low plasma efavirenz concentrations ($p < 0.2$) with 1 degree of freedom (df). In the multivariate analysis, only the viral load maintained statistical significance with a p-value of < 0.001 showing that those with low efavirenz plasma concentrations (< 1 μg/mL) are 11

times more likely to have detectable viral loads of more than 400 copies/mL.

Majority of study participants (86.2%) had not experienced known efavirenz associated adverse drug reactions(ADRs) (CNS and/or skin rash) within the past six months prior to the study. Majority of patients (65.5%) who reported CNS ADRs had efavirenz plasma concentration between 1 and 4 μg/mL. Over 54% of those who reported skin rash within the past six months were found to have efavirenz concentrations within the recommended therapeutic range of 1–4 μg/mL (X^2 ($N = 145$) = 2.61, $p = 0.856$).

Discussion

This study has shown that the overall median for all the participants' efavirenz plasma concentration to be within the recommended therapeutic range, however, there was very high inter-individual variability (111%). The high variability resulted in 16.6% of the patients having sub-therapeutic efavirenz plasma concentrations and

Table 2 Univariable and multivariable logistic regression analysis to assess the risk factors associated with efavirenz plasma concentration below 1 μg//mL among children being treated with efavirenz based cART

Variable	Number of efavirenz samples N	Efavirenz < 1 μg//mL N (%)	Univariate analysis		Multivariate analysis	
			Crude OR (95% CI)	p-value	Adjusted OR (95% CI)	p- value
Sex						
Male	85	11 (12.9)	1		1	
Female	60	13 (21.7)	1.86 (0.77–4.49)	0.168	1.83 (0.68–4.95)	0.232
Age group (years)						
5–10	63	7 (11.1)	1		1	
11–15	82	17 (20.7)	2.09 (0.81–5.41)	0.128	2.07 (0.69–6.15)	0.192
Orphan status						
No	82	11 (13.4)	1			
Yes	63	13 (20.6)	1.67 (0.69–4.05)	0.249		
CD4 (cells/μL)						
> 350	123	17 (13.8)	1		1	
< 350	22	7 (31.8)	2.91 (1.03–8.17)	0.043	0.79 (0.22–2.84)	0.718
Viral Load (copies/mL)						
< 400	105	7 (6.7)	1		1	
> 400	40	17 (42.5)	10.3 (3.84–27.86)	0.000	11.0 (3.66–33.09)	0.000
BMI-for-Age Percentiles						
5th – 85th	99	19 (19.2)	1			
< 5th	46	5 (10.9)	0.51 (0.18–1.47)	0.215		
Height for age						
Normal height	94	17 (18.1)	1			
Moderately stunted	38	5 (13.2)	0.68 (0.23–2.01)	0.493		
Severely stunted	13	2 (15.4)	0.82 (0.17–4.06)	0.811		
Weight for age						
Normal weight	92	15 (16.3)	1			
Moderate malnutrition	32	6 (18.8)	1.18 (0.42–3.37)	0.751		
Severe malnutrition	21	3 (14.3)	0.86 (0.22–3.27)	0.820		

Key: cART combination antiretroviral therapy, *OR* Odds Ratio, *CI* Confidence interval, *BMI* Body mass index

30% with supra therapeutic and potentially harmful plasma concentrations. Virologic failure was very high (70%) among those with sub-therapeutic levels compared to those with therapeutic and supra-therapeutic levels. The probability of having virological failure among those with sub-therapeutic levels was 11 times more compared to those with therapeutic and supra-therapeutic levels.

The median efavirenz levels from this study are comparable to the findings reported in another study whereby a median of 2.8 μg/mL was observed with the samples having been collected 8–20 h post dosing [26]. The proportion of patients found with recommended adequate efavirenz plasma concentrations in this study was 53.1%. This proportion is much lower than that seen in other studies where the proportions of patients within the recommended therapeutic levels ranged from 60 to 71%

[12, 27, 28]. However, a meta-analysis by Bouazza et al. showed that the probability of being within the recommended therapeutic range varied between 56 and 60% regardless of the fixed dose combination [29]. These results are more in keeping with the findings from our study.

We observed a wide range of inter-individual variability of 111% in the plasma concentrations placing a very large proportion of the children outside the therapeutic range of 1–4 μg/mL. Such wide inter-individual variabilities have also been seen by other studies [10, 28, 30]. The variability may be attributed to the growth and development processes which are still ongoing among pediatric patients impacting the maturity of metabolic organs such as liver and kidneys, feeding patterns affecting drug absorption and hence bioavailability, maturation of hepatic enzymes and variation in drug elimination [31, 32]. Variability can furthermore be

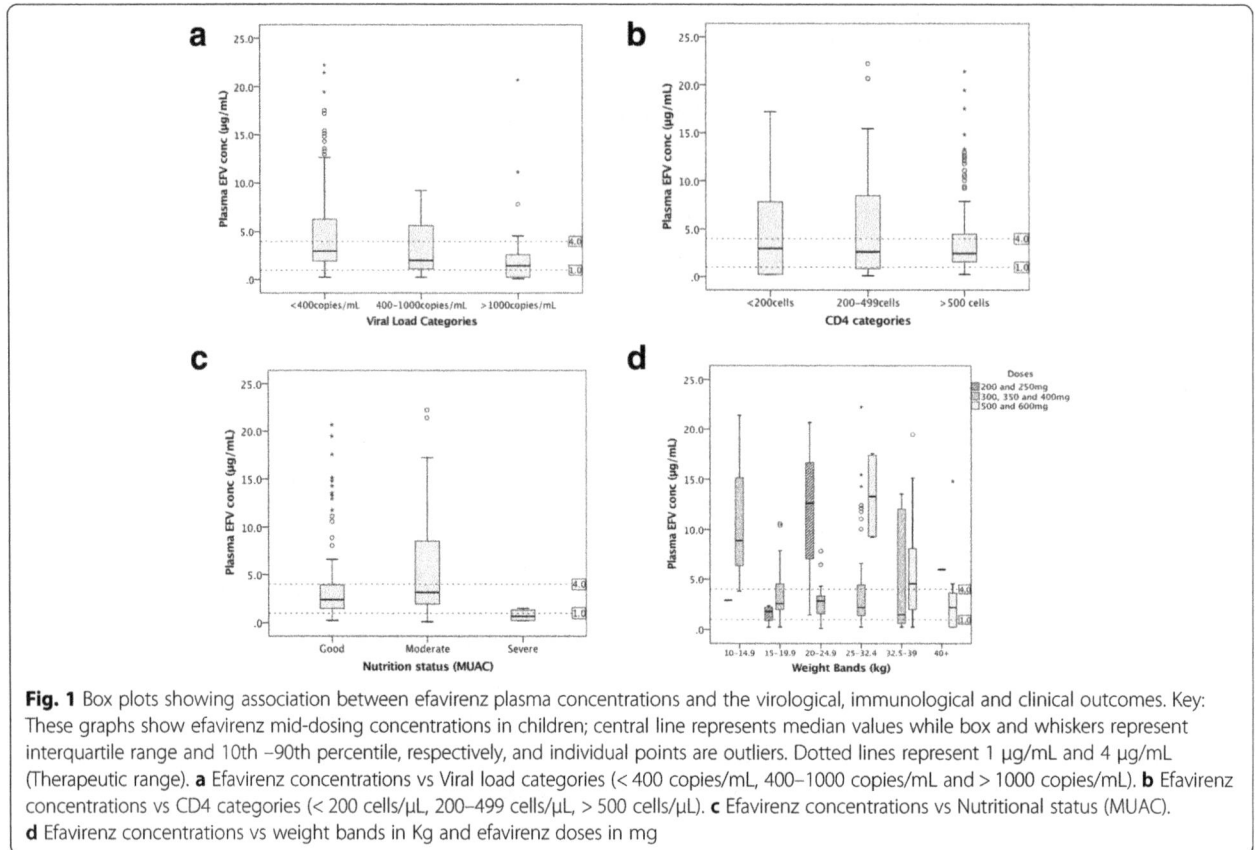

Fig. 1 Box plots showing association between efavirenz plasma concentrations and the virological, immunological and clinical outcomes. Key: These graphs show efavirenz mid-dosing concentrations in children; central line represents median values while box and whiskers represent interquartile range and 10th –90th percentile, respectively, and individual points are outliers. Dotted lines represent 1 μg/mL and 4 μg/mL (Therapeutic range). **a** Efavirenz concentrations vs Viral load categories (< 400 copies/mL, 400–1000 copies/mL and > 1000 copies/mL). **b** Efavirenz concentrations vs CD4 categories (< 200 cells/μL, 200–499 cells/μL, > 500 cells/μL). **c** Efavirenz concentrations vs Nutritional status (MUAC). **d** Efavirenz concentrations vs weight bands in Kg and efavirenz doses in mg

attributed to genetics, particularly single nucleotide genetic polymorphism of the gene for *CYP2B6* enzyme responsible for efavirenz metabolism [33]. Higher mean plasma efavirenz concentrations in Tanzanians were observed compared to Ethiopians, suggesting slow efavirenz metabolism among Tanzanians [34]. This is consistent with our findings in which 30.3% of our study participants were found to have efavirenz plasma concentrations above the recommended therapeutic interval even though these patients had been on efavirenz doses prescribed in accordance with the recommended weight bands. Therefore, based on our findings we believe that some of our study participants might be slow efavirenz metabolizers due to genetic polymorphism leading to higher than recommended plasma concentrations.

Our study found that a significantly strong association exists between efavirenz plasma concentration and virologic response. Out of the 24 participants (16.6%) with sub-therapeutic plasma efavirenz concentrations 17 (70.8%) were found to have poor virologic treatment response compared to only 20.5% and 15.6% of those with therapeutic and supra-therapeutic efavirenz plasma concentrations respectively. Patients with plasma efavirenz concentrations of below 1 μg/mL are 11 times more likely to have detectable viral load levels. Our findings are consistent with findings in other studies which also

found the existence of significant association between efavirenz plasma concentrations and virologic treatment response [15, 35–39]. Various studies have also reported sub-therapeutic concentrations of varying prevalence, relating it to non-adherence to treatment and associating it with poor treatment response [28, 40].

Poor virologic treatment response was observed in 15.6% of participants with supra-therapeutic efavirenz concentrations. Viral resistance may be the reason for these patients to have poor virologic response despite the fact that they were found to have supra-therapeutic concentrations. The high proportion of children with supra-therapeutic efavirenz concentrations suggests that the doses of efavirenz given to our pediatric patients may not be optimal in providing the necessary concentrations for therapeutic needs putting them at a higher risk for CNS toxicity. Supporting our findings with the findings by Mukonzo et al., we believe that our pediatric patients are being given efavirenz at doses larger than their therapeutic needs exposing them to more potential risk of CNS adverse drug reactions (40). These findings also emphasize the importance of monitoring efavirenz plasma concentrations to ensure that pediatric patients whose pharmacokinetics are subject to constant changes due to growth and development benefit maximally from cART.

Clinical response based on weight for age, height for age and MUAC revealed a non-significant association between efavirenz plasma concentration and clinical treatment response. The study by Mutwa et al. conducted in Rwandan children reported that a poor clinical response based on WAZ or HAZ is associated with a poor immunological recovery and virological failure [41].

It is known that children in sub-Saharan Africa have high levels of malnutrition with low weight-and-height for age indicating large proportions of wasting and stunting. Studies within Tanzania and neighboring countries have reported high proportions of poor nutritional status among HIV children [41–43]. Similar proportions have been seen in this study where a large number of children were either stunted or underweight, and among the underweight a significant proportion were wasted. The poor nutritional status of the children could potentially have an impact on the immunological and pharmacological responses to cART.

Conclusion

Our study has demonstrated a wide inter-individual variability in efavirenz plasma concentrations among Tanzanian pediatric patients in routine clinical practice with a little over half of the children within the recommended therapeutic range. Virologic failure is very high in children with sub-therapeutic levels with the probability of having virological failure among those with sub-therapeutic levels being 11 times more compared to those with therapeutic and supra-therapeutic levels. A large proportion of children have poor nutritional status. Children with concentrations outside the therapeutic window pose a risk of treatment failure due to sub-therapeutic plasma concentrations and risk for CNS adverse drug reactions resulting from supra-therapeutic levels. This emphasizes the importance of conducting therapeutic drug monitoring to ensure better treatment success particularly for pediatric HIV patients.

Abbreviations
AIDS: Acquired Immunodeficiency Syndrome; BMI: Body mass index; cART: Combination antiretroviral therapy; CNS: Central Nervous System; CTCs: Care and Treatment Centers; CV: Coefficient of Variation; HAZ: Height for age; HIV: Human immunodeficiency virus; HPLC: High-Performance Liquid Chromatography; ICD: Infectious Disease Center; IRB: Institutional Review Board; MNH: Muhimbili National Hospital; MUAC: Mid upper arm circumference; MUHAS: Muhimbili University of Health and Allied Sciences; NACP: National AIDS control Program; NNRTI: Non-Nucleoside Reverse Transcriptase Inhibitor; NRTI: Nucleoside Reverse Transcriptase Inhibitors; WAZ: Weight for Age; WHO: World health organization

Acknowledgements
This study would not be successful without active involvement of the children and their guardians. We also thank the nurses in those CTCs for assisting in identifying patients and obtaining data from the CTC files and Ms. Dorisia Nanage for running the HPLC analysis.

Funding
This study was a Masters' of Science dissertation research through the Muhimbili University of Health and Allied Sciences. MUHAS had no role with the data collection process or analysis. Likewise, they were not involved in the writing of the report. The authors have had full access of the data, and the decision to submit report for publication.

Authors' contributions
SS and SM designed the study. SS drafted the manuscript and was responsible for the study conduct. NU was involved in laboratory analysis of samples. SS, EN and SM participated in the data analysis and interpretation of the report. All authors were involved in the review of the manuscript. All authors read and approved the final manuscript.

Competing interests
The authors declare that they have no competing interests.

Author details
[1]Health Department, Chamwino District Council, Chamwino, Dodoma, Tanzania. [2]Unit of Pharmacology and Therapeutics, School of Pharmacy, Muhimbili University of Health and Allied Sciences (MUHAS), Dar es Salaam, Tanzania. [3]Management Development for Health (MDH), Dar es Salaam, Tanzania. [4]Department of Clinical Pharmacology, School of Medicine, Muhimbili University of Health and Allied Sciences (MUHAS), Dar es Salaam, Tanzania.

References
1. (WHO). Global update on HIV treatment: Results, Impact and Opportunities.; 2013.
2. Temiye EO, Akinsulie AO, Ezeaka CV, Adetifa IM, Iroha EO, Grange AO, et al. Constraints and prospects in the management of pediatric HIV/AIDS. J Natl Med Assoc. 2006;98(8):1252–9.
3. NACP. National Guidelines For the management of HIV and AIDS. Fourth Edition 2012. 2012. Available from https://aidsfree.usaid.gov/sites/default/files/hts_policy_tanzania.pdf.
4. Organization WH. Technical update on treatment optimization. Use of efavirenz during pregnancy: a public health perspective. Available from http://apps.who.int/iris/bitstream/handle/10665/70920/9789241503792_eng.pdf;jsessionid=2A042C9A9E9A72C58F94731FB9C8C880?sequence=1. 2012.
5. Cain LE, Phillips A, Lodi S, Sabin C, Bansi L, Justice A, et al. The effect of efavirenz versus nevirapine-containing regimens on immunologic, virologic and clinical outcomes in a prospective observational study. AIDS. 2012; 26(13):1691–705.
6. Ngo-Giang-Huong N, Jourdain G, Amzal B, Sang-a-gad P, Lertkoonalak R, Eiamsirikit N, et al. Resistance patterns selected by nevirapine vs. efavirenz in HIV-infected patients failing first-line antiretroviral treatment: a bayesian analysis. PLoS One. 2011;6(11):e27427.
7. Antiretroviral Therapy Cohort C, Mugavero MJ, May M, Harris R, Saag MS, Costagliola D, et al. Does short-term virologic failure translate to clinical events in antiretroviral-naive patients initiating antiretroviral therapy in clinical practice? AIDS. 2008;22(18):2481–92.
8. Pillay P, Ford N, Shubber Z, Ferrand RA. Outcomes for efavirenz versus nevirapine-containing regimens for treatment of HIV-1 infection: a systematic review and meta-analysis. PLoS One. 2013;8(7):e68995.
9. Melvin AJ, Warshaw M, Compagnucci A, Saidi Y, Harrison L, Turkova A, et al. Hepatic, renal, hematologic, and inflammatory markers in HIV-infected children on long-term suppressive antiretroviral therapy. J Pediatric Infect Dis Soc. 2017;6(3):e109–e15.
10. Marzolini C, Telenti A, Decosterd LA, Greub G, Biollaz J, Buclin T. Efavirenz plasma levels can predict treatment failure and central nervous system side effects in HIV-1-infected patients. AIDS. 2001;15(1):71–5.
11. Peacock-Villada E, Richardson BA, John-Stewart GC. Post-HAART outcomes in pediatric populations: comparison of resource-limited and developed countries. Pediatrics. 2011;127(2):e423–41.
12. Puthanakit T, Tanpaiboon P, Aurpibul L, Cressey TR, Sirisanthana V. Plasma efavirenz concentrations and the association with CYP2B6-516G >T polymorphism in HIV-infected Thai children. Antivir Ther. 2009;14(3):315–20.
13. Lee KY, Lin SW, Sun HY, Kuo CH, Tsai MS, Wu BR, et al. Therapeutic drug monitoring and pharmacogenetic study of HIV-infected ethnic Chinese

receiving efavirenz-containing antiretroviral therapy with or without rifampicin-based anti-tuberculous therapy. PLoS One. 2014;9(2):e88497.

14. Stahle L, Moberg L, Svensson JO, Sonnerborg A. Efavirenz plasma concentrations in HIV-infected patients: inter- and intraindividual variability and clinical effects. Ther Drug Monit. 2004;26(3):267–70.

15. Salem AH, Fletcher CV, Brundage RC. Pharmacometric characterization of efavirenz developmental pharmacokinetics and pharmacogenetics in HIV-infected children. Antimicrob Agents Chemother. 2014;58(1):136–43.

16. Burger D, van der Heiden I, la Porte C, van der Ende M, Groeneveld P, Richter C, et al. Interpatient variability in the pharmacokinetics of the HIV non-nucleoside reverse transcriptase inhibitor efavirenz: the effect of gender, race, and CYP2B6 polymorphism. Br J Clin Pharmacol. 2006;61(2):148–54.

17. Bennett DE, Bertagnolio S, Sutherland D, Gilks CF. The World Health Organization's global strategy for prevention and assessment of HIV drug resistance. Antivir Ther. 2008;13(Suppl 2):1–13.

18. Katayev A, Balciza C, Seccombe DW. Establishing reference intervals for clinical laboratory test results: is there a better way? Am J Clin Pathol. 2010; 133(2):180–6.

19. Fletcher CV, Brundage RC, Fenton T, Alvero CG, Powell C, Mofenson LM, et al. Pharmacokinetics and pharmacodynamics of efavirenz and nelfinavir in HIV-infected children participating in an area-under-the-curve controlled trial. Clin Pharmacol Ther. 2008;83(2):300–6.

20. WHO Global Health Database on Child Growth and Malnutrition Blössner. Geneva: Programme of Nutrition; 1997. http://apps.who.int/iris/bitstream/handle/10665/63750/WHO_NUT_97.4.pdf.

21. Mei Z, Grummer-Strawn LM. Standard deviation of anthropometric Z-scores as a data quality assessment tool using the 2006 WHO growth standards: a cross country analysis. Bull World Health Organ. 2007;85(6):441–8.

22. (CDC) CfDCaP. BMI percentile calculator for Child and Teen. Division of Nutrition, Physical Activity and Obesity. Available from https://www.cdc.gov/healthyweight/bmi/calculator.html.

23. Higgins N, Tseng A, Sheehan NL, la Porte CJ. Antiretroviral therapeutic drug monitoring in Canada: current status and recommendations for clinical practice. Can J Hosp Pharm. 2009;62(6):500–9.

24. U.S. Department of Health and Human Services, Food and Drug Administration. Center for Drug Evaluation and Research (CDER). Center for Veterinary Medicine (CVM). 2018. Available from https://www.fda.gov/downloads/drugs/guidances/ucm070107.Pdf.

25. Mukonzo JK, Owen JS, Ogwal-Okeng J, Kuteesa RB, Nanzigu S, Sewankambo N, et al. Pharmacogenetic-based efavirenz dose modification: suggestions for an African population and the different CYP2B6 genotypes. PLoS One. 2014;9(1):e86919.

26. Wintergerst U, Hoffmann F, Jansson A, Notheis G, Huss K, Kurowski M, et al. Antiviral efficacy, tolerability and pharmacokinetics of efavirenz in an unselected cohort of HIV-infected children. J Antimicrob Chemother. 2008; 61(6):1336–9.

27. Mutwa PR, Fillekes Q, Malgaz M, Tuyishimire D, Kraats R, Boer KR, et al. Mid-dosing interval efavirenz plasma concentrations in HIV-1-infected children in Rwanda: treatment efficacy, tolerability, adherence, and the influence of CYP2B6 polymorphisms. J Acquir Immune Defic Syndr. 2012;60(4):400–4.

28. Ren Y, Nuttall JJ, Egbers C, Eley BS, Meyers TM, Smith PJ, et al. High prevalence of subtherapeutic plasma concentrations of efavirenz in children. J Acquir Immune Defic Syndr. 2007;45(2):133–6.

29. Bouazza N, Cressey TR, Foissac F, Bienczak A, Denti P, McIlleron H, et al. Optimization of the strength of the efavirenz/lamivudine/abacavir fixed-dose combination for paediatric patients. J Antimicrob Chemother. 2017; 72(2):490–5.

30. Fabbiani M, Di Giambenedetto S, Bracciale L, Bacarelli A, Ragazzoni E, Cauda R, et al. Pharmacokinetic variability of antiretroviral drugs and correlation with virological outcome: 2 years of experience in routine clinical practice. J Antimicrob Chemother. 2009;64(1):109–17.

31. Neely MN, Rakhmanina NY. Pharmacokinetic optimization of antiretroviral therapy in children and adolescents. Clin Pharmacokinet. 2011;50(3):143–89.

32. Lu H, Rosenbaum S. Developmental pharmacokinetics in pediatric populations. J Pediatr Pharmacol Ther. 2014;19(4):262–76.

33. Liu X, Ma Q, Zhao Y, Mu W, Sun X, Cheng Y, et al. Impact of single nucleotide polymorphisms on plasma concentrations of Efavirenz and Lopinavir/ritonavir in Chinese children infected with the human immunodeficiency virus. Pharmacotherapy. 2017;37(9):1073–80.

34. Ngaimisi E, Habtewold A, Minzi O, Makonnen E, Mugusi S, Amogne W, et al. Importance of ethnicity, CYP2B6 and ABCB1 genotype for efavirenz pharmacokinetics and treatment outcomes: a parallel-group prospective cohort study in two sub-Saharan Africa populations. PLoS One. 2013;8(7):e67946.

35. Nacro B, Zoure E, Hien H, Tamboura H, Rouet F, Ouiminga A, et al. Pharmacology and immuno-virologic efficacy of once-a-day HAART in African HIV-infected children: ANRS 12103 phase II trial. Bull World Health Organ. 2011;89(6):451–8.

36. Sutcliffe CG, van Dijk JH, Bolton C, Persaud D, Moss WJ. Effectiveness of antiretroviral therapy among HIV-infected children in sub-Saharan Africa. Lancet Infect Dis. 2008;8(8):477–89.

37. Brundage RC, Yong FH, Fenton T, Spector SA, Starr SE, Fletcher CV. Intrapatient variability of efavirenz concentrations as a predictor of virologic response to antiretroviral therapy. Antimicrob Agents Chemother. 2004; 48(3):979–84.

38. Lowenthal ED, Ellenberg JH, Machine E, Sagdeo A, Boiditswe S, Steenhoff AP, et al. Association between efavirenz-based compared with nevirapine-based antiretroviral regimens and virological failure in HIV-infected children. JAMA. 2013;309(17):1803–9.

39. Bienczak A, Denti P, Cook A, Wiesner L, Mulenga V, Kityo C, et al. Plasma Efavirenz exposure, sex, and age predict Virological response in HIV-infected African children. J Acquir Immune Defic Syndr. 2016;73(2):161–8.

40. Johnston V, Cohen K, Wiesner L, Morris L, Ledwaba J, Fielding KL, et al. Viral suppression following switch to second-line antiretroviral therapy: associations with nucleoside reverse transcriptase inhibitor resistance and subtherapeutic drug concentrations prior to switch. J Infect Dis. 2014;209(5):711–20.

41. Mutwa PR, Boer KR, Asiimwe-Kateera B, Tuyishimire D, Muganga N, Lange JM, et al. Safety and effectiveness of combination antiretroviral therapy during the first year of treatment in HIV-1 infected Rwandan children: a prospective study. PLoS One. 2014;9(11):e111948.

42. Sutcliffe CG, van Dijk JH, Munsanje B, Hamangaba F, Sinywimaanzi P, Thuma PE, et al. Weight and height z-scores improve after initiating ART among HIV-infected children in rural Zambia: a cohort study. BMC Infect Dis. 2011;11:54.

43. Sunguya BF, Poudel KC, Otsuka K, Yasuoka J, Mlunde LB, Urassa DP, et al. Undernutrition among HIV-positive children in Dar Es Salaam, Tanzania: antiretroviral therapy alone is not enough. BMC Public Health. 2011;11:869.

24

Cardiovascular and microvascular outcomes of glucagon-like peptide-1 receptor agonists in type 2 diabetes: a meta-analysis of randomized controlled cardiovascular outcome trials with trial sequential analysis

Xiaowen Zhang[1†], Fei Shao[1,2†], Lin Zhu[1], Yuyang Ze[1], Dalong Zhu[1*] and Yan Bi[1*]

Abstract

Background: Efficacy trials showed that glucagon-like peptide–1 receptor (GLP1R) agonists reduced metabolic risk factors in addition to glucose lowering, but the cardiovascular and microvascular efficacy of this drug class remains to be determined. We aimed to evaluate the overall cardiovascular and microvascular efficacy of GLP1R agonists by performing a meta-analysis with trial sequential analysis.

Methods: Randomized controlled, cardiovascular outcomes trials including at least 2000 patient-years' follow-up and 100 composite cardiovascular events were included. Trial sequential analysis (TSA) was performed and the quality of evidence was graded.

Results: Thirty-three thousand four hundred fifty-seven patients and 4105 cardiovascular events from 4 large trials were included. GLP1R agonists were associated with a statistically significant reduction in risks for all-cause mortality (hazard ratio [HR]: 0.88, 95% CI: 0.81 to 0.95; number needed to treat [NNT]: 286 person-years), cardiovascular mortality (HR: 0.87, 95% CI: 0.79 to 0.96; NNT: 412 person-years), stroke (HR: 0.87, 95% CI: 0.76 to 0.98; NNT: 209 person-years) and the composite adverse cardiovascular outcome (MACE; HR: 0.91, 95% CI: 0.85 to 0.96; NNT: 241 person-years). The magnitude of benefit on MACE was attenuated in patients with a history of congestive heart failure (HR: 0.96, 95% CI: 0.85 to 1.08 with; HR: 0.87, 95% CI: 0.77 to 1.00 without). The risks for hospitalization for heart failure and myocardial infarction were not significantly different. The quality of the evidence was deemed as moderate to high based on GRADE approach. TSA provided firm evidence for a 10% reduction in all-cause mortality, a 15% reduction in MACE, and lack of a 15% reduction in hospitalization for heart failure, but evidence remains inconclusive for cardiovascular mortality and myocardial infarction. GLP1R agonists numerically reduced the rates for nephropathy but the risk for retinopathy was similar.

Conclusions: Meta-analysis with trial sequential analysis suggested that GLP1R agonists significantly reduced the risk for all-cause mortality and composite cardiovascular outcomes, but the reduction of cardiovascular mortality remains to be confirmed.

Keywords: Glucagon-like peptide-1 receptor agonist, Cardiovascular outcome, Microvascular outcome, Meta-analysis, Trial sequential analysis, Randomized controlled trial

* Correspondence: zhudalong@nju.edu.cn; biyan@nju.edu.cn
†Xiaowen Zhang and Fei Shao contributed equally to this work.
[1]Department of Endocrinology, Affiliated Drum Tower Hospital, Nanjing University School of Medicine, 321 Zhongshan Road, Nanjing, Jiangsu Province 210008, China
Full list of author information is available at the end of the article

Background

Type 2 diabetes mellitus (T2DM) is complex metabolic disorder associated with an increased risk for cardiovascular, microvascular and other complications [1]. The promising glucose-lowering effects as well the microvascular benefits of many anti-hyperglycemic drugs have been well documented, but the cardiovascular benefits of these drugs are uncertain [2–4]. Some hypoglycemic medications may even increase rather than reduce the risk of cardiovascular events [5, 6]. Consequently, the US Food and Drug Administration (FDA) have mandated cardiovascular safety assessments of new diabetes treatments [7, 8]. Incretin-based therapies, which include glucagon-like peptide–1 receptor (GLP1R) agonists and dipeptidyl peptidase–4 inhibitors (DDP-4i), are one of the many new anti-hyperglycemic drugs since the last decade. They have now emerged as popular treatment option for glycemic control because of their excellent performance in reducing body weight, blood pressure and postprandial lipoproteins, in addition to marked glucose lowering [9–11]. Whether these metabolic benefits might translate into cardiovascular and microvascular benefits remains an important issue. Several large-scale randomized controlled trials (RCTs) have addressed this issue but the conclusions were not consistent. In this context, we performed a meta-analysis of randomized controlled trials to investigate the effect of GLP1R agonists on cardiovascular outcomes. We also performed trial sequential analysis (TSA) to reduce type I error in meta-analysis to evaluate whether findings from meta-analyses were conclusive or not.

Methods

We conducted the meta-analysis in accordance with the Preferred Reporting Items for Systematic Reviews and Meta-Analyses (PRISMA) (Additional file 1) and Meta-analysis Of Observational Studies in Epidemiology (MOOSE) guidelines (Additional file 2) [12].

Data sources and searches

We searched MEDLINE, the Cochrane Central Register of Controlled Trials, and EMBASE from their inception to 28 September 2017 without language restrictions. The following keywords were used: glucagon-like-peptide-1 receptor agonists, exenatide, liraglutide, dulaglutide, albiglutide, lixisenatide, semaglutide, taspoglutide, and randomized controlled trial. Reference lists of the identified reports and relevant reviews were also checked for further relevant studies.

Study selection

Two reviewers independently assessed the eligibility of studies. To be included, studies had to 1) be randomized controlled, cardiovascular outcome trials which made direct comparisons of glucagon-like-peptide-1 receptor agonists with placebo or active antidiabetic drugs of other classes; 2) contain at least 2000 patient-years of follow-up and 100 composite cardiovascular events to exclude small trials with unreliable hazard ratios; 3) have cardiovascular outcomes predefined and independently adjudicated; and 4) report at least one of our selected cardiovascular outcomes. Discrepancies, if any, were resolved by consensus by a third independent investigator.

Outcome measures

The primary endpoints were all-cause and cardiovascular death. Secondary endpoints were myocardial infarction, stroke, hospitalization for heart failure, and the major adverse cardiovascular event (MACE) defined as the composite of death from cardiovascular causes, nonfatal myocardial infarction or nonfatal stroke. Microvascular outcomes included nephropathy and retinopathy. We also included efficacy outcomes in the analysis.

Data extraction and quality assessment

Data extraction was performed by two investigators from each trial using clearly defined extraction forms. The following items were recorded: the registry number, type of treatments, number of patients, follow-up duration, patient demographic and clinical data (age, sex, duration of diabetes, baseline HbA1c levels etc.), history of cardiovascular disease (coronary artery disease, heart failure, stroke, and peripheral arterial disease), medications for diabetes and cardiovascular diseases. We also extracted the number of patients with events and the reported hazard ratio of each outcome. The same reviewers independently assessed the quality of each randomized trial according to the Cochrane Collaboration guideline [13].

Grading of evidence

We graded the overall methodological quality of each pooled analysis using the Grading of Recommendations, Assessment, Development and Evaluation (GRADE) approach. The quality of evidence was judged as high, moderate, low or very low, using GRADEpro version 3.6 (GRADEpro GDT).

Data synthesis and statistical analysis

Results of meta-analyses are presented as pooled hazard ratios with their corresponding 95% confidence intervals (CIs). In cases hazard ratios were not available, we used odds ratio instead. We estimated the amount of between-study heterogeneity with the I-square statistic and the $\chi 2$-based Q test [14]. Data were pooled with the fixed-effects model (Mantel-Haenszel method) because the absence of significant heterogeneity across studies, with random-effect models (DerSimonian–Laird method) as complement [15]. The number needed to treat (NNT) was calculated from randomized trials for risk estimates where risk difference was significant, taking into account the exposure time of treatment within each study. Publication bias was evaluated by funnel plots and Egger's tests but these tests had limited ability to adequately assess small-study effects because all involved a small number of trials. Predefined subgroup data for MACE based on a variety of clinical variables were directly extracted from each trial and pooled subgroup analyses were conducted. We did a meta-regression analysis to estimate the effects of several covariates—age, gender, body mass index, HbA1c, duration of diabetes, and the percentage of coronary heart disease, chronic heart failure, chronic kidney disease—

Table 1 Characteristics of included randomized controlled trials

Trial	ELIXA	LEADER	SUSTAIN 6	EXSCEL
Year	2015	2016	2016	2017
No. of patients	6068	9340	3297	14,752
No. of countries	49	32	20	35
No. of study sites	NA	310	230	687
Median duration of follow-up, years	2.1	3.8	2.1	3.2
Median duration of exposure to treatment, years	1.9	3.5	1.8	2.4
GLP1R agonist	Lixisenatide	Liraglutide	Semaglutide	Exenatide
Control	Placebo	Placebo	Placebo	Placebo
Age, years	60.3	64.3	64.6	56.0
Male, %	69.3	64.3	60.7	62.0
Diabetes duration, years	9.3	12.7	13.9	12.0
Body mass index	30.2	32.5	32.8	31.7
Current smoking, %	11.7	NA	NA	11.6
HbA1c, %	7.7	8.7	8.7	8.0
Systolic blood pressure, mmHg	129 ± 17	135.9 ± 17.8	135.6 ± 17.2	NA
Diastolic blood pressure, mmHg	NA	77.2 ± 10.3	77.0 ± 10.0	NA
LDL cholesterol, mg/dL	78.8 ± 35.4	NA	82.3 ± 45.6	NA
History of cardiovascular disease				
Hypertension, %	76.4	NA	92.8	NA
Coronary artery disease, %	100	81.4	60.4	52.9
Heart failure, %	22.4	17.9	24.3	16.6
Stroke, %	5.5	NA	12.4	17.3
Peripheral arterial disease, %	7.7	NA	NA	18.9
Chronic kidney disease, %	23.2	24.7	28.5	21.7
Diabetes medications				
Insulin, %	39.1	44.6	58.0	46.4
Metformin, %	66.3	76.4	73.2	76.8
Sulfonylureas, %	33.2	50.5	42.8	36.6
Thiazolidinediones, %	1.6	6.2	2.3	3.9
DPP-4 inhibitor, %	NA	< 0.1	0.2	15.0
Cardiovascular Medications				
ACEI or ARB, %	85.0	82.8	83.5	80.0
Statin, %	92.7	72.1	72.8	73.5
Anti-thrombotic, %	97.5	74.3	76.3	73.6
Beta-blocker, %	84.5	55.4	57.4	55.8
Aldosterone antagonists, %	NA	5.4	5.9	6.2
NCT No.	NCT01147250	NCT01179048	NCT01720446	NCT02098395

ACEI angiotensin-converting-enzyme inhibitor, *ARB* angiotensin receptor antagonist, *GLP1R* glucagon-like peptide 1–receptor agonist, *LDL* cholesterol: low-density lipoprotein cholesterol, *NA* not available

might have on endpoints with significant association. For the effect estimate, a 2-tailed p value less than 0.05 was considered statistically significant. Analyses were done by using the Stata software, version 12.0 (STATA Corporation, College Station, TX, USA).

TSA could reduce type I error because it combines estimation of required information size with adjusted threshold for statistical significance [16–18]. The required information size was calculated based on a relative risk reduction of 10% in all-cause and cardiovascular mortality and a relative risk reduction of 15% in other outcomes. An overall 5% risk of type I error and a statistical test power of 80% were employed.

Results

Study selection and characteristics

Of 1980 citations initially identified, 71 were retrieved for full-text evaluation and 4 trials (ELIXA, LEADER, SUSTAIN 6, and EXSCEL) met inclusion criteria (Additional file 3: Figure S1) [19–22]. A total of 33,457 patients receiving GLP1R agonists (n = 16,706) or placebo (n = 16,751) were included in the analysis. All 4 trials were large, prospective, multicenter, double-blind, randomized placebo-controlled trials with independent cardiovascular endpoint adjudication and adequate follow-up time (range 6924–47,206 patient-years of follow-up). All trials were performed across multiple countries. The mean age enrolled in all the included trials ranged from 56 to 65 years, the mean duration of diabetes from 9.3 to 13.9 years, the mean HbA1c level from 7.7 to 8.7%, and the mean body mass index ranged from 30.2 to 32.8. Overall, 64% patients were male, 70% had a history of coronary heart disease,

18% had heart failure and 23.5% had chronic kidney disease. 46% patients had concomitant insulin use, 74.4% had metformin, 40% had sulfonylureas; new anti-diabetic drugs such as DDP4i and sodium-glucose cotransporter-2 inhibitors were used in very limited number of patients. Cardiovascular medications and other detailed baseline characteristics of each trial are presented in Table 1. Primary and secondary endpoints, inclusion and exclusion criteria of included randomized controlled trials were presented in (Additional file 3: Table S1).

The method of random sequence generation was reported in all trials. All trials had blinding of personnel and participants. In 2 trials, blinded outcome adjudication was not performed, so they were judged as being of unclear risk of bias. The risk for detection bias, attrition bias, reporting bias and other bias were generally low. All 4 trials were deemed as good quality, with detailed quality assessment summarized in Additional file 3: Table S2.

Total and cardiovascular mortality

There were 1161 deaths among 16,706 patients randomly assigned to receive GLP1R agonists and 1314 deaths among 16,751 patients assigned to placebo. Pooled analysis showed a statistically significant reduction in all-cause mortality with GLP1R agonists compared with placebo (HR: 0.88, 95% CI: 0.81 to 0.95, p = 0.001; Fig. 1); the NNT was 286 person-years' exposure to treatment. No evidence of significant heterogeneity was found (I^2 = 0). TSA showed that although the pooled sample size did not exceed the estimated required information size, the cumulative Z-curve crossed the conventional boundary and also the trial sequential monitoring

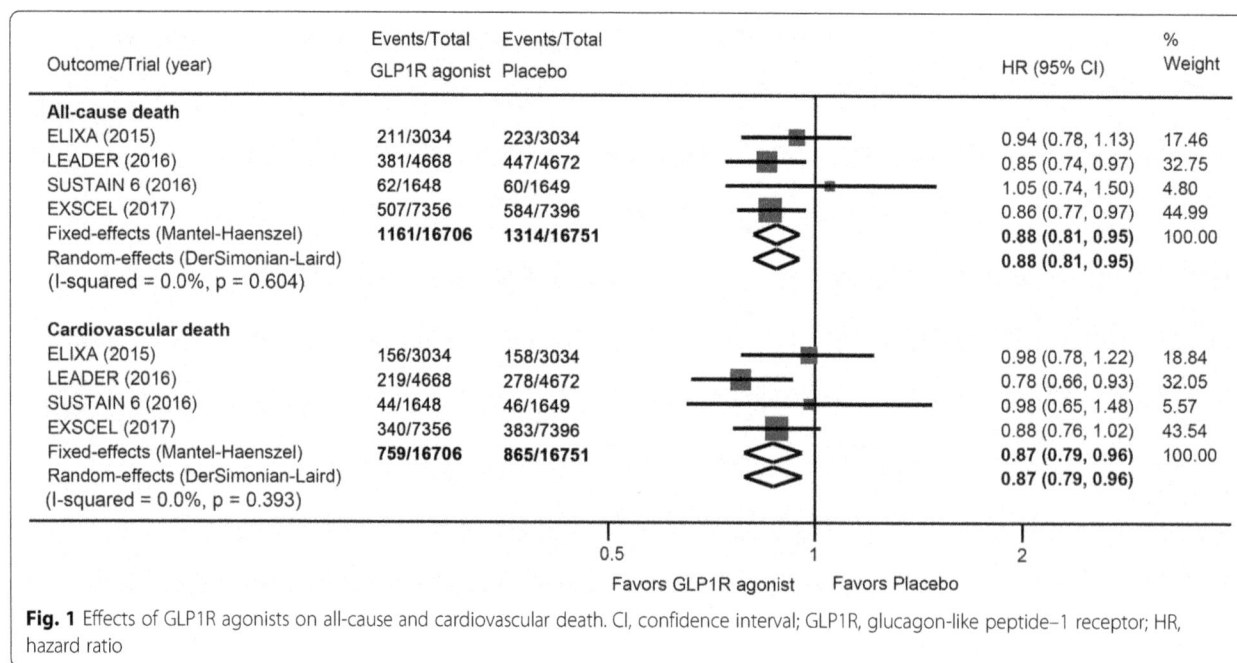

Outcome/Trial (year)	Events/Total GLP1R agonist	Events/Total Placebo		HR (95% CI)	% Weight
All-cause death					
ELIXA (2015)	211/3034	223/3034		0.94 (0.78, 1.13)	17.46
LEADER (2016)	381/4668	447/4672		0.85 (0.74, 0.97)	32.75
SUSTAIN 6 (2016)	62/1648	60/1649		1.05 (0.74, 1.50)	4.80
EXSCEL (2017)	507/7356	584/7396		0.86 (0.77, 0.97)	44.99
Fixed-effects (Mantel-Haenszel)	**1161/16706**	**1314/16751**		**0.88 (0.81, 0.95)**	100.00
Random-effects (DerSimonian-Laird)				**0.88 (0.81, 0.95)**	
(I-squared = 0.0%, p = 0.604)					
Cardiovascular death					
ELIXA (2015)	156/3034	158/3034		0.98 (0.78, 1.22)	18.84
LEADER (2016)	219/4668	278/4672		0.78 (0.66, 0.93)	32.05
SUSTAIN 6 (2016)	44/1648	46/1649		0.98 (0.65, 1.48)	5.57
EXSCEL (2017)	340/7356	383/7396		0.88 (0.76, 1.02)	43.54
Fixed-effects (Mantel-Haenszel)	**759/16706**	**865/16751**		**0.87 (0.79, 0.96)**	100.00
Random-effects (DerSimonian-Laird)				**0.87 (0.79, 0.96)**	
(I-squared = 0.0%, p = 0.393)					

0.5   1   2

Favors GLP1R agonist   Favors Placebo

Fig. 1 Effects of GLP1R agonists on all-cause and cardiovascular death. CI, confidence interval; GLP1R, glucagon-like peptide–1 receptor; HR, hazard ratio

boundary (Fig. 2), providing firm evidence for a 10% reduction in total mortality with GLP1R agonists when compared with placebo.

Of 16,706 patients assigned to GLP1R agonists, 759 experienced cardiovascular death, as did 865 of 16,751 patients with placebo. Overall, there was a statistically significant reduction in cardiovascular mortality with use of GLP1R agonists (HR: 0.87, 95% CI: 0.79 to 0.96, $P = 0.005$) (Fig. 1); the number needed to treat was 412 person-years' exposure to treatment. Similarly, no heterogeneity was detected ($I^2 = 0$). In TSA, the Z-curve crossed the conventional boundary but did not cross the monitoring boundary, indicating a 10% reduction in

cardiovascular mortality with GLP1R agonists was inconclusive and that additional evidence is needed (Fig. 3). The risk for non-cardiovascular death was not significantly different (HR: 0.90, 95% CI: 0.78 to 1.03, $P = 0.11$).

Myocardial infarction and stroke

Meta-analysis did not show statistically significant difference in incidence of myocardial infarction between patients with GLP1R agonists and those with placebo (HR: 0.94, 95% CI: 0.86 to 1.02, $P = 0.143$; Fig. 4). GLP1R agonists were associated with a statistically significant reduction in rates of stroke (HR: 0.87, 95% CI: 0.76 to 0.98, $P = 0.023$; Fig. 4); the number needed to treat was

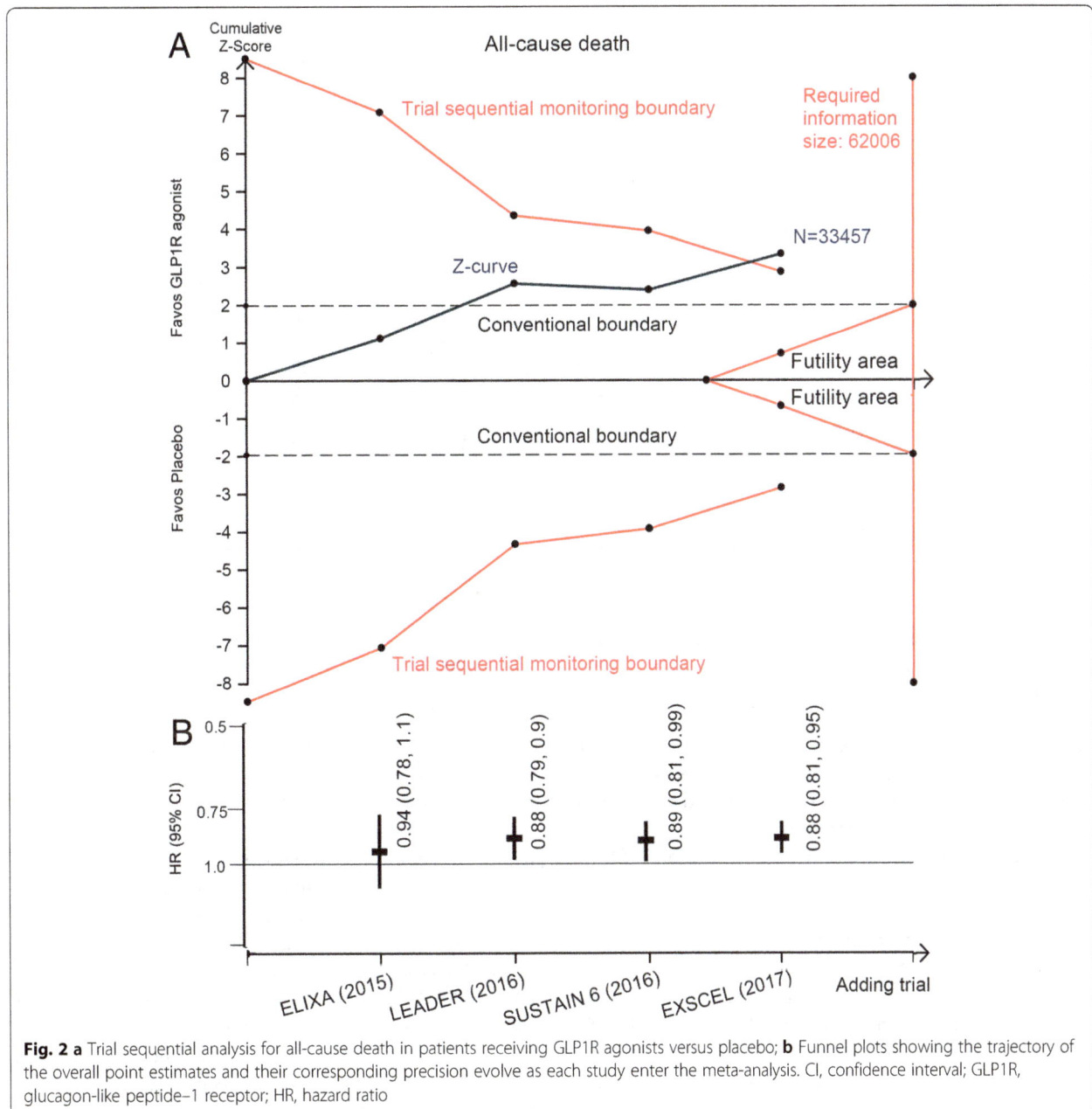

Fig. 2 a Trial sequential analysis for all-cause death in patients receiving GLP1R agonists versus placebo; **b** Funnel plots showing the trajectory of the overall point estimates and their corresponding precision evolve as each study enter the meta-analysis. CI, confidence interval; GLP1R, glucagon-like peptide–1 receptor; HR, hazard ratio

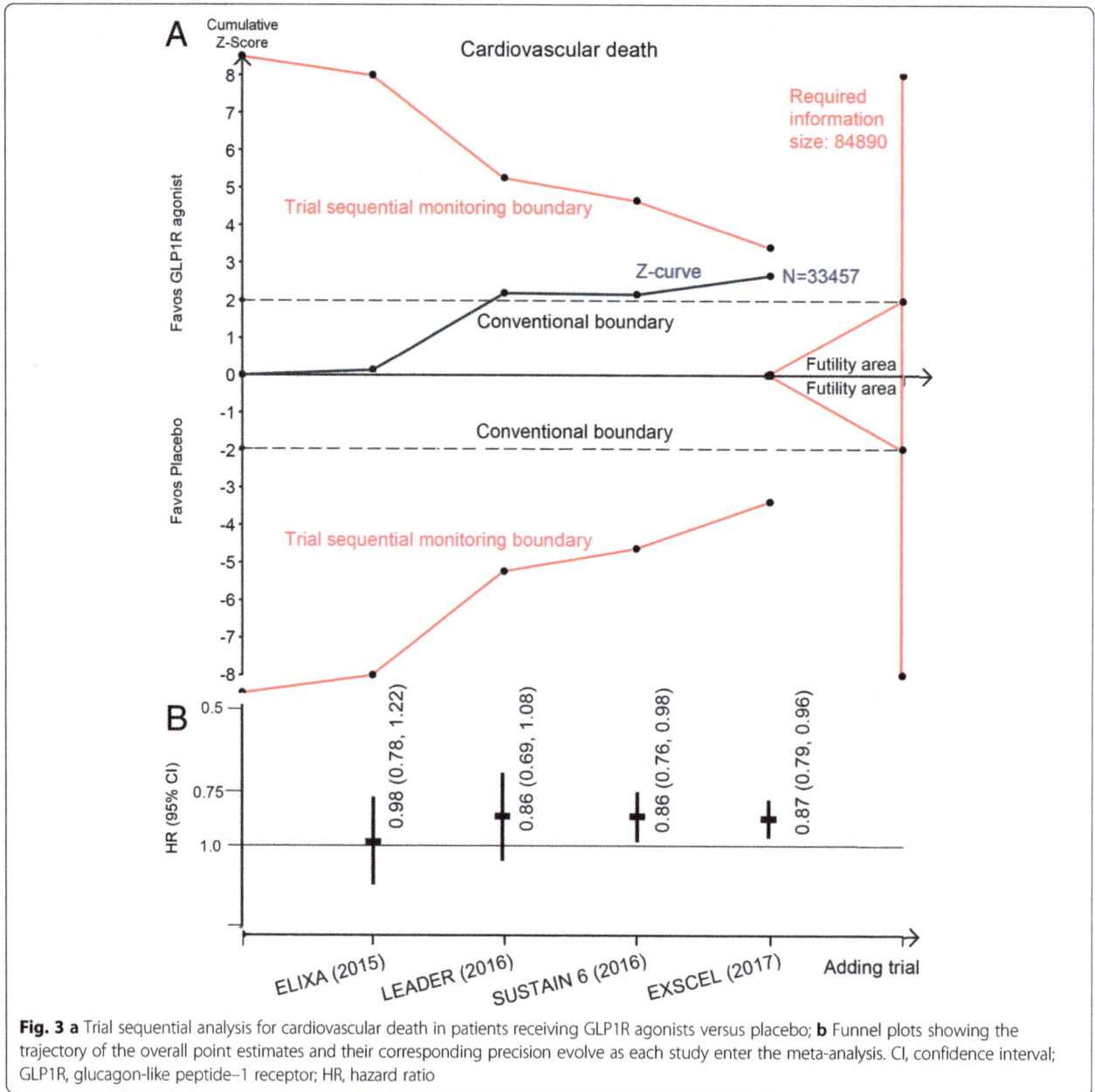

Fig. 3 a Trial sequential analysis for cardiovascular death in patients receiving GLP1R agonists versus placebo; **b** Funnel plots showing the trajectory of the overall point estimates and their corresponding precision evolve as each study enter the meta-analysis. CI, confidence interval; GLP1R, glucagon-like peptide–1 receptor; HR, hazard ratio

209 person-years' exposure to treatment. We did not find significant heterogeneity in both comparisons ($I^2 = $ 24.4% and 28.8 respectively). TSA suggested that a 15% reduction in myocardial infarction and stroke was inconclusive and future trials are needed (Additional file 3: Figures S2 and S3).

Hospitalization for heart failure

There was no significant difference in rate of hospitalization for heart failure between the use of GLP1R agonists and placebo (HR: 0.93, 95% CI: 0.83 to 1.04, $P = 0.203$) (Fig. 4). We did not find evidence of heterogeneity across these trials ($I^2 = 0$). In TSA, the cumulative Z-curve crossed the futility area,

suggesting firm evidence for lack of a 15% relative risk reduction in risk for hospitalization for heart failure (Additional file 3: Figure S4).

Major adverse cardiovascular event

Treatment with GLP1R agonists resulted in a statistically significant reduction in MACE compared with placebo; rates were 11.7% (1961 of 16,706 patients) and 12.8% (2144 of 16,751 patients) respectively (HR: 0.91, 95% CI: 0.85 to 0.96, $P = 0.002$) (Fig. 4). Considerable heterogeneity was detected ($I^2 = 50.1\%$); the number needed to treat was 241 person-years' exposure to treatment. TSA showed that the pooled sample size exceeded the estimated required information size and the cumulative Z-curve

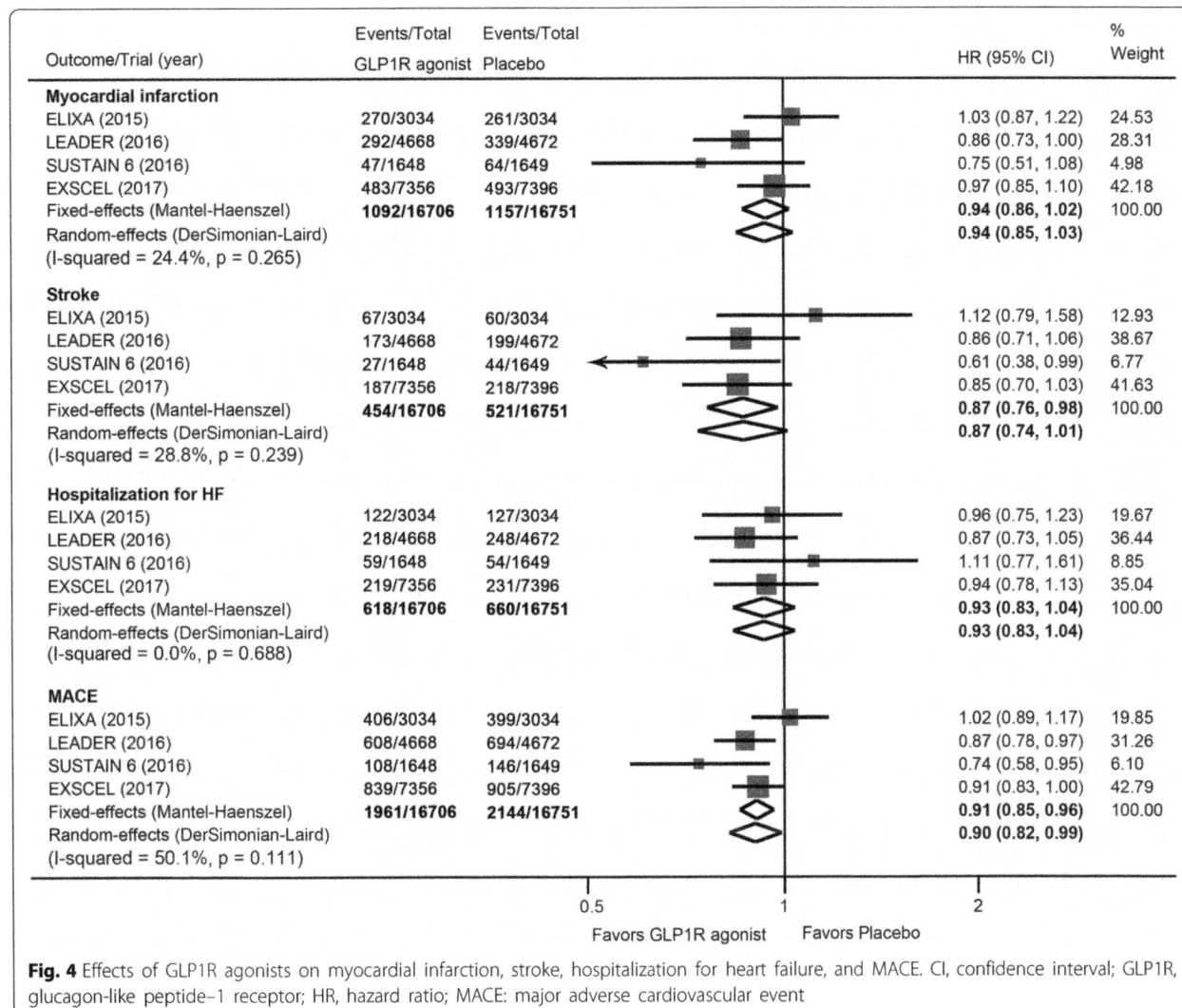

Outcome/Trial (year)	Events/Total GLP1R agonist	Events/Total Placebo	HR (95% CI)	% Weight
Myocardial infarction				
ELIXA (2015)	270/3034	261/3034	1.03 (0.87, 1.22)	24.53
LEADER (2016)	292/4668	339/4672	0.86 (0.73, 1.00)	28.31
SUSTAIN 6 (2016)	47/1648	64/1649	0.75 (0.51, 1.08)	4.98
EXSCEL (2017)	483/7356	493/7396	0.97 (0.85, 1.10)	42.18
Fixed-effects (Mantel-Haenszel)	**1092/16706**	**1157/16751**	**0.94 (0.86, 1.02)**	**100.00**
Random-effects (DerSimonian-Laird)			**0.94 (0.85, 1.03)**	
(I-squared = 24.4%, p = 0.265)				
Stroke				
ELIXA (2015)	67/3034	60/3034	1.12 (0.79, 1.58)	12.93
LEADER (2016)	173/4668	199/4672	0.86 (0.71, 1.06)	38.67
SUSTAIN 6 (2016)	27/1648	44/1649	0.61 (0.38, 0.99)	6.77
EXSCEL (2017)	187/7356	218/7396	0.85 (0.70, 1.03)	41.63
Fixed-effects (Mantel-Haenszel)	**454/16706**	**521/16751**	**0.87 (0.76, 0.98)**	**100.00**
Random-effects (DerSimonian-Laird)			**0.87 (0.74, 1.01)**	
(I-squared = 28.8%, p = 0.239)				
Hospitalization for HF				
ELIXA (2015)	122/3034	127/3034	0.96 (0.75, 1.23)	19.67
LEADER (2016)	218/4668	248/4672	0.87 (0.73, 1.05)	36.44
SUSTAIN 6 (2016)	59/1648	54/1649	1.11 (0.77, 1.61)	8.85
EXSCEL (2017)	219/7356	231/7396	0.94 (0.78, 1.13)	35.04
Fixed-effects (Mantel-Haenszel)	**618/16706**	**660/16751**	**0.93 (0.83, 1.04)**	**100.00**
Random-effects (DerSimonian-Laird)			**0.93 (0.83, 1.04)**	
(I-squared = 0.0%, p = 0.688)				
MACE				
ELIXA (2015)	406/3034	399/3034	1.02 (0.89, 1.17)	19.85
LEADER (2016)	608/4668	694/4672	0.87 (0.78, 0.97)	31.26
SUSTAIN 6 (2016)	108/1648	146/1649	0.74 (0.58, 0.95)	6.10
EXSCEL (2017)	839/7356	905/7396	0.91 (0.83, 1.00)	42.79
Fixed-effects (Mantel-Haenszel)	**1961/16706**	**2144/16751**	**0.91 (0.85, 0.96)**	**100.00**
Random-effects (DerSimonian-Laird)			**0.90 (0.82, 0.99)**	
(I-squared = 50.1%, p = 0.111)				

Favors GLP1R agonist   Favors Placebo

Fig. 4 Effects of GLP1R agonists on myocardial infarction, stroke, hospitalization for heart failure, and MACE. CI, confidence interval; GLP1R, glucagon-like peptide-1 receptor; HR, hazard ratio; MACE: major adverse cardiovascular event

crossed both the conventional boundary and the trial sequential monitoring boundary, indicating that there is firm evidence for a 15% reduction in risk for MACE with GLP1R agonists when compared with placebo (Fig. 5).

Largely consistent results on MACE were found across a number of subgroup analyses. The magnitude of the benefit of GLP1R agonists on MACE was attenuated in patients with a younger age, with a body mass index less than 30, with a history of congestive heart failure (Additional file 3: Figure S5), but the tests for interaction were not significant (Table 2).

Microvascular outcomes

The rates for nephropathy was numerically lower in patients with GLP1R agonists than placebo (648/13680 versus 757/13709, OR: 0.80, 95% CI: 0.60 to 1.06, $P = 0.121$) (Fig. 6). There was no significant difference in risk for retinopathy (370/13680 versus 359/13709, OR: 1.15, 95% CI: 0.83 to 1.60, $P = 0.394$) between the use of

GLP1R agonists and placebo (Fig. 6). Significant heterogeneity was detected across trials in both analyses (I^2 = 83.7% and 73.5% respectively).

Grading of evidence

Based on GRADE summaries (Table 3), we deemed the quality of the evidence to be high for total and cardiovascular mortality and stroke, and moderate for other outcomes. Reasons for rating down were provided in Table 3.

Efficacy outcomes

GLP1R agonists significantly reduced HbA1c level compared with placebo, with a weighted mean difference of -0.57% (95% CI: -0.74 to -0.40) (Fig. 7). GLP1R agonists also significantly reduced body weight (WMD: -2.25 kg; 95% CI: -3.09 to -1.41) and systolic blood pressure (WMD: -1.33 mmHg; 95% CI: -1.80 to -0.86), and increased heart rate (WMD: 2.07 beats per minute; 95% CI: 0.87 to 3.27).

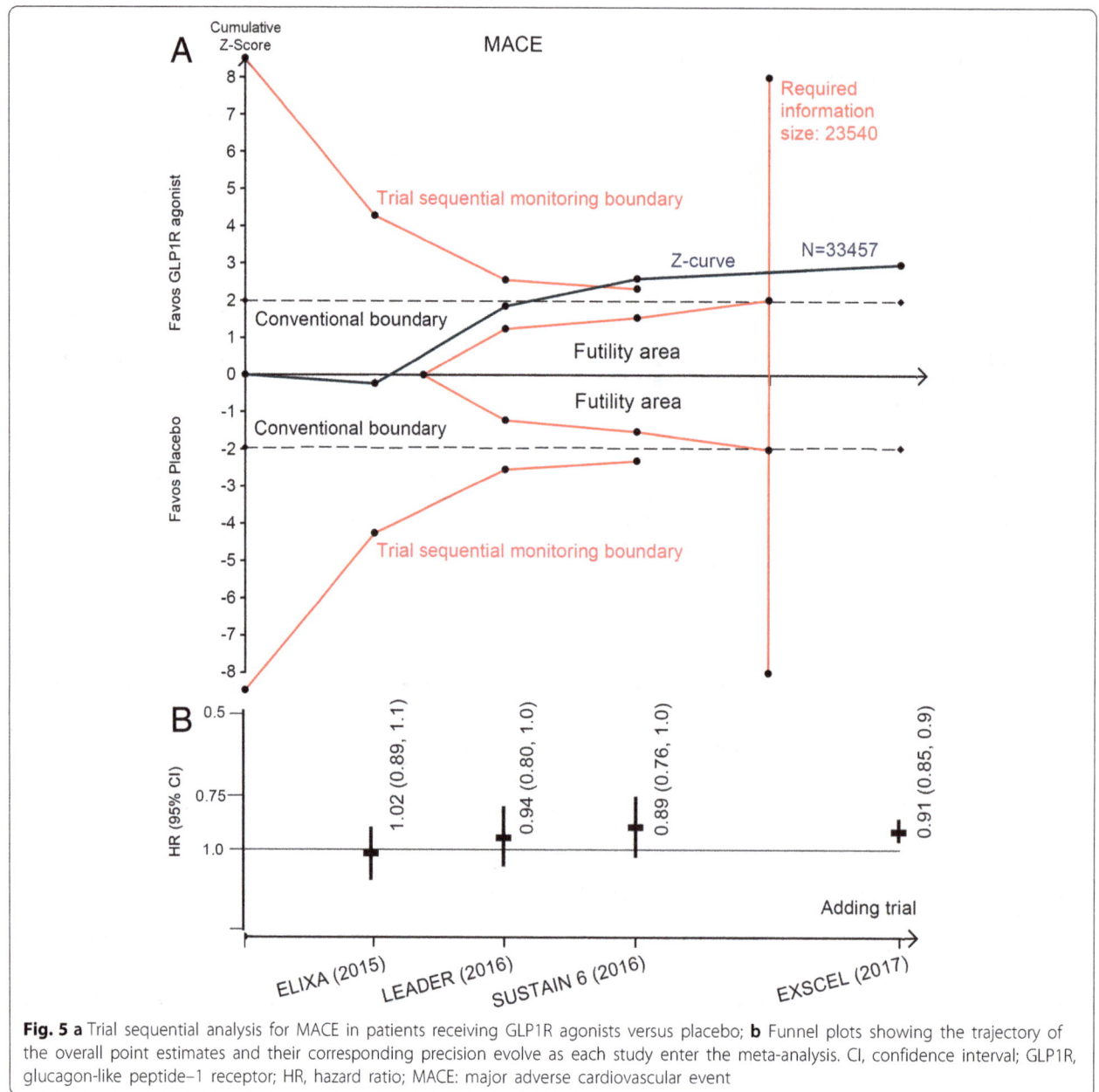

Fig. 5 a Trial sequential analysis for MACE in patients receiving GLP1R agonists versus placebo; **b** Funnel plots showing the trajectory of the overall point estimates and their corresponding precision evolve as each study enter the meta-analysis. CI, confidence interval; GLP1R, glucagon-like peptide–1 receptor; HR, hazard ratio; MACE: major adverse cardiovascular event

Discussion

In this meta-analysis of 33,457 patients and 4105 cardiovascular events from 4 large double-blind, randomized placebo-controlled cardiovascular outcome trials, we showed that 1) GLP1R agonists were associated with a statistically significant reduction in risks for all-cause (high-quality evidence), cardiovascular mortality (high--quality evidence), stroke (high-quality evidence) and the composite outcome of cardiovascular mortality, nonfatal myocardial infarction or nonfatal stroke (moderate-quality evidence); 2) the risks for hospitalization for heart failure and myocardial infarction were not significantly different (moderate-quality evidence); 3) TSA provided firm evidence for a 10% reduction in all-cause

mortality, a 15% reduction in MACE, and lack of a 15% reduction in hospitalization for heart failure with GLP1R agonists compared with placebo, but evidence remains inconclusive for cardiovascular mortality and myocardial infarction; 4) the magnitude of the benefit of GLP1R agonists on MACE was more remarkable in patients without a history of congestive heart failure but attenuated in patients with; 5) GLP1R agonists numerically reduced the rates for nephropathy but the risk for retinopathy was similar; 6) GLP1R agonists showed sustained reduction in HbA1c level and a number of other metabolic risk factors.

Several previous meta-analyses have evaluated the cardiovascular effect of GLP1R [23–25]. Two analyses reported

Table 2 Subgroup analyses for MACE

Subgroups	HR (95% CI)	P value	P value for interaction
Age			
< 60–65 years	0.92 (0.77, 1.10)	0.38	0.58
≥ 60–65 years	0.85 (0.79, 0.93)	0.001	
Gender			
Male	0.91 (0.85, 0.98)	0.02	0.53
Female	0.87 (0.78, 0.98)	0.02	
Race			
White	0.94 (0.88, 1.01)	0.09	0.12
Black	0.77 (0.59, 1.00)	0.05	
Asian	0.78 (0.62, 0.97)	0.03	
Body mass index			
< 30 kg/m^2	0.93 (0.83, 1.05)	0.22	0.69
≥ 30 kg/m^2	0.88 (0.81, 0.96)	0.008	
Glycated hemoglobin level			
< 8.0–8.5%	0.91 (0.83, 1.00)	0.04	0.73
≥ 8.0–8.5%	0.89 (0.82, 0.97)	0.01	
Insulin therapy			
Yes	0.88 (0.81, 0.97)	0.01	0.98
No	0.88 (0.80, 0.98)	0.01	
Duration of diabetes			
< 10–15 years	0.91 (0.81, 1.02)	0.09	0.74
≥ 10–15 years	0.89 (0.82, 0.96)	< 0.01	
History of congestive heart failure			
Yes	0.96 (0.85, 1.08)	0.47	0.27
No	0.87 (0.77, 1.00)	0.05	
Estimated GFR			
≥ 60 mL/min/1.73m^2	0.91 (0.79, 1.05)	0.19	0.82
< 60 mL/min/1.73m^2	0.89 (0.72, 1.09)	0.25	
≥ 30 mL/min/1.73m^2	0.88 (0.82, 0.95)	< 0.001	0.81
< 30 mL/min/1.73m^2	0.87 (0.55, 1.39)	0.57	

CI confidence interval, *GFR* glomerular filtration rate, *HR* hazard ratio, *MACE* major adverse cardiovascular event

no substantial difference in risk for total mortality or the major composite outcomes between GLP1R agonists and control treatments [23, 24]. These analyses were limited to RCTs primarily to evaluate the glucose-lowering efficacy of GLP1R agonists, all with the number of cardiovascular events as few as tens and the number of participants from tens to hundreds. Cardiovascular outcomes in these trials were based on clinician-reported adverse events rather than predefined and independently adjudicated. Another meta-analysis [25] included 3 of the cardiovascular outcome trials. They found that GLP1R agonists were associated with a lower mortality (odds ratio: 0.89; 95% CI: 0.80 to 0.99), but the risk for MACE was not significantly different (odds ratio: 0.88; 95% CI: 0.74 to 1.04). The important EXSCEL trial [22]—the largest trial among the 4

cardiovascular outcome trials was not included in their analysis. Incorporating data from EXSCEL trial to our analysis substantially improved the power of meta-analysis to detect potential difference of rare outcomes (adding another 14,752 patients and 1091 cardiovascular events). Compared with the analysis by Liu and colleagues which only detected total mortality benefit of GLP1R agonists, we extended the benefits to cardiovascular mortality, stroke and the composite MACE. We provided the funnel plots showing the trajectory of the overall point estimates and their corresponding precision evolved as each trial entered the meta-analysis. It can be seen that the benefits on MACE became significant until the EXSCEL trial was included. Another difference was that we employed HR rather than odds ratio in pooled analyses. We chose HR because it

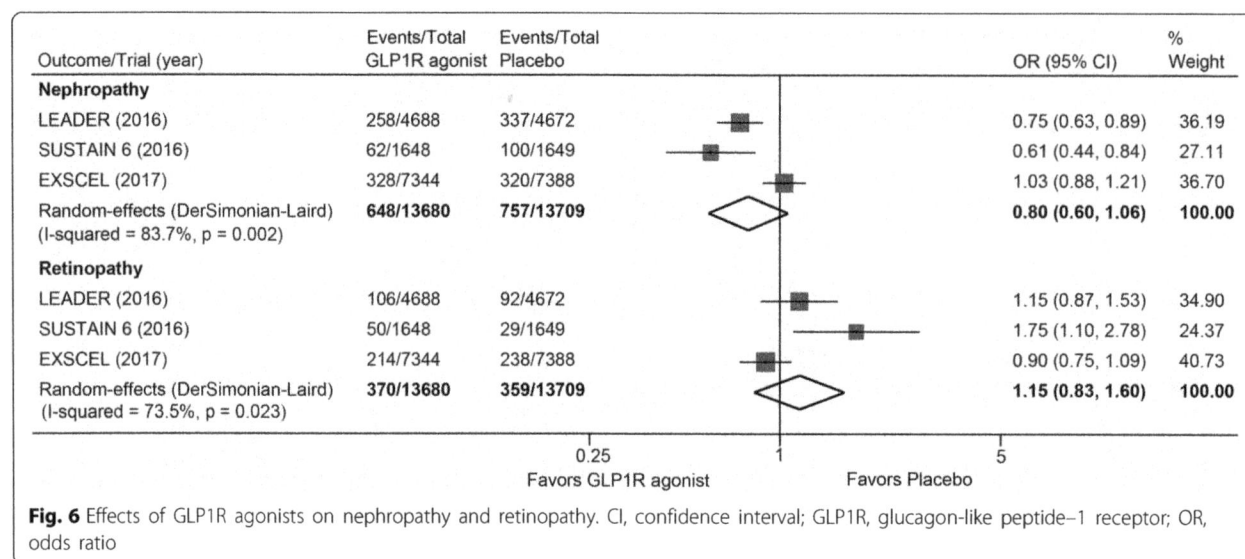

Outcome/Trial (year)	Events/Total GLP1R agonist	Events/Total Placebo		OR (95% CI)	% Weight
Nephropathy					
LEADER (2016)	258/4688	337/4672		0.75 (0.63, 0.89)	36.19
SUSTAIN 6 (2016)	62/1648	100/1649		0.61 (0.44, 0.84)	27.11
EXSCEL (2017)	328/7344	320/7388		1.03 (0.88, 1.21)	36.70
Random-effects (DerSimonian-Laird) (I-squared = 83.7%, p = 0.002)	**648/13680**	**757/13709**		**0.80 (0.60, 1.06)**	100.00
Retinopathy					
LEADER (2016)	106/4688	92/4672		1.15 (0.87, 1.53)	34.90
SUSTAIN 6 (2016)	50/1648	29/1649		1.75 (1.10, 2.78)	24.37
EXSCEL (2017)	214/7344	238/7388		0.90 (0.75, 1.09)	40.73
Random-effects (DerSimonian-Laird) (I-squared = 73.5%, p = 0.023)	**370/13680**	**359/13709**		**1.15 (0.83, 1.60)**	100.00

0.25 Favors GLP1R agonist 1 Favors Placebo 5

Fig. 6 Effects of GLP1R agonists on nephropathy and retinopathy. CI, confidence interval; GLP1R, glucagon-like peptide–1 receptor; OR, odds ratio

allows harmonization of the time-period variability across the trials. Although the direction of results might not be changed using different effect of estimates, the magnitudes of benefit were different. Finally, we determined whether findings from meta-analyses were conclusive by performing TSA and assessed the quality of evidence using the GRADE approach. These comprehensive analyses provide convincing evidence that GLP1R agonists reduce total mortality and MACE.

The US Food and Drug Administration (FDA) requires that all new anti-diabetic drugs must demonstrate good cardiovascular safety with an upper boundary of risk < 1.3. [26] This statement was first raised because a strong

and consistent relationship with increased risk of heart failure was reported to be associated with rosiglitazone [5, 6]. Cardiovascular concern has also latter been raised with DDP-4i [27] particularly for saxagliptin [28] also with regard to the risk of admission to hospital for heart failure. Heart failure, one important diabetes complication with high frequency, morbidity and mortality, has previously been relegated to an inferior position compared with microvascular and macrovascular complications in diabetes [4]. Due to this emerging concern, the FDA has now called to have heart failure systematically assessed in cardiovascular outcome trials of all new glucose-lowering drugs [29]. Our analysis, based on >

Table 3 GRADE assessment of confidence in estimates of effect in randomized trials

Outcome	No. of participants (trials)	Risk of bias	Consistency	Directness	Precision	Publication bias	Quality
MACE	33,457 (4)	No serious limitations	Serious limitations[a]	No serious limitations	No serious limitations	No serious limitations	Moderate
All-cause death	33,457 (4)	No serious limitations	No serious limitations	No serious limitations	No serious limitations	No serious limitations[d]	High
Cardiovascular death	33,457 (4)	No serious limitations	No serious limitations	No serious limitations	No serious limitations	No serious limitations	High
Myocardial infarction	33,457 (4)	No serious limitations	No serious limitations[b]	No serious limitations	Serious limitations[c]	No serious limitations	Moderate
Stroke	33,457 (4)	No serious limitations	No serious limitations[b]	No serious limitations	No serious limitations	No serious limitations	High
Hospitalization for heart failure	33,457 (4)	No serious limitations	No serious limitations	No serious limitations	Serious limitations[c]	No serious limitations	Moderate

GRADE Grading of Recommendations Assessment, Development and Evaluation
[a]Moderate to substantial heterogeneity: $I^2 = 50.1\%$
[b]I^2 = 24.4 and 28.8% respectively. Did not downgrade for mild heterogeneity
[c]95% confidence interval (CI) include important harm and benefit
[d]Did not downgrade even though Egger's test detected a possible publication bias. We did not downgrade because all trials included were large-scale randomized trials and these tests had limited ability to adequately assess small-study effects due to a small number of trials

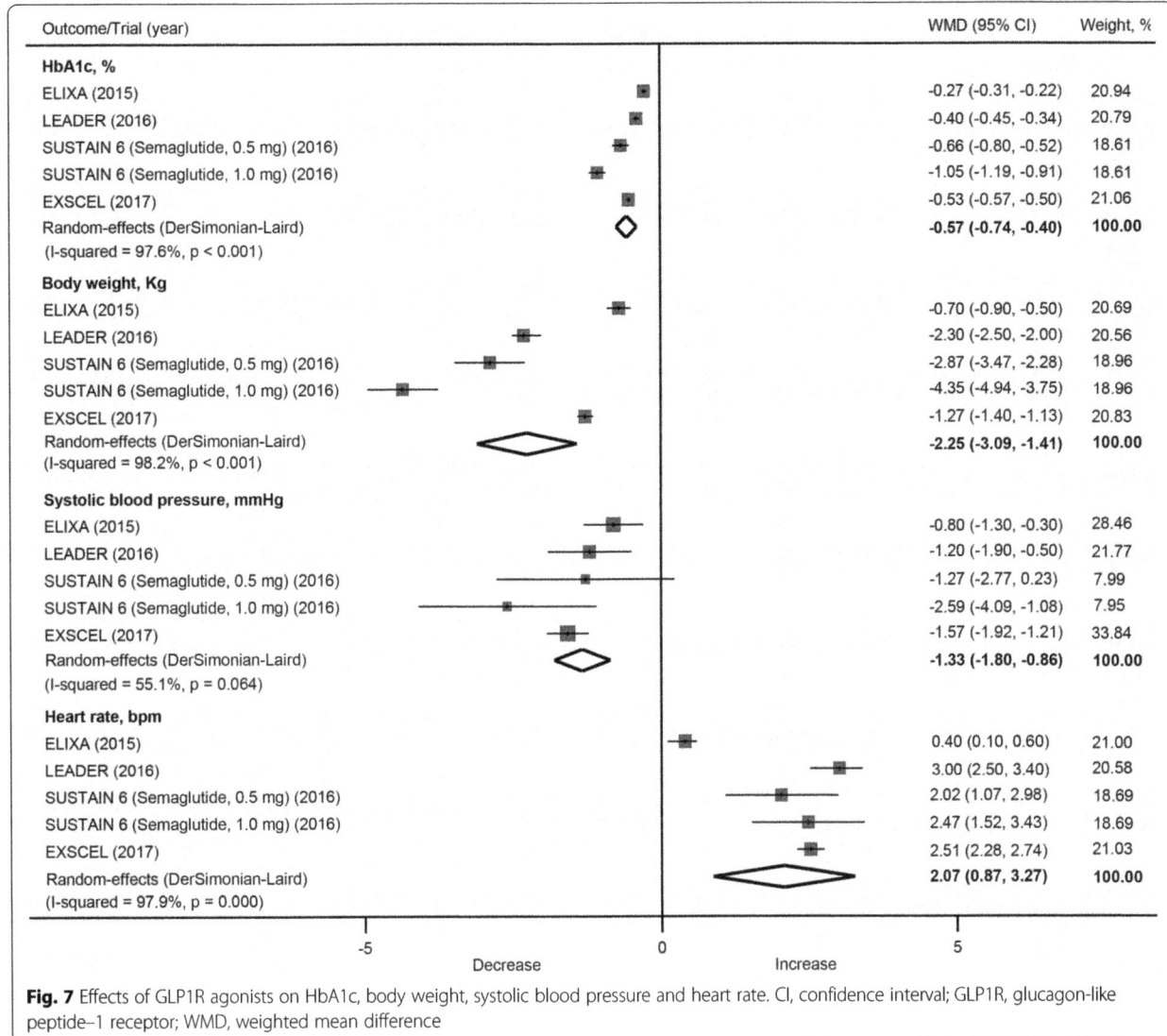

Outcome/Trial (year)		WMD (95% CI)	Weight, %
HbA1c, %			
ELIXA (2015)		-0.27 (-0.31, -0.22)	20.94
LEADER (2016)		-0.40 (-0.45, -0.34)	20.79
SUSTAIN 6 (Semaglutide, 0.5 mg) (2016)		-0.66 (-0.80, -0.52)	18.61
SUSTAIN 6 (Semaglutide, 1.0 mg) (2016)		-1.05 (-1.19, -0.91)	18.61
EXSCEL (2017)		-0.53 (-0.57, -0.50)	21.06
Random-effects (DerSimonian-Laird)		**-0.57 (-0.74, -0.40)**	**100.00**
(I-squared = 97.6%, p < 0.001)			
Body weight, Kg			
ELIXA (2015)		-0.70 (-0.90, -0.50)	20.69
LEADER (2016)		-2.30 (-2.50, -2.00)	20.56
SUSTAIN 6 (Semaglutide, 0.5 mg) (2016)		-2.87 (-3.47, -2.28)	18.96
SUSTAIN 6 (Semaglutide, 1.0 mg) (2016)		-4.35 (-4.94, -3.75)	18.96
EXSCEL (2017)		-1.27 (-1.40, -1.13)	20.83
Random-effects (DerSimonian-Laird)		**-2.25 (-3.09, -1.41)**	**100.00**
(I-squared = 98.2%, p < 0.001)			
Systolic blood pressure, mmHg			
ELIXA (2015)		-0.80 (-1.30, -0.30)	28.46
LEADER (2016)		-1.20 (-1.90, -0.50)	21.77
SUSTAIN 6 (Semaglutide, 0.5 mg) (2016)		-1.27 (-2.77, 0.23)	7.99
SUSTAIN 6 (Semaglutide, 1.0 mg) (2016)		-2.59 (-4.09, -1.08)	7.95
EXSCEL (2017)		-1.57 (-1.92, -1.21)	33.84
Random-effects (DerSimonian-Laird)		**-1.33 (-1.80, -0.86)**	**100.00**
(I-squared = 55.1%, p = 0.064)			
Heart rate, bpm			
ELIXA (2015)		0.40 (0.10, 0.60)	21.00
LEADER (2016)		3.00 (2.50, 3.40)	20.58
SUSTAIN 6 (Semaglutide, 0.5 mg) (2016)		2.02 (1.07, 2.98)	18.69
SUSTAIN 6 (Semaglutide, 1.0 mg) (2016)		2.47 (1.52, 3.43)	18.69
EXSCEL (2017)		2.51 (2.28, 2.74)	21.03
Random-effects (DerSimonian-Laird)		**2.07 (0.87, 3.27)**	**100.00**
(I-squared = 97.9%, p = 0.000)			

-5　　　0　　　5
Decrease　　　Increase

Fig. 7 Effects of GLP1R agonists on HbA1c, body weight, systolic blood pressure and heart rate. CI, confidence interval; GLP1R, glucagon-like peptide-1 receptor; WMD, weighted mean difference

33,000 patients and 4000 cardiovascular events, provided robust reassurance about the cardiovascular safety of GLP1R agonists, showing no increase in risks for hospitalization for heart failure and myocardial infarction. The upper boundary of risk of each individual and composite outcome was far less than 1.3 in our analysis. Our exploratory finding that the magnitude of the benefit of GLP1R agonists on MACE was more remarkable in patients without a history of congestive heart failure but attenuated in patients with remain to be confirmed in future studies. If confirmed, it would have great impact in the selection of patients for GLP1R agonist use.

Moreover, we found that GLP1R agonists instead reduced the risk for a number of cardiovascular outcomes. In our analysis, a 10% risk reduction in all-cause mortality and a 15% reduction in MACE were evident, although a 10% reduction in cardiovascular mortality still remains inconclusive. The relative risk reduction may seem relatively small, however, it should be duly noted that these benefits were observed in a population with the majority, if not all, patients had established cardiovascular disease (CVD) or at high cardiovascular risk in whom other cardiovascular risk factors were well treated. A large portion of patients were taking concomitant cardiovascular protection medications such as renin–angiotensin–aldosterone system inhibitors, β-blockers, statins or ezetimibe, and acetylsalicylic acid etc. Therefore, the cardiovascular protective effect of GLP1R agonists appears to be additive to that of evidence-based cardiovascular pharmacotherapies [30, 31]. Another important finding of our study was that total mortality was significantly reduced with GLP1R agonists. This finding was considered critically important because the common use of evidence-based cardiovascular pharmacotherapies substantially lower the incidence of mortality, which makes potential difference difficult to detect. For instance, more intensive low-density lipoprotein (LDL) cholesterol–lowering therapy with PCSK9 antibodies or ezetimibe did not show benefit in reducing cardiovascular and total mortality, although a reduced composite outcomes was observed [32–34].

Previous guidelines in cardiology did not make a recommendation on the selection of anti-hyperglycemic drugs in diabetes patients with established CVD or at high cardiovascular risk [30, 31]. The recently published cardiovascular outcomes trials of new antidiabetic therapies have provided additional data on cardiovascular outcomes in patients with type 2 diabetes with cardiovascular disease or at high risk for CVD [19–22, 28, 35–38]. The 2018 Standards of Medical Care in Diabetes recommends that in this population, anti-hyperglycemic therapy should begin with metformin and subsequently incorporate an agent proven to reduce major adverse cardiovascular events and cardiovascular mortality (currently empagliflozin and liraglutide) [39]. Our analyses support the recommendation that anti-hyperglycemic drugs should be chosen with preference in diabetes patients with established CVD or at high cardiovascular risk, with GLP1R agonists and also sodium–glucose cotransporter 2 inhibitors [35] as priority, after considering drug-specific and patient factors.

The mechanisms of cardiovascular protection associated with GLP1R agonists are considered multidimensional, which was discussed elsewhere [40]. It may be associated with reduction of body weight, blood pressure, the lipid profile and lowering the risk for hypoglycemia, and amelioration of insulin resistance and inflammation, etc. Although our findings were obtained in the context of no obvious heterogeneity among trials, whether the cardiovascular benefits of GLP1R agonists represent a class effect remains to be definitively established. Other large-scale randomized controlled cardiovascular outcome trials are ongoing, such as the ITCA 650 trial (NCT01455896) with 4000 patients and the REWIND (Researching Cardiovascular Events With a Weekly INcretin in Diabetes, NCT01394952) with 9622 patients (Additional file 3: Table S3). Of note, overexpression of mTOR stimulated GLP-1 production, indicating a link role of mTOR between energy supply and the production of GLP-1 [41]. Indeed, inhibition of mTOR with rapamycin attenuated inflammation, inhibited progression, and enhanced stability of atherosclerotic plaques in animal models [42]. The potential effect of the inhibition of the mTOR pathway in the treatment of cardiovascular diseases warrants further investigation.

Limitations

We acknowledge several limitations. First, the results were analyzed on trial level data but not on patient level data; individual patient-level data could improve the accuracy of the findings. Second, our finding that the magnitude of the benefit of GLP1R agonists on MACE was more remarkable in patients without a history of congestive heart failure but attenuated in patients with an only be considered exploratory and remain to be confirmed in future studies. Third, publication bias tests had limited ability to adequately assess small-study effects because all involved a small number of trials. Fourth, the conclusions were based on diabetes patients with established or high risk for CVD and could be generalized to patients with low cardiovascular risk.

Conclusions

Moderate-to-high quality of evidence suggested that GLP1R agonists did not increase the risk for any of, but instead reduced the risk for a number of cardiovascular outcomes. A 10% reduction in all-cause mortality and a 15% reduction in the composite outcome of cardiovascular death, nonfatal myocardial infarction or nonfatal stroke were evident. In diabetes patients with established CVD or at high cardiovascular risk, GLP1R agonists could be a preferred anti-hyperglycemic agent after considering drug-specific and patient factors. Future studies are needed to confirm the long-term cardiovascular benefits of GLP1R agonists.

Additional files

Additional file 1: PRISMA checklist. (DOCX 22 kb)

Additional file 2: MOOSE checklist. (DOC 71 kb)

Additional file 3: Figure S1. Flow diagram of study selection; Table S1. Primary and secondary endpoints, inclusion and exclusion criteria of included randomized controlled trials; Table S2. Risk of bias of included randomized controlled trials; Figure S2. Trial sequential analysis for myocardial infarction in patients receiving glucagon-like peptide-1 receptor agonists versus placebo; Figure S3. Trial sequential analysis for stroke in patients receiving glucagon-like peptide-1 receptor agonists versus placebo; Figure S4. Trial sequential analysis for hospitalization for heart failure in patients receiving glucagon-like peptide-1 receptor agonists versus placebo; Figure S5. Analysis of MACE based on patients with or without a history of congestive heart failure; Table S3. Characteristics of large ongoing randomized controlled trials evaluating cardiovascular efficacy of GLP-1 receptor agonist. (DOCX 1010 kb)

Abbreviations

CIs: Confidence intervals; CVD: Cardiovascular disease; DDP-4i: Dipeptidyl peptidase–4 inhibitors; FDA: Food and Drug Administration; GLP1R: Glucagon-like peptide–1 receptor; GRADE: Grading of Recommendations, Assessment, Development and Evaluation; HR: Hazard ratio; LDL: Low-density lipoprotein; MACE: Major adverse cardiovascular event; NNT: Number needed to treat; PRISMA: Preferred Reporting Items for Systematic Reviews and Meta-Analyses; RCTs: Randomized controlled trials; T2DM: Type 2 diabetes mellitus; TSA: Trial sequential analysis

Funding

This work was supported by National Natural Science Foundation of China (81800752), Natural Science Foundation of Jiangsu Province (BK20170125), Jiangsu Provincial Key Medical Discipline (ZDXKB2016012), and the Key Research and Development Program of Jiangsu Province of China (BE2015604 and BE2016606). The funders had no role in the study design, data collection and analysis, writing of the report, and decision to submit the article for publication.

Authors' contributions

XZ conceived the study, selected studies and extracted the data, analyzed and interpreted the data, and wrote the first draft of the manuscript. FS selected studies and extracted the data, analyzed and interpreted the data, and wrote the first draft of the manuscript. LZ and YZ contributed to the study protocol and analyzed and interpreted the data. DZ and YB conceived the study, interpreted the data, and wrote the first draft of the manuscript. All authors read and approved the final manuscript.

Competing interests

The authors declare that they have no competing interests.

Author details

[1]Department of Endocrinology, Affiliated Drum Tower Hospital, Nanjing University School of Medicine, 321 Zhongshan Road, Nanjing, Jiangsu Province 210008, China. [2]Department of Endocrinology, Nanjing Drum Tower Hospital Clinical College of Traditional Chinese and Western Medicine, Nanjing University of Chinese Medicine, 321 Zhongshan Road, Nanjing, Jiangsu Province 210008, China.

References

1. Di Angelantonio E, Kaptoge S, Wormser D, Willeit P, Butterworth AS, Bansal N, et al. Association of cardiometabolic multimorbidity with mortality. JAMA. 2015;314:52–60.
2. Gerstein HC, Miller ME, Genuth S, Ismail-Beigi F, Buse JB, Goff DJ, et al. Long-term effects of intensive glucose lowering on cardiovascular outcomes. N Engl J Med. 2011;364:818–28.
3. Patel A, MacMahon S, Chalmers J, Neal B, Billot L, Woodward M, et al. Intensive blood glucose control and vascular outcomes in patients with type 2 diabetes. N Engl J Med. 2008;358:2560–72.
4. Gilbert RE, Krum H. Heart failure in diabetes: effects of anti-hyperglycaemic drug therapy. Lancet. 2015;385:2107–17.
5. Nissen SE, Wolski K. Effect of rosiglitazone on the risk of myocardial infarction and death from cardiovascular causes. N Engl J Med. 2007; 356:2457–71.
6. Singh S, Loke YK, Furberg CD. Thiazolidinediones and heart failure: a teleo-analysis. Diabetes Care. 2007;30:2148–53.
7. Holman RR, Sourij H, Califf RM. Cardiovascular outcome trials of glucose-lowering drugs or strategies in type 2 diabetes. Lancet. 2014; 383:2008–17.
8. Goldfine AB. Assessing the cardiovascular safety of diabetes therapies. N Engl J Med. 2008;359:1092–5.
9. Waldrop G, Zhong J, Peters M, Rajagopalan S. Incretin-based therapy for diabetes. what a cardiologist needs to know J Am Coll Cardiol. 2016;67: 1488–96.
10. Eliasson B, Moller-Goede D, Eeg-Olofsson K, Wilson C, Cederholm J, Fleck P, Diamant M, Taskinen MR, Smith U. Lowering of postprandial lipids in individuals with type 2 diabetes treated with alogliptin and/or pioglitazone: a randomised double-blind placebo-controlled study. Diabetologia. 2012;55:915–25.
11. Eng C, Kramer CK, Zinman B, Retnakaran R. Glucagon-like peptide-1 receptor agonist and basal insulin combination treatment for the management of type 2 diabetes: a systematic review and meta-analysis. Lancet. 2014;384:2228–34.
12. Moher D, Liberati A, Tetzlaff J, Altman DG. Preferred reporting items for systematic reviews and meta-analyses: the PRISMA statement. Ann Intern Med. 2009;151:264–9. W64
13. Higgins JPT, Altman DG, Sterne JAC. Assessing risk of bias in included studies. In: Higgins JPT, Green S, editors. Cochrane handbook for systematic reviews of interventions. Version 5.1.0 [updated March 2011]. The Cochrane Collaboration; 2011. http://handbook-5-1.cochrane.org/. Accessed 28 Sept 2017.
14. Higgins JP, Thompson SG, Deeks JJ, Altman DG. Measuring inconsistency in meta-analyses. BMJ. 2003;327:557–60.
15. Mantel N, Haenszel W. Statistical aspects of the analysis of data from retrospective studies of disease. J Natl Cancer Inst. 1959;22:719–48.
16. Wetterslev J, Thorlund K, Brok J, Gluud C. Trial sequential analysis may

17. establish when firm evidence is reached in cumulative meta-analysis. J Clin Epidemiol. 2008;61:64–75.
17. Pogue JM, Yusuf S. Cumulating evidence from randomized trials: utilizing sequential monitoring boundaries for cumulative meta-analysis. Control Clin Trials. 1997;18:580–93.
18. Brok J, Thorlund K, Wetterslev J, Gluud C. Apparently conclusive meta-analyses may be inconclusive--trial sequential analysis adjustment of random error risk due to repetitive testing of accumulating data in apparently conclusive neonatal meta-analyses. Int J Epidemiol. 2009;38:287–98.
19. Marso SP, Daniels GH, Brown-Frandsen K, Kristensen P, Mann JF, Nauck MA, et al. Liraglutide and cardiovascular outcomes in type 2 diabetes. N Engl J Med. 2016;375:311–22.
20. Pfeffer MA, Claggett B, Diaz R, Dickstein K, Gerstein HC, Kober LV, et al. Lixisenatide in patients with type 2 diabetes and acute coronary syndrome. N Engl J Med. 2015;373:2247–57.
21. Marso SP, Bain SC, Consoli A, Eliaschewitz FG, Jodar E, Leiter LA, et al. Semaglutide and cardiovascular outcomes in patients with type 2 diabetes. N Engl J Med. 2016;(19):1834–44.
22. Holman RR, Bethel MA, Mentz RJ, Thompson VP, Lokhnygina Y, Buse JB, et al. Effects of once-weekly exenatide on cardiovascular outcomes in type 2 diabetes. N Engl J Med. 2017;377:1228–39.
23. Ding S, Du YP, Lin N, Su YY, Yang F, Kong LC, Ge H, Pu J, He B. Effect of glucagon-like peptide-1 on major cardiovascular outcomes in patients with type 2 diabetes mellitus: a meta-analysis of randomized controlled trials. Int J Cardiol. 2016;222:957–62.
24. Monami M, Dicembrini I, Nardini C, Fiordelli I, Mannucci E. Effects of glucagon-like peptide-1 receptor agonists on cardiovascular risk: a meta-analysis of randomized clinical trials. Diabetes Obes Metab. 2014;16:38–47.
25. Liu J, Li L, Deng K, Xu C, Busse JW, Vandvik PO, Li S, Guyatt GH, Sun X. Incretin based treatments and mortality in patients with type 2 diabetes: systematic review and meta-analysis. BMJ. 2017;357:j2499.
26. US Department of Health and Human Services, Food and Drug Administration, Center for Drug Evaluation and Research. Guidance for industry: diabetes mellitus— evaluating cardiovascular risk in new antidiabetic therapies to treat type 2 diabetes. Available: https://www.fda.gov/downloads/Drugs/GuidanceComplianceRegulatoryInformation/Guidances/UCM071627.pdf. Accessed 28 Sept 2017.
27. Li L, Li S, Deng K, Liu J, Vandvik PO, Zhao P, et al. Dipeptidyl peptidase-4 inhibitors and risk of heart failure in type 2 diabetes: systematic review and meta-analysis of randomised and observational studies. BMJ. 2016:i610.
28. Scirica BM, Bhatt DL, Braunwald E, Steg PG, Davidson J, Hirshberg B, et al. Saxagliptin and cardiovascular outcomes in patients with type 2 diabetes mellitus. N Engl J Med. 2013;369:1317–26.
29. McMurray JJ, Gerstein HC, Holman RR, Pfeffer MA. Heart failure: a cardiovascular outcome in diabetes that can no longer be ignored. Lancet Diabetes Endocrinol. 2014;2:843–51.
30. O'Gara PT, Kushner FG, Ascheim DD, Casey DJ, Chung MK, de Lemos JA, et al: 2013 ACCF/AHA guideline for the management of ST-elevation myocardial infarction: a report of the American College of Cardiology Foundation/American Heart Association task force on practice guidelines. J Am Coll Cardiol 2013;61:e78–140.
31. Montalescot G, Sechtem U, Achenbach S, Andreotti F, Arden C, Budaj A, et al. 2013 ESC guidelines on the management of stable coronary artery disease: the task force on the management of stable coronary artery disease of the European Society of Cardiology. Eur Heart J. 2013;34:2949–3003.
32. Ridker PM, Revkin J, Amarenco P, Brunell R, Curto M, Civeira F, et al. Cardiovascular efficacy and safety of bococizumab in high-risk patients. N Engl J Med. 2017;(16):1527–39.
33. Sabatine MS, Giugliano RP, Keech AC, Honarpour N, Wiviott SD, Murphy SA, et al. Evolocumab and clinical outcomes in patients with cardiovascular disease. N Engl J Med. 2017;(18):1713–22.
34. Cannon CP, Blazing MA, Giugliano RP, McCagg A, White JA, Theroux P, et al. Ezetimibe added to statin therapy after acute coronary syndromes. N Engl J Med. 2015;372:2387–97.
35. Zinman B, Wanner C, Lachin JM, Fitchett D, Bluhmki E, Hantel S, et al. Empagliflozin, cardiovascular outcomes, and mortality in type 2 diabetes. N Engl J Med. 2015;373:2117–28.
36. Neal B, Perkovic V, Mahaffey KW, de Zeeuw D, Fulcher G, Erondu N, et al. Canagliflozin and cardiovascular and renal events in type 2 diabetes. N Engl J Med. 2017;(7):644–57.
37. White WB, Cannon CP, Heller SR, Nissen SE, Bergenstal RM, Bakris GL, et al.

Alogliptin after acute coronary syndrome in patients with type 2 diabetes. N Engl J Med. 2013;369:1327–35.

38. Green JB, Bethel MA, Armstrong PW, Buse JB, Engel SS, Garg J, et al. Effect of sitagliptin on cardiovascular outcomes in type 2 diabetes. N Engl J Med. 2015;373:232–42.

39. Standards of Medical Care in Diabetes—2018. Diabetes Care. 2018; Supplement 1:S1–155.

40. Nauck MA, Meier JJ, Cavender MA, Abd El Aziz M, Drucker DJ. Cardiovascular actions and clinical outcomes with glucagon-like peptide-1 receptor agonists and dipeptidyl peptidase-4 inhibitors. Circulation. 2017; 136:849–70.

41. Xu G, Li Z, Ding L, Tang H, Guo S, Liang H, Wang H, Zhang W. Intestinal mTOR regulates GLP-1 production in mouse L cells. Diabetologia. 2015;58: 1887–97.

42. Tarantino G, Capone D. Inhibition of the mTOR pathway: a possible protective role in coronary artery disease. Ann Med. 2013;45:348–56.

25

One-year mortality among hospital survivors of cholinesterase inhibitor poisoning based on Taiwan National Health Insurance Research Database from 2003 to 2012

Min-Chun Chuang[1,2†], Chih-Hao Chang[3,4,5†], Chung Shu Lee[3,4,5], Shih-Hong Li[3,5], Ching-Chung Hsiao[5,6], Yueh-Fu Fang[3,4,5] and Meng-Jer Hsieh[1,7*] [iD]

Abstract

Background: Acute cholinesterase inhibitor (CI) poisoning, including organophosphate and carbamate poisoning, is a crucial problem in developing countries. Acute intoxication results in a cholinergic crisis, neurological symptoms, or respiratory failure. However, the short-term and long-term outcomes of CI poisoning are seldom reported.

Methods: Data from the National Health Insurance Research Database were used to investigate the outcomes after organophosphate and carbamate poisoning. Patients who were hospitalized for a first episode of acute CI poisoning between 2003 and 2012 were enrolled in this study. Outcomes of acute CI poisoning with or without mechanical ventilation were analyzed.

Results: Among 6832 patients with CI poisoning, 2010 developed respiratory failure requiring mechanical ventilation, and the other 4822 patients did not require mechanical ventilation. The hospital mortality rate was higher in patients requiring mechanical ventilation than in those not requiring mechanical ventilation (33.3% versus 4.7%, $p < 0.0001$). In patients with respiratory failure with mechanical ventilation, the patients without pneumonia had higher mortality rate than those with pneumonia. (36.0% versus 19.9%, $p < 0.0001$). The 1-year mortality rate the survivors of CI poisoning was 6.7%. Among 5932 survivors after cholinesterase inhibitor poisoning, the one-year mortality rate in patients with mechanical ventilation during hospitalization was higher than those without mechanical ventilation during hospitalization (11.4% versus 5.4% respectively, p < 0.0001).

Conclusions: The one-year mortality rate of survivors after CI poisoning was 6.7%. Meanwhile, age, pneumonia, and mechanical ventilation may be predictive factors for the one-year mortality among the survivors after CI poisoning. Diabetes mellitus was not a risk factor for hospital mortality in patients with CI poisoning.

Keywords: Organophosphates intoxication, Intensive care unit, Respiratory failure, Mechanical ventilation

* Correspondence: mengjer@cgmh.org.tw
†Min-Chun Chuang and Chih-Hao Chang contributed equally to this work.
[1]Department of Pulmonary and Critical Care Medicine, Chiayi Chang-Gung Memorial Hospital, No. 6, Sec. West, Chia-Pu Road, Pu-Tz City, Chiayi 613, Taiwan
[7]Department of Respiratory Care, Chang-Gung University, Taoyuan City, Taiwan
Full list of author information is available at the end of the article

Background

Organophosphates (OP) have been used as pesticides in countries where considerable agricultural activities are performed for more than 50 years. The acute intoxications caused by cholinesterase inhibitors (CI), including organophosphates and carbamates (CM), is a major problem, either by accidental ingestion or due to suicide attempts [1].

Both organophosphates and carbamates are potent cholinesterase inhibitors capable of causing severe cholinergic toxicity following cutaneous exposure, inhalation, or ingestion [2]. Cholinesterase inhibitors act by inhibiting acetylcholinesterase, which causes the accumulation of acetylcholine within synaptic clefts, resulting in the overstimulation and disruption of neurotransmission in both the central and peripheral nervous systems. The cholinergic overload leads to characteristic muscarinic, nicotinic, and central nervous system symptoms, including bradycardia, miosis, lacrimation, salivation, bronchorrhea, bronchospasm, urination, emesis, and diarrhea [3]. Respiratory failure following acute CI poisoning is a multi-factorial process; it includes depression of the central nervous system, neuromuscular weakness, excessive respiratory secretions, bronchoconstriction, and pneumonia [4, 5].

The standard therapeutic strategy for cholinesterase inhibitor poisoning includes decontamination, atropine, oximes, benzodiazepines and supportive care. Atropine and oximes are used to counteract the cholinergic symptoms, and benzodiazepines are used to prevent seizure activities [6]. However, the high mortality rate of acute CI poisoning ranges from 10 to 50%, even in the setting of highly sophisticated intensive care [7–12]. Few studies have reported the following outcome after organophosphate intoxication. In this study, we assessed the outcomes of OP and CM poisoning by using data from the National Health Insurance Research Database (NHIRD).

Methods

Ethics statement

The study protocol was approved by the Institutional Review Board of Chang-Gung Medical Foundation (No. 104-8058B). Research was conducted in accordance with the 1964 Declaration of Helsinki and its later amendments. All personally identifiable information was encrypted prior to the release of the Taiwanese NHIRD (https://nhird.nhri.org.tw/en/). Consequently, patient consent was waived for this study.

Data source

This retrospective longitudinal study used data from the NHIRD, which is released and managed by the Taiwan National Health Research Institute. The National Health Insurance program is a mandatory social insurance program established by the Taiwanese government. It has provided comprehensive health care for all Taiwanese citizens since March 1, 1995, and currently covers 23.7 million enrollees, representing approximately 99.0% of the national population. The NHIRD comprises enrollment files, claims data, catastrophic illness files, and a drug prescription registry. It represents one of the largest nationwide healthcare service databases in the world.

Patients and outcome

Patients who were hospitalized with a first diagnosis of OP and CM poisoning [International Classification of Diseases, Version 9, Clinical Modification (ICD-9-CM) code 989.3] between January 2003 and December 2012 were enrolled as the study subjects. The baseline comorbidities of the subjects were retrieved from the inpatient claims data. The following comorbidities were defined: diabetes mellitus (DM; ICD-9-CM code 250), hypertension (ICD-9-CM codes 401–405), coronary artery disease (ICD-9-CM codes 410–414), cerebrovascular accident (ICD-9-CM codes 430–438), asthma (ICD-9-CM codes 493), liver failure (ICD-9-CM codes 570), chronic obstructive pulmonary disease (ICD-9-CM codes 491, 492, and 496), and chronic renal failure (ICD-9-CM code 585). The exclusion criteria were 1) patients younger than 18 years ($n = 89$) and 2) subjects with missing data for sex ($n = 7$). All citizens in Taiwan are mandatory to participate in National Health Insurance program, and death was defined as the date of withdrawal from the insurance system according to the NHIRD data. In the previous study, the prognostic factors in organophosphate poisoning such as mechanical ventilation (MV) [10, 13], pneumonia [14], renal failure [9], and some medical comorbidities (diabetes mellitus, coronary artery disease, cerebrovascular accident, hypertension), [15] have been reported. These clinical variables were included in the analysis of mortality rate. Non-invasive ventilation was not included in the study.

Statistical analysis

Data are expressed as mean ± standard deviation for continuous variables and as frequency and percentage for categorical variables. Chi-square tests were used for categorical variables, and Student t tests were used for continuous variables. Cox proportional hazard regression model was used to identify possible risk factors for mortality rate in patients with cholinesterase inhibitor poisoning intoxication. The variables used in the univariate COX proportional hazard regression model were age, sex, common comorbidities, medication, pneumonia, hemodialysis, and mechanical ventilation. The variables with P values < 0.05 in the univariate model were used in the multivariate analysis. Survival curves were plotted by using the Kaplan–Meier approach and were compared through the log rank test. All statistical analyses were performed by using MedCalc, version 12.5 (MedCalc Software, Ostend, Belgium). Two-tailed p values less than 0.05 were considered statistically significant.

Results

Baseline characteristics of these patients with CI poisoning are shown in Table 1. From January 2003 to December 2012, 6832 patients were hospitalized with a diagnosis of CI intoxication. The mean age of the patients was 55.39 ± 16.44 years, and 2038 (29.3%) patients were female. Among these patients, 29.4% had respiratory failure and received mechanical ventilation during hospitalization. The overall hospital mortality rate in patients with OP and CM intoxication was 13.2%.

Table 2 shows the demographic and clinical characteristics of the survivors versus nonsurvivors of OP and CM poisoning. Age, sex, and the comorbidities of hypertension, chronic renal failure, and hyperlipidemia were significantly different between the survivors and nonsurvivors. A higher percentage of the nonsurvivors were given with atropine, pralidoxime (PAM), hemodialysis, and mechanical ventilation than the survivors. The hospital days was higher in survivors than in non-survivors (9.61 ± 11.43 vs. 6.58 ± 12.31, < 0.0001).

Table 1 Characteristics of patients with acute cholinesterase inhibitor poisoning (N = 6832)

Characteristics	
Age, mean ± SD, years old	55.39 ± 16.44
Female Sex, N (%)	2038 (29.8)
Comorbidities	
Diabetes mellitus, N (%)	773 (11.3)
Hypertension, N (%)	909 (13.3)
Coronary artery disease, N (%)	192 (2.8)
Cerebrovascular accident, N (%)	177 (2.6)
Chronic renal failure, N (%)	53 (0.8)
Chronic obstructive pulmonary disease, N (%)	111 (1.6)
Asthma, N (%)	45 (0.7)
Liver failure, N (%)	30 (0.4)
Interventions	
Atropine use, N (%)	3653 (53.5)
Pralidoxime use, N (%)	3479 (50.9)
Hemodialysis, N (%)	124 (1.8)
Mechanical ventilation, N (%)	2010 (29.4)
Pneumonia, N (%)	492 (7.2)
Hospital mortality, N (%)	900 (13.2)
Hospital days, mean ± SD	9.21 ± 11.60

Data are presented as mean ± SD or N (%)

Among 6832 patients with CI poisoning, 2010 patients developed respiratory failure requiring mechanical ventilation, and the other 4822 patients were did not require mechanical ventilation. The hospital mortality rate was higher in patients with mechanical ventilation than in those without mechanical ventilation (33.3% versus 4.7%, p < 0.0001; Table 3). Besides, patients with mechanical ventilation had more hospital days than patients without mechanical ventilation (15.42 ± 16.33 vs. 6.62 ± 7.54, < 0.0001).

Table 4 shows the results for the univariate and multivariate analysis of variables associated with hospital mortality in patients with CI intoxication. Age, liver failure, atropine, hemodialysis, and mechanical ventilation were positively correlated with the hospital mortality rate. But hypertension, pneumonia, and PAM use were also negatively correlated with the hospital mortality.

In Table 5, we applied univariate analysis to predict one-year mortality in survivors after CI poisoning. According to univariate analysis, age, diabetes mellitus, PAM use, hemodialysis, mechanical ventilation, and pneumonia during hospitalization were significant predictors of one-year mortality in patients with CI poisoning. After adjusting for these factors in a multivariate Cox regression analysis. Age, pneumonia, and mechanical ventilation were independent risk factors for one-year mortality among survivors of cholinesterase inhibitor poisoning.

Figure 1 illustrates the Kaplan–Meier survival curves indicating that the patients with OP intoxication who underwent mechanical ventilation exhibited a significantly higher hospital mortality rate (p < 0.0001) than did those who did not undergo mechanical ventilation.

The 1-year survival rate of the survivors of CI poisoning was 93.3%. Among the 5932 survivors of CI poisoning, 1339 (22.6%) underwent mechanical ventilation during hospitalization and 152 (11.4%) died within 1 year. By contrast, 246 (5.4%) of the remaining 4593 survivors who did not require mechanical ventilation died within 1 year. Figure 2 shows that the 1-year cumulative survival rates differed significantly between survivors who underwent mechanical ventilation and those who did not undergo mechanical ventilation during admission (p < 0.0001).

Discussion

This is the first nationwide population-based study with a relatively large number to investigate the one-year mortality of survivors after CI poisoning. Chronic renal failure, hemodialysis, and respiratory failure requiring mechanical ventilation were significantly associated with a poor outcome. For those survivors after CI poisoning, the one-year mortality rate of survivors after CI poisoning was 6.7%, and age, pneumonia, and mechanical ventilation were independent risk factors for one-year mortality among survivors of cholinesterase inhibitor poisoning. A recent

Table 2 Comparison of clinical characteristics between survivors and non-survivors of cholinesterase inhibitor poisoning (N = 6832)

	Non-survivors (N = 900)	Survivors (N = 5932)	95% CI of difference between means or percentages	P value
Age, mean ± SD, years old	62.18 ± 15.48	54.36 ± 16.34	6.682 to 8.959	< 0.0001
Female Sex, N (%)	306 (34.0)	1732 (29.2)	1.49 to 8.2%	0.0033
Comorbidities				
Diabetes mellitus, N (%)	117(13.0)	656 (11.1)	−0.38 to 4.4%	0.0867
Hypertension, N (%)	78 (8.7)	831 (14.0)	3.09 to 7.28%	< 0.0001
Coronary artery disease, N (%)	17 (1.9)	175 (3.0)	−0.097 to 2.02%	0.0727
Cerebrovascular accident, N (%)	32 (3.6)	145 (2.4)	0.0045 to 2.68%	0.0506
Chronic renal failure, N (%)	20 (2.2)	33 (0.6)	0.71 to 2.8%	< 0.0001
Chronic obstructive pulmonary disease, N (%)	16 (1.8)	95 (1.6)	−0.64 to 1.34%	0.6967
Asthma, N (%)	3 (0.3)	42 (0.7)	−0.25 to 0.75%	0.195
Liver failure, N (%)	11 (1.2)	19 (0.3)	0.27 to 1.86%	< 0.0001
Atropine use, N (%)	698 (77.6)	2955 (49.8)	0.55 to 4.69%	< 0.0001
Pralidoxime use, N (%)	564 (62.7)	2915 (49.1)	10.1 to 17.02%	< 0.0001
Hemodialysis, N (%)	59 (6.6)	65 (1.1)	3.94 to 7.34%	< 0.0001
Mechanical ventilation, N (%)	671 (74.6)	1339 (22.6)	48.83 to 55.01%	< 0.0001
Pneumonia, N (%)	85 (9.4)	407 (6.9)	0.55 to 4.69%	0.0052
Hospital days, mean ± SD	6.58 ± 12.31	9.61 ± 11.43	−3.846 to −2.225	< 0.0001

CI, Confidence interval; Data are presented as mean ± SD or N (%)

prospective population-based cohort study in Unite State showed hospital mortality of pneumonia was 6.5%, but the one-year mortality was up to 30.6%. [16] The result is similar in our study that pneumonia is a predictive factor for the one-year mortality after CI poisoning.

Several strengths of this study are worth highlighting. First, this was a nationwide population-based study, meaning that a relatively large number of CI intoxication patients were included, and this sample was considered representative of the general population. Second, the study cohort was largely selected from a computerized database comprising all Taiwanese CI intoxication patients diagnosed between January 1, 2003, and December 31, 2012, thus decreasing the potential for selection bias.

The disease burden of OP and CM toxicity differs between Taiwan and most western countries [17]. Because OP and CM are easily accessed and highly lethal, this type of toxicity is one of the most frequent causes of poisoning in Taiwan [18]. Previous epidemiologic data of 1985–2006 indicate that most cases of OP exposure involve a single OP (80.37%), and the overall mortality rate is 12.71% [8], which is similar to that (13.2%) in our study.

Respiratory failure is one of the most important complications of CI poisoning. This may be due to respiratory muscle weakness, aspiration, hypersecretion, pneumonia, sepsis, or acute respiratory distress syndrome. [4]. A retrospective study of 155 patients reported that 59% of patients with CI poisoning developed respiratory failure [14].

In our study, 29.4% of patients had respiratory failure with mechanical ventilation. The mortality rate was 33.4% among the patients who were mechanically ventilated, whereas it was 4.7% among the patients who were not mechanically ventilated. (95% CI of the difference between percentages was 26.54 to 30.89%, $p < 0.0001$) These findings demonstrate that CI intoxication patients who require mechanical intubation had a higher mortality rate than those without mechanical intubation. This information aids clinical physicians in realizing that respiratory failure is a useful prognostic indicator in patients with CI poisoning.

In the previous reports, several prognostic factors were associated with CI poisoning, including age, serum cholinesterase and bicarbonate levels, and acute physiology and chronic health evaluation II scores [12, 19]. A retrospective study of 118 patients with OP poisoning reported that the DM status did not increase mortality [20]. This result is consistent with our findings that diabetes is not associated with both hospital mortality and one-year mortality. Sungur revealed that among patients with OP insecticide poisoning, the mortality rate was 50% in patients requiring mechanical ventilation and 21% in those not mechanically ventilated [11]. In the current nationwide study of 6832 patients, the hospital mortality rate was 33.4% among those with mechanical ventilation. A recent study demonstrated that acute renal failure was associated with mortality in organophosphorus poisoning. [9]. Our study showed that

Table 3 Comparison of the clinical characteristics in patients with or without mechanical ventilation (N = 6832)

	With mechanical ventilation (N = 2010)	Without mechanical ventilation (N = 4822)	95% CI of difference between means or percentages	P value
Age, mean ± SD, years old	58.37 ± 16.38	54.15 ± 16.31	3.376 to 5.076	< 0.0001
Female sex, N (%)	654 (32.5)	1384 (28.7)	1.38 to 6.25%	0.0016
Diabetes mellitus, N (%)	259 (12.9)	514 (10.7)	0.5 to 3.97%	0.0081
Hypertension, N (%)	205 (10.2)	704 (14.6)	2.68 to 6.05%	< 0.0001
Coronary artery disease, N (%)	59 (2.9)	133 (2.8)	−0.75 to 1.04%	0.6865
Cerebrovascular accident, N (%)	76 (3.8)	101 (2.1)	0.79 to 2.71%	0.0001
Chronic renal failure, N (%)	24 (1.2)	29 (0.6)	0.098 to 1.21%	0.0110
Chronic obstructive pulmonary disease, N (%)	29 (1.4)	82 (1.7)	−0.41 to 0.92%	0.4426
Asthma, N (%)	13 (0.6)	32 (0.7)	−0.39 to 0.5%	0.937
Liver failure, N (%)	13 (0.6)	17 (0.4)	−0.16 to 0.67%	0.094
Atropine use, N (%)	1577 (78.5)	2076 (43.1)	33.06 to 37.67%	< 0.0001
Pralidoxime use N (%)	1453 (72.3)	2026 (42.0)	27.84 to 32.7%	< 0.0001
Hemodialysis, N (%)	83 (4.1)	41 (0.9)	2.32 to 4.19%	< 0.0001
Pneumonia, N (%)	322 (16)	170 (3.5)	10.83 to 14.25%	< 0.0001
Hospital mortality rate, N (%)	671 (33.4)	229 (4.7)	26.54 to 30.89%	< 0.0001
Hospital days, mean ± SD	15.42 ± 16.33	6.62 ± 7.54	8.224 to 9.358	< 0.0001

CI, Confidence interval; Data are presented as mean ± SD or N (%)

when patients with CI poisoning received hemodialysis during hospitalization, the hospital mortality rate was higher (OR; 6.332, 95% confidence interval: 4.419–9.074).

In our study, the prescription percentage of PAM and atropine was significantly higher in nonsurvivors than in survivors. This could be due to one of the two following reasons. First, the survivors may have experienced less CI toxicity and may have had less severe clinical symptoms. Therefore, PAM and atropine were not prescribed, according to clinical judgement. Second, most of the survivors may have experienced CM intoxication. Because PAM is not suggested for use in CM intoxication,

Table 4 Clinical variables associated with hospital mortality in patients with organophosphate and carbamate poisoning analyzed by multivariate Cox regression (N = 6832)

Parameter	Univariate analysis HR (95% CI)	P value	Multivariate analysis HR (95% CI)	P value
Age	1.022 (1.018–1.026)	< 0.0001	1.020 (1.015–1.024)	< 0.0001
Female Sex	1.148 (0.999–1.318)	0.0506		
Diabetes	1.076 (0.885–1.306)	0.4635		
Hypertension	0.629 (0.497–0.794)	< 0.0001	0.615 (0.485–0.779)	0.0001
Coronary artery disease	0.582 (0.360–0.941)	0.0273	0.485 (0.300–0.785)	0.0751
Cerebrovascular accident	1.179 (0.828–1.679)	0.3607		
Chronic renal failure	2.634 (1.690–4.105)	< 0.0001	1.449 (0.893–2.351)	0.1330
Chronic obstructive pulmonary disease	0.875 (0.534–1.436)	0.5980		
Asthma	0.544 (0.175–1.688)	0.2920		
Liver failure	2.693 (1.486–4.882)	0.0011	2.348 (1.293–4.264)	0.0050
Atropine	2.406 (2.054–2.818)	< 0.0001	1.951 (1.628–2.337)	< 0.0001
Pralidoxime	1.184 (1.032–1.359)	0.0161	0.591 (0.506–0.691)	< 0.0001
Hemodialysis	2.520 (1.929–3.291)	< 0.0001	1.454 (1.087–1.946)	0.0117
Pneumonia	0.754 (0.600–0.947)	0.0154	0.480 (0.382–0.603)	< 0.0001
Mechanical ventilation	5.160 (4.426–6.014)	< 0.0001	4.684 (3.976–5.517)	< 0.0001

CI, Confidence interval; Data are presented as mean ± SD or N (%)

Table 5 Clinical variables associated with one-year mortality in patients with organophosphate and carbamate poisoning analyzed by multivariate Cox regression (*N* = 5932)

Parameter	Univariate analysis HR (95% CI)	*P* value	Multivariate analysis HR (95% CI)	*P* value
Age	1.019 (1.013–1.026)	< 0.0001	1.016 (1.009–1.022)	< 0.0001
Female Sex	0.844 (0.674–1.056)	0.1385		
Diabetes mellitus	1.335 (1.006–1.771)	0.0451	1.185 (0.891–1.575)	0.2437
Hypertension	0.962 (0.722–1.282)	0.7923		
Coronary artery disease	1.110 (0.639–1.930)	0.7110		
Cerebrovascular accident	1.026 (0.548–1.923)	0.9360		
Chronic renal failure	1.932 (0.722–5.174)	0.1900		
Chronic obstructive pulmonary disease	1.293 (0.642–2.604)	0.4722		
Asthma	1.071 (0.344–3.337)	0.9062		
Liver failure	0.796 (0.112–5.658)	0.8194		
Atropine	0.992 (0.814–1.207)	0.9321		
Pralidoxime	1.367 (1.121–1.668)	0.0020	1.102 (0.892–1.362)	0.3669
Hemodialysis	2.443 (1.304–4.576)	0.0053	1.678 (0.890–3.163)	0.1095
Pneumonia	2.860 (2.196–3.725)	< 0.0001	1.962 (1.477–2.605)	< 0.0001
Mechanical ventilation	2.199 (1.796–2.692)	< 0.0001	1.722 (1.371–2.162)	< 0.0001

CI, Confidence interval; Data are presented as mean ± SD or N (%)

the percentage of PAM use may have been lower in the survivors.

The findings of this study should also be interpreted in light of its limitations. First, serum laboratory data were not available in the NHIRD. Thus, we could not obtain the level of acetylcholinesterase activity, which is a direct biomarker for toxicity of organophosphorus. However, not all hospitals check acetylcholinesterase activity to

the patients. Second, we could not categorize the precise intensity of the intoxication because NHIRD may not provide the detailed clinical course, such as clinical symptoms, the cause of intoxication (exposure to organophosphate or carbamates), the dose of toxin, the dose and length of antidote, or time to doctors. Third, the present study is a retrospective cohort study. Despite the meticulous design and control of some confounding

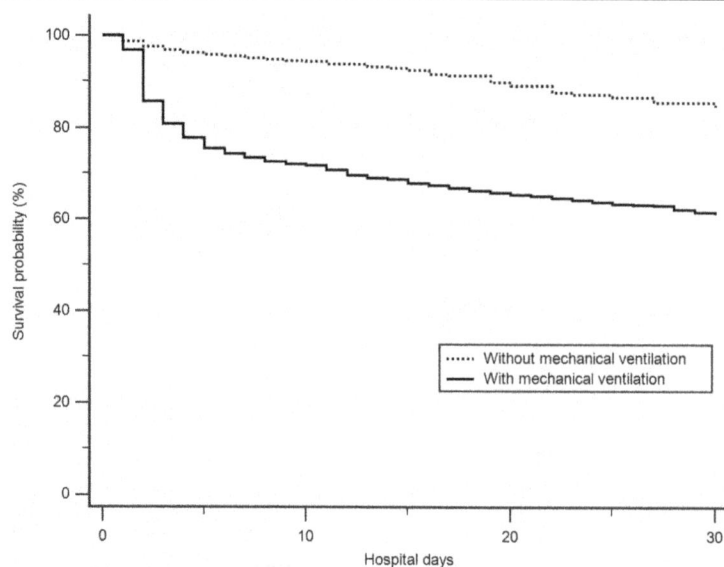

Fig. 1 Kaplan-Meier survival curve for the patients with mechanical ventilation and without mechanical ventilation during hospitalization (*N* = 6832, Logrank test *P* < 0.0001)

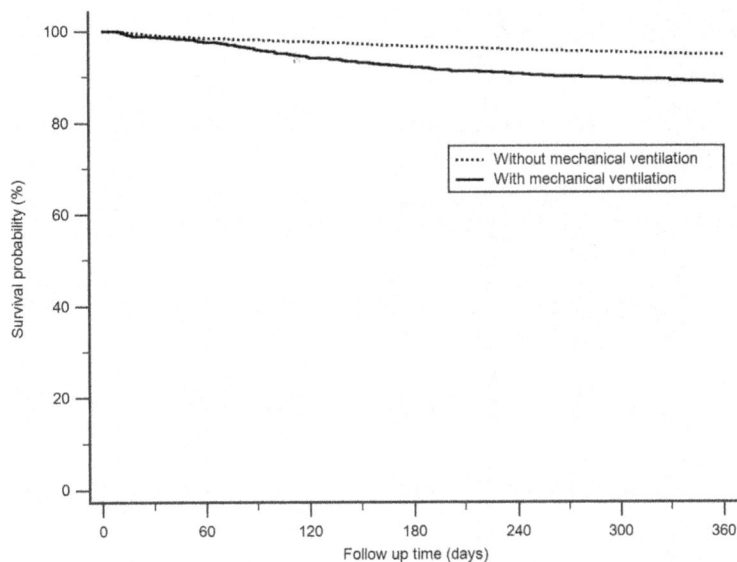

Fig. 2 Kaplan-Meier survival curve of the survivors after organophosphate and carbamate poisoning, one year follow up ($N = 5932$, logrank test, $P < 0.0001$)

factors, biases could remain because of possibly unmeasured or unknown confounding factors. We were unable to consider the severity of the diseases, which reduced our chances of showing the severity related effects of co-morbidities. Finally, causes of death for the patients cannot be reported in the study because we have no death certificate databases.

Conclusions

Among the survivors of CI poisoning, the one-year mortality rate was 6.7%. For the survivors after CI poisoning, age, pneumonia, and mechanical ventilation may be predictive factors for the one-year mortality. In addition, DM was not a risk factor for death in patients with CI poisoning.

Abbreviations

CAD: coronary artery disease; CI: cholinesterase inhibitor; CM: carbamates; CNS: central nervous system; COPD: chronic obstructive pulmonary disease; CVA: cerebrovascular accident; DM: diabetes mellitus; NHIRD: National Health Insurance Research Database; OP: organophosphate; PAM: pralidoxime

Acknowledgements
We thank Mr. Ching-Ter Chang in Chang Gung University, for validating and confirming all the statistics in this study.

Funding
This study did not receive any specific grant from funding agencies in the public, commercial, or not-for-profit sectors.

Authors' contributions
MCC and MJH took responsibility for the accuracy of the data analysis. MCC, CHC, and CSL drafted the manuscript. MCC, CHC, and CCH were responsible for the primary data analysis. YFF and MJH conceived the study and participated in its design. SHL and YFF performed the interpretation of the results. All authors read and approved the final manuscript.

Competing interests
All authors state that they have no conflicts of interest.

Author details
[1]Department of Pulmonary and Critical Care Medicine, Chiayi Chang-Gung Memorial Hospital, No. 6, Sec. West, Chia-Pu Road, Pu-Tz City, Chiayi 613, Taiwan. [2]Graduate Institute of Clinical Medical Sciences, College of Medicine, Chang Gung University, Taoyuan City, Taiwan. [3]Department of Pulmonary and Critical Care Medicine, Linkou Chang-Gung Memorial Hospital, Chang-Gung medical foundation, Taoyuan City, Taiwan. [4]Division of Pulmonary and Critical Care, Department of Internal Medicine, Saint Paul's Hospital, Taoyuan City, Taiwan. [5]Chang-Gung University College of Medicine, Taoyuan City, Taiwan. [6]Department of Nephrology, Chang Gung Memorial Hospital, Taoyuan City, Taiwan. [7]Department of Respiratory Care, Chang-Gung University, Taoyuan City, Taiwan.

References
1. Eddleston M, Phillips MR. Self poisoning with pesticides. BMJ. 2004; 328(7430):42–4.
2. Lamb T, Selvarajah LR, Mohamed F, Jayamanne S, Gawarammana I, Mostafa A, Buckley NA, Roberts MS, Eddleston M. High lethality and minimal variation after acute self-poisoning with carbamate insecticides in Sri Lanka - implications for global suicide prevention. Clin Toxicol (Phila). 2016;54(8): 624–31.
3. Rusyniak DE, Nanagas KA. Organophosphate poisoning. Semin Neurol. 2004; 24(2):197–204.
4. Hulse EJ, Davies JO, Simpson AJ, Sciuto AM, Eddleston M. Respiratory complications of organophosphorus nerve agent and insecticide poisoning. Implications for respiratory and critical care. Am J Respir Crit Care Med. 2014;190(12):1342–54.
5. Eddleston M, Mohamed F, Davies JO, Eyer P, Worek F, Sheriff MH, Buckley NA. Respiratory failure in acute organophosphorus pesticide self-poisoning. QJM. 2006;99(8):513–22.
6. Jokanovic M. Medical treatment of acute poisoning with organophosphorus and carbamate pesticides. Toxicol Lett. 2009;190(2):107–15.
7. Gunduz E, Dursun R, Icer M, Zengin Y, Gullu MN, Durgun HM, Gokalp O.

Factors affecting mortality in patients with organophosphate poisoning. J Pak Med Assoc. 2015;65(9):967–72.

8. Lin TJ, Walter FG, Hung DZ, Tsai JL, Hu SC, Chang JS, Deng JF, Chase JS, Denninghoff K, Chan HM. Epidemiology of organophosphate pesticide poisoning in Taiwan. Clin Toxicol (Phila). 2008;46(9):794–801.

9. Banday TH, Tathineni B, Desai MS, Naik V. Predictors of morbidity and mortality in organophosphorus poisoning: a case study in rural Hospital in Karnataka, India. N Am J Med Sci. 2015;7(6):259–65.

10. Noshad H, Ansarin K, Ardalan MR, Ghaffari AR, Safa J, Nezami N. Respiratory failure in organophosphate insecticide poisoning. Saudi Med J. 2007; 28(3):405–7.

11. Sungur M, Guven M. Intensive care management of organophosphate insecticide poisoning. Crit Care. 2001;5(4):211–5.

12. Kang EJ, Seok SJ, Lee KH, Gil HW, Yang JO, Lee EY, Hong SY. Factors for determining survival in acute organophosphate poisoning. Korean J Intern Med. 2009;24(4):362–7.

13. Acikalin A, Disel NR, Matyar S, Sebe A, Kekec Z, Gokel Y, Karakoc E. Prognostic factors determining morbidity and mortality in organophosphate poisoning. Pak J Med Sci. 2017;33(3):534–9.

14. Wang CY, Wu CL, Tsan YT, Hsu JY, Hung DZ, Wang CH. Early onset pneumonia in patients with cholinesterase inhibitor poisoning. Respirology. 2010;15(6):961–8.

15. Huang HS, Hsu CC, Weng SF, Lin HJ, Wang JJ, Su SB, Huang CC, Guo HR. Acute anticholinesterase pesticide poisoning caused a long-term mortality increase: a Nationwide population-based cohort study. Medicine. 2015; 94(30):e1222.

16. Ramirez JA, Wiemken TL, Peyrani P, Arnold FW, Kelley R, Mattingly WA, Nakamatsu R, Pena S, Guinn BE, Furmanek SP, et al. Adults hospitalized with pneumonia in the United States: incidence, epidemiology, and mortality. Clinical infectious diseases : an official publication of the Infectious Diseases Society of America. 2017;65(11):1806–12.

17. Satoh T, Hosokawa M. Organophosphates and their impact on the global environment. Neurotoxicology. 2000;21(1–2):223–7.

18. Yang CC, Wu JF, Ong HC, Hung SC, Kuo YP, Sa CH, Chen SS, Deng JF. Taiwan National Poison Center: epidemiologic data 1985-1993. J Toxicol Clin Toxicol. 1996;34(6):651–63.

19. Sun IO, Yoon HJ, Lee KY. Prognostic factors in cholinesterase inhibitor poisoning. Med Sci Monit. 2015;21:2900–4.

20. Liu SH, Lin JL, Shen HL, Chang CC, Huang WH, Weng CH, Hsu CW, Wang IK, Liang CC, Yen TH. Acute large-dose exposure to organophosphates in patients with and without diabetes mellitus: analysis of mortality rate and new-onset diabetes mellitus. Environ Health. 2014;13(1):11.

Permissions

List of Contributors

Isabelle Guay, Simon Boulanger, Charles Isabelle, Eric Brouillette, Kamal Bouarab and François Malouin
Centre d'Étude et de Valorisation de la Diversité Microbienne (CEVDM), Département de biologie, Faculté des sciences, Université de Sherbrooke, 2500 Boul. Université, Sherbrooke, QC J1K 2R1, Canada

Félix Chagnon and Eric Marsault
Département de pharmacologie, Faculté de médecine et des sciences de la santé, Université de Sherbrooke, 3001, 12 th avenue Nord, Sherbrooke, QC J1H 5N4, Canada

Anum Saqib
Department of Pharmacy, The Islamia University of Bahawalpur, Bahawalpur, Punjab, Pakistan

Muhammad Rehan Sarwar
Department of Pharmacy, The Islamia University of Bahawalpur, Bahawalpur, Punjab, Pakistan
Akhtar Saeed College of Pharmaceutical Sciences, Lahore, Pakistan

Sadia Iftikhar
Akhtar Saeed College of Pharmaceutical Sciences, Lahore, Pakistan

Muhammad Sarfraz
College of Pharmacy, Al Ain University of Science and Technology, Al Ain, Abu Dhabi, UAE

Sun Young Kyung, Jin Young Yoon, Eun Suk Son, Yu Jin Kim, Jeong Woong Park and Sung Hwan Jeong
Department of Internal Medicine, Gachon University Gil Medical Center, 21 Namdong-daero 774, Namdong-gu, Incheon 21565, Republic of Korea

Dae Young Kim
Department of Biological Science, College of Bio-nano Technology, Gachon University, Seongnam-daero 1342, Seongnam, South Korea

Sileshi Tadesse
Yekatit 12 Hospital Medical College, Addis Ababa, Ethiopia

Haile Alemayehu and Tadesse Eguale
Aklilu Lemma Institute of Pathobiology, Addis Ababa University, Addis Ababa, Ethiopia

Admasu Tenna
Department of Internal Medicine, School of Medicine, College of Health Sciences, Addis Ababa University, Churchill Avenue, Addis Ababa, Ethiopia

Getachew Tadesse
Department of Biomedical Sciences, College of Veterinary medicine and Agriculture, Addis Ababa University, Debrezeit, Ethiopia

Tefaye Sisay Tessema
Institute of Biotechnology, College of natural and Computational sciences, Addis Ababa University, Addis Ababa, Ethiopia

Workineh Shibeshi
Department of Pharmacology and Clinical Pharmacy, School of Pharmacy, College of Health Sciences, Addis Ababa University, Churchill Avenue, Addis Ababa, Ethiopia

Karen Roksund Hov, Bjørn Erik Neerland and Torgeir Bruun Wyller
Oslo Delirium Research Group, Department of Geriatric Medicine, Oslo University Hospital, Oslo, Norway
Institute of Clinical Medicine, University of Oslo, Oslo, Norway

Vegard Bruun Wyller
Institute of Clinical Medicine, University of Oslo, Oslo, Norway
Department of Paediatrics, Akershus University Hospital, Lørenskog, Norway

Anders Mikal Andersen
Department of Pharmacology, Oslo University Hospital, Oslo, Norway

Øystein Undseth
Department of Acute Medicine, Oslo University Hospital, Oslo, Norway

Alasdair M. J. MacLullich
Edinburgh Delirium Research Group, Geriatric Medicine, University of Edinburgh, Edinburgh, UK

Eva Skovlund
Department of Public Health and Nursing, Norwegian University of Science and Technology, Trondheim, Norway

Eirik Qvigstad
Department of Cardiology, Oslo University Hospital, Oslo, Norway

Yuhong Li, Qi Ren, Lingyan Zhu, Yingshu Li, Jinfeng Li, Yiyang Zhang, Guoying Zheng, Tiesheng Han and Fumin Feng
Hebei Province Key Laboratory of Occupational Health and Safety for Coal Industry, School of Public Health, North China University of Science and Technology, No.21 Bohai Road, Tangshan 063210, People's Republic of China

Shufeng Sun
College of Nursing and Rehabilitation, North China University of Science and Technology, Tangshan 063210, China

Pimradasiri Srijiwangsa and Saranyoo Ponnikorn
Chulabhorn International College of Medicine, Thammasat University, (Rangsit Campus), Pathum Thani 12121, Thailand

Kesara Na-Bangchang
Chulabhorn International College of Medicine, Thammasat University, (Rangsit Campus), Pathum Thani 12121, Thailand
Center of Excellence in Pharmacology and Molecular Biology of Malaria and Cholangiocarcinoma, Chulabhorn International College of Medicine, Thammasat University, Pathum Thani, Thailand

Nan Chen, Qiujie Zhang, Li-wei Liu, Fei Yu and Xin Yu
Department of Geriatrics, Qilu Hospital of Shandong University, Jinan, Shandong, China

Kuan-xiao Tang
Department of Geriatrics, Qilu Hospital of Shandong University, Jinan, Shandong, China
Present Address: Department of Geriatrics, Qilu Hospital of Shandong University, No. 107, Wenhua Xi Road, Jinan, Shandong 250012, People's Republic of China

Jian-bo Zhang
Department of Emergency, Qilu Hospital of Shandong University, Jinan, Shandong, China

Yun-peng Zhao
Department of Orthopedics, Qilu Hospital of Shandong University, Jinan, Shandong, China

Li-yan Li
Department of Endocrinology and Metabolism, First People's Hospital of Jinan City, Jinan, Shandong, China

Tao Peng
Department of Nephrology, Qilu Hospital of Shandong University, Jinan, Shandong, China

Feng Huang
Institute of Cardiovascular Diseases and Guangxi Key Laboratory Base of Precision Medicine in Cardio-cerebrovascular Diseases Control and Prevention, The First Affiliated Hospital of Guangxi Medical University, Nanning, Guangxi 530021, P. R. China

James Henry Obol, Peter Akera, Pamela Ochola Atim and Felix Kaducu
Department of Public Health, Faculty of Medicine, Gulu University, Gulu, Uganda

Sylvia Awor
Department of Obstetrics and Gynaecology, Faculty of Medicine, Gulu University, Gulu, Uganda

Ronald Wanyama
Department of Biochemistry, Faculty of Medicine, Gulu University, Gulu, Uganda

Kenneth Luryama Moi
Department of Medical Microbiology and Immunology, Faculty of Medicine, Gulu University, Gulu, Uganda

Bongomin Bodo
Department of Paediatrics and Child Health: Faculty of Medicine, Gulu University, Gulu, Uganda

Patrick Olwedo Odong
District Health Office, Amuru District Local Government, Gulu, Uganda

Emmanuel Otto Omony
District Health Office, Agago District Local Government, Agago, Uganda

Hussein Oria
Department of Pharmacy, School of health Sciences Makerere University, Kampala, Uganda

David Musoke
Department of Pharmacology, Faculty of Medicine, Gulu University, Gulu, Uganda

Melissa Palmer, Lee Jennings, Caleb Bliss and Patrick Martin
Global Development Lead Hepatology, Shire, 300 Shire Way, Lexington, MA 02421, USA

Debra G. Silberg
Shire International GmbH, Zahlerweg 10, 6301 Zug, Switzerland

Peter Kardos
Group Practice, Center for Allergy, Respiratory and Sleep Medicine, Red Cross Maingau Hospital, Frankfurt am Main, Germany

Kai-Michael Beeh
insaf Respiratory Resarch Institute, Wiesbaden, Germany

Ulrike Sent Tobias Mueck and Heidemarie Gräter
Medical Affairs Consumer Healthcare, Sanofi-Aventis Deutschland GmbH, Frankfurt-Hoechst, Germany

Martin C. Michel
Department of Pharmacology, Johannes Gutenberg University, Obere Zahlbacher Str. 67, 55131 Mainz, Germany

Jun Yuan
Department of Cardiology, The People's Hospital of Guangxi Zhuang Autonomous Region, Nanning 530021, Guangxi, China

Min Li, Min Xu and Xin Gao
Department of Nephrology, The 88th Hospital of PLA, Taian, People's Republic of China

Wei Liu
Department of Medicine, The 88th Hospital of PLA, Taian, People's Republic of China

Amsalu Bokore and Belay Korme
Nekemte referral hospital, Nekemte, Ethiopia

Getu Bayisa
Wollega University, Nekemte, Ethiopia

Natalie Eaton, Hélène Cabanas, Cassandra Balinas, Anne Klein, Donald Staines and Sonya Marshall-Gradisnik
School of Medical Science, Griffith University, QLD, Gold Coast, Australia
The National Centre for Neuroimmunology and Emerging Diseases, Menzies Health Institute Queensland, Griffith University, QLD, Gold Coast, Australia

Ling-Ling Chang
Department of Chemical and Materials Engineering, Chinese Culture University, Shih-Lin, Taipei 11114, Taiwan, Republic of China

Wan-Song Alfred Wun
Fertility Specialists of Houston, Houston, TX 77054, USA

Paulus S. Wang
Department of Physiology, School of Medicine, National Yang-Ming University, Taipei 11221, Taiwan, Republic of China
Department of Medical Research and Education, Taipei Veterans General Hospital, Taipei 11217, Taiwan, Republic of China
Medical Center of Aging Research, China Medical University Hospital, Taichung 40402, Taiwan, Republic of China
Department of Biotechnology, Asia University, Taichung 41354, Taiwan, Republic of China

O. Awodele, W. A. Badru, A. A. Busari, O. E. Kale, T. B. Ajayi and R. O. Udeh
Toxicology Unit, Department of Pharmacology, Therapeutics and Toxicology, College of Medicine, University of Lagos, PMB 12003, Idi-Araba Campus, Lagos, Nigeria

P. M. Emeka
Department of Pharmaceutical Sciences, College of Pharmacy, King Faisal University Hofuf, Hofuf, Kingdom of Saudi Arabia

Noura El-Ahmady El-Naggar and Sara M. El-Ewasy
Department of Bioprocess Development, Genetic Engineering and Biotechnology Research Institute, City of Scientific Research and Technological Applications, Alexandria, Egypt

Sahar F. Deraz
Department of Protein Research Genetic Engineering and Biotechnology Research Institute, City of Scientific Research and Technological Applications, Alexandria, Egypt

Ghada M. Suddek
Department of Pharmacology and Toxicology, Faculty of Pharmacy, Mansoura University, Mansoura, Egypt

Monica Danial and Mohamed Azmi Hassali
Discipline of Social and Administrative Pharmacy, School of Pharmaceutical Sciences, Universiti Sains Malaysia, 11800 Minden, Penang, Malaysia

Loke Meng Ong
Clinical Research Center (CRC) Penang General Hospital, 10990 Jalan Residensi, Pulau Pinang, Malaysia

Amer Hayat Khan
Discipline of Clinical Pharmacy, School of Pharmaceutical Sciences, Universiti Sains Malaysia, 11800 Minden, Penang, Malaysia

Xiaojun Zhuo, Shenyu Ouyang, Pei Niu and Mou Xiao
Department of Cardiology, Affiliated Changsha Hospital of Hunan Normal University, The Fourth Hospital of Changsha, Changsha 410006, Hunan, People's Republic of China

Bi Zhuo
Department of Pharmacology, People's Hospital of Laibin, Laibin 546100, Guangxi, People's Republic of China

Michael Wan, Marion Elligsen and Lesley Palmay
Department of Pharmacy, Sunnybrook Health Sciences Centre, 2075 Bayview Avenue, Toronto, ON M4N 3M5, Canada

Sandra A. N.Walker
Department of Pharmacy, Sunnybrook Health Sciences Centre, 2075 Bayview Avenue, Toronto, ON M4N 3M5, Canada
Leslie Dan Faculty of Pharmacy, University of Toronto, 144 College Street, Toronto, ON M5S 3M2, Canada
Division of Infectious Diseases, Sunnybrook Health Sciences Centre, 2075 Bayview Avenue, Toronto, ON M4N 3M5, Canada
Sunnybrook Research Institute, Sunnybrook Health Sciences Centre, 2075 Bayview Avenue, Toronto, ON M4N 3M5, Canada

Jerome A. Leis
Division of Infectious Diseases, Sunnybrook Health Sciences Centre, 2075 Bayview Avenue, Toronto, ON M4N 3M5, Canada
Sunnybrook Research Institute, Sunnybrook Health Sciences Centre, 2075 Bayview Avenue, Toronto, ON M4N 3M5, Canada
Department of Medicine, Sunnybrook Health Sciences Centre, 2075 Bayview Avenue, Toronto, ON M4N 3M5, Canada
Faculty of Medicine, University of Toronto, 1 King's College Circle, Toronto, ON M5S 1A8, Canada

ElaineMartin
Present address: Elaine Martin, Trillium Health Partners, 100 Queensway W, Mississauga, ON L5B 1B8, Canada

Selemani Saidi Sungi
Health Department, Chamwino District Council, Chamwino, Dodoma, Tanzania

Eliford Ngaimisi
Unit of Pharmacology and Therapeutics, School of Pharmacy, Muhimbili University of Health and Allied Sciences (MUHAS), Dar es Salaam, Tanzania

Nzovu Ulenga
Management Development for Health (MDH), Dar es Salaam, Tanzania

Philip Sasi and Sabina Mugusi
Department of Clinical Pharmacology, School of Medicine, Muhimbili University of Health and Allied Sciences (MUHAS), Dar es Salaam, Tanzania

Xiaowen Zhang, Lin Zhu, Yuyang Ze, Dalong Zhu and Yan Bi
Department of Endocrinology, Affiliated Drum Tower Hospital, Nanjing University School of Medicine, 321 Zhongshan Road, Nanjing, Jiangsu Province 210008, China

Fei Shao
Department of Endocrinology, Affiliated Drum Tower Hospital, Nanjing University School of Medicine, 321 Zhongshan Road, Nanjing, Jiangsu Province 210008, China
Department of Endocrinology, Nanjing Drum Tower Hospital Clinical College of Traditional Chinese and Western Medicine, Nanjing University of Chinese Medicine, 321 Zhongshan Road, Nanjing, Jiangsu Province 210008, China

Min-Chun Chuang
Department of Pulmonary and Critical Care Medicine, Chiayi Chang-Gung Memorial Hospital, No. 6, Sec. West, Chia-Pu Road, Pu-Tz City, Chiayi 613, Taiwan
Graduate Institute of Clinical Medical Sciences, College of Medicine, Chang Gung University, Taoyuan City, Taiwan

Meng-Jer Hsieh
Department of Pulmonary and Critical Care Medicine, Chiayi Chang-Gung Memorial Hospital, No. 6, Sec. West, Chia-Pu Road, Pu-Tz City, Chiayi 613, Taiwan
Department of Respiratory Care, Chang-Gung University, Taoyuan City, Taiwan

Shih-Hong Li
Department of Pulmonary and Critical Care Medicine, Linkou Chang-Gung Memorial Hospital, Chang-Gung medical foundation, Taoyuan City, Taiwan
Chang-Gung University College of Medicine, Taoyuan City, Taiwan

Chih-Hao Chang, Chung Shu Lee and Yueh-Fu Fang
Department of Pulmonary and Critical Care Medicine, Linkou Chang-Gung Memorial Hospital, Chang-Gung medical foundation, Taoyuan City, Taiwan
Division of Pulmonary and Critical Care, Department of Internal Medicine, Saint Paul's Hospital, Taoyuan City, Taiwan

Chang-Gung University College of Medicine, Taoyuan City, Taiwan

Ching-Chung Hsiao
Chang-Gung University College of Medicine, Taoyuan City, Taiwan

Department of Nephrology, Chang Gung Memorial Hospital, Taoyuan City, Taiwan

Index

R
Randomized Controlled Trial, 52, 123, 255
Renal Insufficiency, 46, 80-81, 87
Respiratory Failure, 27, 269-272, 275-276
Rituximab, 158-161, 163, 165-166
Rivaroxaban, 134-142

S
S. Epidermidis, 2, 5-6
Small Colony Variant, 10-11
Staphylococcus Aureus, 1-2, 11, 36-38, 42-43, 238, 242-245
Stent Thrombosis, 92, 94, 96-99, 101, 134-138, 140, 142, 226-228, 234
Supra-therapeutic Dose,, 184

Surgical Site Infection, 36-40, 43, 242

T
Ticagrelor, 135-136, 141-142, 226-228, 230, 233, 235-236
Tomatidine, 1-3, 6, 10-11
Toxicological Profile, 184
Trimethoprim, 36, 38, 40-41
Triple Antiplatelet Therapy, 92-93, 95, 101-102, 142, 226-228, 235
Trough Concentration, 44, 47, 52, 237-238, 243

V
Vancomycin, 37, 237-245
Volixibat, 111-116, 118-123